Common Foundation Studies *in* NURSING

For Churchill Livingstone:

Senior Commissioning Editor: Jacqueline Curthoys
Project Development Manager: Mairi McCubbin
Design Direction: George Ajayi, Judith Wright

Common Foundation Studies *in* NURSING

Edited by

Neil Kenworthy MBA BEd RGN RMN
Management and Training Consultant, Lincoln, UK

Gillian Snowley MEd BSc(Hons) DipNurs(Lond) RGN
Formerly Deputy Dean, Faculty of Health, University of Hull, Hull, UK

Cynthia Gilling MA BEd(Hons) RGN RM RNT
Formerly Head of School of Health and Community Studies, King Alfred's College of
Higher Education, Winchester, UK

THIRD EDITION

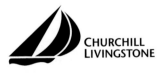
CHURCHILL LIVINGSTONE

EDINBURGH LONDON NEW YORK PHILADELPHIA ST LOUIS SYDNEY TORONTO 2002

CHURCHILL LIVINGSTONE
An imprint of Harcourt Publishers Limited

⚓ is a registered trademark of Harcourt Publishers
Limited

First published 1992
Second edition 1996
Third edition 2002

ISBN 0 443 07034 2

British Library Cataloguing in Publication Data
A catalogue record for this book is available from the British
Library

Library of Congress Cataloging in Publication Data
A catalog record for this book is available from the
Library of Congress

Note
Medical knowledge is constantly changing. As new
information becomes available, changes in treatment,
procedures, equipment and the use of drugs become
necessary. The editors, the contributors and the
publishers have taken care to ensure that the information
given in this text is accurate and up to date. However,
readers are strongly advised to confirm that the information,
especially with regard to drug usage, complies with the
latest legislation and standards of practice.

The
publisher's
policy is to use
**paper manufactured
from sustainable forests**

Printed in Spain

Contents

Contributors *vii*
Preface *ix*

SECTION 1

Nursing and the context of nursing
practice 1

1 **Introduction: what is nursing?** 3
Introduction to the development of the
nursing profession; Introduction to the
branch programmes; After qualifying,
what next?; Conclusion

2 **The context of practice** 41
Introduction; The history of the National
Health Service; The structure of the
National Health Service; Policy
developments since 1997; The National
Plan; The social care sector and partnership
with the NHS; The independent sector;
The contribution of nursing: making a
difference; Conclusion

3 **Ethics** 77
Understanding what is meant by nursing
ethics; Values as the basis for moral thought
and action; Ethical theory as a basis for
moral thought and action; Caring as the
basis for moral thought and action; Making
moral decisions in nursing practice;
Prescription for ethical reasoning, decision
making and action

4 **Legal issues** 113
Importance of the law; Sources of law;
Legal forums; Criminal law; Civil law;
Documentation

5 **Managing cultural diversity in care** 129
Introduction; What is culture?; Transcultural
care; Providing culture sensitive care; Good
practice in transcultural care; Conclusion

SECTION 2

Theory supporting nursing care 147

6 **The physiological basis of nursing** 149
The cell; The sustenance of life;
Homeostasis and the body systems

7 **The psychological basis of nursing** 197
The contribution of psychology to nursing;
Nature, nurture and human behaviour;
Acknowledging people as individuals;
Making assessments; Using memory
effectively; Problem solving; Stress;
Conclusion

8 **The sociological basis of nursing** 225
Introduction; Sociological theory; Health as
a social construct; Health beliefs;
Socialisation; Social roles and role sets;
Culture; Social policy; Community care;
Primary health care: a new direction;
Conclusion

SECTION 3

Fundamental nursing principles and skills 251

9 **The nurse as a communicator** 253
The importance of communication in nursing; The complexity of communication and the potential for misunderstanding; What is communication?; Self and communication; Matching communication to different contexts; Conclusion

10 **The nurse as health promoter** 279
Introduction; The Ottawa Charter; New strategies; An integrated approach; Psychology and health promotion; Health promotion and health education; Health education models; Health for everyone

11 **Accountability in practice** 309
Nursing as a profession; Changes in the concepts of professionalism; Accountability and the nurse; The Code of Professional Conduct; The role of the statutory bodies; Professional organisations and trade unions; The international setting; Conclusion

12 **Evidence-based practice** 331
Nursing research; Types of research; The research process; Ethical issues; Research as part of nursing knowledge and practice; Conclusion

13 **Nursing theory and nursing care** 365
Introduction; How and where does care take place?; Concepts, theories, models and care pathways; Record keeping; Conclusion

14 **Safe nursing practice** 391
Introduction; Adopt a questioning approach; Inform your practice with up-to-date knowledge and evidence; Know your limitations; Be aware of hazards in the environment; Remember that prevention is the key; Take prompt action in the case of an emergency; Communicate effectively; Report concerns

15 **Caring for the person with pain** 457
Introduction; Classifying the experience of pain; The physiology of pain; Assessing pain

16 **Palliative care and care of the dying** 483
Causes of death in the UK today; History of care of the dying; The palliative care approach; Facing the possibility of death; Palliative care and managing the symptoms; Managing the last days of life; Bereavement; The stress of caring for the dying

Index 509

Contributors

Andrew M. Betts MEd RMN AdvDipCouns CPNCert CertEd
Health Lecturer, School of Nursing, University
of Nottingham, Nottingham, UK
9   *The nurse as a communicator*

Helen Caulfield LLB MA
Solicitor, Royal College of Nursing, London, UK
4   *Legal issues*

Mark Darley BA MA RGN
Operational Services Manager, Faculty of
Health, South Bank University, Romford, UK
2   *The context of practice*

Pat A. Downer MA PGCEA RGN RNT RSCN DN PWT
Formerly Director of Studies, Specialist
Practice in Health Care, University of Surrey,
Guildford, UK
13   *Nursing theory and nursing care*

Diana Forster BA MSc RGN RM RHV RNT
Independent Writer and Consultant in Health
Psychology and Health Promotion,
London, UK
10   *The nurse as health promoter*

Cynthia Gilling MA BEd RGN RM RNT
Formerly Head of School of Health and
Community Studies, King Alfred's College of
Higher Education, Winchester, UK
 1   *Introduction: what is nursing*
11   *Accountability in practice*

Kevin Gormley BA MSc RGN RMNONC RCNT RNT
Nurse Lecturer, Queen's University of Belfast,
Belfast, Northern Ireland
8   *The sociological basis of nursing*

Benjamin Gray BA PhD
Research Fellow, Faculty of Health,
South Bank Hospital, Redwood College of
Health Studies, Harold Wood Hospital,
Romford, UK
12   *Evidence-based practice*

Tracey Heath MSc BSc PGDipEd RGN
Lecturer and Senior Nurse, School of Nursing,
University of Hull, Hull, UK
14   *Safe nursing practice*

Christine L. Henry DN DipPallCare RGN ENB931 285 FETC
Scunthorpe General Hospital, Scunthorpe,
North Lincolnshire, UK
16   *Palliative care and care of the dying*

Linda Husband BScN MSc PhD SRN SCM HV
Lecturer, School of Nursing, University of Hull,
Hull, UK
15   *Caring for the person with pain*
16   *Palliative care and care of the dying*

Neil Kenworthy MBA BEd RGN RMN
Management and Training Consultant,
Lincoln, UK
1   *Introduction: what is nursing?*

Pam Smith PhD MSc BNurs RHN HVCert DNCert RNT
Professor of Nursing, South Bank University,
Redwood College of Health Studies,
Romford, UK
12   Evidence-based practice

Gillian Snowley BSc MEd DipNurs(Lond) RGN
Formerly Deputy Dean, Faculty of Health,
University of Hull, Hull, UK
1   Introduction: what is nursing?
6   The physiological basis of nursing

Alison Spires BSc MSc DipNEd RGN RM RCNT
Senior Lecturer, Adult Nursing, South Bank
University, London, UK
5   Managing cultural diversity in care

Pamela Taylor BSc DipN RGN RGN ENB199, A33, 998
Deputy Manager, Minor Injuries Unit, Finchley
Memorial Hospital, London, UK
14   Safe nursing practice

Isabelle Whaite MA SPSN CertEd RGN RM RCNT
Principal Lecturer in Nursing, Department of
Primary and Community Nursing, University
of Central Lancashire, Faculty of Health,
Preston, UK
3   Ethics

John A. Wilkinson BSc MSc RGN RMN DipN DipNEd
ENB100
Assistant Director: Education and Practice,
Peterborough Hospitals NHS Trust,
Peterborough, UK
7   The psychological basis of nursing

Preface

This popular textbook has been meeting the needs of new entrants to nursing studies since publication of the first edition in 1992. This third edition, a decade later, has been prompted by the significant changes that have occurred in recent years to the structure and content of nursing education that prepares students for entry to the professional register.

The recommendations of the Commission for Nursing and Midwifery Education, chaired by Sir Leonard Peach in 1999, and their subsequent implementation by Council have meant a number of alterations and additions to the curriculum, together with a reduction in the length of the Common Foundation programme to one year. This new edition of *Common Foundation Studies in Nursing* sets out to help students meet the new 'competencies' required by the United Kingdom Central Council as they complete their first year of the course.

As in all editions of this book, the long-standing concept of the nurse as a 'knowledgeable doer' is promoted, along with the belief that nursing must recognise the individuality of the patient and be health focused. Contributors to the text are either specialists in their own field or people closely involved in the preparation and delivery of nursing courses.

There have been some structural alterations to this third edition, most noticeably a different section structure and the removal of the section introducing the different client groups, which gave students an overview of nursing care of adults, children and persons with mental illness and learning difficulties. This aspect of health care provision is far from neglected, however, but is now incorporated into all chapters of the text using case examples and interactive opportunities for the student. Increased use of case studies reflects all settings for care and there is a definite focus on practice and practical skills.

Section 1: Nursing and the context of nursing practice answers the question, 'What is nursing?' It is an introduction to nursing and the main client groups, as well as exploring such issues as the changing expectations of society, the changing roles of nurses and new technology.

The current structure of the health service is also discussed, exploring care-provision pathways, priorities in health care and the contribution of the multidisciplinary team. Additionally, there are chapters on the professional role of the nurse, with particular emphasis on ethics in health care, legal issues and a completely new chapter addressing the management of cultural diversity in health care.

Section 2: Theory supporting nursing care updates the chapters on the physiological, psychological and sociological bases of care. The genetic revolution is a new feature of the physiology chapter and stress has now been incorporated into the psychology chapter.

Section 3: Fundamental nursing principles and skills is a large section of the book, consisting of eight chapters. The chapter on 'Safe nursing practice' is completely new, covering a wide range of safety topics from lifting, skin care, infection control and resuscitation to accuracy of recording, client consent and patient dignity/ confidentiality. Other chapters in this section cover communication, health promotion, account-ability, research/evidence-based practice, pain, and palliative care and care of the dying.

All chapters are well referenced and provide ample case examples and open learning activities.

The editors and contributors recognise that entrants to nursing courses come from back-grounds giving a diversity of knowledge, age and experience but believe that the text will be of value to all in their transition from new students to completion of the first year's studies.

2001

Neil Kenworthy
Gillian Snowley
Cynthia Gilling

ACKNOWLEDGEMENTS

The editors would like to extend particular thanks to those authors who contributed to the original chapters in the second edition and whose work has provided the foundation for the current volume:

Alison Barnes
Margaret Clarke
Terttu Corbett
Peter Draper
Roger Ellis
Jon Evans
Eva Garland
Bob Gates
Christopher Goodall

Jane Hodges
Sally Huband
Stephanie Kirby
Rob Newell
Peter Nicklin
Gill Pharaoh
Mary Walker
Mary Watkins

1

Nursing and the context of nursing practice

SECTION CONTENTS

1. Introduction: what is nursing? 3

2. The context of practice 41

3. Ethics 77

4. Legal issues 113

5. Managing cultural diversity in caring 129

1

Introduction: what is nursing?

Neil Kenworthy   Gillian Snowley
Cynthia Gilling

CHAPTER CONTENTS

Introduction to the development of the nursing profession 4
    Women and healing 4
    Social change and health 5
    The new Poor Law 1834 5
    The legacy of Florence Nightingale 5
    The Nightingale School 6
    Nurse registration and the drive for professionalism 7
    Nursing developments during the 20th century 8
    Pre-registration nursing programmes 9
    UKCC competencies for the Common Foundation Programme 9
    Being a nursing student 10
    Patients and clients 10

Introduction to the branch programmes 10
    Nursing adults 10
        Medical nursing 11
        Surgical nursing 11
        Critical care nursing 12
        Care of the elderly 14
        Future trends in adult care 14
    Children's nursing 14
        Changing patterns of children's health and illness 15
        Changes in the provision of health care for children 16
        Caring for children in hospital 16
        Caring for children in the community 16
        The role of the children's nurse 16
        Other aspects of children's nursing 18
        The future of children's nursing 18
    Learning disability nursing 18

    Defining and assessing for learning disability 19
    Causes of learning disability 20
    Incidence and prevalence of learning disability 20
    Historical overview of learning disability care 21
    The role of the learning disability nurse 22
    The future of learning disability nursing 22
    Mental health nursing 22
    Historical overview of mental health care 23
    Images of mental illness: fear and stigma 24
    Approaches to mental health and illness 24
    The medical model and physical treatments 24
    Psychological treatments 25
    Settings for care 25
    The role of the mental health nurse 25
    The future of mental health nursing 26

After qualifying, what next? 27
    Actual and predicted changes for nursing in 2001 and beyond 27
    Possible career options 28
    Further qualifications? 29
    A modern career framework 30
    Lifelong learning 31
    Preceptorship 32
    PREP and portfolios 32

Conclusion 33

References 33

Further reading 34

Appendix 1 35

As many of the earliest schools of nursing in this country are now celebrating their centenaries, it is opportune to reflect on how they, and nursing as a career, began. Many well-known and not so well-known names have helped to shape the career of nursing as we know it today, but although these nurses have fought for professional registration and pushed forward changes in practice, research and education, external influences have often had the greatest impact. Recently, both the political agenda and the public have forced changes in health care, whereas in the past few hundred years social change had a greater influence.

This chapter:
- describes the development of the nursing profession from early times to the present day, including the traditional role of women in healing and the influence of early reformers
- outlines the various client groups cared for by nurses (adults, children, patients with learning disability and patients with mental illness), and the care practices for each group, as well as the specific role of the nurse in each speciality and future trends
- looks at the changing context of nursing today, likely future changes, and the need for continuing professional education.

INTRODUCTION TO THE DEVELOPMENT OF THE NURSING PROFESSION

The image of the nurse and the history of nursing are inextricably intertwined. Davies (1980) asserts that nursing cannot be seen in a vacuum, but must be considered within its social context. To understand the issues that influence nursing today and that have implications for the future, it is necessary to understand the historical background to those issues.

Images of nursing are often synonymous with images of women, as women have traditionally formed – and still do form – the majority of the nursing workforce. The history and development of nursing is linked to the developing role of women in society.

Women and healing

The first records of women and health care are from ancient Egypt when women formed part of a highly organised and respected female healing tradition that centred on the worship of Isis, the restorer of life and source of healing herbs. Such women were instrumental in passing on their knowledge to the physicians of Classical Greece. Famous names such as Aristotle and Hippocrates, (between 460 BC and 320 BC), who were central to the development of philosophy and medical ethics, come to mind, but it is interesting that at this time women were forbidden to study medicine. The Romans, with their extensive and sophisticated water systems, were obviously interested in health and health care but women such as Hygeia were seen as subservient helpers to the male health care promoters.

It was the advent of Christianity during the first century AD and its subsequent spread across Europe that promoted the nursing role. With the emphasis on good works and charity, the church organised women or deaconesses to visit the sick and needy. During the Middle Ages the first hospitals began to appear across Europe and in England, usually on the routes pilgrims took, but those who looked after the sick in these foundations were the brothers and sisters from the various religious orders.

From the 14th to the 16th centuries, the Renaissance saw significant religious, economic and social change. This stimulated a questioning approach, led by the German monk Martin Luther, that challenged the Catholic Church. Eventually, by 1530, Europe was divided into two faiths, Protestant and Catholic, and in England Henry VIII took the opportunity the Reformation provided to break with Rome. This was followed by the dissolution of the monasteries with the associated closure of their very beneficial infirmaries.

The new Protestant attitude to health and illness was to see suffering as very much the will of God. There was much less emphasis on the intervention of the saints and the Virgin Mary in healing and the role of carers was seen as less valuable.

Social change and health

The 16th and 17th centuries also saw major ideological, social and economic changes influencing care of the sick. A rising population heralded lack of jobs and a subsequent rise in social unrest, poverty and vagrancy. In 1601 the very first Poor Law Act had been passed which was to become the anchor of social policy for the next 300 years. This Act was designed to operate through the parishes where money was collected to help the poor and needy. Almshouses and hospitals for the poor were built.

During the 18th century a number of private schools designed for the better teaching of surgeons, and which were the forerunners of today's medical schools, were established in London. Medical students were taught at these institutions and medical students performed many tasks that later came to be nursing duties. Matrons were appointed by the governors and were responsible for household affairs, including the linen room and the control of female staff. Nurses were of lower status and mainly lived outside the hospital. Those who lived in usually slept in small rooms off the wards (later to be converted into sisters' sitting rooms or ward offices, which some of today's nurses will still remember!). Nurses received some money and an allowance of beer, since water in those days was unfit to drink.

The new Poor Law 1834

With the increasing momentum of the Industrial Revolution, the old systems of social relief for the poor and sick were becoming overstretched. In 1832 a commission was set up to investigate the workings of the Poor Law. The man associated mostly with this work was Sir Edwin Chadwick (1800–1890). For Chadwick, poverty, poor health and crime were all forces that stopped the realisation of the full potential of national production.

The report was therefore dominated by the notion that most paupers were able-bodied. In 1834 the Poor Law Amendment Act came into force. This saw the building of the first workhouses for the poor, sick and needy. However, conditions inside the workhouses were often worse than the most intolerable conditions to be found in the outside world – the aim supposedly being to deter idleness. The commission recommended that the categories of children, the sick, the insane and the able-bodied be separated, with strict segregation of the sexes. However, more often than not they were all mixed up together. The workhouses became objects of fear, only to be resorted to as the last desperate measure. During this time the sick poor were nursed by elderly pauper women who were often somewhat physically and intellectually limited in their ability to care for the sick. Within 40 years it became obvious that the care of the sick in the workhouses needed reform. New infirmaries were built, known as Poor Law Hospitals, and these were allowed to admit and train probationer nurses. Many of these hospitals are still with us and used for elderly care and some older patients remember these buildings as workhouses. Although they were incorporated into the National Health Service (NHS) in 1948, the stigma of the Poor Law remained with them for many years. The term 'probationer nurse' also remained as the name for a nurse in training until the term 'student' was introduced in the late 1950s.

During the course of the 19th century, attitudes towards the poor changed, and poverty came to be seen not as a result of idleness but often due to sickness or other circumstances. It was generally felt that there should be greater protection for the less fortunate members of society.

The legacy of Florence Nightingale

No account of the development of nursing would be complete without the mention of Florence Nightingale (1820–1910). Florence Nightingale achieved celebrity status in her own lifetime through her work in the Crimean War, but this was only two years of her long and busy life. Many notable books have been written about her and these are well worth reading to see how her influence is still with nursing today (see Further reading).

Florence Nightingale was born of wealthy middle class parents who were religious with strict Victorian ideals. She had the benefit of a good education and was able to converse easily with many leading social and political figures of the day. She developed an interest in social issues and began to study public health reports and commissions, in which she was to become an expert. Her parents refused to allow her to train as a nurse at the Salisbury Infirmary near the family home in Hampshire, but she was later allowed to undertake 3 months training in Kaiserworth, Germany, in a hospital staffed by deaconesses. In 1853 she was appointed superintendent of the Establishment for Gentlewomen during Illness, Harley Street, London. During her time there she revolutionised its management, installing piped hot water, lifts and many labour-saving devices. She was emphatic on the need for nurses to concentrate on nursing tasks, rather than domestic duties. As a result of her position, she started lobbying her old friend Sidney Herbert – a statesman who was later to become Minister at War – on the need for nursing reform.

After the battle of the Alma, at the beginning of the Crimean War, reports in the press criticised British medical facilities for the wounded. In response, Florence was appointed by Sidney Herbert to supervise the introduction of female nurses into the military hospitals in Turkey. Thirty-eight nurses had been interviewed and recruited in the 2 weeks prior to leaving England. In November 1854 Miss Nightingale arrived in the Scutari barracks only to find that the military doctors would not allow her nurses into the hospital. Ten days later, however, the casualties poured in from the battle of Inkerman and the nurses were fully stretched at their work! Miss Nightingale's persistence, her powerful connections at home and her control of a large budget all contributed to her being able to turn around the deplorable conditions into something resembling a therapeutic institution. She applied sanitary principles, and although she was mistaken in her understanding of the spread of infection,

improved ventilation and less overcrowding undoubtedly contributed towards reducing the mortality rate of the wounded. Miss Nightingale's personal dynamism was reflected in the long hours she worked. She contracted Crimean fever but recovered and returned to work, determined to improve the conditions for the soldiers. She recognised their human dignity and they in return held her in high esteem.

On her return to England, Florence set about campaigning to improve the health of the army. The 1860 Royal Commission resulted in the establishment of an Army Medical School and improvements in barracks and army hospitals. Florence provided the commission with a formidable collection of statistics. For this achievement she became the first woman to be elected a Fellow of the Statistical Society. She developed a revolutionary new way of collecting statistics, known as Model Forms. Several London hospitals and government departments later adopted these. Many nurses today regard Florence Nightingale as the first research nurse in the UK.

Another nurse and healer who contributed to the welfare of allied soldiers in the Crimean War was Mary Seacole, of mixed Scottish and Jamaican descent. Although she was experienced in the treatment of fevers and wound care, the authorities in England rejected Mary's services. Of her own volition, she visited the battlefields, dispensing comfort and provisions to the wounded. In 1856 she returned, bankrupt, to England. She published a book about her travels, one of the few published writings of any black woman before the 20th century. She was helped financially by fundraising attempts by the soldiers she had nursed and finally by a pension from Queen Victoria. Until her centenary in 1981, Mary was forgotten, but renewed interest in her and her achievements has resulted in a nursing award named after her.

The Nightingale School

While Miss Nightingale was in the Crimea, Sidney Herbert had set up a committee to collect money from a grateful nation in the form of a fund (known as the Nightingale Fund) to enable her to train nurses. St Thomas's Hospital eventually became the site for the new Nightingale Nursing School.

Florence had envisaged a nursing school similar to a medical school, but the medical officer insisted that the probationers, as assistant nurses, would be under the supervision of the matron, a Mrs Wardroper. Despite only a few of the probationers lasting the 4-year contract, publicity for the school was good. By the 1870s many of the London teaching hospitals were laying the foundations of a training school along Nightingale lines.

Pressure from ladies wishing to nurse and the demand for trained nurses led Miss Nightingale to devote more time to the school. She introduced the grade of special probationer that was intended for ladies. They paid £30 for their board and lodgings but received the same training as the ordinary probationers who paid nothing. At the end of the year, they expected to be appointed to superior positions as ward sisters, matrons or lady superintendents. A systematic form of lectures and examinations for the probationers was introduced when a new medical officer was appointed. All this helped the school gain a good reputation and soon Miss Nightingale was exporting her best sisters to set up schools and take charge of hospitals and infirmaries. The fund also undertook to train nurses for home nursing. Florence worked with William Rathbone, a wealthy shipping magnate in Liverpool, who donated a new building in his home city as a school to train nurses to care both at home and in hospital.

Nursing and hygiene certainly improved under the Nightingale system, and a career structure for nurses was established, opening up nursing as a respectable occupation for middle class women.

Nurse registration and the drive for professionalism

The success of the Nightingale reforms led to a rapid increase in the number of training schools. Lady probationers added prestige, and as more middle class people became hospital patients there was a demand for more and better nurses. Advances in medical science such as antiseptic surgery and anaesthesia, pioneered by Lister, Pasteur and Simpson, also demanded a more conscientious type of nurse. Middle class women saw nursing as a worthy career, and at this time only teaching or the newly developing Civil Service offered any alternative.

By the 1880s the new nurse leaders were beginning to ask whether nursing should be tested by public examination and that only those passing this examination be entered on a register and be entitled to call themselves a nurse. Medical practitioners had been required to do this by the provisions of the 1858 Medical Act and there had been a significant improvement in standards. Miss Nightingale and Miss Luckes, matron of the London Hospital, were against registration, believing it was a waste to train every nurse with a uniform training for each different type of nursing.

The main protagonist was Ethel Gordon Manson who at the age of 24 was appointed matron of St Bartholomew's Hospital, London. Her experience convinced her of the need for a uniform training to raise standards and guarantee a professional status for nursing. Her marriage to Dr Bedford Fenwick in 1887 allowed her to continue in the struggle for state registration supported by her husband, who was a political activist. Her fight for registration was to take her the best part of the next 30 years.

The Bedford Fenwicks took over the publication the *Nursing Record*, which then changed to the *British Journal of Nursing*. Mrs Bedford Fenwick was editor, a post she held for nearly 50 years. She used this journal to gain support for her ideas. From the turn of the century until 1914, registration bills were introduced into Parliament but were blocked.

It was the impact of the changes during the First World War that eventually hastened the registration debate. Young women volunteered to nurse for the war effort. With a short basic training, these Voluntary Aid Detachment (VAD) nurses were sent to assist trained nurses, and in their uniforms with red crosses on their aprons were called nurses. It was the threat of these women diluting nursing that united nurses in favour of registration. Even at the last minute there was still not complete agreement, and the new Minister for Health had to step in and draft his own bill.

In 1919 the Nurses Registration Act was passed. Each country was to set up a register of qualified nurses and compile a syllabus for instruction and for examination. Mrs Bedford Fenwick became state registered nurse (SRN) no. 1 on the register for England and Wales. In 1921 the General Nursing Council (GNC) was set up, and this included a disciplinary committee which had the power to remove those felt to be unfit to remain on the register.

The register comprised several parts, the main part containing the names of all nurses satisfying the conditions of admission to the register. There were supplementary parts for:

- male nurses
- mental nurses
- children's nurses
- fever nurses
- nurses trained in the care of mental defectives.

Internal discipline and the protection of the public, two important tenets of professional identity, were in the hands of the GNC. However, nurses had given the right to control the standards of entry and the requirements of basic training to the government, and this regulation is one of the most crucial characteristics of professional status. It was another 60 years before this control was regained.

Nursing developments during the 20th century

During the 1930s there was widespread dissatisfaction within nursing over recruitment, pay and conditions. A series of reports offered constructive remedies but the outbreak of the Second World War meant that all proposals were shelved. With the advent of war, nursing became part of the complex machinery of the Home Front. Recruitment was still a problem, as many potential nurses preferred to join the military services. In 1943 the pay of nurses was put on a level with

that of teachers and as a temporary measure a grade of assistant nurse was introduced. This was to become the grade of state enrolled nurse (SEN) and this was envisaged as a bedside nurse working under the supervision of an SRN. The distinction gradually became eroded. Many SENs found themselves with no clear definition of their role, they felt exploited and they had no career structure. This 'temporary' training continued for the next 40 years! During the 1980s and 90s, enrolled nurses were provided with opportunities to convert to registered nurses and the enrolled nurse training was finally abolished.

During the 1960s there was an attempt to give nursing more say in policy decisions by introducing a formal management structure into nursing. The report of the Committee on Senior Nursing Staff (Salmon Report) based nursing management on three tiers, ward sisters/charge nurses being the lowest or first line managers, accountable to nursing officers and senior nursing officers. Many nurses did not take readily to these new roles, and progression to nursing officer posts usually meant leaving clinical work. There was no obvious career pathway for those who wanted to stay in the clinical setting.

In 1979 a new Nurses, Midwives and Health Visitors Act was passed, and the United Kingdom Central Council for Nursing Midwifery and Health Visiting (UKCC) and four national boards were established. In 1986 the UKCC put forward its proposals for a new preparation of nurses (known as Project 2000), which included such radical changes as not counting the students as part of the nursing workforce, putting the training programme at the academic level of a diploma and having a common entry for all types of nursing speciality, with a common foundation programme of 18 months before pursuing the chosen speciality (see page 9 for further details).

At the same time, the NHS was undergoing major reorganisation with the introduction of a general management culture, eventually culminating in the development of Trusts which were expected to function as businesses under the umbrella of guidance from the NHS national and regional executive bodies. Alongside these political and organisational changes within the health care field, the knowledge base of nursing had grown, to keep pace with the considerable advances in medicine. This meant new approaches were rapidly needed for delivering care. Patients knew more and demanded more. The nursing process and primary nursing, backed up by research-based theory, contributed to a more individualised, patient-orientated approach to care. The routine so treasured by the Nightingale nurses had been replaced by individual care plans agreed between patient and nurse.

The power and influence of nursing may appear to have been reduced during the reforms of the last 20 years with the loss of 'the matron'. In reality, though, nurses are becoming powerful leaders not just of nursing but also of general health care delivery, and career opportunities are significantly more varied than they were 50 years ago. However, it is important that in taking on new responsibilities nurses should not lose the essentials, the core skills of nursing that have been cherished over the centuries.

Pre-registration nursing programmes

At the time of writing, most student nurses will have entered nursing on a 3-year, full-time diploma course. Some will be undertaking a degree programme, again usually full-time. All nursing courses are now run within the university sector, but strong links with the NHS, social services and other care providers are maintained in relation to the practice experience which all student nurses must have. Whether at diploma or degree level, the course is 50% theoretical study and 50% in the practice setting. The first year is the Common Foundation Programme (CFP), recently reduced from 18 months to 1 year, which is the foundation on which all further nursing preparation is based. During this time you should have experience in all four nursing branches/specialities, in order to give you some insight into the branch of nursing you wish to study and in which you wish to qualify. They are:

- nursing adults
- nursing children

- mental health nursing
- learning disability nursing.

The actual programmes of nursing education have recently undergone another major review by both the government and the UKCC. In *Making a Difference* (DoH 1999), the Department of Health outlines the government's plans to expand the nursing workforce, to strengthen nursing leadership, to widen access to nurse education and to increase the practical components of the first year with longer practice placements than in the previous Common Foundation Programme. As a result, all universities will now be running this new programme, with flexible modes of entry to the profession, fast-tracking for some students, and opportunities to 'bank' academic credit and use vocational qualifications gained for parts of the course if a student leaves before completion of the full course. The UKKC report *Fitness for Practice* (UKCC 1999) also revealed significant concerns in the profession regarding some aspects of nurse education and so put forward its recommendations for what is now today's route into the nursing profession.

UKCC competencies for the Common Foundation Programme

The UKCC outlined the requirements to be achieved at the end of the Common Foundation Programme and the competencies required on registration, and these are printed in full at the end of this chapter (Appendix 1). If successful, at the end of the course you will be qualified to nurse within your chosen speciality in either the hospital or community setting. The UKCC uses the term 'competence' to describe 'the skills and ability to practise safely and effectively without the need for direct supervision' (UKCC 1999). The main areas of study required to achieve these competencies will be:

- professional, ethical and legal issues
- the theory and practice of nursing
- the context in which health and social care is delivered
- organisational structures and processes
- communication

- social and life sciences relevant to nursing practice
- frameworks for social care provision and care systems.

All these areas will be introduced to you during the CFP.

Being a nursing student

It can be quite difficult being a nursing student in a university setting. In order to achieve the number of hours required in theory and practice to register as a nurse, the programmes are very full and have less flexibility and freedom than other university courses. This is particularly so in the last 2 years when you will be undertaking more practical work and be part of the nursing team and doing shift-work. Chapters 3, 4 and 11 emphasise the importance of ethics, the law and the accountability and responsibility nurses must take on if they are to uphold the safety and trust that is given to them by patients and clients. Part of training to be a nurse is assimilating the attitudes and values of the nursing profession in a way that can profoundly influence the thinking, personality and lifestyle of the individual concerned. Being a good nurse not only demands theoretical knowledge and practical expertise, but also growth in moral experience or practical wisdom (Thompson et al 1994).

Patients and clients

You will come across both these terms. 'Patients' are usually those who are physically sick and in hospital or at home and requiring medical treatment, whereas the term 'clients' is usually reserved for those who are either mentally ill or require psychological or social care. You will obviously meet patients who are acutely ill in hospital, for example someone having had a heart attack (myocardial infarction) or having been admitted for surgery in hospital, and people with chronic conditions, such as arthritis, in the community. You should experience the care of children, mothers and babies in both hospital and community settings. Clients with mental health problems and people with learning disability will

be encountered mainly in community, social care and home settings.

People now have a greater access to medical knowledge through the media, literature and the internet. Consequently their expectations are greater and, rightly, they wish to be more involved in the planning of the treatment they will receive. Nurses can empower patients and clients by involving them in planning their care (see Ch. 13).

All nurses must learn to manage the professional values of equity and fairness when dealing with patients and clients. This is a commitment to health for all, irrespective of class, creed, age, gender, sexual orientation, culture or ethnic background. Chapter 5 explores this area further, and points to ways in which nurses can manage care in a multicultural society.

INTRODUCTION TO THE BRANCH PROGRAMMES

To assist you in deciding which branch you would like to undertake, the following section is designed to give a brief outline of the client group likely to be cared for within each branch and the care practices for that particular group. The specific role of the nurse for each speciality and future trends are also outlined.

NURSING ADULTS

The greatest number of nurses in practice care for adults (those who are over 16 years of age) and this is the branch of nursing which most people know as 'general nursing'. However, this branch encompasses many different specialities and subspecialities, some of which will be considered here. Adults today will be seeking and receiving care in a variety of settings, ranging from health centres to hospitals (private and NHS), clinics or clients' homes. Those adults in hospital will be requiring support in their sick role. The nurse will be involved in providing psychological support as well as meeting the individual's physical needs in what, for most, is the acute phase of their illness. Adults requiring terminal care will receive this in a variety of settings, including hospitals, hospices or their own homes.

Traditionally, hospitals have been the main setting for adult care, but patterns of care have changed as patterns of disease have changed. There have been, and continue to be, considerable advances in science and technology affecting health care provision. High-tech areas such as operating theatres are unrecognisable from those of 20 years ago, cardiac surgery is now an everyday occurrence, and organ transplants are performed frequently. Prosthetic surgery (e.g. hip replacement) is now very sophisticated and benefits many. All these advances have affected the role of the nurse caring for adults across the care settings. Present policies for care provision mean shorter acute hospital admissions with longer periods of convalescence in the community.

The care of adults is usually considered under medical specialities that take place in both hospital and community settings. So the major nursing care groups are:

- medical nursing, which will include the nursing of infectious diseases
- surgical nursing
- critical care nursing
- elderly care nursing.

Students of the adult branch will gain experience with most of these groups and, of course, care of the elderly is a certain feature of all types of adult nursing today. Many acute care patients are elderly.

Medical nursing

Medical nursing generally takes place in hospital, although many people in the community require the specialist skills of the medical nurse. These skills include effective communication and close observation for signs of pain, breathlessness, abnormal body temperature, altered colour, or mental distress. In extreme circumstances, lifesaving interventions such as cardiopulmonary resuscitation may be required. Many individuals requiring medical nursing have heart and lung disorders, with chest pain and breathlessness being common symptoms. Myocardial infarction (Case

Case example 1.1 Care of the patient following myocardial infarction

Ted, a 42-year-old chemical engineer, is married with two teenage children. He enjoys the occasional game of squash, is a little overweight and smokes. While doing some alterations to the house, he collapsed, complaining of severe chest pain. His wife rang for the GP and an ambulance, and Ted was subsequently admitted to the local coronary care unit (CCU).

The nurse will be involved in Ted's care in the CCU or later in the medical ward. In the CCU the nurse will encourage Ted to rest (giving him psychological support), in order to reduce his cardiac activity. She will monitor the administration of analgesics, anti-arrhythmics, vasodilators and other drugs, usually via an intravenous cannula.

Observations will include monitoring the electrocardiogram (ECG), noting any arrhythmias, and taking pulse and blood pressure readings. The nurse should be competent to observe for signs of shock, recognise an impending cardiac arrest and, if required, initiate cardiopulmonary resuscitation.

The nurse's role will also include ensuring that Ted is free from pain. She should be aware of his basic nursing needs and any anxieties he has in relation to his condition. The patient's fears should be discussed openly, and he should be given information and reassurance. This aspect of the nursing role will be continued on the medical ward as Ted begins to adapt to a new lifestyle. In this phase of treatment, the nurse will be involved in educating him and encouraging him to adopt healthy eating patterns, to reduce or stop smoking, and to exercise regularly once recovery is complete.

example 1.1), heart failure, bronchitis, emphysema and asthma (Case example 1.2) are some of the commonest disorders in medical wards.

Patients with endocrinological disorders, the commonest being diabetes mellitus, will be encountered by the adult branch student and Case example 1.3 describes the role of the nurse in this situation. Other patient groups include those with rheumatoid arthritis and those with infectious diseases, and both groups may well now be cared for in specialist units.

Surgical nursing

Surgical nursing is a rapidly changing area of care with advanced technology introducing new techniques which reduce the trauma to the

Case example 1.2 Care of the patient during an acute asthmatic attack

Simon, aged 14, was admitted to the ward at 10.00 p.m. He had a history of asthma since he was a little boy, but controlled the condition well using an inhaler. He was accompanied by his mother, who was a nurse, but has not practised for some time. Skin tests showed Simon is allergic to the house dust mite. He looked anxious and pale and was having great difficulty in getting his breath. The houseman immediately gave intravenous hydrocortisone to reduce bronchial inflammation and thereby ease breathing.

The nurse's role in Simon's care will initially be to sit with him and his mother, giving them calm reassurance while the drug takes effect. Later on, by talking to the mother, the nurse may assess her understanding of her son's allergy and determine whether she has taken all possible steps to reduce Simon's contact with house dust mites.

Case example 1.3 Care of the patient with newly diagnosed diabetes mellitus

Jean, aged 32, has just returned from a camping holiday with her husband and two small children. While on holiday she became thirsty and rather tired, but attributed this to the hot weather. Her husband returned from his first day back at work to find her slumped in a chair, unconscious. She was admitted to the accident and emergency department of the local hospital, where diabetes mellitus was diagnosed. She was then transferred to the ward for treatment. Following an intravenous infusion of dextrose and insulin, she soon felt much better.

Initially, the nurse's role will be to monitor Jean's blood and urine glucose levels by taking blood samples and testing the urine. Care of the intravenous infusion, with the addition of glucose, will need to be carefully regulated. As Jean recovers, the nurse will need to explain how to adjust to living with diabetes. Jean will need to know how to administer her own injections, how to care for herself with respect to diet, weight and likely infections, and what to do when she has had insufficient glucose or insulin.

patient and reduce the amount of time spent in hospital. Patients undergoing operations previously with admission times of 10–14 days can now expect to be discharged in 24–48 hours; thanks to advances such as keyhole surgery. This type of surgery is now widely available, reducing

the need for major invasive techniques. Examples are laparoscopic cholecystectomy (gall bladder removal) and arthroscopic meniscectomy (removal of cartilage in the knee joint). Many patients are now admitted for day case surgery, for example cataract removal, removal of nasal polyps, minor gynaecological operations and simple hernia repairs, all of which until recently warranted at least a few days in hospital, if not longer.

These changes have resulted in a role change for the surgical nurse. The high turnover of patients means that the care will almost always be for the 'high-dependency' patients, a great number of whom will require specialist care. It also means that the nurse is less able to build up a rapport with patients, although they and their families need significant consideration when everything occurs so swiftly. Planning for discharge is crucial because many of these patients require acute care in the community and remain dependent in their own homes for much longer.

Nurses working in surgical care have a vital role to play in preparing the patient, both physically and psychologically, for forthcoming surgery, and in maintaining safety and adequate pain control following the operation. There may be considerable technical care required. The most common operations likely to be encountered by the adult branch student are abdominal, rectal, orthopaedic, gynaecological and breast. Case examples 1.4 and 1.5 give some indication of the role of the nurse for those having major surgery.

It is probable that the adult branch student will gain some experience in the operating theatre and anaesthetic room, where the emphasis on patient safety is paramount. It is very helpful in understanding the factors which affect a patient's postoperative comfort and eventual recovery to have seen what happened during the surgery itself.

Critical care nursing

Critical care nursing usually takes place in specialised units which might include:

- intensive therapy units (ITUs)
- coronary care units (CCUs)
- spinal injury units

Case example 1.4 Care of the patient following mastectomy

Juliette is a 45-year-old nurse manager of a busy surgical unit. Having been a capable and innovative ward sister for a number of years at the same hospital, she is well respected by junior and senior staff. Following the discovery of a lump in her breast, a diagnosis of cancer is confirmed, and Juliette has been advised by the surgeon that a mastectomy is indicated. Juliette lives alone but has a number of friends.

If there is no specialist nurse available to help mastectomy patients, the nurse on the ward will fulfil this function. Nursing intervention will include discussing with Juliette her hopes and fears and her reaction to taking on the role of patient. This may include some consideration of the ways in which being in familiar surroundings is or is not a comfort. Involvement of a close friend in these conversations could be suggested.

Postoperatively, the nurse will be responsible for care of the drainage tube and the wound. At this time, she will need to be aware of Juliette's possible reaction to the scar and to a change in body image. The nurse should know what is available in the way of reconstruction appliances and clothes for women who have had a mastectomy.

Case example 1.5 Care of the patient with a colostomy

John, a 45-year-old solicitor, is married and has two teenage children. He was diagnosed as having cancer of the rectum, and, in view of the pathology report, it was considered that the best treatment for him would be an abdominoperineal resection of the rectum, resulting in a permanent colostomy. The operation was successful, and John was soon discharged home. In the hospital, there was no stoma care nurse. The nurses seemed very busy, so he was reluctant to ask questions regarding caring for the colostomy.

The community nurse will need to show John how to attach his appliance and care for the skin surrounding the colostomy. Advice on diet should help to regulate the action of the colostomy so that John can confidently go out in public. He will need to know how to dispose of the contents and the bag both at home and in public places. He may be anxious about odour and should be advised on special deodorants. He may also wonder whether he can play sports and whether his sex life will be affected. The nurse will need to be able to assess and discuss such fears, and help John to regain sufficient confidence to enjoy sports and resume sexual relations with his wife. Helping the patient to regain confidence in these and other areas is perhaps the most important and rewarding aspect of stoma care nursing.

- burns units
- renal units
- neurosurgical units
- accident and emergency units.

Critical care nursing is that which is required by individuals admitted as emergencies or transferred following major surgery or other treatments. Nurses working in such units require the ability to make quick decisions in life-threatening situations and require a high order of knowledge of physiology and psychology in order to judge patients' responses in any given emergency. They will also be trained and skilled in using special emergency clinical equipment. It may often be a stressful environment, and multidisciplinary teamwork is the norm for good practice. Case example 1.6 describes a possible scenario in critical care nursing.

Case example 1.6 Critical care nursing of a tracheostomy patient (contributed by Pamela Taylor)

Anthony, a 38-year-old builder's labourer, fell 30 ft from some scaffolding, sustaining multiple fractures and a subdural haematoma. Initially, he was intubated and attached to a ventilator so that his respiratory function could be monitored. After a week he was breathing spontaneously, but as access to his chest was still required to remove secretions, a tracheostomy was performed.

Some of the main aspects of Anthony's care related to the tracheostomy. He still required oxygen; this was humidified and supplied through an adaptor set connected to the tracheostomy tube. Regular suction was required to remove secretions. Anthony initially produced large amounts of infected secretions, which were greenish in colour and very tenacious. The observations of the nurse were critical at all times. Anthony's neurological and chest condition improved following a course of antibiotics; subsequently, the tracheostomy tube was changed. As his blood oxygen levels began to improve, he no longer required oxygen. When Anthony's swallowing reflex returned, he was tempted with fluids and a little soft diet. As this was successful, his tracheostomy tube was closed off for short periods until he was finally breathing on his own.

In Anthony's case, the physical nursing care required initially took priority over psychological and social care. Care was concentrated on establishing and sustaining respiration. Correct administration of oxygen and knowledge of the nursing skills required in caring for a tracheostomy were essential. The nursing model chosen to guide care reflected this priority in needs.

Care of the elderly

More attention is now being paid to the specific care required by elderly people. In the 1980s pioneering work in this area of practice was carried out at Burford Hospital, Oxford (Pearson 1988), and this set the scene for positive developments nationally.

Elderly patients may be admitted to medical or surgical wards for assessment and they often present with multiple pathologies, for example diabetes with hypertension and anaemia. New techniques in anaesthesia and a reduction in operating times means that many more elderly people can undergo surgery without undue risk.

However, an increasing number of people are now living into their late 80s and 90s. The very elderly perhaps have different needs from those who are, say, 10 years younger, and specialist nurses are able to design programmes of care to meet the needs of this group of patients.

All students will spend time working with elderly patients and should take every opportunity to discover the creative and exciting programmes of care that can make caring for the older person such a rewarding experience.

One of the commonest causes of acute disability in the older person is cerebrovascular accident (stroke), and all student nurses are likely to be involved in care for stroke patients from a very early stage in training. The rehabilitation of these patients presents one of the major and most complex challenges to adult branch nurses (Case example 1.7).

Future trends in adult care

The UK has an ageing population. The incidence of chronic illness will increase at the same time as the number of the supporting younger population decreases. This means ever growing demands on the health care system. Technological advances mean ever shorter acute in-patient episodes of care and significant increases in care in the community with an accompanying change in the role of the adult branch nurse.

 Case example 1.7 Care of the dysphasic stroke patient

Joseph is 75 years old. He has been married for 30 years, has two children and two grandchildren, and is now retired from self-employment as a carpenter. He was diagnosed 10 days ago as having had a cerebrovascular accident, which has left him with weakness in his left arm and difficulty in speaking. He is finding communicating very frustrating. His wife says that he is an extremely private and independent person. Unfortunately, he now finds himself unable to eat, drink or attend to his toilet needs without assistance.

The nurse's role will be to help Joseph to regain some degree of independence in the activities of daily living. In planning a programme of care with him, the nurse can take the opportunity to establish a communication system with Joseph, for example a key words board with which he can indicate his needs. Enhancing the patient's ability to communicate is arguably the most important and challenging aspect of caring for stroke victims, and one in which patience is paramount. Time and gentleness are required to give Joseph long enough to gesticulate and make sounds; the temptation to speak for him or to make swift assumptions about what he wants must be resisted. The patient must never be treated like a child or like someone who is incapable of understanding. He will be desperately frustrated and anguished and must be given time to express himself. He requires everything that is best in nursing.

CHILDREN'S NURSING

Children's nursing has seen major developments since the 1960s and paediatric nurses can be proud of their achievements in being at the forefront of humanising hospitals. These changes have been introduced as paediatric nurses have continued to explain that children are not 'small adults' and that they have physical, psychological and social needs different from those of adults. Paediatric philosophies of care have been developed from the work of major psychologists and by various national and international reports, including the United Nations' list of children's rights (UN 1987), which was adopted by the British government in 1991 (Box 1.1). The National Association for the Welfare of Children in Hospital (which is now Action for Sick Children) has also worked with the professionals to improve the care and facilities for children in hospital. In 1985, it produced a charter which has

---

Box 1.1   United Nations declaration of the rights of the child (abbreviated)

1. The right to equality, regardless of race, colour, religion, sex or nationality.
2. The right to healthy mental and physical development.
3. The right to a name and nationality.
4. The right to sufficient food, housing and medical care.
5. The right to special care if handicapped.
6. The right to love, understanding and care.
7. The right to free education, play and recreation.
8. The right to immediate aid in the event of disasters and emergencies.
9. The right to protection from cruelty, neglect and exploitation.
10. The right to protection from persecution and to an upbringing in the spirit of worldwide brotherhood and peace.

Box 1.2   National Association for the Welfare of Children in Hospital (NAWCH) charter for children in hospital

1. Children shall be admitted to hospital only if the care they require cannot be equally well provided at home or on a day basis.
2. Children in hospital shall have the right to have their parents with them at all times, provided that this is in the best interests of the child. Accommodation should therefore be offered to all parents, and they should be helped and encouraged to stay. In order to share in the care of their child, parents should be fully informed about ward routine and their active participation encouraged.
3. Children and/or parents shall have the right to information appropriate to age and understanding.
4. Children and/or parents shall have the right to informed participation in all decisions involving their health care. Every child shall be protected from unnecessary medical treatment and steps taken to mitigate physical or emotional distress.
5. Children shall be treated with tact and understanding and at all times their privacy shall be respected.
6. Children shall enjoy the care of appropriately trained staff, fully aware of the physical and emotional needs of each age group.
7. Children shall be able to wear their own clothes and have their own personal possessions.
8. Children shall be cared for with other children of the same age group.
9. Children shall be in an environment furnished and equipped to meet their requirements, and which conforms to recognised standards of safety and supervision.
10. Children shall have full opportunity for play, recreation and education suited to their age and condition.

---

now been adopted in many European countries (Box 1.2). Today, of course, much medical and nursing care of children takes place in the community and this is dealt with later.

Changing patterns of children's health and illness

Children's health has improved dramatically over the past 100 years, mainly due to changes in social conditions, public health measures and better nutrition. Today, deaths of children from malnutrition and from infectious and diarrhoeal diseases are seen only in developing countries. At the beginning of the 19th century, however, diseases such as tuberculosis, rheumatic fever and polio were common, with children staying in hospital for long periods of time. Although many diseases in children have decreased over the years, some are on the increase, the most significant being in the number of children suffering from asthma and diabetes. Children's wards admit significant numbers of children with cancer and leukaemia. The prognosis has improved a great deal but many children require periods in hospital for treatment. Genetic disorders, such as cystic fibrosis, are another cause of childhood morbidity. The child with cystic fibrosis, the most common serious inherited disease, will often require periods in hospital to treat infection or improve nutritional status.

Children and accidents

After the age of 1 year, the most common cause of death for children and adolescents is accidents. Not only are they a significant cause of death, but they can also result in permanent disability. Many children die from accidents each year, and many attend accident and emergency departments. Young children being cared for at home may suffer accidents such as poisonings, burns and scalds and falls. As the child gets older, he is exposed to the wider environment, and the most common cause of death is that of a child pedestrian who is involved in a traffic accident.

Changes in the provision of health care for children

Prior to the 19th century, sick children were nursed at home. There were no facilities specifically for children and admission to adult hospitals ran the risk of cross-infection. In the mid-19th century Dr Charles West founded the first children's hospital, Great Ormond Street. This stimulated the foundation of other children's hospitals and many hospitals allocated specific wards for the care of children. At this time, there were no facilities for mothers to stay or visit a sick child, and consequently, parents were separated from their sick children for long periods, with only minimal visiting hours. Gradually it was recognised that children were suffering as a result of this deprivation of parental comfort. The Platt Report (Ministry of Health 1959), the work of John Bowlby (1971) and other psychologists, and the formation of the pressure group the National Association for the Welfare of Children in Hospital (NAWCH) led to changes in the way in which children were treated (see Box 1.2). Other reports emphasised that, wherever possible, children should be treated at home and that hospital admissions should be kept short. This has been assisted by the advent of day surgery and the expansion of paediatric community nursing.

Caring for children in hospital

Most children who are admitted to hospital will be cared for in a children's ward in an acute general hospital. Children's wards were among the first to encourage free visiting for relatives and to ensure that children wore their own clothes while in hospital. Most paediatric units have abolished the traditional nurses' uniform in favour of something less formal and less threatening to young children. There will be facilities for children to play and for parents to stay overnight with their child. Schooling is catered for.

Staffing of children's wards and adequate numbers of paediatric nurses in areas such as accident and emergency and intensive care units has been the subject of major scrutiny over the past 10 years. It is now recognised that children should be nursed by specialist staff wherever they are receiving care and so paediatric nurses will be seen working in accident and emergency departments, outpatients' departments, intensive care units and some specialist surgical wards where there are just one or two beds for children. Student nurses may expect to gain experience in any or all of these areas.

Caring for children in the community

Certain members of the primary health care team work specifically with children. The health visitor is responsible, in conjunction with the GP, for monitoring growth, carrying out developmental assessments and encouraging families to have their children immunised. The health visitor also has a key role in health promotion and early identification of problems within the family. She is in the prime position to work with parents to reduce the numbers of accidents occurring to children.

Paediatric community nurses may be attached to the acute hospital services and follow up children on discharge (Case example 1.8). Others may be more specialised and help with specific cases, such as children who may require fairly intensive care (for example, they may be oxygen dependent or have a tracheostomy). As the demand for the service increases and the benefits become apparent, the number of paediatric community nurses is increasing, and child branch student nurses may be able to spend more time working with them.

The role of the children's nurse

Children who require health care have the right to have their parents with them at all times, unless it is not in their best interests. Children's nursing is therefore family centred, and the nurse needs to work with the whole family in order to meet the needs of the sick child. Children are dependent on adults even when they are well, and parents can be encouraged to give the

Case example 1.8

Martin is a paediatric community nurse attached to a children's unit. James, one of the children for whom Martin is currently caring, is aged 18 months and has been diagnosed as having diabetes mellitus.

He was initially stabilised in hospital on insulin twice daily. His mother was taught to give his injections but was still quite apprehensive when James was discharged after 3 days. She is also having problems, as James helps himself to biscuits and cakes from the other children's plates if she is not watchful. She is also finding it very traumatic to have to monitor James's blood sugar.

Martin's role is to support and advise James's mother as she comes to terms with his condition. He is monitoring James's blood sugars and is able to contact the doctor should there be a need to alter the dose of insulin. James's mother requires extra support when he develops a viral infection and refuses to eat; Martin is then able to increase his visiting to the family to prevent James being admitted to hospital.

---

day-to-day care that they would give their child at home. In addition, parents can be taught by the paediatric nurse to give more specialised care. The complexity of care that the parents give should be decided by the nurse and the parents together. Initially, the parents might require teaching in specific areas with support from the nurse. The benefits of the parents remaining as the main carer are that:

- The child is likely to feel more secure when cared for by a familiar person.
- The parents can contribute to the well-being of the child and can support him when he needs them most.
- The parent's ability to undertake much of the care can contribute to an early discharge for the child.

This approach has led to the development of paediatric models of care which recognise the unique relationship between the nurse, the parent and the child.

The children's nurse will need to have the knowledge, skills and attitudes to care for children in a variety of settings. Some of these are illustrated in Case example 1.9.

Case example 1.9

Emma was born with an imperforate anus and went to theatre at the age of 24 hours for the formation of a colostomy, which she will need until she is old enough to have special surgery. She is Simon and Jane's first baby and is being cared for on the neonatal unit. Jane wished to breastfeed Emma but needed help to get feeding established, as, to begin with, Emma had an intravenous infusion. At first, both Simon and Jane were frightened of caring for Emma's colostomy.

In the initial stages, the paediatric nurse needed to be able to observe Emma closely, as she had had an anaesthetic and could have developed respiratory problems. Because of her age, she is vulnerable to cold and infection. There could also be problems with the colostomy, and the nurse needed to observe the stoma closely to ensure that there was a good blood supply. Babies have small circulating blood volumes, so the nurse needed to observe the intravenous infusion closely to ensure that Emma received the correct amount of fluid. The nurse therefore needs to have *special skills related to paediatric nursing*. She also needs to understand the anxiety felt by Simon and Jane and support them during the time that they are in hospital, thus being a *counsellor* to the parents.

When Emma was first admitted, a junior doctor made several attempts to site an intravenous infusion. Emma became very distressed and, after the third attempt, the nurse intervened and suggested that the doctor get some assistance. Postoperatively, the nurse is aware that Emma is in pain; however, she has not been prescribed any analgesia as the anaesthetist feels that the dangers of using analgesia for neonates outweigh the benefits. The paediatric nurse contacts the surgical registrar, who does prescribe for pain relief. The paediatric nurse is here acting as an *advocate*.

When Emma has made progress, the nurse teaches Jane how to breastfeed and how to give normal baby care. As Jane becomes more confident, the nurse teaches her how to change the colostomy bag. The nurse is acting as a *teacher*.

Prior to Emma's discharge, the nurse will contact the paediatric community nurse, who will visit the ward and develop a relationship with the family prior to discharge. She will ensure that there is continuity of care and that Jane does not feel unsupported when she first gets home. The ward nurse will also contact Emma's health visitor, so that she is prepared for the discharge. In this way, the nurse is acting as a *liaison* between the hospital and the community.

After discharge, the parents will need to know where they can obtain colostomy bags, and they have also asked to meet other parents with babies with a similar condition. The paediatric nurse thus acts as a *resource adviser*.

Other aspects of children's nursing

Intensive care and special care baby units

Paediatric nurses work in these areas, usually following further specialist courses. Premature babies and babies who have had problems before or during birth are cared for in special care baby units (SCBUs) and sometimes the care may require total life support. Other sick children need intensive care for a variety of reasons, especially following major surgery, such as cardiac or trauma surgery. Unless the child is admitted to a specialised unit, it is likely that this kind of intensive care will be provided in an adult intensive care unit.

Special needs of adolescents

Although it is increasingly recognised that adolescents have needs different from those of adults or small children, there are few special units as the general opinion is that there are insufficient numbers requiring hospital treatment to justify this. Adolescents are usually learning to adapt to a different body image, which can make them very self-conscious. They need privacy and are also very threatened by anything likely to affect their appearance. They identify strongly with their peer group and need their support and contact. Some adolescents may be facing important exams that require space and a quiet place to study away from the bustle of the ward. Happily, many acute hospital managers are now making available separate facilities for adolescents requiring in-patient care and child branch students will usually gain some experience of nursing these patients.

Children with special needs

These children may be hospitalised for a variety of reasons, for example with an acute illness or for surgery. They may be admitted because they are failing to thrive at home and need investigation, or they may be admitted to give parents some respite for a short period. Children who have been abused also sometimes require hospital care for immediate protection and care of injuries. These children are often emotionally damaged and require special care and understanding.

Terminally ill children

The death rate in children is, fortunately, low. However, it is likely that the children's nurse will come into contact with the terminally ill at some time. The death of a child is always hard to face, as it seems to contravene the normal laws of nature. This issue is covered in Chapter 16.

Child protection and the 'at risk' register

It was only in the 1960s that child abuse was recognised as a problem, although it has been occurring throughout history. After the inquiry into the death of Maria Colwell in 1973, which identified flaws in the system, an 'at risk' register was introduced. This ensured that the name of any child suspected of having been abused would be on a register, so that if there were further suspicions, professionals could identify any previous incidents and the case would be followed up. Children's nurses must be fully aware of any local policies and procedures that should be followed if there is any suspicion of abuse or if the nurse is caring for a child who is known to have been abused.

The future of children's nursing

Children's nursing is alive and well as a speciality and paediatric nurses have a responsibility to ensure that it remains so. Children have a right to be nursed by an appropriately qualified nurse, whether at home or in hospital. Technological advances and shorter stays in hospital now mean that children who are in hospital are likely to be acutely ill. The role of the children's nurse in the community is expanding, involving more teams and greater specialisation, so that fewer children are admitted to hospital at all.

LEARNING DISABILITY NURSING

'Learning disability' is a term with contemporary usage in the UK to describe a group of people

Activity 1.1

The following terms are also used to describe people with a learning disability:

- learning difficulty
- mentally subnormal
- mentally retarded
- mentally impaired
- spastic
- idiot
- imbecile
- moron
- cretin
- Benny

1. Are you aware of other terms that have general usage?
2. Which of these terms do you think is the most acceptable to people in general?
3. Do you think that any of the terms create a negative image of this group of people?

Case example 1.10

Lucy was born in 1967, following a normal pregnancy and labour. She was the youngest of three sisters. It soon became apparent to the family that Lucy was not reaching the normal developmental milestones. At this time, Lucy was referred to a paediatrician at the local general hospital, who diagnosed her as suffering from a mild mental handicap. The paediatrician advised the parents to 'take her home, give her plenty of love, but do not expect too much from her'. During her childhood, Lucy found it difficult to mix well with other children. Her slowness and the distinctive delay in her speech caused much teasing and bullying. Her parents decided that it would be better for Lucy if she were to attend a 'special school'. Lucy thrived in this environment; she learned to read and write, and was able to undertake basic calculations in mathematics. At 16 years of age, Lucy attended a boarding school for 2 years, where she took a simple catering course that was designed to prepare her for future employment.

However, when Lucy returned home, numerous problems arose. She had become a confident, assertive young woman. Her mother still wanted the 'old' Lucy. Her mother encouraged Lucy to stay in her room to do jigsaw puzzles, colour picture books and play her collection of pop tapes. Soon Lucy developed aggressive outbursts that escalated over a period of time into vicious attacks on members of her family. Her mother sought the advice of their GP, who referred them to a community learning disability team. After a series of visits from a community learning disability nurse, Lucy articulated a desire to leave home. With the reluctant support of her parents, Lucy left home and moved into a small community home for people with a learning disability. She now lives in a four-bed-roomed house run by her local authority, with three other people who also have a learning disability. She attends a local resource centre run by the local authority from Monday to Friday. She attends college once a week to update her catering course; she hopes this will enable her to leave the resource centre as she hopes to find a full-time job in a hotel. In addition, she now has a full social life and a boyfriend, and visits her family about once a month at her old home.

with significant developmental delay that results in arrested or incomplete achievement of the 'normal' milestones of human development. These milestones relate to intellectual, emotional, social and spiritual aspects of development. Significant delays in one or more of these may lead to a person being described as having a learning disability. Until recently, the term mental handicap was much more frequently used, but was replaced because it was felt it portrayed a negative image of people with disability. In the USA the term retardation is widely used for the classification of learning disability. Activity 1.1 lists some other terms that are used.

In 1985 Gostin estimated there were 110 000 people with a severe learning disability in England, and more than 350 000 with a mild disability. This represents a significant section of society that is entitled to access to the resource of a skilled, specialist nurse, who is able to meet their health needs.

Defining and assessing for learning disability

The term learning disability means different things to different people. In reading Case example 1.10 you may have some difficulty in deciding whether or not Lucy has a learning disability. How one decides whether an individual has a learning disability is, in fact, quite complex.

The most common criteria used for identifying learning disability are social competence and intellectual ability, but these are not without their problems. For instance people with a chronic mental health problem may be socially incompetent because they are not able to adapt to the changing

Table 1.1 Some examples of the causes of learning disability at different periods in human development

	Possible cause	Example
Prenatal	Chromosome abnormality	Down's syndrome
	Damaged genes	Recessive phenylketonuria
		Dominant tuberous sclerosis
	Illness during pregnancy	Toxaemia
	Environment and nutrition	Substance abuse
	Infections	Rubella, toxoplasmosis
Perinatal	Developmental abnormality	Prematurity
	Birth injury	Cerebral palsy
Postnatal	Infections	Encephalitis
	Physical	Non-accidental injury
	Toxins	Heavy metals (e.g. lead), drug reactions
	Deprivation	Maternal deprivation
	Trauma	Road accident

demands of society, but do not have a learning disability. People with problems of communication, hearing and vision may have some degree of social incompetence and yet do not have a learning disability.

Intelligence tests are generally agreed to provide a relatively objective measure of the intellectual ability of an individual. Despite their limitations, which include cultural bias and poor predictive ability, if they are used appropriately and by properly trained technicians they are generally thought to provide an indication of learning disability. If the results are then used in conjunction with the criterion of social competence, this enables the most accurate definition of learning disability within an individual.

Causes of learning disability

Learning disability is not an illness and so cannot be cured by medical or nursing intervention. However, the condition of learning disability can be greatly ameliorated by appropriate support and care.

Known and unknown causes of learning disability can occur during the pre-, intra- and postnatal periods of human development.

It is not surprising, given the long gestation period in humans, that a major proportion of learning disability results from the prenatal period. It should be remembered that during this period the embryo and fetus are particularly vulnerable to damage from a variety of factors. Equally, all the possible complications and trauma that surround birth make the infant particularly vulnerable to perinatal (up to 28 days after birth) causes of learning disability. Lastly, the growing child is a vulnerable member of society who, without careful attention to both physical and psychological care, may be susceptible to the possibility of developing a learning disability. Some specific conditions associated with learning disability are shown in Table 1.1.

A high proportion of learning disability used to be recorded as being idiopathic (of unknown cause), for example, by some unknown effect of birth trauma. Recent advances in the use of non-invasive methods of imaging the brain while still in utero have helped us to understand how a reduction in blood flow in the brain can result in learning disability. Some types of learning disability cases were in the past presumably labelled as learning disability caused by birth trauma whereas in fact they may have been the result of pathological disorders prior to birth. In addition, work in the study of genetics is providing new insights into a wide variety of disorders that were previously recorded as idiopathic.

Incidence and prevalence of learning disability

Calculating the incidence of learning disability is extremely difficult, because there is no way of detecting the vast majority of infants who have a learning disability at birth. Only the obvious manifestations of learning disability at birth – for example Down's syndrome, with its physical characteristics – can be detected. This early diagnosis gives the ability to calculate the incidence of this disorder. Where there is no obvious physical manifestation, one must wait for delay in a child's development to ascertain whether he has a learning disability.

It is more appropriate, therefore, in learning disability, to talk about prevalence. Prevalence is concerned with an estimation of the number of people with a condition, disorder or disease as a proportion of the general population. If one uses the IQ as an indicator of learning disability, one is able to calculate that 2–3% of the population have an IQ below 70, which represents a large segment of society. Given that a large number of people with such an estimated IQ never come into contact with a caring agency, it is more common to refer to the 'administrative prevalence' – i.e. the number of people who are provided with some form of service from caring agencies. On this basis, there is a general consensus that the overall prevalence of moderate and severe learning disability is approximately 3–4 per 1000 of the general population. Within this group it is not uncommon to find multiple disability, including physical and/or sensory disability as well as behavioural difficulties. It is this group of people who require lifelong support in order for them to achieve and maintain a valued lifestyle. It has often and long been complained that people with a learning disability are not afforded the same rights as other citizens. Careful measurement of prevalence is one way of ensuring that people with special needs are provided with special resources when they are required.

Historical overview of learning disability care

Prior to the 20th century, people with a learning disability were dealt with in the same manner as those with a mental health problem. It was not until 1904 that a Royal Commission was set up to advise on the needs of the 'mentally defective'

population. This commission resulted in the 1913 Mental Deficiency Act which advised that:

- people who were mentally defective needed protection from society and indeed from themselves
- all mentally defective people should be identified and brought into contact with caring agencies
- mentally defective people should not be condemned because of their condition
- a central organising body should be established to work with the local caring agencies who would be responsible for the care of individual people.

The Act introduced compulsory certification of 'defectives' admitted to institutions, and clearly served to segregate people with a learning disability from the rest of society. As a consequence, large institutions (often called asylums) were built. The management and care of people with learning disability was with the local authorities and stayed this way until they came under the control of the NHS in 1948.

The next major piece of legislation was the 1959 Mental Health Act, which replaced previous terminology with the term mental sub-normality and severe mental sub-normality. The Act required local authorities to provide both day and residential care for people with a learning disability, and made provision for voluntary attendance at a hospital rather than compulsory certification, but still perpetuated the need for mental health legislation for people with learning disability. A series of scandals in the 1960s regarding the care of people with learning disabilities in the large institutions resulted in the publication in 1971 by the DHSS of the document *Better Services for the Mentally Handicapped*. This document promoted a model of community care with a significant reduction in hospital beds and a corresponding increase in local authority provision. The following years saw the closure of learning disability hospitals and care being transferred to the community. The National Health Service and Community Care Act in 1990 made local authorities responsible for acting as lead providers of care packages for people with learning disabilities.

Many people with learning disability now live in small homes with high levels of independence, no longer segregated from wider society. However, there are some people who, because of their particular behavioural problems, require much more structured and supervised care which is provided in special settings with skilled staff.

The role of the learning disability nurse

The role of the learning disability nurse in enabling the person with a learning disability to reach his own 'balance and highest potential' is vitally important to this segment of society. In a sense, the role of the learning disability nurse is no different from that of any other speciality of the family of nursing. But the nurse in learning disability works within a multidisciplinary team in a variety of settings. For example, nurses within the speciality can be found working in learning disability hospitals, community learning disability teams, community homes run by local authorities or NHS Trusts and special schools, as well as private and voluntary sectors. The nurse in learning disabilities is becoming increasingly specialised in caring for people with special needs. These include:

- people with a profound learning disability and/or multiple physical, sensory, motor disabilities
- people with a learning disability who also have a mental health problem
- people with a learning disability who present their carers with behavioural problems
- people with a learning disability who have offended in law.

Regardless of the context or the setting in which the learning disability nurse works, or the specific needs of the person or people being cared for, the nurse will need to develop a number of skills. These skills can then be exercised in order to promote an independent and valued lifestyle for people with a learning disability.

Specifically, the role of the learning disability nurse is to promote:

- the health of the person with a learning disability

- communication and interpersonal skills, including alternative methods of communicating
- independence through teaching life skills
- advocacy and self-advocacy through advocacy programmes
- the philosophy of normalisation
- the rights, risks and responsibilities associated with being a citizen
- dignity and respect
- leisure, recreation and stimulation
- meaningful work opportunities
- lifelong learning
- working in partnerships with families
- harmonious working relationships within the multidisciplinary team for the enhanced care of a person with a learning disability.

If nurses in learning disability are able to fulfil such a role, they are clearly able to make an important contribution to the achievement of the optimal health of those with a learning disability.

The future of learning disability nursing

This is developing in a context very different from the one with which many experienced nurses are familiar. The work has moved to a clearly focused community approach more quickly than for some other nursing specialities. The nurse is also having to become more specialised in caring for people with very special needs, as those with less profound problems are now living with greater independence and integration into society. Learning disability branch student nurses will undoubtedly have the opportunity to experience all ranges of care in a wide variety of settings.

MENTAL HEALTH NURSING

The individual with mental health problems is nowadays viewed not so much as a patient suffering from an illness, but rather as a person with difficulties that need to be tackled in order to achieve as full a life as possible.

Psychiatry and mental health care have undergone great changes in the UK during the last century. Today, treatment will involve a range of ideas that emphasise the psychological and social needs of clients, and is most likely to occur in the communities in which clients have to face their difficulties, rather than in a remote institution. Apart from this shift towards social care, the great debate in psychiatry and mental health care has covered the appropriateness and effectiveness of treatment. Treatments have come and gone during the latter part of the 20th century, as some, such as major tranquillisers and behaviour therapy, have resulted in important changes in the well-being of mentally distressed people, while others, such as insulin coma, institutionalised care and psychoanalytical treatment, have been shown either to be detrimental to clients or to confer little or no benefit. One significant development has been the rise in importance of the mental health nurse, and the enlargement of her role in care and treatment of those experiencing mental distress.

To describe those suffering from psychological distress as being mentally ill has become increasingly unfashionable, except in the medical profession. Nurses, in particular, have preferred to speak of 'people with mental health problems' and to describe themselves as 'mental health nurses'. Certainly, there is little evidence for an organic basis for many so-called mental illnesses, and some critics of psychiatry have preferred to separate these difficulties, which are sometimes referred to simply as 'problems with living', from mental problems that do have obvious organic causes, such as dementia and drug-induced and toxic states.

Historical overview of mental health care

Once again it is helpful to look at the history of mental health care when attempting to understand present treatments, assumptions and attitudes. There are references in the Bible to both mild and severe mental distress. In the UK, medical care began to become systemised in the 16th century. At this time, practitioners made little distinction between disorders of the body and mind, and similar treatments were likely to be applied to people suffering from physical or mental distress. These treatments were often both ineffective and unpleasant, involving bloodletting and purging. Diagnosis of differing mental illnesses was rudimentary, the major distinction being between mania and melancholia.

Towards the end of the 17th century, incarceration of the mentally ill in public and private 'madhouses' became the dominant mode of care. The standard of care in these institutions was apparently uniformly poor, consisting of inadequate physical surroundings and diet, erosion of liberty and harsh treatments. This state of affairs continued until the end of the 18th century, when more enlightened philosophies prevailed. As a result of dissatisfaction with mental health care, William Tuke, a wealthy Quaker, founded in 1795 The Retreat in York, which based its care on 'moral' treatment. Moral treatment is based on the notion that mentally ill people have control over their behaviour and can, with the help and example of others, exercise that control, with a resulting improvement in their mental well-being. Records show these tactics worked well.

The medicalisation of mental distress brought immense power to change people's experience of such disorders. Initially some medical interventions were of dubious value, but the approach did lead to research taking place, and eventually powerful and effective treatments were developed. In particular, two new groups of drugs – antidepressants and major tranquillisers – changed the face of psychiatry and mental health nursing in the space of a few years. The drugs often had unpleasant or dangerous side-effects, but they exerted a powerful influence on mood and behaviour. Nurses became carers rather than custodians. Patients were less often admitted to hospital, and if admitted were discharged back into the community with greater rapidity.

Approaches to mental health in the UK today often combine a range of approaches to the client. Although medical treatment still dominates, research into the role of social circumstances in the genesis and maintenance of mental distress and illness has been recognised. This has had a considerable influence in clinical practice, particularly by those who pursue psychosocial models of care. These attempts at a more integrated approach to care will often involve a team of professionals, including psychologists, occupational therapists, counsellors and nurses, as well as psychiatrists.

Images of mental illness: fear and stigma

There can be no doubt that mental distress, particularly when severe, gives rise to fear and stigma. Mental distress continues to be associated, in the public mind, with unpredictability, violence and bizarre behaviour, while in reality those experiencing mental distress are more likely to be quiet, withdrawn and fearful of others. On the rare occasion when disturbed or frightening behaviour does occur, it is taken to be potent evidence both of the dangerous nature of mentally distressed people and for the need to ensure their increased supervision, usually in institutions. This fear is often fuelled by the media, and it is not surprising that the public have confused and inaccurate ideas about mental illness.

Approaches to mental health and illness

This is an area that needs to be explored, discussed and debated by the student learning to be a mental health nurse, and is a topic beyond the scope of this brief introduction to mental health nursing. However, the main approaches are summarised in Table 1.2. The dominant view of mental distress is still medical, with drug treatment being commonplace. But there are several other important approaches to understanding and treating mental illness and all main methods are discussed briefly below.

The medical model and physical treatments

Drug treatments

As noted above, the introduction of effective drug treatments to psychiatry transformed the lives of those suffering from mental distress. The most significant therapeutic innovation was the use of tranquillisers (phenothiazines and butyrophenones) in psychotic illnesses, particularly schizophrenia. Their action in the treatment of schizophrenia is by blocking the transmission of dopamine, a neurotransmitter thought to be implicated in the odd beliefs and sensations that characterise the illness. When given by injection as a long-acting preparation, clients are able to live a relatively normal life in the community. Although this represents a huge improvement in the care of schizophrenics, two major difficulties

Approach	Characteristics
Medical model	Uses the same general approach as for physical medicine. Stresses the role of physical causes of mental distress. Emphasises drug treatment
Sociological approach	Emphasises the role of society in creating and contributing to mental distress. Stresses the importance of labelling mentally ill people as deviant
Cognitive-behavioural	Stresses the role of learning in contributing to both difficulties and their resolution. Does not acknowledge differences in the causation of problematic and non-problematic experiences
Psychoanalysis	Asserts that mental distress is symptomatic of unconscious internal conflicts, usually from childhood
Humanism	Emphasises human needs, particularly for esteem and self-actualisation. Distress is consequent upon thwarting of these needs
Anti-psychiatry	Sees mental distress as a sane response to an insane world. Suggests that mental illness is an experience to be lived rather than a problem to be solved

Table 1.2   Characteristics of main approaches to mental health

have been found. First, a number of individuals do not remain stable on these powerful drugs, and, second, the drugs themselves give rise to profound side-effects, for which further medication is required. This can often lead to difficulties with clients adhering to treatment.

The other group of drugs are the antidepressants – tricyclics and monoamine oxidase inhibitors (MAOIs). Like tranquillisers, these drugs work on chemical messengers in the brain, namely noradrenaline and serotonin. While there is evidence that these drugs do have considerable effect in lifting mood, both groups also have serious side-effects, lessening the likelihood of client adherence. This is particularly so with the MAOIs, for which a special diet is required. Furthermore, the use of these drugs in isolation leaves issues in the client's life, which may have contributed to the depression, untouched.

Electroconvulsive therapy (ECT)

ECT remains a highly controversial treatment. When first introduced in 1938, it was used indiscriminately and at high frequency for a huge variety of complaints. Its reputation as a dangerous, frightening treatment, with impairment of memory as a side-effect, led to fear among patients and the public. Much of the controversy that still surrounds ECT today is based on misunderstanding of how it is currently practised. ECT is now a highly specific treatment used as a final resort in certain kinds of depression, where its usefulness is well recognised. A brief electric shock is passed through the brain. The patient is given a general anaesthetic so feels no pain. The risks associated with ECT are similar to those associated with any general anaesthetic, and the main side-effect is of short-term memory loss. The role of the nurse is to care for patients before and throughout the procedure until they are conscious, and to give careful supervision for a period after treatment.

Psychological treatments

Psychological approaches have had a great deal of impact on mental health work, and, within the specialist services, it would be unusual to find a mental health team that did not possess a heavy commitment to psychological interventions. Very often the nurse is involved in these interventions and Table 1.3 summarises the main features of several key psychological approaches to treatment.

Settings for care

Over the past 20 years the large institutions that used to care for many hundreds of mentally ill patients have been closed and new smaller acute units have been built. These units may offer in-patient facilities, day care facilities and occupational therapy, and are mainly run by mental health nurses. Acutely distressed clients are cared for as in-patients, either because there are severe concerns about their ability to care for themselves, or about their desire to harm themselves or others, or because the nature of their treatment requires close observation. For most, the stay in a hospital or unit will be very brief. Consequently much mental health nursing is now carried out in GP clinics, in community mental health centres or in the client's own home. Care in the community is thought to disrupt the individual's life much less than admission to hospital, and continuing to carry on a normal life also helps in confronting problems where they occur. Thus, community mental health nursing is at the core of the role of the mental health nurse. Therefore preparation for discharge will be a significant part of care planning for those nurses working in the hospital setting. The development of the community psychiatric nurse (CPN) was almost entirely due to the greater effectiveness of drug treatments for mental illness. Their current therapeutic and preventative roles have developed from these origins.

The role of the mental health nurse

Mental health nurses (registered mental nurse, or RMN) often regard the creation of relationships with their clients as the core of their work. Although many nurses have undertaken courses in particular forms of therapy, these specific

Table 1.3 Major psychological approaches to mental distress

Approach	Features
Psychodynamic psychotherapy	Derived from psychoanalysis Involves eliciting and examining underlying conflicts Little evidence of effectiveness Little practised by nurses Remains an influential theoretical approach in psychiatry
Humanistic therapies and counselling (client-centred approach)	Based on the work of Carl Rogers Emphasises qualities of the therapist (warmth, empathy, respect) Emphasises human uniqueness and growth Influential and widely practised by nurses Little evidence of effectiveness in serious mental distress
Cognitive-behaviour therapy	Derived from conditioning theory and cognitive psychology Emphasises present problems and learning coping tactics Widely applicable and effective in serious mental distress Not yet widely accepted among nurses
Groupwork	Can be practised for any of the above therapies, sharing their therapeutic approaches and strengths and weaknesses Can involve simple support Very popular in mental health settings Has been practised by nurses (and others) with little training and support
Complementary/alternative therapies	Not specifically psychological Many different approaches, but all emphasise the 'whole' person Little evidence of effectiveness Widely practised but unregulated Rapidly increasing in popularity in nursing

interventions are firmly grounded in the relationships nurses build with their clients.

Mental health nursing always involves the use of interpersonal skills to engage the client, gain information, respond to emotions and help in initiating behavioural change. In counselling, these skills are used in a more structured way, usually in the context of a formal, developing and helping relationship in which the nurse helps the client to explore his emotions and behaviours.

Cognitive-behaviour therapy is a comparatively new approach, characterised by an emphasis on the client's problems in the present, and concentrating on maintaining factors rather than attempting to find supposed causes in the past.

During therapy, clients are taught to recognise unproductive thoughts and behaviours that give rise to difficulty, to challenge them and to practise new and more adaptive behaviours.

The future of mental health nursing

As we have seen, there has been a steady move towards community care for people experiencing mental distress. Successive government reports have stressed the need for this community-based approach (DHSS 1989).

However, support for the initiative has not been universal. As well as unease among communities about having long-stay psychiatric hospital patients relocated into their midst, user and care groups have campaigned vociferously against hospital closures, often claiming that closure will result in an increased burden on families.

The plight of mentally distressed people among the nation's prison population and the homeless has also given rise to heated debate, and nurses are currently developing roles to address the needs of homeless people experiencing mental distress. However, there is no clear evidence that these problems, although undoubtedly severe, are related to hospital closures and community care.

Mental health care faces considerable challenges in the future. In particular, examination of the needs of ethnic minorities, women, older people, children and offenders with mental health problems has only begun to be addressed. The Butterworth Report (DoH 1994) focuses on these challenges and highlights the need for a flexible response to future mental health needs and the role of nurses in rising to these opportunities.

A key element in NHS reforms has been the recognition that service users and carers have an important role in determining the care they receive. As a result, nurses have seen the necessity for helping users to exercise that right to involvement. Of all the challenges likely to be presented to the mental health nurse in the future, this expansion of their relationships with clients and carers is perhaps most crucial, and represents a culmination of the shift in the role of the mental health nurse from custodial attendant to partner in care.

AFTER QUALIFYING, WHAT NEXT?

Most newly qualified nurses are likely to begin their career within their chosen speciality, although, in this first decade of the 21st century, significant numbers will not work in hospitals or even within the NHS, as the earlier sections of this chapter indicate. Wherever you choose to work, it is critical to appreciate that gaining your nursing qualification is only the 'end of the beginning' of learning to nurse. The social,

political, economic and technological developments are changing the context in which nurses are working today, and the pace of change is expected to increase rather than slow down. The concept of a registered nurse who can practise the full range of nursing skills from the day of qualification is unrealistic and the newly qualified nurse should receive support in the form of supervised practice for a period following first employment. This, and the need for continuing professional education, is covered later in the chapter.

Actual and predicted changes for nursing in 2001 and beyond

At the time of writing, it is clear that the context of care is changing rapidly and that its delivery is likely to be unrecognisable within the next 10 years. Special reports on nursing (DoH 1999, UKCC 1999) and other writers (e.g. Nicklin & Kenworthy 2000) give descriptions of these changes and the challenges they pose for nursing. These can be summarised as follows:

- The growth of electronic communications is a major development, and expanding rapidly, so that the general public using health care services is now better informed and can gain ready access via the internet to information about diagnosis, treatment choices and care possibilities. Better informed users will expect that the professional nurse will be able to explain the research base for the care given, whereas most patients were not, until recently, able to be equally knowledgeable in the decisions made about their care.

- Communications technology advances and the development of Tele-medicine means that diagnosis will no longer always need attendance at an outpatient clinic when a visual image of an injury or disorder can be diagnosed by a doctor many miles away. This means that clinics may become nurse-led or may even not be necessary as GPs consult 'down-line' with experts far away.

- The explosion of technology has meant major changes in practice, particularly in surgery, so that 'keyhole' endoscopic operations now require only day-case attendance for patients rather than 10–14 day in-patient episodes. This means huge patient turnover in day units and a massive increase in community care for respite and convalescence. It also means that many straightforward operations will not be carried out in traditional hospital settings but can be conducted within primary care settings in surgeries where consultants already see patients and conduct minor surgery. The effect of this on hospital care may be that only specialised and complex acute work, such as transplant surgery, critical care, some aspects of cancer care and advanced technique medicine or surgery will need to be carried out in these settings. Nursing work and place of work will, likewise, alter, and the traditional hospital nurse's role is set to change.

• In mental health and learning disability, there has already been a major shift from care in huge, isolated institutions to smaller community units and homes run in partnership between the health, social services and private sectors. Modern life also brings an increasing awareness and incidence of substance abuse, mainly among young people, and an increase of serious mental illness which adds pressure to 'the system' and challenges nurses in every sector of health care.

Users of mental health and learning disability services, and their families, are gaining an increasingly loud voice in the nature and quality of care provided and this decade should see considerable developments of imaginative care programmes for these clients.

• The demographic profile of our society means that the elderly, and the disorders of old age, will become increasingly prevalent. Hospital care for the elderly is increasingly concerned with acute illness, while rehabilitation services and day care are community based and shared with social services and the independent sector.

• Disease remains unpredictable. HIV and AIDS remains a serious problem for health professionals, and other bacterial and virus problems which challenge the most austere antibody regimens are emerging. Bovine spongiform encephalopathy (BSE) and Creutzfeldt–Jakob disease (CJD) and other food-related disorders have only just begun to challenge society.

• The expanding knowledge of genetics and its application leaves the health care world on the edge of possible breakthrough developments in diagnosis, prevention and treatment of many disorders. This is likely to affect the nature of care in every area.

• The economics of health care provision remains a constant struggle for whichever political party is in power and it must now be seen as an increasingly international issue. In the UK, the nurse, along with other health professionals, will undoubtedly be required to carry out a wider range of activities than in the past with little or no increase in resources.

All of the above issues mean that the role of the nurse is changing, in some cases quite dramatically and in every case there can no longer be an expectation that the newly qualified nurse will go into a 'job for life'. Changes also require more effective multidisciplinary teamwork and nurses will be required to work flexibly and collaboratively with a range of professionals and agencies. This is as much a challenge for staff in other disciplines as it is for nurses but nurses are well placed to foster teamwork and this will become increasingly important for high quality health care.

Changes ahead will almost certainly mean further training and education for qualified nurses, and often a willingness to change work setting or even employer in order to work with the same patient/client group. But the possession of a registered nurse qualification will usually mean that the prospects of full employability are good if the nurse is adaptable to the changing circumstances just described.

Possible career options

While most qualified nurses will still work in the NHS in hospital or community settings, the range of opportunities in social services and the independent sector is increasing. Mental health, learning disability and elderly care nursing work has expanded into these sectors prolifically over the past 10 years and the registration and quality control of services is highly regulated. There are now excellent career development opportunities as all the care sectors are trying to work together to meet political and public demand for a seamless service. The expansion of the private acute care sector is notable and independent sector hospitals, such as BUPA and Nuffield hospitals, are subject to rigorous quality control by the NHS and associated organisations. The registered nurse is a valuable member of the care team in all of these settings and the need for professional support and development is now recognised in settings outside of the NHS.

Other career opportunities for the qualified nurse include working in occupational health, perhaps in industry and the business sector, nursing in the armed forces, working abroad (although there may be requirements for further professional assessment to meet another country's registration demands) and working in the commercial sector as a nursing adviser for a range of activities or products.

Further qualifications?

The majority of nurses today qualify at the level of a higher education diploma in addition to their nursing registration. Many will wish to continue further study to the level of a first degree following initial qualification and employment. All universities which offer nursing education will be able to advise prospective students about the range of programmes available for part-time top-up to degree level. It is often possible, and certainly desirable, to combine academic studies with further professional learning at an advanced level as part of career progression in any of the professional settings described previously. In some cases this is mandatory – for example, to become a specialist, advanced practitioner.

It is now possible to become qualified as a specialist practitioner in all branches of nursing for both hospital and community work. In the past, it has always been necessary to undertake further education and training to become a health visitor (public health nurse), district nurse (home care nurse) or community psychiatric nurse. To become a specialist community nurse today in any branch of nursing, health visiting or school nursing, further education and practice at degree

level is required. In addition to these community nursing qualifications, it is now recognised that further specialist education and qualification is required in every area of practice so nurses can now consider specialising in, for example:

- critical care of the adult
- critical care of the newborn or children
- acute care of the elderly
- coronary care
- palliative care
- dealing with challenging behaviours in the field of learning disability
- mental health nursing of children and adolescents
- substance abuse.

These are just a few examples of specialist areas in which advanced qualifications can now be obtained. There are many more, and details are normally available from the local university nursing education department or the training manager in the workplace. Support for time and funding for undertaking these courses is always a matter for discussion with the workplace manager who is likely to be supportive if the new learning is beneficial and essential to the care required in the area.

For some nurses, there is a desire to change direction completely and move into a different branch of nursing altogether. Now that there is a common foundation programme for all initial nurse education, it is possible, within the regulations, to undertake just the new branch programme. However, this is not always easy in practice because of workforce planning requirements and the inability of managers to release valuable staff to take a course in another speciality which will ultimately take them away for good. It will usually be possible if the nurse does not require a salary for the duration of the new programme. Some qualified general nurses wish to pursue a career in midwifery and this is still possible to do as an 18-month post-registration programme. However, midwifery is becoming, increasingly, a first level direct-entry programme at degree level.

It is, of course, possible that nurses will wish to use their first professional and academic qualification as the basis for a move into another health or social care profession. Careers in clinical psychology, social work, the professions allied to medicine (e.g. physiotherapy, occupational therapy, language therapy, podiatry, radiography), pharmacy, biomedical sciences and medicine may be options. Other avenues available could include nursing research, management or education with their equivalent paths to further qualifications.

So, qualified nurses have many opportunities for gaining further qualifications and for career progression. But it is not essential to gain all these extra qualifications to be a highly valued member of a health or social care team and readers should not feel overwhelmed by the range of options and opportunities described here. Many nurses are content not to pursue continuing career progression through formal qualifications and promotion. Instead they will enjoy 'horizontal' careers which enable them to use their professional skills to the full. However, it is important to recognise that initial qualification will not be enough to sustain any nurse for the whole of a career and professional development and updating will be an absolute essential.

A modern career framework

At the time of writing, the UK Department of Health has just announced plans for a new career framework for nurses to provide 'more satisfying and rewarding careers' (DoH 1999).

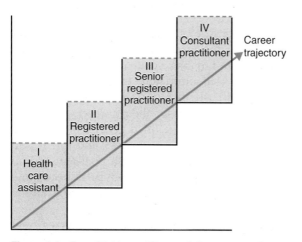

Figure 1.1 From 'Making a difference', Department of Health (1999).

The new structure for the NHS is to replace 'clinical grading' (introduced in the 1990s and accompanied by major problems in implementation for reasons of perceived, and possibly actual, inequity) with a four-stage framework which is shown at Figure 1.1.

The new framework incorporates the recently announced new nurse, midwife and health visitor 'consultant' posts. The post of nurse consultant is to provide an opportunity for experienced and highly qualified nurses to remain in practice if they wish to do so, without having to move into management, education or other careers to enhance their pay. Nurse, midwife and health visitor consultants are to have responsibility in four main areas: expert practice; professional leadership; education; research leading to service development. The weight in any one area will vary according to the specific post but all consultants will spend at least half of their working time in practice. This is a new development for nursing and one which excites many in a profession where career advancement has usually meant leaving clinical practice.

So, the overview of the career framework for nursing from pre-nursing to consultant is shown at Table 1.4. While this framework is planned for use within the NHS, nurses working elsewhere will usually find comparable responsibilities and rates of pay for the same level of experience, expertise and qualifications. The appropriate level of experience and academic/professional qualification is shown in the table and it will be noted that at the higher levels of work, qualifications other than those specifically for nursing may be required. For example, higher level management or research qualifications may be necessary at consultant level. However, in most services the role of clinical leadership still rests with the ward/departmental sister or charge nurse and their equivalents in community and other settings. Leadership here is critical to the quality of care delivered, the morale of staff and the learning climate for students. Many student nurses today will aspire to be the equivalent of a ward sister, a well recognised but sometimes undervalued role and one which is likely to remain for many years despite the major changes occurring in health

	Typically people here will, at a minimum, be competent...	**Typically posts will include...**	**Typically people here will have been educated and trained to...**
Table 1.4	The new career framework for nurses, midwives and health visitors (DoH 1999)		
I	... to provide basic and routine personal care to patients/clients and a limited range of clinical interventions routine to the care setting under the supervision of a registered nurse, midwife or health visitor	... cadets and health care assistants and other clinical support workers	... National Vocational Qualification levels 1, 2 or 3
II	... to do the above and exercise clinical judgement and assume professional responsibility and accountability for the assessment of health need, planning, delivery and evaluation of routine direct care, for both individuals and groups of patients/clients; direct and supervise the work of support workers and mentor students	... both newly registered nurses and midwives and established registered practitioners in a variety of jobs and specialities in both hospital and community and primary care settings	... higher education diploma or first degree level, hold professional registration and in some cases additional specialist-specific professional qualifications
III	... to do the above and assume significant clinical or public health leadership of registered practitioners and others, and/ or clinical management and/or specialist care	... experienced senior registered practitioners in a diverse range of posts including ward sisters/ charge nurses, community nurses, midwives, health visitors and clinical nurse specialists	... first or masters degree level, hold professional registration and in many cases additional specialist-specific professional qualifications
IV	... to do the above and provide expert care, to provide clinical or public health leadership and consultancy to senior registered practitioners and others and initiate and lead significant practice, education and service development	... experienced and expert practitioners holding nurse, midwife or health visitor consultant posts	... masters or doctorate level, hold professional registration and additional specialist-specific professional qualifications commensurate with standards proposed for recognition of a 'higher level of practice'

care. Table 1.4 gives an idea of its recommended position in the hierarchy of nursing!

Lifelong learning

As already stated, the rapid changes in health care and modes of delivery mean that nurses are constantly required to revise their role and update knowledge and skills. Registration is just the beginning of a career of continuous updating. The UKCC's standards for education and practice (1993) make this explicit when they require:

• Newly registered nurses to complete a period of about 4 months' support under the guidance of a preceptor to ensure that practitioners do not take on too much responsibility too soon or inappropriately. During this period of role transition, practitioners are accountable for their professional practice.

• Practitioners to maintain and develop their professional knowledge and competence through a minimum of 5 study days every 3 years.

• Nurses to formally notify their intention to practise every 3 years, providing details of qualification and area of practice when initially registered. These details are required when re-registering, re-entering practice after a break of 5 years or more, or changing area of practice using a different registerable qualification. (Midwives notify their intention to practise annually.)

• Completion of an approved return to practice programme and assessment of professional competence following a break in practice of 5 years or more.

- Practitioners to maintain a personal professional portfolio to include experience, developments and achievements. The profile should be a dynamic means of recording career progress and contain details of continuing education, assessment of development needs and plans to meet these needs.

This is echoed by the Department of Health in *Making a Difference* (DoH 1999):

We expect every nurse, midwife and health visitor to understand fully the obligations associated with professional registration and accountability. They should practise in accordance with the UKCC Code of Professional Conduct and related guidance. We expect them to maintain and improve their professional knowledge and competence – at the very least to the minimum required during each registration cycle – and to acknowledge any limitations in knowledge and competence, undertaking new or expanded responsibilities in accordance with current guidance about the scope of professional practice.

The continuing professional development of the registered nurse is a joint responsibility between the nurse and the employer. The nurse has the right to expect training opportunities to be available and employers should require nurses to keep up to date and be re-skilled, if necessary, for the work they are required to do. One of the newest requirements by the NHS (1999) is that all staff working in the NHS should have a personal development plan by 2001; this is to ensure that staff continue their professional development and update their knowledge and skills. Although many nurses now work outside the NHS, the same principles apply in order for nurses to remain on the professional register.

Chapter 2 outlines the importance of professional development within the framework of clinical governance in the NHS, and Chapter 11 describes the place of professional development within the UKCC Code of Conduct for the profession.

Preceptorship

Part of the experience of a student nurse is to be supported in the practice component of training by an experienced, qualified nurse – usually called a mentor – who usually also takes part in the assessment of the student's practical work. It has now been recognised that the newly qualified registered nurse also requires practical supervision and support for the first 6–12 months following registration and so a 'preceptor' should be assigned to the 'probationer' nurse. The lack of confidence of many newly qualified nurses is sometimes compounded by senior staff who expect newly registered nurses to be able to do everything! This has never been expected of doctors, who are required to serve a 'house' year before being admitted to the register. A period of preceptorship is now the equivalent for nurses and is normally provided. The key elements of preceptorship are to provide the newly qualified nurse with a role model, education about practice issues and feedback on performance, but there is no requirement for formal assessment within the process. Preceptors will normally be qualified nurses in the same speciality and will have about 2 years' experience and, probably, a teaching and assessing qualification in addition to their nurse registration. The purpose of preceptorship is to assist in the transition from student to registered nurse and to help the new nurse to gain confidence and expertise in the new role.

PREP and portfolios

As mentioned earlier in this chapter, and as detailed in Chapter 11, nurses have a statutory duty to remain competent within their sphere of practice and unless this is achieved they are unable to remain on the register (UKCC 1993). At re-registration, which is required every 3 years following initial registration, nurses have to sign to declare that they have met their post-registration education and practice (PREP) requirements. The PREP standard requires the recording of all continuing professional development over the past 3 years *and* that the nurse has continued in practice for at least 100 days over the past 3 years.

The portfolio

The method of compiling evidence of learning and achievements in professional development is the nurse's individual professional portfolio. In many cases student nurses will be encouraged to begin a portfolio from the first day of training, so that it becomes a natural accompaniment to work and learning thereafter. Since the NHS is now requiring all staff to have personal development plans, the nurse's portfolio will assist greatly and should probably be acceptable as it is, in meeting this new demand. Many employers have developed their own portfolio packs for staff and many others are available commercially. Of course, it is possible for nurses to develop their own portfolio folders to accommodate the requirements of PREP and the live register.

A successful portfolio, for PREP and possibly other demands, will enable nurses to demonstrate that they have:

- reviewed their competence within the present work setting (this might be achieved through showing evidence of reflective practice)
- set personal objectives for professional development, normally with the assistance of the supervisor or line manager
- developed an action plan for learning, gaining new experience and skills
- implemented the plan, with evidence of courses, study days, new experiences achieved
- reviewed what happened and how progress has been made
- recorded study time and learning outcomes.

Of course, this is just an example of how a portfolio might be constructed. There will be many varieties in use in work settings, but all should have a common theme of recording and reflecting on progress. At first, this may seem a daunting process, but making simple jottings of particular events and experiences, and the learning that resulted, is how portfolios can be built up. Daily recordings will not be necessary for the purpose of PREP, but significant events and achievements will be valuable. Beyond the requirements for PREP, many employers are now asking applicants to submit their portfolio with the application form and to discuss it as part of the selection process.

CONCLUSION

All students of nursing are encouraged to find out something about the 'heritage' of nursing and its birth as a recognised profession. There is no doubt that knowing something of the history of nursing assists in understanding some of the challenges, obstacles and opportunities of today's world of nursing. The year 2001 sees the beginning of a national change of pre-registration nursing education, which is described here and elsewhere in the book. The 21st century also begins with some dramatic changes in the nature of medicine, health care and patterns of delivery and this pace is set to increase. There has never been a time when the most appropriate preparation of nurses and continuing professional development was so vital for the safe and effective practice of nursing.

REFERENCES

Baly M 1995 Nursing and social change, 3rd edn. Routledge, London
Bowlby J 1971 Attachment and loss. Penguin, Harmondsworth, vol 1
Davies C (ed) 1980 Rewriting nursing history. Croom Helm, London
Department of Health 1989 Caring for people: community care in the next decade and beyond. Cmnd 849. HMSO, London
Department of Health 1992 Social care for adults with learning disabilities. Mental Handicap LAC (92) 15. HMSO, London
Department of Health 1994 Working in partnership: a collaborative approach to care [Report of the Mental Health Nursing Review team: the Butterworth Report]. HMSO, London
Department of Health 1999 Making a difference: strengthening the nursing, midwifery and health visiting contribution to health and health care. DoH, London
DHSS 1971 Better services for the mentally handicapped. HMSO, London
Gostin L 1985 The law relating to mental handicap in England and Wales. In: Craft M, Bicknell J, Hollin S, Mental handicap: a multidisciplinary approach. Baillière Tindall, London
Ministry of Health 1959 The welfare of children in hospital [the Platt Report]. HMSO, London
National Association for the Welfare of Children in Hospital 1985 Charter. NAWCH, London
Nicklin P, Kenworthy N 2000 Teaching and assessing in nursing practice: an experiential approach. Baillière Tindall and Royal College of Nursing, London

Pearson A 1988 Primary nursing: nursing in the Burford and Oxford Development Units. Chapman and Hall, London

Thompson J, Melia K, Boyd K 1994 Nursing ethics. Churchill Livingstone, Edinburgh

UKCC 1993 Standards for post-registration education. RL 8 (93). UKCC, London

UKCC 1999 Fitness for practice: the UKCC Commission for Nursing and Midwifery Education. UKCC, London

United Nations 1987 United Nations convention on the rights of the child. HMSO, London

FURTHER READING

Alexander M F, Fawcett J N, Runciman P J (eds) 1994 Nursing practice: hospital and home – the adult. Churchill Livingstone, Edinburgh

Baly M 1986 Florence Nightingale and the nursing legacy. Croom Helm, London

Barber P (ed) 1987 Mental handicap: facilitating holistic care. Using Nursing Models series. Hodder and Stoughton, London

DHSS 1985 The role of the nurse for people with a mental handicap. Ref. CNO 855. HMSO, London

English National Board for Nursing, Midwifery and Health Visiting 1994 The nursing of children; a resource guide. ENB, London

Goffman E 1961 Asylums: essays on the social situation of mental patients and other inmates. Anchor, New York

UKCC 1992 A guide for students of nursing and midwifery. UKCC, London

UKCC 2001 The PREP handbook. UKCC, London

Warner M, Longley M, Gould G, Picek A 1998 Healthcare futures 2010. Welsh Institute for Health and Social Care, University of Glamorgan, Pontypridd, Wales

Appendix 1 UKCC competencies (2000) for the end of the common foundation year and for entry to the register (UKCC 1999)

Domain	Outcomes to be achieved for entry to the branch programme	Competencies for entry to the register
Professional and ethical practice	Discuss in an informed manner the implications of professional regulation for nursing practice • demonstrate a basic knowledge of professional regulation and self-regulation • recognise and acknowledge the limitations of one's own abilities • recognise situations which require referral to a registered practitioner Demonstrate an awareness of the UKCC's *Code of professional conduct* • commit to the principle that the primary purpose of the registered nurse is to protect and serve society • accept responsibility for one's own actions and decisions Demonstrate an awareness of, and apply ethical principles to, nursing practice • demonstrate respect for patient and client confidentiality • identify ethical issues in day-to-day practice Demonstrate an awareness of legislation relevant to nursing practice • identify key issues in relevant legislation relating to mental health, children, data protection, manual handling, and health and safety, etc. Demonstrate the importance of promoting equity in patient and client care by contributing to nursing care in a fair and anti-discriminatory way • demonstrate fairness and sensitivity when responding to patients, clients and groups from diverse circumstances • recognise the needs of patients and clients whose lives are affected by disability, however manifest	Manage oneself, one's practice, and that of others, in accordance with the UKCC's *Code of professional conduct*, recognising one's own abilities and limitations • practise in accordance with the UKCC's *Code of professional conduct* • use professional standards of practice to self-assess performance • consult with a registered nurse when nursing care requires expertise beyond one's own current scope of competence • consult other health care professionals when individual or group needs fall outside the scope of nursing practice • identify unsafe practice and respond appropriately to ensure a safe outcome • manage the delivery of care services within the sphere of one's own accountability Practise in accordance with an ethical and legal framework which ensures the primacy of patient and client interest and well-being and respects confidentiality • demonstrate knowledge of legislation and health and social policy relevant to nursing practice • ensure the confidentiality and security of written and verbal information acquired in a professional capacity • demonstrate knowledge of contemporary ethical issues and their impact on nursing and health care • manage the complexities arising from ethical and legal dilemmas • act appropriately when seeking access to caring for patients and clients in their own homes Practise in a fair and anti-discriminatory way, acknowledging the differences in beliefs and cultural practices of individuals or groups • maintain, support and acknowledge the rights of individuals or groups in the health care setting • act to ensure that the rights of individuals and groups are not compromised • respect the values, customs and beliefs of individuals and groups • provide care which demonstrates sensitivity to the diversity of patients and clients

(Cont'd)

Appendix 1 (*Continued*)

Domain	Outcomes to be achieved for entry to the branch programme	Competencies for entry to the register
Care delivery	Discuss methods of, barriers to and the boundaries of effective communication and interpersonal relationships • recognise the effect of one's own values on interactions with patients and clients and their carers, families and friends • utilise appropriate communication skills with patients and clients • acknowledge the boundaries of a professional caring relationship Demonstrate sensitivity when interacting with and providing information to patients and clients Contribute to enhancing the health and social well-being of patients and clients by understanding how, under the supervision of a registered practitioner, to: • contribute to the assessment of health needs • identify opportunities for health promotion • identify networks of health and social care services Contribute to the development and documentation of nursing assessments by participating in comprehensive and systematic nursing assessment of the physical, psychological, social and spiritual needs of patients and clients • be aware of assessment strategies to guide the collection of data for assessing patients and clients and use assessment tools under guidance • discuss the prioritisation of care needs • be aware of the need to reassess patients and clients as to their needs for nursing care Contribute to the planning of nursing care, involving patients and clients and, where possible, their carers, demonstrating an understanding of helping patients and clients to make informed decisions • identify care needs based on the assessment of a patient or client	Engage in, develop and disengage from therapeutic relationships through the use of appropriate communication and interpersonal skills • utilise a range of effective and appropriate communication and engagement skills • maintain and, where appropriate, disengage from professional caring relationships which focus on meeting the patient's or client's needs within professional therapeutic boundaries Create and utilise opportunities to promote the health and well-being of patients, clients and groups • consult with patients, clients and groups to identify their need and desire for health promotion advice • provide relevant and current health information to patients, clients and groups in a form which facilitates their understanding and acknowledges choice/individual preference • provide support and education in the development and/or maintenance of independent living skills • seek specialist/expert advice as appropriate Undertake and document a comprehensive, systematic and accurate nursing assessment of the physical, psychological, social and spiritual needs of patients, clients and communities • select valid and reliable assessment tools for the required purpose • systematically collect data regarding the health and functional status of individuals, clients and communities through appropriate interaction, observation and measurement • analyse and interpret data accurately to inform nursing care and take appropriate action Formulate and document a plan of nursing care, where possible in partnership with patients, clients, their carers and family and friends, within a framework of informed consent • establish priorities for care based on individual or group needs • develop and document a care plan to achieve optimal health, habilitation, rehabilitation based on assessment and current nursing knowledge

- participate in the negotiation and agreement of the care plan with the patient or client and with their carer, family or friends, as appropriate, under the supervision of a registered nurse
- inform patients and clients about intended nursing actions, respecting their right to participate in decisions about their care

Contribute to the implementation of a programme of nursing care, designed and supervised by registered practitioners

- undertake activities which are consistent with the care plan and within the limits of one's own abilities

Demonstrate evidence of a developing knowledge base which underpins safe nursing practice

- access and discuss research and other evidence in nursing and related disciplines
- identify examples of the use of evidence in planned nursing interventions

Demonstrate a range of essential nursing skills, under the supervision of a registered nurse, to meet individuals' needs, which include: maintaining dignity, privacy and confidentiality; effective communication and observational skills, including listening and taking physiological measurements; safety and health, including moving and handling and infection control; essential first aid and emergency procedures; administration of medicines; emotional, physical and personal care, including meeting the need for comfort, nutrition and personal hygiene

Contribute to the evaluation of the appropriateness of nursing care delivered

- demonstrate an awareness of the need to assess regularly a patient's or client's response to nursing interventions
- provide for a supervising registered practitioner, evaluative commentary and information on nursing care based on personal observations and actions
- contribute to the documentation of the outcomes of nursing interventions

- identify expected outcomes, including a time frame for achievement and/or review in consultation with patients, clients, their carers and family and friends and with members of the health and social care team

Based on the best available evidence, apply knowledge and an appropriate repertoire of skills indicative of safe nursing practice

- ensure that current research findings and other evidence are incorporated in practice
- identify relevant changes in practice or new information and disseminate it to colleagues
- contribute to the application of a range of interventions to support patients and clients and which optimise their health and well-being
- demonstrate the safe application of the skills required to meet the needs of patients and clients within the current sphere of practice
- identify and respond to patients and clients' continuing learning and care needs
- engage with, and evaluate, the evidence base which underpins safe nursing practice

Provide a rationale for the nursing care delivered which takes account of social, cultural, spiritual, legal, political and economic influences

- identify, collect and evaluate information to justify the effective utilisation of resources to achieve planned outcomes of nursing care

Evaluate and document the outcomes of nursing and other interventions

- collaborate with patients and clients and, when appropriate, additional carers to review and monitor the progress of individuals or groups towards planned outcomes
- analyse and revise expected outcomes, nursing interventions and priorities in accordance with changes in the individual's condition, needs or circumstances

(Cont'd)

Appendix 1 (*Continued*)

Domain	Outcomes to be achieved for entry to the branch programme	Competencies for entry to the register
	Recognise situations in which agreed plans of nursing care no longer appear appropriate and refer these to an appropriate accountable practitioner • demonstrate the ability to discuss and accept care decisions • accurately record observations made and communicate these to the relevant members of the health and social care team	Demonstrate sound clinical judgement across a range of differing professional and care delivery contexts • use evidence-based knowledge from nursing and related disciplines to select and individualise nursing interventions • demonstrate the ability to transfer skills and knowledge to a variety of circumstances and settings • recognise the need for adaptation and adapt nursing practice to meet varying and unpredictable circumstances • ensure that practice does not compromise the nurse's duty of care to individuals or the safety of the public
Care management	Contribute to the identification of actual and potential risks to patients, clients and their carers, to oneself and to others and participate in measures to promote and ensure health and safety • understand and implement health and safety principles and policies • recognise and report situations which are potentially unsafe for patients, clients, oneself and others	Contribute to public protection by creating and maintaining a safe environment of care through the use of quality assurance and risk management strategies • apply relevant principles to ensure the safe administration of therapeutic substances • use appropriate risk assessment tools to identify actual and potential risks • identify environmental hazards and eliminate and/or prevent where possible • communicate safety concerns to a relevant authority • manage risk to provide care which best meets the needs and interests of patients, clients and the public
	Demonstrate an understanding of the role of others by participating in inter-professional working practice • identify the roles of the members of the health and social care team • work within the health and social care team to maintain and enhance integrated care	Demonstrate knowledge of effective inter-professional working practices which respect and utilise the contributions of members of the health and social care team • establish and maintain collaborative working relationships with members of the health and social care team and others • participate with members of the health and social care team in decision making concerning patients and clients • review and evaluate care with members of the health and social care team and others
		Delegate duties to others, as appropriate, ensuring that they are supervised and monitored • take into account the role and competence of staff when delegating work • maintain one's own accountability and responsibility when delegating aspects of care to others • demonstrate the ability to coordinate the delivery of nursing and health care

Demonstrate literacy, numeracy and computer skills needed to record, enter, store, retrieve and organise data essential for care delivery

Demonstrate key skills
- literacy: interpret and present information in a comprehensible manner
- numeracy: accurately interpret numerical data and their significance for the safe delivery of care
- information technology and management: interpret and utilise data and technology, taking account of legal, ethical and safety considerations, in the delivery and enhancement of care
- problem solving: demonstrate sound clinical decision making which can be justified even when made on the basis of limited information

Personal and professional development

Demonstrate responsibility for one's own learning through the development of a portfolio of practice and recognise when further learning is required
- identify specific learning needs and objectives
- begin to engage with, and interpret, the evidence base which underpins nursing practice.

Acknowledge the importance of seeking supervision to develop safe nursing practice

Demonstrate a commitment to the need for continuing professional development and personal supervision activities in order to enhance knowledge, skills, values and attitudes needed for safe and effective nursing practice
- identify one's own professional development needs by engaging in activities such as reflection in, and on, practice and lifelong learning
- develop a personal development plan which takes into account personal, professional and organisational needs
- share experiences with colleagues and patients and clients in order to identify the additional knowledge and skills needed to manage unfamiliar or professionally challenging situations
- take action to meet any identified knowledge and skills deficit likely to affect the delivery of care within the current sphere of practice

Enhance the professional development and safe practice of others through peer support, leadership, supervision and teaching
- contribute to creating a climate conducive to learning
- contribute to the learning experiences and development of others by facilitating the mutual sharing of knowledge and experience
- demonstrate effective leadership in the establishment and maintenance of safe nursing practice

The context of practice

Mark Darley

CHAPTER CONTENTS

Introduction 42
   Background 42

The history of the National Health Service 43

The structure of the National Health Service 45
   The Health Act 1999 47
   The 1999 Act and professional
     self-regulation 47
   The NHS Executive function 48
   Health authorities 48
   National Health Service Trusts 49
   Primary care groups and Trusts 49
   Community health councils 50

Policy developments since 1997 50
   Clinical governance 50
   Evidence-based practice 52
   Continuing professional development 52
   Risk management 53
   NHS organisations and professional
     regulation 54
   Regulation and performance in the
     medical profession 55
   The practitioner perspective on clinical
     governance 57

The National Plan 58
   Introduction 58
   Background 58
   The announcement of the National
     Plan 58
   Resourcing the National Plan 59
   The key elements of the National Plan 59
   Reaction to the National Plan 61

Structural changes to NHS bodies and
   organisation embodied in the National
   Plan 62
Concluding comments on the National
   Plan 63

The social care sector and partnership with the NHS 63
   Background 63
   The partnership between the NHS and
     local government 65
   The local government White Paper
     1997 65
   The strategic context for public health 66
   The health improvement programme 66

The independent sector 69

The contribution of nursing: making a difference 70
   Recruitment and retention 71
   Professional education 72

Conclusion 73

References 74

Further reading 75

The purpose of this chapter is to put into context the setting in which health care is provided in the UK as we enter the 21st century. The chapter aims to:

- provide brief details about the historical context and background to the development of the National Health Service (NHS) as a precursor to providing a more detailed insight into health policy from 1997 onwards, including an outline of the current structure and political imperatives that govern the NHS
- outline changes in such areas as policy for nursing, public health and partnership with social services, as these inform much of government thinking on health and service development.

INTRODUCTION

The relevance of this chapter to the new student in the nursing and midwifery professions focuses on the increasing requirement for all practitioners to be aware of the main influences on their everyday working lives. While some would argue that the decision to train as a nurse or midwife is in a large part prompted by a desire to care for people, it is no longer feasible in an increasingly political world to do this in isolation from the political and policy influences that shape the world in which we work. It is for this reason that the modern nursing and midwifery student needs to understand the context of care in order to remain informed, up to date and, ultimately, competent. It is hoped, therefore, that the issues and subjects raised in this chapter will be informative and provide a sound base from which students can build a deeper understanding of the context of care and its relevance to their work.

Inevitably, any discussion on health policy in the UK will centre on the policy objectives of the particular government in power. There is little doubt that the development of the NHS has always been influenced by the political complexion of the prevailing government. Consequently, it is impossible to separate the development of the service from politics and, increasingly, the political intervention or influence of the government of the day on the development of the NHS has become more acute as time has passed. It is for this reason that the elements of this chapter which seek to describe the way in which the NHS is developing in the very early part of this new century, along with government-inspired efforts to work more closely with other welfare state agencies, might appear to be a thinly veiled exposition of government policy. This is not intentional as the text merely reflects the relationship that exists between politics and health care in modern Britain.

Background

Since the last edition of this book (Kenworthy, Snowley and Gilling 1996), the National Health Service has celebrated its 50th anniversary. This anniversary roughly coincided with the election of a Labour government in 1997 which in itself heralded a period of significant change for the service as first Frank Dobson and latterly Alan Milburn, as Secretaries of State for Health, have worked to understand the nature of the NHS and then propose reforms which, in their view, will make it 'modern and dependable'.

During the first 2 years of this Labour government, a number of major policy papers were published which were intended to provide the framework for, and develop the shape of, service provision for the ensuing 5–10 years. Among these key papers were *The New NHS: Modern, Dependable* (DoH 1997), *A First Class Service: Quality in the New NHS* (DoH 1998a), *The New NHS – Working Together: Securing a Quality Workforce for the NHS* (DoH 1998b), *Saving Lives: Our Healthier Nation* (DoH 1999a) and *Making a Difference: Strengthening the Nursing, Midwifery and Health Visiting Contribution to Health and Healthcare* (DoH 1999b). This series of major policy White Papers, in addition to the many Health Service Circulars (HSCs) which are issued almost daily from the Department of Health, have signalled the intent of the government to radically reform the National Health Service to enable it to meet the rigorous targets that have been set (Rivett 1998).

In common with most governments, the Labour government of 1997 was concerned with the level of funding required to support the NHS and how this money was spent. Although it was widely recognised during the election of 1997 that the service was facing an increasingly large financial crisis, and a crisis of morale among its staff, it was at least 2 years before the government admitted that a more radical approach to funding was necessary. A rethink took place following initial pledges to maintain the spending targets of the previous administration. This led to a fundamental spending review which in itself prefaced the publication of the *National Plan* (DoH 2000) – a plan for investment for the National Health Service – in August 2000.

One of the most fundamental questions that faces a so-called developed nation is that of how best to fund and provide an effective and comprehensive health care service for its citizens. During the years of the Conservative government in power between 1979 and 1997, the radical approach of introducing the concepts of the free market and the principles of commercial enterprise were to the fore. Although the assumption that health care should be provided in the main from public taxation was never challenged, the relationship between the independent sector and the public sector was blurred to the point where more and more private capital was being invested in the National Health Service and more joint ventures – called the 'private finance initiative' (PFI) – were embarked upon. Although the Labour government promised to rid the NHS of the 'internal market', as it was called, it did not entirely dispense with the idea of using private capital. This is evident from its continued enthusiasm for PFIs to fund and build new hospitals. Indeed some proposals go so far as to provide clinical services also.

Among economists and policy analysts there appears to be no consensus as to the best way of funding and providing a health care system in a modern industrial economy. The key consideration seems to focus on taking full account of a nation's cultural, social and political environment and then tailoring a health care system that best suits this. Consequently, while there are many who would look to the USA as an example of an outstanding health care system, there are just as many who would suggest that this system only works from a cultural perspective in America and therefore cannot be grafted onto the cultural, social and political environment that exists in, for example, the UK. A simple polarisation of debate between privately funded or insurance-based health care and publicly funded or 'socialised' health care only partially describes the reality in any country.

It is clear to many that although there are many imperfections and problems associated with providing a health care system which is funded almost entirely from public taxation and which is comprehensive and free at the point of delivery, there is little resolve to alter or change these founding principles. Aneurin Bevan, as the prime architect of the NHS, would recognise the National Health Service as it is structured today, in that it is based squarely on the principles that he engendered. What would be different would be the organisational structures that govern the flow of resources from Parliament down to individual hospitals and health care settings, in addition to the strategic decision-making structures which influence the future provision of services. What follows describes the major features of health care in the UK at the beginning of the 21st century allied to brief discussions of major issues associated with the development of the NHS and partnerships with other sectors of the welfare state and independent sector.

THE HISTORY OF THE NATIONAL HEALTH SERVICE

As has been previously stated, it is important to understand the history of the National Health Service as a way of developing an appreciation of the context within which health care is provided in the UK.

The National Health Service was founded in 1948 as a way of ensuring that the British public would never have to go back to the kind of health care provision that existed prior to the Second World War. The prime concern of Aneurin Bevan, and of the Labour government of which he was a member, was to ensure that health care was universal, free at the point of delivery and paid for primarily out of central taxation. Resourcing the service in this way was a major departure from previous arrangements which largely focused on charitable contributions, local taxes, direct charges and insurance schemes. A classic pre-war issue was a fee payable for consulting a GP. This has been opposed since 1948 but it is interesting to note that GPs are campaigning for its reintroduction in response to the publication of the National Plan in 2000 (Webster 1988).

The National Health Service was established by the National Health Service Act of 1946. The Act deemed that Parliament holds the Secretary of State for Health to account for all aspects of the service and the way in which resources are deployed. Parliament is also able to call members of the service to account when important issues are investigated or inquiries are held.

Charles Webster, a major historian of the National Health Service, noted that Bevan was unable to achieve a consensus on how the service should be organised. He consequently decided to maintain the compartmentalised approach which saw the continued existence of an acute and primary care sector with a residual public health function which would focus on preventative and health promotion. As Webster maintains, the strongest aspect of Bevan's National Health Service was the power vested in the acute sector as represented by hospitals, and, especially, consultant doctors. Almost 70% of available resources were invested in this area of the NHS, which ultimately was focused around providing for the needs of medical consultants who sat at the top of a huge clinical professional pyramid, commonly known as 'the Firm'.

Interestingly, although many would take the view that underfunding has been a problem that has afflicted the National Health Service only in the last 20 years, this phenomenon has much deeper roots. As far back as 1951, the Guillebaud Committee was set up to investigate the unrelenting demand for health services which Bevan had not wholly foreseen. The prevailing view at the time of the setting up of the NHS was that initially there would be a massive draw on resources as the system established itself, but that this would then tail off as health care problems were ameliorated and the requirement for services dropped. What happened in fact was that demand for services started at a high level and continued to increase. The Guillebaud Committee therefore concluded that the resourcing of the service was a problem that had not necessarily been foreseen and that it would be difficult to maintain a level of funding which would adequately provide the services people demanded.

Although the National Health Service experienced a number of reorganisations and policy initiatives which changed the way in which hospitals were managed, and increased the involvement of nurses in particular in the provision and management of services, it was not until the election of the Thatcher government in 1979 that the most profound efforts were made to reconsider the very nature of the NHS and the ways in which it was funded, organised and provided.

One of the most significant developments following the election of the Conservative government in 1979 was the independent inquiry into the management of the National Health Service led by Roy Griffiths who, at the time, was the managing director of the Sainsburys supermarket chain. The main findings of the Griffith Management Inquiry Team suggested to the government that the NHS suffered from a lack of well defined and clearly focused management. One of the most famous pronouncements of the Griffiths Inquiry was that had Florence Nightingale walked into one of the hospitals of the day, she would have found it difficult to identify who was in charge.

One of the major outcomes of the so-called Griffiths Report was to move away from what had been consensus management in the NHS – which had existed up to 1983 – towards a stronger commitment to what was known as 'general management' (Strong and Robinson 1988). The result of this was that a series of regional, district and unit general managers in the NHS were established to exercise overall control of the sector of the health service they were responsible for. Although this produced much consternation among the clinical professions, most notably in the nursing profession, who felt largely excluded from senior levels of management due to the low number of nurses that were appointed to these jobs, their establishment did enable the NHS to develop a more businesslike approach to its work.

The general management posts evolved, following the NHS review of 1989, into chief executive posts with overall management responsibility for National Health Service Trusts. Chief executives were assisted in this work by a board of directors which comprised a chairman, executive directors and non-executive directors. This board of directors oversaw the establishment and development of the National Health Service Trusts with the intention of enabling the new organisations to oversee the operation of the newly established internal market. This 'market' was conceived to bring greater competition, efficiency and financial savings to the National Health Service. The consequence was that NHS Trusts were established essentially in competition with one another, which in turn led to a number of Trusts developing somewhat aggressive approaches to the establishment and maintenance of what they perceived as their market. Reaction from the clinical professions and elsewhere within the National Health Service suggested that, although some perceived the internal market as bringing benefits to the NHS, in the main the internal market was not well received. Consequently, when the Labour government was elected in 1997, it pledged to abolish the internal market. Despite doing this, many of the structural changes made by the Conservative government were retained or modified.

In view of the high esteem in which the service is generally held by members of the British public, it would be politically unthinkable for any government to consider abolishing the National Health Service and replacing it with an insurance-based or privately funded system. Although the government of Margaret Thatcher was widely believed to want to privatise the National Health Service, any real policy initiative to do this was never successfully considered outside of the cabinet office. Instead, a number of far reaching managerial and organisational changes were made, leaving a legacy typified by the establishment of NHS Trusts, the replacement of regional health authorities with regional offices, and a much stronger focus on what many have termed the 'new public management' based on an internal market and strong focus on businesslike approaches to service provision and management. Probably the most significant human embodiment of this service was the establishment of chief executives for all health authorities and Trusts. From the perspective of the nursing profession, this was an important development to which nursing leaders reacted. The government ultimately conceded that each Trust board had to include a director of nursing among the five executive directors that a chief executive was allowed to appoint.

The post of executive director of nursing (and quality) is very differently configured from Trust to Trust, but there can be little doubt that the existence of such a post has had a profound effect on developing the profile of nursing in hospital organisation and management. This has laid the foundations for many of the developments contained in the initiatives proposed by the Labour government since 1997 and ultimately enshrined in the National Plan of 2000. Although early research was carried out by Professor Jane Robinson and colleagues at the University of Nottingham on the effectiveness and nature of chief nurse or director of nursing role, there has been little research done since to properly quantify what the contribution of these posts has been (Robinson and Legrand 1994, Robinson and Strong 1987).

THE STRUCTURE OF THE NATIONAL HEALTH SERVICE

Although many people consider the National Health Service to be an organisation which covers all areas of the UK as one body, this is in fact not true. Separate National Health Services effectively exist for the four countries of the

United Kingdom. Consequently, Departments of Health exist for the Northern Ireland Office (with social services), the Scottish Office and the Welsh Office, in addition to the existence of a Department of Health for England. Each Department of Health has a separate chief nursing and chief medical officer, all of whom have an influence on developing local policy differences which apply in each country in response to major policy initiatives for the whole of the National Health Service (Merry 2000). Consequently, when, for example, a major policy document such as *Making a Difference: Strengthening the Nursing, Midwifery and Health Visiting Contribution to Healthcare* (DoH 1999b) is launched for the nursing profession, it is important to appreciate that slightly different documents exist for each of the four countries, in order to ensure that the policy is relevant to local organisational, legal and cultural conditions. The boundaries and regions are shown in Figure 2.1 and the broad structure of the NHS is outlined in Figure 2.2.

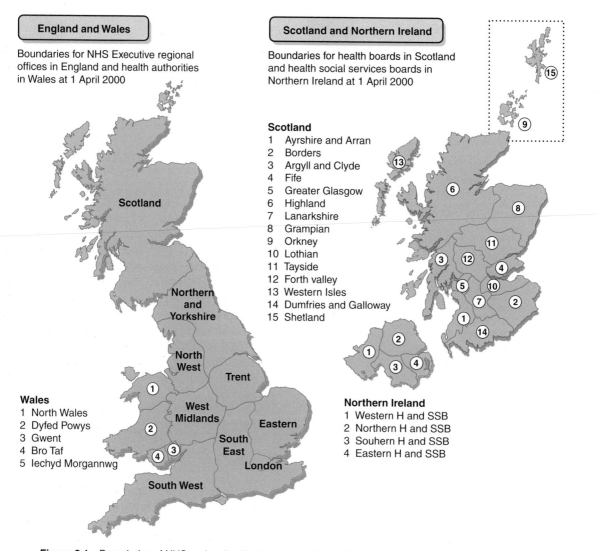

England and Wales

Boundaries for NHS Executive regional offices in England and health authorities in Wales at 1 April 2000

Scotland

Northern and Yorkshire

North West

Trent

West Midlands

Eastern

South East

London

South West

Wales
1 North Wales
2 Dyfed Powys
3 Gwent
4 Bro Taf
5 Iechyd Morgannwg

Scotland and Northern Ireland

Boundaries for health boards in Scotland and health social services boards in Northern Ireland at 1 April 2000

Scotland
1   Ayrshire and Arran
2   Borders
3   Argyll and Clyde
4   Fife
5   Greater Glasgow
6   Highland
7   Lanarkshire
8   Grampian
9   Orkney
10 Lothian
11 Tayside
12 Forth valley
13 Western Isles
14 Dumfries and Galloway
15 Shetland

Northern Ireland
1 Western H and SSB
2 Northern H and SSB
3 Souhern H and SSB
4 Eastern H and SSB

Figure 2.1   Boundaries of NHS regional authorities in the UK and Northern Ireland. (Based on Merry 2000.)

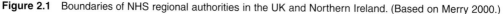

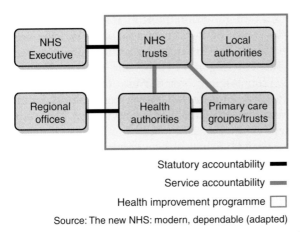

Statutory accountability ▬

Service accountability ▬

Health improvement programme ☐

Source: The new NHS: modern, dependable (adapted)

Figure 2.2   The structure of the new National Health Service (adapted from DoH 1999).

The Health Act 1999

The operation of the National Health Service has always been governed by an Act of Parliament which sets out the main structures of the service and its purposes. Following its election in 1997 and subsequent announcement of reforms of the National Health Service, in June 1999 the government received royal assent for the current Health Act. Essentially the Act implements the provisions outlined in the government White Paper *The New NHS: Modern, Dependable* which was published in 1997. The Act also outlines how the National Health Service will differ in the four countries of the UK. The main elements of the Act are as follows:

- GP fundholding will be abolished and replaced by primary care groups (PCGs) and primary care trusts (PCTs).
- Health improvement programmes will be established which will govern the development of local health care.
- The Act includes powers to develop more profound partnerships between the National Health Service, social services and local government. This will be achieved by changing the ways in which money will move between the different sectors and how the constituent agencies can also work together.
- High security hospitals can be formed as National Health Trusts.

- The statutory body, the Commission for Health Improvement, is established with the role of monitoring quality in the health service.
- All NHS Trusts have a statutory duty to improve the quality of care which is ultimately exercised by the chief executive.
- Powers are included in the Act to monitor the price of drugs within the NHS.
- Powers are included in the Act for an NHS tribunal to dismiss doctors or other clinicians who commit fraud.

A series of patient-centred services are also provided for in proposals contained in the Act: these include walk-in high street health centres, better health care partnerships between GPs, dentists, pharmacists, optometrists, etc. Also proposed were: increased use of day surgery in health centres, greater variety in services available in one place and health checks and advice sessions in new clinics, some of which may be provided in places of easier access for the public.

The 1999 Act and professional self-regulation

One of the major issues that affects clinical professionals has been the ongoing discussion surrounding the way in which the professions are regulated. Traditionally, the medical, nursing and professions allied to medicine have had their own regulatory bodies such as the GMC and the UKCC. These bodies managed systems of professional self-regulation as a means of protecting the public (Box 2.1). Although not widely appreciated by members of the profession, the only way a government in the past has been able to make changes to this system has been through the enactment of primary legislation. A significant change brought about by the 1999 Act has been the establishment of new powers for the Secretary of State to use the councils of the relevant bodies to make significant changes to, for example, education, disciplinary matters, registration or any other aspect of regulatory function. This will be significant in that it reduces the amount of time required to make important changes in the

---

Box 2.1   Professional self-regulation

The concept of professional self-regulation has existed in the UK for a great many years. This concept applies to the way in which the nursing and medical professions, and professions allied to medicine, regulate their affairs in the interests of protecting the public. Broadly speaking, the intention of these bodies is to ensure that the public can be guaranteed that the care they receive from a clinical professional is of the highest quality offered by someone who is being prepared as a result of completing a pre-ordained programme of education to a particular standard. All regulatory bodies are established by an Act of Parliament which, until the publication of the 1999 Health Services Act, could only be changed through primary legislation.

Regulatory bodies have a number of features in common. These are:

- The maintenance of a register of names of those attaining the right to be represented on the professional register.
- The administration of disciplinary and investigatory procedures to ensure that practitioners, about whom they receive a complaint, can in instances where negligence is proven, be removed from the register or cautioned.
- The development of educational policy aimed at ensuring that programmes leading to professional registration ensure that practitioners are competent and fit for practice.
- The maintenance of international relations to ensure that practitioners wishing to work in the UK meet European Community standards and that UK practitioners wishing to work abroad are able to meet the standards of other countries.

They work closely with government on a range of other policy and practice issues including the commissioning of research and the setting up of inquiries and investigations where required.

---

regulation of health care professionals, while also making their governance more flexible and responsive to the needs of society. In the light of a number of significant scandals in the medical world, in particular during 1999 and into 2000, these powers were seen as being a particularly important part of the government's plans to modernise the National Health Service and bring the way in which the professions govern themselves and relate to the public more up to date.

The NHS Executive function

In England, the National Health Executive (NHSE) provides the most senior level of executive management within the National Health Service. This is part of the Department of Health and has responsibility for managing the eight regional offices of England. These are: Eastern Region, London Region, North West Region, Northern and Yorkshire Region, South East Region, South West Region, Trent Region and West Midlands Region (see Fig. 2.1).

The NHSE has until recently been managed by a chief executive, although proposals are currently being made for this role to be combined with executive responsibility in a new post which will be appointed towards the end of 2000.

The NHSE in England has a chief medical officer and chief nursing officer who are responsible for major policy developments in those clinical areas. This is also the case for the executive functions within Wales, Northern Ireland and Scotland, although one major difference in Northern Ireland is that the executive function prevails over the provision of social care as well as health care.

The structure of the senior level of executive responsibility in Wales means that an NHS directorate has been established which is directly responsible to the National Assembly for Wales. The directorate prevails over five health authorities, 16 NHS Trusts and 22 local health groups.

In Scotland, a management executive exists which is responsible to the Scottish Parliament. The executive oversees the work of 15 health boards which in turn manage the work of primary care Trusts, acute hospital Trusts and all other health services within Scotland.

As already noted, Northern Ireland is slightly different in that a Department of Health and Social Services has been set up with a health and social service executive providing the most senior level of executive management. This oversees the work of four health and social services boards which in turn look after the work of GP fundholders, health and social services agencies and health and social services Trusts.

Health authorities

In England there are 99 health authorities which each, on average, serve a population of about

500 000 people. Each health authority has a chief executive and executive team who must include a finance director and a director of public health. These people are normally appointed by the chair and non-executive directors of the health authority, who together comprise the board of directors.

The role of health authorities is largely strategic in nature and includes:

- Assessing health needs for the local population.
- Developing strategy to meet the assessment of local health care need which, since the election of the government in 1997, has been drawn together as a health improvement programme (HIMP). The HIMP is not developed in isolation as local interest groups have an opportunity to contribute also.
- Using the HIMP as a template, the health authority is in a position then to determine what health care services are provided for the local population and where these are located.
- Ensuring that allocation of resources to all aspects of the local health care economy is done in such a way as to meet the overall strategic aims of the authority and provide the best levels and quality of care to the local population. Health authorities also have a responsibility to maintain surveillance of public health and develop strategies for the prevention and control of communicable diseases.
- Responding to nationally derived standards to develop high quality and efficient delivery of services. This response will normally be framed as locally relevant standards with locally agreed targets to ensure that the health authority is best placed to meet government objectives.
- Supporting the establishment of primary care groups and assisting those who wish to develop as primary care Trusts.

In addition to outlining the responsibilities health authorities exercise on behalf of the NHSE, it is also important to point out that all groups funded by them are ultimately accountable to the health authority and through to the National Health Executive for the way in which they provide their services in individual organisations.

Health authorities thus will play a key role in aiding the government to achieve its key objectives for the public health. This was supported in the National Plan through the announcement of improved primary care facilities in deprived areas, more screening programmes for women and children, more smoking cessation programmes and work to improve the diet of 4–6-year-olds in schools. Much of this will be expressed in health authority Health Improvement Programmes (described later in the chapter) and through improved partnership with social care or local government agencies. The health and health and social care boards in Scotland and Northern Ireland carry largely similar responsibilities.

National Health Service Trusts

In common with health authorities, each National Health Service Trust has a board of directors who are responsible for managing and overseeing the work of the Trust and ensuring that it meets requirements placed on it in terms of financial probity and the quality of clinical care. Each Trust has a chief executive and at least five executive directors who must include a director of finance, a medical director and a director of nursing. As with health authorities, each Trust has a chair and a series of non-executive directors who will be included in the appointment process for the executive directors. The posts of chair and non-executive director are appointed by the Secretary of State for Health.

Since 1997, the number of Trusts has fallen from about 440 to 374. The mergers which caused this reduction were premised on the belief that they would provide more effective health care for the population they serve in addition to becoming more financially efficient. These are important considerations, as NHS Trusts receive the majority of their income from agreements negotiated with health authorities and local primary care groups and the need to constantly assure value for money and clinical effectiveness is paramount.

Primary care groups and Trusts

One of the major innovations of the Conservative government up to 1997 was to enable groups of general practitioners to come together and form 'fundholding' practices. This led in some instances to a number of accusations being made about the development of a two-tier service which ran against the founding principles of the National Health Service. It was widely believed that people who were cared for in the community by a fundholding practice could possibly gain quicker and better access to acute services than those whose doctor was not a fundholder. While the argument and debate about this continued up to the general election of 1997, it did not take the Labour government long to change the whole basis for the provision of community care through the general practitioner, thereby putting an end to the debate.

The response of the Labour government was to establish primary care groups (PCGs) which cover on average between 50 000 and 250 000 people. As with Trusts, a board is responsible for managing the work of the PCG and this will typically be made up of four to seven general practitioners, one or two community nurses, a social services representative, a lay member, a health authority non-executive member and the chief executive. The role of a PCG covers three key functions:

1. the improvement of health throughout the community
2. the development of primary and community health care services
3. commissioning secondary services from local acute trusts.

PCGs are effectively sub-committees of health authorities, to whom they are accountable.

Since the 1997 election, a further level of primary provision has been developed in the form of primary care Trusts (PCTs). PCGs are enabled to attain the status of a PCT by applying to their health authority to have responsibility for commissioning services at what is called level three or level four. PCTs started to appear from April 2000 onwards. In keeping with the trends throughout the rest of the National Health Service, level four PCTs have an executive which is mostly made up of clinical professionals. In addition, a board exists which has a chair, five lay members, three professional members taken from the executive, a chief executive and a finance director. Provision for a further level of primary care Trust with joint responsibility for commissioning both health and social care services was proposed in the National Plan announced in August 2000.

Community health councils

Until their abolishment was announced as part of the National Plan, community health councils (CHCs) represented the views of the public in the running and work of the National Health Service. They were statutory bodies with a membership drawn from voluntary organisations, local authorities and the community at large. Although the government places a great emphasis on the importance of community involvement in decision making and the management of the National Health Service, and in particular the patient perspective, the National Plan has made it clear that community health councils will no longer exist. However, at the time of writing, this decision is being challenged in the House of Lords. They are to be replaced by a patient advocacy service and patient forums which are discussed in more detail later in this chapter.

POLICY DEVELOPMENTS SINCE 1997

A range of new policies have emerged under the auspices of the Labour government of 1997. What follows are brief descriptions of these initiatives with comments on their relevance to practice and the context of care.

Clinical governance

Among the many policy initiatives conceived by the Labour government, perhaps one has both captured the imagination of clinical professionals working in the National Health Service while, at the same time, presenting a range of problems as to its exact meaning and influence on clinical services. Clinical governance, as this initiative has become known, was announced in the government White Paper entitled *A First Class Service: Quality in the New NHS* (DoH 1998a). The principles which underpin the government's perspective on clinical governance were outlined in this paper and then further amplified in a Health Service Circular which was distributed to NHS Trusts in the early part of 1999.

Perhaps the most critical matter to grasp when considering clinical governance was that the initiative announced the government's intention to put clinical quality at the centre of NHS Trust and community health care providers' business. Previously, the prime consideration of NHS Trusts was to ensure that financial matters were being properly managed in accordance with the requirements of the government and the existing Act of Parliament. Although many Trusts quite rightly placed a great emphasis on clinical developments and professional development among staff, there was no requirement to report this to the Trust board or to make it a feature of the annual report. Clinical governance was intended to change this.

Since its announcement, clinical governance has also spawned a plethora of conferences and study days intended to assist clinical staff in their ability to understand what clinical governance means, how it impacts on their practice and how it can be established within the service. The fact that these study days and conferences are needed suggests that the concept of clinical governance is not altogether easy to grasp. Indeed many of the functions already being carried out within Trusts prior to the announcement of clinical governance suggested that it was in many respects already happening. The important point about clinical governance is that it draws together a range of often disparate functions within an NHS Trust under a common umbrella and gives them a title that everyone within the service can identify with.

Essentially, clinical governance brings together the following important functions within NHS Trusts:

- continuing quality improvement focused on clinical services
- effective risk management (including controls assurance and health and safety)

- effective use of evidence-based practice
- effective management of complaints about clinical services and management of any subsequent legal activity
- establishment and development of an effective system of continuing professional development for the majority of clinical staff
- establishment of systems to monitor performance of clinical professionals and, where necessary, to either act at the earliest point when professional practice is deemed to fall below an accepted standard, or ensure that the correct procedures are observed when negligence is identified.

It is clear from the above list that many of the functions identified were already taking place prior to the development of clinical governance as a concept. Indeed many of these would impact on the work of practitioners wherever they were employed within a health service organisation. As has been stated, the important consideration here is to understand that clinical governance for the first time brought these matters together. Indeed many directors of nursing working throughout the NHS had these responsibilities as part of their directorate, and it often became a natural consideration to ask the director of nursing to lead clinical governance.

It is clear that many aspects of clinical governance focus on the work of doctors, although this is not exclusively the case. It was often noted throughout the early stages of implementing clinical governance that the word 'clinician', which is used regularly throughout policy documents, should not relate to doctors alone. This said, it became increasingly important to ensure that the medical profession was properly appraised of developments with clinical governance and, more importantly, that they were in support of these developments. The consequence of this was that, in the majority of cases, Trusts decided to ask the medical director and director of nursing to work together to ensure that an effective system of clinical governance was developed within the Trust and that this had relevance and meaning to all clinical professional groups. It is also worth remembering that in so doing, the medical director and director of nursing had to ensure not only that all members of the professions allied to medicine were included in activities to establish clinical governance, but also that its influence on practice was relevant to them too.

Another important consideration in relation to clinical governance was the fact that the government made it absolutely clear in its introductory comments on the policy that this would be a 10-year programme of improvement within the NHS. The importance of this assertion lies in the fact that many people had observed over time that politically inspired policies often looked to the short term and did not enable services to develop over the medium to long term. The government stated from the outset that it did not expect rapid results with clinical governance but hoped that its establishment over 2–3 years would in time produce the kind of result which would lead to improved clinical services and quality of care. While the service implements clinical governance, two bodies, the National Institute for Clinical Excellence (NICE) and the Commission for Health Improvement (CHI), have been set up to set national clinical standards and to monitor them. Their roles are outlined in Boxes 2.2 and 2.3.

Evidence-based practice

Developments have taken place over previous years with the intention of ensuring that the quality of research and evidence at the disposal of clinicians was such that it could drive improvements in practice. Developments such as the Centre for Dissemination at the University of York and the Cochrane Database were all intended to ensure that practitioners working within the NHS could access high-quality information when developing their services or clinical care. It was evident that one of the problems of this system was that there was no effective means of ensuring that it actually influenced practice in reality. More often than not, the information was regarded as esoteric and research-focused in nature and many practitioners struggled to make it relevant to their individual work. The impact of clinical governance in this respect was that Trusts were required to put into place systems that not

---

Box 2.2 **The National Institute for Clinical Excellence**

The National Institute for Clinical Excellence (NICE) started work on the 1 April 1999. NICE has three main functions which include:

1. appraisal of new and existing health care technologies
2. the production of clinical guidelines
3. further development of clinical audit and confidential enquiries.

NICE was established as a special health authority in order to offer advice to all health care professionals in England and Wales on a range of issues relating to the introduction of new medications and technologies which influence both the cost and efficiency of health care provision.

Like other organisations in the National Health Service, NICE has a chairman (at the time of writing, this was Professor Michael Rawlings). The board of NICE includes seven non-executive directors and four executive directors. The latter group includes a chief executive, a clinical director, director of communications and a finance director. In addition to the above, a group made up of representatives from patient and care groups, the health care professions, the health care industry and the secretariat forms what is known as the NICE Partners Council.

The role of NICE ultimately, within the government's policy framework for improving quality within the National Health Service, is to set standards for the service.

The equivalent organisation to NICE in Scotland is the Scottish Health Technology Assessment Centre (SHTAC).

---

only produced information on which development could be based but also put into place systems which enabled them to disseminate information around the organisation to ensure that practice was of a uniformly high level of quality and consistent with practice throughout the majority of the profession. In addition to the systems already mentioned, Trusts are already in receipt of information from the government based on the findings of major confidential inquiries and, more recently, the deliberations of the National Institute for Clinical Excellence.

Continuing professional development

An area that has often concerned practitioners has been the availability of resources to enable

The Commission for Health Improvement (CHI) was established on 1 November 1999 as a statutory body included in the 1999 Health Act. Its key aims are to reduce perceived variations in clinical quality throughout the NHS and work to reduce and eliminate malpractice. Its main functions include:

- leading at a national level on the development of clinical governance throughout the NHS
- scrutinising locally produced arrangements for clinical governance
- conducting national and local review on work to establish and implement NICE guidelines and national service frameworks
- working with the NHS on identifying serious problems with clinical services at an early stage
- managing and working with external inquiries into major incidents within the NHS.

The commission has a chair and director of health improvement. In addition to these two posts, CHI has among its 14 members an appointment from the National Assembly for Wales. The board is made up of health service professionals, academics and lay members. Supporting the board are 40 permanent staff with an additional 200–300 staff drawn from a range of clinical professions within the NHS who are seconded to the commission to participate in reviews.

CHI was established to carry out a rolling programme of reviews of clinical governance and clinical quality arrangements within local Trusts. In addition to this, it is able to carry out spot checks in Trusts where major problems are perceived to exist. These can be notified by clinical professionals, patients or members of the public.

Whereas NICE sets standards for the NHS, CHI is largely responsible for monitoring those standards and working to develop improvements.

The parallel organisation in Scotland is the Clinical Standards Board, which was set up on 1 April 1999.

them to develop their clinical practice and carry forward their education. In its pronouncements on clinical governance and its desire to modernise the National Health Service, the government made it very clear that investment in continuing professional development was seen as an absolute priority for the NHS. Within the provisions for clinical governance, Trusts were required by April 2000 to have in place continuing professional development plans for the majority of clinical staff. These plans might typically look forward over a 1-, 2- or 3-year period

during which practitioners would agree with their manager or a senior clinical colleague a plan for developing clinical competencies in addition to accessing the necessary educational programme to enable them to achieve these. Once again, clinical governance was important in that it provided a framework within which such activity could be planned. In the past, a planned approach to clinical governance was largely dependent on the individual whim of senior managers or directors of nursing.

The importance of ensuring that continuing professional development is appropriately planned and invested in impacts on the service in a number of areas. First, it provides a signal to newly qualified staff that their education will be valued by the organisation when they join the permanent staff. Second, staff will be encouraged to access education which enables them to improve their clinical practice rather than collecting qualifications for their own sake. Third, there is always a desire to ensure that public money which is invested in the education of National Health Service staff is properly spent and that value for money is achieved. By ensuring that the majority of staff are covered by a continuing professional development plan, NHS Trusts are assisted in their own planning processes in that they can commission via the local education consortium, on a year-to-year basis, the education they need for their staff rather than relying on guesswork, which has often previously been the case. Finally, the importance to practitioners of effective and planned continuing professional development is that they can be assisted in their career development by basing their approach to continuing professional development on either using a mentor or using effective clinical supervision.

Risk management

For many years the concept of risk management has been used by organisations – the insurance industry and the airline industry among others – to assess the likelihood of an adverse event happening and to estimate how this would impact on the organisation and its market. Accurate risk management allows, for example, commercial enterprises to focus their investment programmes in areas that are likely to prevent the occurrence of serious adverse incidents and insurance companies to assess the nature of premiums they should charge when insuring particular activities.

The notion of risk assessment has become increasingly important within the NHS, especially since the removal of Crown immunity during the 1990s suggested that NHS organisations would be exposed to greater claims and increased litigation. The importance of effective risk management within, for example, a National Health Service Trust, has thus now become apparent to all.

Risk management applies not only to traditional areas of risk in the non-clinical arena but increasingly to the identification analysis and control of risk associated with clinical care. The majority of NHS Trusts now have membership of the Clinical Negligence Scheme for Trusts (CNST), which is a system for assisting Trusts to identify and manage their risk in a proactive fashion in order to limit the exposure of the organisation to litigation. It is important to view risk management as a proactive or positive phenomenon rather than a negative one. The relevance of risk management to clinical governance is that it can now be effectively incorporated into systems to achieve clinical governance. This is done by working with clinicians, for example, to focus on quality and clinical standards as a way of ensuring that the prospects for untoward incidents or mistakes occurring is reduced to an absolute minimum.

At the time of writing, the potential bill to the NHS for litigation has breached the £1 billion per annum level. It is therefore increasingly important that all staff in the service understand their contribution to effective risk management, and that members of the Trust board accept their responsibility for ensuring that risk management throughout the organisation is being properly approached. The concept of controls assurance has been extended from financial matters to matters relating to quality with a consequent responsibility being placed on the board and ultimately the chief executive to be wholly accountable and answerable for all matters relating to risk management and quality.

NHS organisations and professional regulation

It has been stated elsewhere in this chapter that professional regulation has received considerable attention from the government. While changes to Acts of Parliament and the structures that govern professional self-regulation are being carried forward, an additional responsibility at Trust level for regulation was contained within proposals for clinical governance.

Although clinical governance is often seen to focus on issues relating to quality, it is potentially easy to forget that Trusts also have a responsibility for establishing a monitoring system which relates to the clinical care offered by the professionals they employ. It is important to note at this juncture that this does not relate only to doctors but also to the work of nurses, midwives, health visitors and all professions allied to medicine. Trusts will be required over time to develop a system which enables them to monitor the professional and clinical capabilities of their staff as a means of allowing them to identify any concerns or problems and deal with these at the earliest possible point. In so doing, it is important that fears among some clinical professionals that there will be a culture of 'naming and shaming' are not only allayed, but that such a process is seen to be prevented in practice.

It is acknowledged that this is one of the most difficult areas for Trusts to make progress in and it may be one of the reasons why the government has acted subsequent to the publication of its proposals on clinical governance to strengthen its influence on national structures for regulating clinical professionals. Despite this, it will still remain a key responsibility for directors of nursing, medical directors and heads of professions allied to medicine to ensure that all clinical professionals working within their areas remain up to date, can access clinical professional development activities and have the means to express their concerns relating to clinical practice in a confidential and professionally safe manner. Trusts, if they can establish systems to do this, will then be able to demonstrate to bodies such as the Commission for Health Improvement, when they visit an organisation to monitor progress with clinical governance arrangements, that they are fully aware of the competence and skills of their clinical professionals in addition to any issues that may arise from this.

Regulation and performance in the medical profession

Between 1998 and 2000 a number of high-profile cases relating to the professional conduct of doctors and associated disciplinary matters received coverage in the media. Around the same time, the Government attempted to influence the regulation and monitoring of professional performance of doctors through clinical governance. While clinical governance covered the professional regulation of all clinical professionals working within the National Health Service, there was renewed focus on the conduct of doctors as public attention considered how well doctors were regulated and whether their professional body, the General Medical Council (GMC), ensured that doctors were 'fit for practice' and, where necessary, sanctioned them when practice fell below required standards.

The GMC responded by producing a document in September 2000 entitled 'Revalidating Doctors: Ensuring Standards, Securing the Future'. This document outlined proposals for revalidation of doctors throughout their career to protect the public from poorly performing doctors, while promoting good medical practice; thereby enabling the public to have greater confidence in doctors. The GMC's proposals suggested that good doctors could prove they were offering high-quality care, while enabling those doctors who fall below required standards to improve their practice. There was also a suggestion that the proposals might protect doctors from 'unfounded' criticism of their fitness to practice. This to refers to defensiveness traditionally encountered from the medical profession at suggestions that it establish open scrutiny of practice. The proposals of the GMC are set out in Figure 2.3.

The process of revalidation, as proposed, is set out in stages as follows.

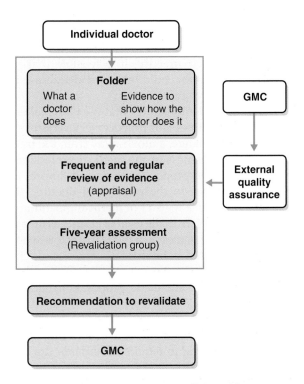

Figure 2.3   The revalidation process. (Adapted from GMC 2000).

Stage 1. A profile of performance will be constructed, wherein information about a doctor's practice and work to update and improve practice will be collected. Doctors will be expected to collect information relating to the pattern of their performance, continuing professional development, involvement in critical incidents and whether complaints or compliments have been made about their practice.

Stage 2. A five-year assessment is proposed wherein, at the end of the revalidation cycle, a doctor will be required to submit his/her folder for assessment by the GMC. The GMC will review this folder using a group of established medical and lay people, known as the 'revalidation group'. After this a certificate will be produced recommending the doctor as either 'fit for practice' or indicating that the doctor's registration should be referred for further consideration by established GMC processes.

Stage 3. This outlines action the GMC will take upon being notified that a doctor has not reached the required standard. For those doctors required to revalidate their practice, it is feasible that a doctor's registration could be suspended, erased or made subject to conditions.

This process demonstrates that the GMC takes revalidation of fitness for practice very seriously. This welcome change, a move away from the traditional defensiveness of the medical profession should, when the proposals are agreed, improve public confidence in the practice of doctors. It will also produce a register of medical practitioners in the UK, which can be used to assure, as far as possible, that the names on it relate to doctors who practice to required standards.

In addition to the work of the GMC, the Department of Health made proposals to tackle poor performance. These proposals are aimed at supporting Trusts, Primary Care Groups (and Trusts) and other service areas to ensure that doctors not performing to required standards can be dealt with sympathetically and fairly. Consequently, the Government has proposed that, where problems arise with the practice of a doctor, an initial view should be taken as to which proposed category the problem falls into, prior to action being taken. The four categories are as follows:

1. Doubts or concerns about clinical performance would lead to referral to an assessment or support centre. This is a new body.

2. Misconduct of a personal nature, such as theft, sexual or racial harassment or violence would be dealt with under the local employer's internal disciplinary procedures.

3. Failure to fulfill contractual commitments, such as not turning up for clinics or undertaking private work to the detriment of NHS responsibilities. Failure to work effectively as a member of the clinical team would also be dealt with by the employer.

4. Serious clinical problems or mistakes which warrant immediate referral to the GMC, without taking the step of referral to an assessment or support centre.

The assessment or support centres, outlined in point 1 above, are the major new Government proposal. Centres will be set up around the country, with the aim of 'offering impartial support to a doctor and local employer by offering advice on what action should be taken in a particular situation'. Each centre would have a Medical Director and Board of Governors with a non-medical Chair. It is proposed that strong non-medical participation in the assessment process is important. The outcomes the centre might recommend include:

- the doctor returning to practice with an assurance that there are no problems
- the doctor returning to practice with monitoring arrangements in place
- a period of re-education and retraining, followed by re-assessment
- re-skilling in a different field of medical practice, followed by re-assessment
- referral to the GMC
- referral for medical treatment
- referral back to the employer or health authority with a report that assesses the problems as serious and intractable
- in addition to the points above, a referral or notification to the Commission for Health Improvement and relevant NHS Executive Regional Office could be made, with the recommendation that a review be necessary due to wider organisational problems relating to the service concerned.

Clearly the Government is attempting to assist Trusts and local service providers in their efforts to deal with problems relating to medical practice. It is widely recognised that, although clinical governance made a serious attempt to do this, there are a number of problems at local level because doctors feel unable to sit in judgement on their colleagues when, in many cases, they have personal or professional relationships causing a conflict of interest. The key advantage of the proposals suggested by the Government is the attempt to take the process out of the service-based setting and into an arena where impartial and properly informed judgements can be made. The proposals by the Government were made public in November 1999 and are likely to come into effect during 2001.

The practitioner perspective on clinical governance

Much of what has been said on clinical governance in this section of the chapter might appear to the average clinical practitioner as managerially orientated. Indeed, one of the key issues in the establishment of clinical governance is that Trusts need to ensure that it is established at clinical level, rather than being a 'top down' initiative. Once clinical governance is properly established within a Trust, there should be particular features which are readily and easily recognisable to clinical practitioners working throughout the organisation.

First and foremost among these tangible aspects of clinical governance should be systems established within the organisation to monitor and improve the quality of clinical care. While systems to achieve this have existed for many years, they are now assuming greater importance as Trusts bring their work in line with government thinking. Quality can be approached in a number of ways:

• An organisation-wide approach to quality where an outside agency such as the Health Quality Service (HQS) of the King's Fund is invited in to examine quality and work with the Trust to develop ways of improving clinical care, or a Trust-wide system such as Total Quality Management (TQM) or some other system which the Trust develops and establishes for itself is used.
• The development of clinical indicators which measure performance and improvement in aspects of clinical care. These must be relevant to individual directorates or clinical specialities as overseen by the clinical director and/or senior nurse or senior health care professional. If clinical indicators of this nature are to have relevance, they will need to be developed in close liaison with all clinical practitioners so that the aspects of practice being measured are not only realistic but also meaningful to practitioners.
• Collection and collation of information relevant to patient charter standards or other government-inspired initiatives.

All of the above will probably be recognisable by a majority of clinical practitioners. They will at some time or other have contributed to the development of indicators or have assisted with the collection and collation of information. This in itself raises another issue which is important in the development of clinical governance. As with most initiatives, the availability of appropriate and adequate resources to make the initiative happen is very important. It was noticeable in the early pronouncements on clinical governance that the government did not necessarily anticipate that the establishment of clinical governance would require additional or extra resources. As part of the work to establish clinical governance, Trusts throughout England were asked to carry out a baseline assessment which was then reported to their relevant Regional Office.

The experience of many Trusts working to gather the information for the baseline assessment for their regional office in 1999 was that while the majority of staff saw the establishment of clinical governance as laudable, many commented on the need for additional resources to make it happen. Invariably this focused on developing computer systems and methods of collecting and processing information. Additionally, it was widely felt that unless the quality of information collected in relation to clinical governance was high, then the decisions and deliberations which would be based on the output of this information might be flawed. The consequence of this was that many Trusts suggested that, in addition to appointing people with specific responsibilities for coordinating clinical governance, it was also important to invest in audit clerks who would be largely responsible for ensuring that information that was put into systems was of a high quality and dependable.

One other area that received a great deal of attention during the early phases of clinical governance was the impact that it would have on existing systems for clinical audit. In the majority of NHS Trusts, a clinical audit committee existed which was usually chaired by a senior medical practitioner within the organisation. Additionally, many audit committees included senior nurses, members from the professions allied to medicine and researchers. It was observed that over time clinical audit had developed a largely medical focus and that the projects which were agreed each year by the Trust and then funded by the health authority were as much the result of the whim of individuals as of any organisational need. An important outcome from establishing clinical governance was that clinical audit started to become much more focused on the clinical objectives and needs of individual clinical directorates. Consequently, a clinical director might, with his key staff, identify two or three areas that would require auditing in a period of time and focus resources on these. From the perspective of individual practitioners working within a ward or clinical area, this consideration was important, as they could have confidence in the knowledge that audit activity was focused on the needs of the clinical area and not something whose relevance, in many cases, was difficult to relate to their individual practice.

THE NATIONAL PLAN

Introduction

After the election of May 1997 the Labour government published a range of policy initiatives intended to achieve its stated aim of modernising the National Health Service, thereby bringing it up to date and making it 'fit for purpose' as the UK entered the 21st century. These initiatives were mentioned earlier in this chapter. This section focuses on the National Plan for the National Health Service (DoH 2000) which was announced in August 2000 by the Secretary of State for Health, Alan Milburn, MP.

Background

Towards the end of 1999 and into the earlier part of 2000, the Labour government expressed increasing frustration with media attention and public opinion which focused on the widely held view that the NHS was failing to provide good care. Stories about falling standards, the malpractice of doctors, low morale among nursing and other staff in the service and the dirty and poorly-maintained state of Britain's hospitals were

rife and regularly appeared in the media. The response of the Labour government was to announce that it would be publishing a National Plan for the National Health Service which would gather together all its previously published initiatives and focus these on a range of issues and initiatives intended, in its view, to bring the service into the 21st century. The plan focused on investment and reform.

A range of activities (including major national and professional conferences, the distillation of professional opinion from a cross-section of people working within the NHS, and an extensive public relations exercise in which half a million questionnaires were distributed to the general public) provided the information the government felt it needed to produce a National Plan. These activities provided people with an opportunity to express their opinions about the service and what they perceived to be the priorities for its continued development and improvement.

The announcement of the National Plan

The culmination of these exercises was the National Plan announced by Mr Milburn. Interestingly, the Prime Minister, Tony Blair, took an intense interest in the development of the National Plan and even went so far as to leak the plan to the Commons shortly before the summer recess in 2000. It was commonly understood that Mr Blair had taken a deep personal interest in the plan as the National Health Service is something which the Labour Party holds very close to its heart. In leaking the document to the Commons, Mr Blair outlined his 'Five Challenges' (Box 2.4) and noted that this was 'the first time that Government has looked long and hard at all aspects of the NHS'. He went on to say NHS staff were 'magnificent but they had been working flat out in a system still organised as it was in 1940s, when today patients and staff expect and demand a wholly different type of service for the new world in which we live'. The intention of Mr Blair and his colleagues was therefore clear. The service was to be fundamentally reformed and the systems of the NHS would be refocused around the primacy and the needs of patients or clients. The National Plan, like that for clinical governance announced in 1998, would be a 10-year plan which promised to focus on long-term solutions for 'removing the outdated practices and perverse incentives that have prevented the best from becoming the norm'. If the government was to be believed, the National Plan would be no overnight quick fix. Rather, it would focus on medium- to long-term solutions for serious concerns afflicting the service.

One of the key considerations of the National Plan was the admission on the part of the government that hospitals and the NHS cannot be effectively managed from Whitehall. The government promised a new relationship between the Department of Health and the National Health Service at local level based on 'the principles of subsidiarity'. The term 'subsidiarity' has become very familiar from the politics of the European Community, where the executive responsibility of the European Parliament can only be exercised in many instances once the local perspective of member states has been taken into account. It remains to be seen whether or not this principle can work effectively within the National Health Service, especially with a government that bases so much of its work on national standards and uniformity which are assessed against targets set and controlled centrally. The important point to consider here is whether or not politicians can resist the temptation to 'meddle' if, for whatever

reason, they perceive the reforms are not moving quickly enough for their needs.

Resourcing the National Plan

The National Plan also followed a massive injection of resources from the Chancellor of the Exchequer which promised to bring the level of finance provided for the National Health Service up to the European average as a percentage of the gross national product. An announcement was made indicating that the expenditure on the NHS would increase by an average of 6.3% year on year. Table 2.1 sets this out in more detail.

Although the government signalled its intention to manage the National Health Service at 'greater arms length', individual NHS Trusts and health authorities will be required to meet demanding targets which, if they fail to achieve them, will lead to the prospect of being publicly named and shamed. At the time of writing, several Trusts had already received visits from teams sent in by the government to deal with failures to reduce waiting lists. This followed 'naming and shaming' in the national press.

The key elements of the National Plan

Access to services and care issues

Maximum waiting times for operations will fall to 6 months, with outpatient appointment waiting times being reduced to 3 months by 2005. From 2002, people whose operation is cancelled on the day of surgery for non-clinical reasons will be provided with another date within the month or offered payment to access private treatment. By 2004, no one should wait more than 4 hours for treatment in an accident and emergency department. In addition, access to a GP will be promised within 48 hours, or a primary care professional within 24 hours.

Finally, letters about care will be copied to patients and patients' views will influence the level of resources Trusts get, although the mechanism for this is, the time of writing, unclear.

Table 2.1 Resources for the National Plan

	1999/00 (out-turn)	2000/01 (plan)	2001/02 (plan)	2002/03 (plan)	2003/04 (plan)	Average annual real terms increase %
Net NHS expenditure (£ million)	40 066	44 234	47 964	52 026	56 424	
% real terms increase		8.0	5.8	5.8	5.8	6.3

The cash increases announced in the budget are:

2000/01	£1.4 billion
2001/02	£2.6 billion
2002/03	£4.1 billion
2003/04	£4.4 billion

When the additional money, announced in the budget, is added to the increase already planned as part of the comprehensive spending review, the actual year-on-year cash growth available to the NHS over the 4 years is:

2000/01	£4.2 billion
2001/02	£3.7 billion
2002/03	£4.1 billion
2003/04	£4.4 billion

Extra beds

As a response to the widely held view that beds in the National Health Service have reduced to too low a level, the National Plan promises an extra 7000 beds by 2004. The provision of these beds will be divided into 2100 for general and acute services with the rest being provided in intermediate care. Further work on what intermediate beds are and how this service will be provided will be communicated through subsequent Health Service Circulars. It was also indicated that up to 100 new hospitals will be built by 2010 as part of a renewed focus on the existing private finance initiatives to ensure the beds will be housed in modern facilities where possible.

The extended role of nurses

All nurses will be able to access professional development to extend their role if they so choose. By 2004, half will be expected to dispense medicines, nurse consultant posts will rise to 1000, support staff will have learning accounts and a leadership learning centre will be established to develop future managers and 'matron' roles. Some £280 million is earmarked to support this work.

Numbers of doctors and nurses

The plan promised 7500 more consultants, 2000 general practitioners and up to 20000 extra nurses and 6500 more therapists for the National Health Service. In addition to bolstering these numbers, the plan made significant pronouncements on extending the powers of nurses to prescribe medications, admit patients to health care and discharge patients home.

Finally, 1000 new places at medical schools were announced to support the growth in consultant numbers on a longer-term basis. In support of the proposed increase in numbers for other professions, plans to establish 100 on-site nurseries were also announced.

Consultant contracts

Following extensive debate about the amount of private practice being carried out by some NHS consultants, the plan promised to tie newly appointed senior doctors into working for the NHS for up to 7 years. Although this measure is likely to be unpopular among some sections of the medical fraternity, the government has endeavoured to make it more palatable by improving the existing merit scheme of bonus payments for senior doctors.

Primary health care Trusts

Although plans to develop primary care groups into primary care Trusts have been in existence for some time, the National Plan announced a new level of Trust which could commission health and social services together. In the government's view, this was an important initiative in that it 'will prevent patients – particularly old people – falling in the cracks between the two services'.

National performance fund

A fund approaching some £500 million will be provided with an average of £5 million for each health authority per year as a means of rewarding those authorities which are deemed to be successful in meeting government targets. Those authorities which fail to measure up in this new regime will be required to work with regional offices to use these funds once plans for improvements have been agreed. This policy supports the wish of the government to manage the service less through the Department of Health by developing the concept of 'earned autonomy' for health authorities and Trusts.

Clinical service development

By 2004, some 20 diagnostic and treatment centres will be established to do routine short-stay or day surgery. Rapid access chest pain clinics will also be set up by 2003. The intention behind this initiative is to reduce the pressure on hospitals that were recognised in the plan as struggling to reduce existing waiting lists. Cancer screening programmes will be increased, as will the availability of cancer drugs to end the 'post code lottery' of access for drug treatment.

Community health councils

Community health councils will be abolished and a patient advocacy service set up in their place. Each hospital, Trust or primary care organisation, will have a patient forum. The membership will be drawn from a wide range of groups including patient survey and local pressure groups, patient groups or voluntary organisations. However, this decision is being challenged in the House of Lords at the time of writing.

The private sector

Although working with the private sector has always been a controversial matter, the National Plan made clear its intention for the National Health Service to work closely with the private sector in future in respect to the use of operating theatres, intensive care beds and developing a more structured approach to 'intermediate' care. A £900 million funding package to support the development of intermediate care was announced. A national framework will be drawn up to govern the nature of the working relationship between the two sectors which, it is intended, will help the two to work together more effectively and efficiently. This will include work to define 'intermediate' care more clearly in addition to defining responsibilities.

Investment in equipment

£300 million will be invested in equipment for cancer, kidney and heart disease services. This is to include 50 new magnetic resonance imaging (MRI) scanners and 200 new CT scanners throughout the UK.

Estates issues

Prior to the publication of the National Plan, many comments about the National Health Service centred on the dire state of Britain's hospitals. The plan therefore announced the provision of £30 million for a 'nationwide cleanup campaign' which was to start straightaway with the intention of tidying patient areas, lavatories and accident and emergency departments.

Reaction to the National Plan

Although sceptics take the view that the National Plan signals yet more central control from the government, many commentators working both within the NHS and outside hope the plan will provide a coherent framework for the modernisation and development of the service.

While some areas of resistance could be predicted, it is expected that the plan will garner strong support from among the nursing profession. This belief is founded on the fact that the National Plan provides significant extra resources for the National Health Service and has used advice and contributions from the Royal College of Nursing and trade unions to frame policy. It also focuses heavily on how nurses can make a far greater contribution to clinical practice by either extending their skills and ultimately becoming nurse consultants (although these posts were not announced as part of the National Plan), or taking advantage of new plans for nurses to access medical training without having to start from the beginning if they make the decision to train as doctors in mid-career. It will be interesting to see if this aspect of the plan has any significant impact on either the number of doctors being trained or the nature of their background. While it clearly made sense for the government to provide for those who wish to make a mid-career break and enter medicine, it is also worth noting that as with other clinical professions experiencing significant difficulties in recruiting to their ranks, measures such as this might do little more than deplete those ranks further. If nothing else, proposals such as this signify the readiness of the government to be radical in its thinking and to challenge professional barriers and perceptions that have existed for decades.

Structural changes to NHS bodies and organisation embodied in the National Plan

A number of changes were proposed as part of the National Plan to those organisations that exist within the National Health Service or which have an impact on its operation. These include:

- The development of a modernisation agency which will incorporate a national patient access team and clinical governance support unit. This will work with regionally based team to 'roll out' the National Plan over the next 10 years.

- Leadership centres will be established by 2001 to improve access to development programmes that are work based and thereby easier to access for existing health care professionals. Although these centres clearly are aimed at clinical professionals occupying existing senior appointments, the intention to include non-executive directors and chairs of trusts was also made clear.

- In response to criticisms about increased politicisation of non-executive appointments at Trusts, an arms-length agency or commission will be established to choose non-executive Trust and health authority directors. The chairmen of regional health authorities will also be replaced by eight commissioners whose job will be to appoint and support Trust board members.

- A national independent panel to advise on hospital closures and reorganisations will be established.

- A national clinical assessment authority, which will be empowered to develop the assessment of a doctor's performance following a complaint, will be set up.

- A coordinating body will be established to oversee the working of regulatory bodies including those for nursing, midwifery and health visiting, medicine, dentistry and the professions allied to medicine. The intention of this body is to ensure that these organisations work more closely together in the future.

- A citizen's council will be established to work with and advise the National Institute of Clinical Excellence on its work in investigating the efficacy of medications and treatments.

- A patient advocacy and liaison service will be established with a presence in every NHS Trust. The service will have direct access to chief executives of Trusts. This is not dissimilar to pre-existing complaints systems where the chief executive in many Trusts manages the collation of information on the progress of complaints and relates this directly to complainants. The clear difference in this respect is the fact that all Trusts will have to provide this level of service now that the principle has been established as a national norm.

- A national agency entitled NHS Plus will be established to sell occupational health services to employers.
- A team will be set up to ensure that action plans to clean up hospitals are put into place.
- A public/private partnership will be established called NHS Lift with the express purpose of developing primary care buildings and facilities.
- A national treatment agency will be established to bring together resources for services to drug misusers.
- A medical education standards board will be set up in order to combine the existing separate functions for educational standards relevant to general practitioners and hospital doctors.

Concluding comments on the National Plan

The National Plan was clearly the government's response to widely expressed concerns among the public and the media about the perceived failings of the National Health Service. As an institution, the National Health Service is held in high esteem by all sections of British society. Politically, it was inconceivable that any government, especially a Labour government, could allow a situation to continue whereby morale within the service and confidence in the service among members of the public would be allowed to decline. A National Plan, therefore, was the sort of response that could be expected from a government with left-of-centre political allegiances. Its success depends not only on the goodwill and hard work of the many thousands of health care professionals and support workers who are employed by the National Health Service, but also on the ability of politicians to enable the service to use the resources at its disposal to develop solutions to the problems facing it. If the government and the Secretary of State for Health do not resist the temptation to interfere too much, it is very likely that the National Plan will be increasingly seen as restrictive rather than enabling. The challenge, therefore, for the government is to enable the plan to liberate the considerable creative talents of clinical, managerial and support staff now that they have a cohesive vision for the development of the service and the resources to achieve this. Finally, the plan will also need to harness and engage public/patient/client opinions and views to be certain that a creative 'partnership' is built between the public and service to produce an improved NHS.

THE SOCIAL CARE SECTOR AND PARTNERSHIP WITH THE NHS

Background

One of the key principles on which health and social policy is being built in the UK in the early years of the 21st century is that of developing effective and meaningful working partnerships between health and social care agencies. These partnerships can also exist between professions within the same service, sectors of a service, or between the services themselves. What follows is a brief overview of how the NHS and the social care sector are being encouraged through explicit government policies to work more closely together in the interest of producing better health care outcomes. Much of this policy is based on the belief that good health is not simply a function of how the NHS acts or provides its services, but is linked to social and economic factors also.

Since the publication of the Black Report in 1980 a debate has taken place in the UK about what influences good health. This debate has often centred around the use of words such as 'inequality' on the one hand or 'differences' on the other. Since 1997 the government has explicitly accepted the notion that matters such as poverty, equality of housing and 'social exclusion' all influence the quality of an individual's health. One of the major outcomes of this change in government thinking has been the assertion that the National Health Service and social care services run by local government will be required to produce strategies which complement one another more closely in the provision of major services for vulnerable or needy groups in society, such as the elderly, for example.

In 1985 the Audit Commission carried out a review of community care services for elderly people. One of its main conclusions was that the management of these services rarely showed effective coordination between health, housing and social services. In addition, it concluded that resources were squandered as a result of this failure to manage or coordinate services. A later Audit Commission report, in 1996, went on to indicate that services for a far wider range of individuals, including those with mental illness, physical handicaps and learning disabilities, were similarly uncoordinated in addition to being seriously under-resourced. The second Audit Commission report was conducted against a background where a major policy initiative in the form of the 1990 NHS and Community Care Act, intended to remedy a number of the deficiencies in the provision of community care, had existed for 6 years.

Despite all the effort of the government to influence the development of care management systems and other methods of ensuring that services for vulnerable groups in the community were effectively provided, the key issue of bringing together how the National Health Service and the social care sector work had not been successfully tackled. There was undoubtedly progress, much of which was focused on how professionals involved in providing services attempted to change the systems they operated to provide care. It was noticeable that although much rhetoric had focused on increasing the involvement of patients, carers and clients in the development of care packages intended to meet their needs, it was often stated by these groups that they had not noticed much change in terms of their involvement since the inception of the Act in 1990. It was clear to many observers that further work had to take place to require the National Health Service and the social care sector to work more closely, and so bring together a profound and clearly evident division between these two important areas of public service.

Finally, also in 1996, the King's Fund published a review of joint commissioning of health and social care over a 3-year period (Leathard 2000). Although many deficiencies were identified, a number of achievements were noted. These included:

- improved mental health assessments in the community achieved by multidisciplinary teams
- better coordinated and comprehensive services for individuals with learning disabilities
- clear improvements in the provision of respite care
- establishment of home bathing service which greatly assists clients and carers
- some improvement in the provision of those with particular housing needs.

Despite these welcome advances, it was evident that while a great deal was being said about how the various agencies could work together, progress was somewhat slow. Experience among those working at the service level indicated that the willingness to collaborate or form partnerships was often lacking, and that attempts to bring disparate agencies together would often fail in the absence of strong and committed leadership from management.

Another issue which influenced the potential for success in terms of inter-agency working was that of differing approaches to models of care. The majority of people working in the social care sector were committed to what they perceived as a 'social care' model for services which was based on the professional perception of a client's needs which often included client input into these perceptions. And although many doctors deny awareness of what is often termed the 'medical model', it was widely perceived among professionals working in the social care sector that the NHS approach to service provision was often based on such a model. National Health Service approaches often used the notion of dysfunction or illness as a basis for the way in which services were organised or provided. Often this was premised on what clinical professionals deemed necessary to meet a need or provide a service. This said, this model was not universally accepted throughout the NHS and although professionals working in this sector do not always subscribe to it, the fact that the model was perceived to exist by other groups meant that it was often difficult to get different sectors to work together.

In the face of the ongoing difficulties in getting local government, which largely controlled the social services sector, and the National Health Service to work together, the Labour government when elected in 1997 renewed its commitment to bringing these two sectors together in more meaningful partnerships for the future.

The partnership between the NHS and local government

With the view that health and equality are largely a product of social, economic and environmental factors gaining official sanction at government level, the foundations were laid for developing partnerships between the National Health Service and local government providers of social care.

In parallel with this new emphasis on partnership, the government carried on its theme of modernising public services into the work of local government. The notion of private finance initiatives, for example, which were initiated by the previous government, are increasingly proposed for the financing of local government projects. Additionally, what was often termed as achieving value for money in the National Health Service has become 'best value' in local government circles. Finally, resources are to be made available for specific projects as long as certain objectives are achieved or standards met. Similar criteria are to be applied to the NHS when Trusts and other organisations within the service wish to access particular earmarked or 'pooled' funding.

The local government White Paper 1997

The local government White Paper published in 1997 outlined the government's views on the modernisation of local government. It contained suggestions or proposals for improved political structures intended to streamline the decision-making process through the introduction of small executive committees working in 'cabinet style' overseen or monitored by locally based scrutiny committees. The White Paper also underlined the government's commitment to improving the way in which local councils focus on their community representation role.

An important proposal contained within the White Paper provided the basis for local government to work more closely with the National Health Service in developing, for example, health improvement programmes (HIMPs) and their own community plans jointly. While the new duty required of local government was for a renewed emphasis on social, economic and environmental well-being of local community, it is envisaged that this responsibility will be one of the main driving influences in establishing the new joint planning framework for health and social care which will focus on wider and better partnership between the two sectors. The concept of the health improvement programme is outlined in greater detail elsewhere in this chapter. This said, the requirement for local government to develop community plans as part of their 'community leadership role' provides yet more opportunity for the two sectors to work together.

The separate nature of funding 'streams' for health and social care initiatives and projects has often been a stumbling block in the efforts to develop meaningful partnerships. The 1999 Health Act proposed the development of pooled budgets which would act as the precursor for integrated services across large parts of the National Health Service and local government. The consequence of this is that the health improvement plans of local health authorities and the community plans of local government will be brought together to achieve the government's objectives, once operational difficulties can be surmounted.

Other areas where local government and the National Health Service are expected to work together include the following:

• The development within primary care groups (PCGs) of representatives from local social services. It is expected that similar arrangements will exist for those PCGs that become primary care Trusts (PCTs).

- The development of regeneration strategies in specific localities where poverty or social and economic degeneration have occurred premised on better partnerships between health and social services.
- Greater emphasis on how local government and the National Health Service tackle health inequality and the links to improving public health by focusing on environmental matters, the value of education and its links to employment, improved transport infrastructure and developments in the quality of housing stock.
- Partnerships will also be premised on the fact that national priorities guidance will be issued by the government which represent the first time that both sectors will have their shared national responsibilities defined.
- Partnerships will be developed for the implementation of national service frameworks for mental health and work to establish a similar framework for older people.
- The establishment of health action zones in 26 localities which will focus on matters relating to the social exclusion of poorer people, through ensuring that services provided by the National Health Service and local government are properly coordinated.
- The use of partnership grants to enable the two sectors to work together to avoid unnecessary hospital admission, develop better discharge policies, develop a greater emphasis on promoting independent living among clients and for the effective management of emergency pressures on both services.
- A greater emphasis on providing more information and support for carers will be developed through partnerships between the two sectors.
- The setting up of the National Care Standards Commission to regulate a number of care services.
- Both sectors would be involved in schemes to underpin the establishment of joint management development between the two sectors and common performance measures for determining the success of management within the National Health Service and local government.

The strategic context for public health

The government's intention to promote the responsibility of local government in leading community focused initiatives was paralleled in the National Health Service through the publication of *Saving Lives: Our Healthier Nation* (DoH 1999a), a White Paper which identified a statutory duty for health authorities to take the lead in improving public health through direct action on health inequalities. The strategic framework within local government is the community plan.

Both sectors therefore needed to ensure that, in developing their relative plans, consultation took place with colleagues in each sector to ensure that the key objectives of one supported the other. Thus, the intention of the government to ensure that all sectors with an influence on improving well-being and health for local communities is fully recognised and properly put into action.

Boxes 2.5–2.7 outline recent government action to improve the health of the population and address health inequalities through the policies explained in *Our Healthier Nation* and *Saving Lives*, and the establishment of the Social Exclusion Unit.

The health improvement programme

The health improvement programme (HIMP) for an area will be produced as a direct result of collaboration and cooperation between NHS Trusts, local primary care groups, representatives of local government and the health authority responsible for developing the plan. The resultant plan is signed off by primary care group and Trust chairs, all of which is underpinned by a document known as the Service and Financial Framework (SAFF) which describes the way in which the HIMP will be organised and funded. All signatories are therefore bound by the plan and have to account to the health authority for any undertaking that they agree to carry forward.

From a more detailed perspective, a Health Service Circular (HSC1998/167) entitled *Health Improvement Programmes: Planning for Better*

Box 2.5   *Health of the Nation* becomes *Our Healthier Nation*

The Conservative government in 1992 published a White Paper entitled *The Health of the Nation*. Essentially this White Paper identified five broad areas which were to be the focus of government-inspired action to improve the state of public health. These five areas were:

1. coronary heart disease and strokes
2. cancers
3. mental illness
4. HIV/AIDS and sexual health
5. accidents.

While it was clear that many welcomed the new focus on discrete areas of action for improving public health, a number of concerns were expressed. For instance, while coronary heart disease and strokes were high on the government's list of priorities, there was little effort to stop tobacco advertising or try and break the link between smoking and poor health. Also, the document contained little or no recognition of the fact that poverty or social deprivation might be explicitly linked to an individual's health.

Following its election in 1997, the Labour government made its intention clear to review the work started by the previous government. In February 1998 it published a consultation paper, *Our Healthier Nation*, which in keeping with the government's desire to modernise the NHS into the 21st century, set out two key aims for England. These were:

- to improve the health of the population by increasing the length of people's lives and the number of years free from illness
- to improve the health of the poorest members of society and to narrow what was perceived as the health gap.

In a similar fashion to the Conservative government's White Paper, *Our Healthier Nation* identified four priority areas, expressed in terms of targets to be met by the year 2010. These included:

1. heart disease and stroke: to reduce the death rate from heart disease and stroke-related illness among people under 65 by up to one third
2. accidents: to reduce accidents by at least one fifth
3. cancers: to reduce the death rate from cancer among people under 65 years by one fifth
4. mental health: to reduce the death rate from suicide and undetermined injury by one sixth.

The number of main targets in the Labour government document had been reduced from five to four. The missing target was that of addressing problems relating to sexual health. However, included in the proposals for making a significant difference in the state of public health were such things as health schools, which would promote a range of initiatives focusing on matters such as diet, exercise, improved academic achievement and improved attitudes towards cigarettes, alcohol, drugs and sexual relations. The notion of healthier workplaces was to be developed whereby the government could influence the standards of health and safety as part of employment rights, while also attempting to address issues relating to stress at work. Finally, healthier neighbourhoods would be developed where work would be carried forward on dealing with perceived health inequalities with particular reference to the health of older people.

Similar documents were published in Scotland with targets being set for coronary heart disease and stroke, cancer, dental and oral health, accidents and teenage pregnancy. In Wales, the Secretary of State announced a consultation document which focused on the idea of health and well-being which would be based on sustainable communities, a more healthy lifestyle and an improved environment. While no explicit target areas were set, the consultation paper did suggest a 5-year research programme which would inform the government on the most effective way of breaking what was perceived as the cycle of poor health in Wales. This research would also underpin the development of targets for health inequalities and health determinants.

Box 2.6   The White Paper *Saving Lives*

In July 1999, a White Paper entitled *Saving Lives* (DoH 1999a) was published as a further exposition of government thinking on ways to improve the state of the nation's health. Separate consultation and guidance had been issued on matters relating to anti-smoking proposals and *Saving Lives* also set a number of targets intended to reduce deaths from heart disease, cut the death rate of all cancers in those under 75, cut the suicide rate, reduce death rates from accidents, set up first aid programmes for 11 and 16 year olds, extend the nurse-led NHS Direct telephone helpline, set up expert patient programmes to help people manage their illnesses and set up public health observatories in each NHS region to identify and monitor local needs and trends.

A range of innovative and ground-breaking proposals were put forward to ensure that these targets could be met, including such things as improving access to facilities in health centres and the workplace with shopping areas being targeted as potential sites for health facilities.

Box 2.7 Social exclusion

In 1998 the government established its Social Exclusion Unit. The establishment of this unit provided further evidence that the government was serious in its efforts to investigate matters which influence health that go beyond the nature of health services provided through the NHS. Included in the work of the unit were improving housing and assisting people to find work more easily. It was the view of the unit that poor people had become concentrated in particular areas of the country, and it was hoped that by putting together proposals which could motivate children at school or improve the access of poorer people to services, in addition to developing family support, some of the factors that influence the health of poor people in poor areas might be improved.

Finally, the unit expressed a desire for a range of agencies within society to work more closely together in order to produce positive influences on the health of the poorer members of society. These proposals focused on ways in which all levels of government could work with local businesses, the voluntary and statutory agencies to develop initiatives which would address the problems of poor health and poverty. Taken in conjunction with proposals announced in the National Plan in 2000 for health agencies and social care agencies to work together, it is possible to conclude that matters relating to inequalities in health and the poor health of less well-off members of society might start to be addressed. This belief is based on the idea that policy thinking at the highest political levels is now accepting the fact that poor health is influenced by many factors and cannot be addressed from the perspective of the National Health Service alone.

Health and Better Health Care outlines the key requirements for inclusion in an acceptable health improvement programme. These are:

- the development of a strategic framework focused on national and local priorities set against measurable targets
- explicit reference to the development of needs assessment
- explicit reference to what is termed 'resource mapping'
- the inclusion of local joint investment plan and the Service and Financial Framework (SAFF)
- a description of how the HIMP was prepared and what arrangements are in place for ensuring that broad-based involvement in future health improvements plans is guaranteed

- that the health improvement plan should be easily accessible to members of the community irrespective of ability.

Work carried out by the King's Fund focused on whether health improvement programmes had begun to show evidence of working together between the two sectors and on what issues were being approached. In mirroring national priorities for health care, it was unsurprising to see, for example, that coronary heart disease/stroke, mental health, cancer and care of older people ranked among the first four categories that most health improvement plans included. In addition to these categories, children and adolescents, accidents, substance misuse, waiting lists and times, primary care, dental health, sexual health, physical disability, hospital service and social determinants of health were other areas included in health improvement plans in descending order of frequency. This work further identified the fact that while these issues were included in the majority of health improvement programmes, references to the requirement for supporting service and financial framework and evidence of how the objectives set within the plans were to be monitored were somewhat scant. Encouragingly, the majority of health improvement programmes surveyed by the King's Fund team mentioned partner organisation and the majority referred to joint work with local authorities or with local NHS Trusts. Finally, joint investment plans were referred to in only 19 of the 36 cases surveyed.

It is clear that while there seems to be wide agreement on the kinds of issues to be included in a health improvement programme, there is still some way to go before health authorities can demonstrate effectively through their plans that they are working closely with partners in local government to fulfil the health services' obligation to improving the public health. The King's Fund team, for example, expected to see in the health improvement programmes produced in 2000 onwards:

- continued evidence of public consultation
- clearer commitments by stakeholders to specific work programmes
- a central place for PCGs

- more detailed health needs assessment and resource mapping data
- specific targets for measurable improvement.

In addition to the points identified above, the team also made a request for health authorities to prepare clearer and more easily digestible summaries of their health improvement programmes so that a wider range of people within local communities could read them and understand them.

THE INDEPENDENT SECTOR

The growth and development of the independent health care sector in the UK has always been somewhat dependent upon prevailing attitudes about its relationship with the National Health Service. During the Conservative administration up to 1997 attempts were made to increase the influence and role of the independent sector, particularly in relation to acute care. In the main, this concentrated on providing a tax break for those who took out private health care insurance, or encouraging companies to develop policies for health care insurance for their employees.

Although the independent health care sector in the UK has rarely provided above 5% of all acute care, for example, it has traditionally provided much of the residential and nursing home care for elderly people. There has been a great deal of reorganisation within the acute sector of the independent health care industry with one or two organisations consolidating their presence within the market. Providers of acute health care would include, for example, BUPA and Nuffield Health Care. A number of foreign owned organisations have managed hospitals within the UK over recent years although their presence is not so evident now.

With the provisions of the National Plan being made public in 2000, it became increasingly clear that the Labour government wished to see greater partnership between the National Health Service and the independent health care sector. In relation to acute care this largely focuses on using the spare capacity within the acute hospitals of the independent sector to assist the National Health Service to meet many of its waiting list targets. This might, for example, focus on the provision of a number of minor surgical procedures, orthopaedic procedures such as replacing knees, shoulders and other joints, and some cardiac procedures. In addition to this, it is clear that the government's views on developing what it calls intermediate care will also involve much closer working between the National Health Service and the independent sector. Before this can be successfully achieved, a good deal of work needs to be done on determining an exact definition of the term 'intermediate care' and how this will be provided for within and between the two sectors.

Based on an initial reading of the National Plan, the government has signalled its intention to develop the number of beds available for people, particularly elderly people, who do not require the care and support offered in an acute facility but are potentially too ill to be properly cared for in a convalescence or nursing home. This area between these two types of care appears to be what the government would like to refer to as 'intermediate care'. It is anticipated, therefore, that this proposed development in care will see a good deal of expansion in the first decade of the 21st century.

Finally, an important area of the independent health care sector is that of nursing homes which provide care for elderly people. The majority of nursing homes are private organisations providing care for elderly people. In addition to these homes there are a number of homes that provide care to people with psychiatric illnesses or those with learning disabilities. All of these homes are regulated by having to obtain a licence granted by the local health authority. In gaining such a licence, the home in question will have to adhere to regulations relating to the number of trained and untrained staff employed by the home and the number on duty at any particular time. The homes themselves comply with all statutory regulations. Naturally, assurances will be offered about the quality of care offered to patients. The health authority will in all cases carry out an initial inspection prior to the granting of a licence and then carry out regular checks after that. If a member of the public doubts the quality of service being offered then the health authority will, in response to any questions about care, carry out spot checks without notice. It is also worth noting that some homes are 'dual registered' with the health authority and the local social services department. This is another area where partnership between the two sectors is evident in that they both have to make sure that common standards apply and are adhered to.

THE CONTRIBUTION OF NURSING: MAKING A DIFFERENCE

In among the wide range of policy pronouncements made by the Labour government after 1997 was a major White Paper which focused on the nursing, midwifery and health visiting professions. Prior to this, a nursing strategy intended to provide a policy framework for the development of nursing within the National Health Service had been launched and developed in the early part of the 1990s. The new document, entitled *Making a Difference: Strengthening the Nursing, Midwifery and Health Visiting Contribution to Health and Health Care* (DoH 1999b), intended to show how this government valued the contribution of nurses to health care in a variety of settings. The publication of this White Paper also bore testament to the fact that the Labour government of 1997 appeared to be more disposed to listening to nursing advice from within the profession than previous governments.

Making a Difference was launched in July 1999 by the then Secretary of State for Health, Frank Dobson, and the soon to retire Chief Nursing Officer and Director of Nursing for England, Dame Yvonne Moores. Within its 82 pages the document set out the reasons why the Labour government valued the contribution of nurses to the National Health Service, in addition to making pronouncements on new nursing, recruitment, developments in education and training, proposals for a new career framework, the improvements of working lives, strengthening leadership, modernising professional self-regulation and working in new ways. The scope of the document was vast and covered almost every aspect of the professional life of nurses, midwives and health visitors working in the UK. (As has been noted elsewhere in this chapter, *Making a Difference* was essentially a document intended to relate to nurses, midwives and health visitors working in England; Wales, Scotland and Northern Ireland produced their own versions.)

It was noted that, at the time of publication, some 332 000 nurses, midwives and health visitors were employed in England alone. Their contribution to the National Health Service was considered to be crucial to the government's ability to succeed in its plans to modernise the National Health Service and improve public health. Set against these pronouncements, the document made it clear that the context within which care was being delivered was changing rapidly, as it had been for some time.

Although the controversy relating to health inequalities has been raging for many years, it was noted that people were generally living longer and healthier lives. The inevitable consequence of this is that more people survive beyond the ages of 75 and 85, leading to an increased demand for high quality nursing care. This care needs to be provided in acute settings but also, increasingly, within the community and in what latterly has become known as the 'intermediate care' arena. This will see the National Health Service working closely with the independent sector to ensure that care is available to all elderly people living within the UK. Statistics suggest that over 26% of households in the UK are single people, the likelihood being that many are without a social network and will be in need of specific nursing care to enable them to remain in their homes late into their lives. It was made clear that this places a responsibility on the professions to adapt their practice to be able to meet this need.

In common with other areas of policy development, the idea of working across boundaries is to the fore in this document. The assertion is made that mortality rates for major causes of death are highest in poorest areas of society, with morbidity linked to unemployment, poor nutrition, poverty and poor housing being particularly high also. Consequently, nurses are expected to develop approaches to care that cross organisational boundaries between the acute and community sectors as well as between the National Health Service and local community care services.

A further major perspective in epidemiology mentioned in the document suggests that nurses will need to meet the challenges of the rise in chronic non-communicable diseases, obesity, mental illness and new infectious diseases with a greater emphasis on integrated care, chronic disease management, disease prevention and working to support individuals to maintain healthy lifestyles. Indeed one of the other major pronouncements that arose out of the publication of *Making a Difference* was that a new grade of nurse, the nurse consultant, would be appointed throughout the National Health Service. It is interesting to note that many of the nurse consultants appointed since the publication of *Making a Difference* have tended to be in the areas mentioned in the early part of the document, often covering such areas as substance abuse, care of the elderly, breast care, innovative roles in caring for people with mental illness and the development of roles that impact on public health.

Another innovation which was announced in *Making a Difference* was the launch of NHS Direct. This impacted not only on the nursing, midwifery and health visiting professions but also provoked considerable reaction from other sectors of the National Health Service. As with many other aspects of government policy, the assertion that technology is driving massive change within society was used as the justification for developing a service which was, in the main, staffed and run by nurses with the intention of providing information technology-based advice to members of the public on health issues via the telephone. While some sections of the medical profession, for example, found such a service threatening to their professional integrity, it was envisaged that the establishment of NHS Direct would make an impact as a result of making important information on health care issues readily available to members of the public. It remains to be seen whether this service will ultimately produce the effect of reducing the number of unnecessary referrals to, for example, general practitioners.

Recruitment and retention

Both the Royal College of Nursing and the trade union Unison have been saying for some time that recruitment and retention issues within the nursing, midwifery and health visiting professions are approaching crisis point. The government recognised this and alluded to it in some detail in *Making a Difference*. The direct result of this recognition is the investment by government of considerable extra resources to raise the number of nurses entering training and, in addition, work with the professions to widen the entry gate into nursing so that a broader range of people can access professional training.

Making a Difference also goes on to outline government proposals for developing career structures and linking this to competency-based pay rates which, at the time of writing, have yet to be finalised.

Essentially, the government proposed a career framework based on four levels of practice:

- Level 1: health care assistant
- Level 2: registered practitioner
- Level 3: senior registered practitioner
- Level 4: consultant practitioner.

The payment bands to be contained within these four levels of practice will in time replace the grading structure that has existed within the nursing profession since 1988. It is hoped to agree a detailed pay structure that will reward professional development and the acquisition of tangible skills relevant to the clinical area in which the practitioner works, and that, as a result, it will become possible to maintain effective retention within the profession and avoid the kind of deadlock that has occurred within many clinical services whereby people become trapped in their pay grade. It is evident that this is viewed as a very important piece of work but one that is not without its difficulties and this may explain why, some 2–3 years after the publication of *Making a Difference*, the new career structure and pay scales for nurses have not been agreed.

Professional education

One of the most important aspects of *Making a Difference* is the commitment of the government to developing the education and training system to produce more nurses, midwives and health visitors 'fit for practice'. When Frank Dobson was Secretary of State for Health for the National Health Service, it became increasingly clear that he was frustrated by the way in which nursing had, in his view, moved away from the practical skills base and a focus on caring skills towards a more academically based curriculum. While the debate as to how far this was true took place within the profession, the Secretary of State signalled his intention to make changes. The outcome of this was that the United Kingdom Central Council for Nursing, Midwifery and Health Visiting (UKCC) established an Education Commission to look at pre-registration training within the UK with the remit of putting forward a series of proposals to adjust the balance within professional training. Programmes would be required to demonstrate a stronger practical foundation allied to greater emphasis on clinical practice placements and the achievement of clinical competencies prior to the point of registration.

The UKCC Education Commission shared common objectives with government's priorities as identified in *Making a Difference*, to the effect that:

- a more flexible career pathway into and within nursing and midwifery education would be developed
- the level of practical skills within training programmes would be increased
- nurse and midwifery training systems would become more responsive to the needs of the National Health Service.

The outcome of the work of the Commission was the publication in 2000 of a series of pre-registration competencies which must be achieved prior to an individual being admitted to the nursing or midwifery register (Box 2.8). Following on from the publication of these competencies, a number of pilot sites were announced throughout England where new approaches to using a

---

Box 2.8   UKCC requirements for pre-registration nursing programmes

Following the deliberations of the UKCC Education Commission and discussions with the government, the UKCC produced a document in May 2000 which outlined its requirements for pre-registration nursing programmes. Students admitted to the professional register will have to have achieved a series of professional competencies arranged into the following domains:

- Professional and ethical practice
- Care delivery
- Care management
- Personal and professional development.

In assisting students to achieve these competencies, institutions offering programmes intended to prepare nurses for entry onto the register will be required to provide a knowledge base which explores the following 'contemporary theoretical perspectives':

- Professional, ethical and legal issues
- The theory and practice of nursing
- The context in which health and social care is delivered
- Organisational structures and processes
- Communication
- Social and life sciences relevant to nursing practice
- Frameworks for social care provision and care systems.

The intention of these competencies is to ensure that graduates of new pre-registration nursing programmes will be 'fit for purpose' in that they will have achieved the required competencies which the UKCC described as 'the skills and ability to practise safely and effectively without the need for direct supervision'.

---

practical competency-based approach to nurse and midwifery education could be tested. At the time of writing, plans to establish these pilot sites were close to completion with the first cohort of students close to being admitted. (A more detailed overview of key changes in education and training for nurses, midwives and health visitors is contained in Chapter 1 of this book.)

The important thing to bear in mind when considering all these changes to the way in which nurses and midwives are educated is that the changes will have a profound impact on the context of care. Assertions that nursing and midwifery education has become too academically biased will be challenged by the new programme which, with the wider entry gate into professional training, will enable a far broader section of society to be represented within the profession who, in turn, will be prepared in such a way as to enable the National Health Service to meet the care needs of the public in different settings and in different ways.

If, as is intended, the quality and consequently the context of care is to be changed and improved, this will require the National Health Service not only to be able to recruit increasing numbers of people into the professions, but also to retain them. One of the major aspects of *Making a Difference* which has a bearing on this is the idea that the government will work increasingly to improve the working lives of nurses, midwives and health visitors. Key among the government's proposals is a requirement on the part of Trusts and health service employers to develop family-friendly policies to enable people with family or care commitments to balance their working lives with their home lives. Trusts will also need to work with regional offices and health authorities to promote better communication throughout the National Health Service to raise awareness of good practice in relation to improving working conditions, and practical support for front line managers to develop more effective systems of self-rostering, particularly where improved IT support is required.

These policies also extend to ensuring that racism within the NHS is dealt with and that the number of black and ethnic minority nurses working in the system reflects more effectively the make-up of society, especially at senior management levels. In common with a number of other policy assertions, the government makes clear its view that staff involvement in Trust activities will be required.

Finally, a commitment is made to strengthening leadership within the nursing, midwifery and health visiting professions, in part as a response to a belief among government ministers that the role of the ward sister had been eroded to the point where it was often difficult to ascertain who was in charge of a ward or clinical area or who coordinated the services there. *Making a Difference* was explicit in expressing

the desire for a greater emphasis on the leadership development of sisters and charge nurses and this has been further amplified in the publication of the National Plan in 2000 where the role of the ward sister/charge nurse has been likened to a 'mini-matron'. The concept of the matron itself carries a number of negative connotations which hark back to the health service of the 1950s and 1960s and it is to be hoped that liberal use of this term will not prove counter-effective.

The result of these assertions should be that continuing professional development systems within Trusts and community services will be established to enable people working at the level of sister or charge nurse to develop their leadership skills in addition to new programmes being developed to ensure that these people can access high quality programmes. This will enable them to progress and ultimately, should they so wish, make a meaningful choice later in their career as to whether they wish to stay at that level or progress to nurse consultant or a senior management role such as director of nursing.

CONCLUSION

This chapter has endeavoured to provide an overview of the broad policy framework within which health care is provided within the UK. As has been observed, it is only possible to do this when set against a complete appreciation of the influence of politics on the provision of health care in this country. The outline in this chapter of government policy in relation to health care should enable the reader to understand the major factors that influence health and how these have, to a large degree, built on reforms and change brought about by previous governments. The exercises suggested in Activity 2.1 should further assist students to understand the context of their everyday working practice. In addition to this political backdrop, some insight has been offered into the way in which these policies will impact on the work of practitioners and the way in which they provide care as we enter the 21st

Activity 2.1

The following simple exercises can be carried out by students as a means of developing a deeper understanding of practice in context with particular emphasis on the relevance to their everyday work:

1. Professional self-regulation

During ward visits it is always worth looking out in staff workstations or communal areas to see if information relating to the work of the UKCC is displayed. Why not, for example, ask qualified colleagues if they know where information on regulatory matters is available? Do they see it as being supportive to them in their everyday practice? Finally, it is also worth asking qualified staff about their understanding of links between the clinical governance arrangements for the hospital or practice area and professional self-regulation.

2. Joint working

If the opportunity arises to work in a clinical area where social care agencies and health services interact or work together, it is worth looking for signs as to how the requirement to develop more meaningful partnerships impacts on the everyday work of individual practitioners.

3. Clinical governance

When working on clinical placement, it would be of importance to first check for readily identifiable signs that the Trust or clinical area is communicating information in support of clinical governance to all members of staff. Having established this, it would also be worthwhile to talk to qualified staff about what clinical governance means to them and how this impacts on everyday practice. What evidence do you see that clinical governance is making a difference? What evidence do you see that all practitioners have an opportunity to make an input into arrangements for clinical governance as a means of benefiting practice?

4. Continuing professional development

Students will be aware from their studies that the relevance of continuing professional development or, in some instances, lifelong learning, is constantly being stressed. While this is relatively straightforward to understand in the higher education environment, what, for example, are the arrangements in Trusts or clinical areas to assist staff with their continuing professional development needs? What structures exist, for example, and what assurances would you, as a prospective member of qualified staff, be given in relation to your continuing professional development needs? Gaining answers to these questions might well influence whether you would want to work in a particular area or not.

5. Making a difference

The importance of the White Paper *Making a Difference* has been stressed throughout this chapter.

Can you discern evidence at clinical level of the impact of this policy on the working lives of the nurses and midwives you meet? Are staff familiar with the main elements of *Making a Difference*? What practical difficulties exist at service level with respect to bringing the main elements of *Making a Difference* into being?

century. The world of health care appears to be changing constantly and all clinical practitioners working within the National Health Service need to be aware of major changes and what these will mean to them in their everyday work. As is apparent in reading this chapter, it is not only the language of health care that is changing, but also the balance of influence between professionals and members of the public.

REFERENCES

Department of Health 1997 The new NHS, modern dependable. Stationery Office, London

Department of Health 1998a A first class service: quality in the new NHS. Department of Health, Leeds

Department of Health 1998b The new NHS – working together: securing a quality workforce for the NHS. Department of Health, London

Department of Health 1998c Partnerships in action: new opportunities for joint working between health and social services. Department of Health, London

Department of Health 1999a Saving lives: our healthier nation. Department of Health, London

Department of Health 1999b Making a difference: strengthening the nursing, midwifery and health visiting contribution to health and health care. Department of Health, London

Department of Health 1999c Supporting doctors, protecting patients: a consultation paper on preventing, recognising and dealing with poor clinical performance of doctors in the NHS in England. Department of Health, London

Department of Health 2000 The national plan: a plan for investment, a plan for reform. Department of Health, London

General Medical Council 2000 Revalidating doctors: ensuring standards, securing the future. General Medical Council, London

Kenworthy N, Snowley G, Gilling C 1996 Common foundation studies in nursing. Churchill Livingstone, London

Leathard A 2000 Healthcare provision: past present and into the 21st century. Stanley Thornes, Cheltenham

Merry P (ed) 2000 Wellard's NHS handbook 2000/01. JMH Publishing, Wadhurst

Rivett G 1998 From cradle to grave: 50 years of the NHS. King's Fund, London

Robinson R, Legrand J 1994 Evaluating the NHS reforms. King's Fund Institute, London

Robinson J, Strong P 1987 Professional nursing advice after Griffiths: an interim report. Nursing Policy Studies Centre, University of Warwick, Coventry

Strong P, Robinson J 1988 New model management: Griffiths and the NHS. University of Warwick Nursing Policy Studies Centre, Warwick

Webster C 1998 The National Health Service: a political history. Oxford University Press, Oxford

FURTHER READING

The history of nursing and nursing policy

These titles provide more detail on how nursing has developed up to and beyond the start of the NHS, along with selected writing on critical developments in the history of the profession. This provides a wider context for the student to aid understanding of how nursing fitted in to the wider political and social background. In addition these texts show how nursing was affected by politics and influenced by those who occupied its senior ranks during throughout the history of the NHS.

Abel-Smith B 1960 A history of the nursing profession. Heinemann, London

Department of Health and Social Security 1972 Report of the Committee on Nursing (Chair: A Briggs). DHSS, London

Dingwall R, Rafferty A, Webster C 1988 An introduction to the social history of nursing. Routledge, London

Glennerster H, Owens, Gatiss S, Kimberley A 1988 The nursing management function after Griffiths: a study in the North West Thames region. London School of Economics and North West Thames Regional Health Authority, London

Venner P 1984 From novice to expert: excellence and power in clinical nursing practice. Addison Wesley, Menlow Park

United Kingdom Central Council for Nursing, Midwifery and Health Visiting 1986 Project 2000: A new preparation for practice. UKCC, London

United Kindom Central Council for Nursing, Midwifery and Health Visiting 1990 The post-registration education and practice project (PREPP). UKCC, London

The history and development of the NHS and health policy

These texts provide valuable insight into detailed thinking on the development and achievements of the NHS. The student may also gain an insight into important policy developments which have shaped the way the NHS works today as well as developing a better understanding of why key initiatives such as the National Plan came about.

Allsop J 1984 Health policy and the National Health Service. Longman, London

Carrier J, Kendall I 1986 NHS mangement and the Griffiths Report. In: Brenton M, Ungerson C (eds) The year book of social policy in Britain 1985–6. Routledge and Kegan Paul, London

Honigsbaum F 1979 The division in British medicine: a history of the separation of general practice from hospital care 1911–1968. Kogan Page, London

Ham C 1982 Health policy in Britain. Macmillan, London

Johnson N (ed) 1995 Private markets in health and welfare: an international perspective. Berg, Oxford

Klein R 1983 The politics of the National Health Service. Longman, London

Klein R (ed) 1998 Implementing the White Paper: pitfalls and opportunities. King's Fund, London

Le Grand J, Robinson R 1984 Privatisation and the welfare state. Allen and Unwin, London

Lugon M, Secker-Walker J 1999 Clinical governance: making it happen. Royal Society of Medicine, London

Ovretveit J, Mathias P, Thompson T 1997 Interprofessional working for health and social care. Macmillan, London

Powell M 1999 New Labour, new welfare state? Policy Press, Bristol

Robinson R 1990 Competition and health care: a comparative analysis of UK plans and US experience. King's Fund, London

Secretary of State for Scotland 1997 The Scottish Health Service: ready for the future. Cm. 3614. Stationery Office, Edinburgh

Welsh Office 1998 Putting patients first. Cm. 3841. Stationery Office, Cardiff

3

Ethics

Isabelle Whaite

CHAPTER CONTENTS

Understanding what is meant by nursing ethics 78
Ethics is thinking and doing 78
Ethics is a complex process of enquiry 79
Values and beliefs 80
Caring: a key value 80
Personal value choices 81
Facts and values as evidence for moral decisions 82
Ethics and the practice of nursing 84
The context of health care 84
Ethical dimensions of care 85
Professional values in nursing practice and ethics 86
The patient is the central focus for what nurses do 87

Values as the basis for moral thought and action 87
Formation of values 87
Personal value systems 88
Learning values through observation, reasoning and experience 89
Model for value clarification 90

Ethical theory as a basis for moral thought and action 91
Philosophical medical ethics as a basis for nursing ethics 91
Devising ethical theory 91
The bioethical model 91
Deontology as a foundation for medical and nursing ethics 91
Utilitarianism as a foundation for medical and nursing ethics 93

Deontology and utilitarianism compared 95
Principles of biomedical ethics 95
The principle of autonomy 96
The principle of justice 96

Caring as the basis for moral thought and action 97
Virtue ethics: a revival 99

Making moral decisions in nursing practice 100
Studies in moral development 100
Influences on the ethical decision-making process 101
The nature and issues of power within relationships 102
Confidentiality 102
What is confidential information? 102
Breaching confidentiality and informed consent 103
Some ethical issues 104
Fair and antidiscriminatory practice 104
What are rights? 105
Upholding rights 105
The patient as citizen has rights 106
Understanding difference 106

Prescription for ethical reasoning, decision making and action 108

References 110

Further reading 112

In their everyday practice, nurses constantly encounter situations that demand an ethical response. To help nurses to clarify their thinking in this area and achieve a 'beginning level' of ethical practice competence, this chapter aims to:

- arrive at an understanding of the term 'nursing ethics'
- investigate the moral values underpinning nurses' actions, and their relationship to the facts
- consider ethics with respect to various aspects of nursing practice
- explore ethical theory and its underlying philosophical approaches
- examine how moral decisions may be made in practice.

UNDERSTANDING WHAT IS MEANT BY NURSING ETHICS

The paucity of research on the subject means that little is known about the quality of nurses' experiences in the practice of nursing ethics. Nurses have yet to tell their own stories about their experiences which would enable the true essence of nursing ethics to be fully understood. In nursing, while there would seem to be agreement about the desirability of including nursing ethics in the curriculum (Gallagher & Boyd 1991, UKCC 1999), there are uncertainties about the true nature of nursing ethics and what constitutes skilled decision making (Allmark 1995). This chapter will explore the meaning of nursing ethics as we understand it at present, question its utility as a basis for nurses' decision making and behaviour in practice and consider the relevance of the study of ethics for the nurse and for practice.

Through theoretical learning and personal exploration this chapter will offer the nurse an opportunity to acquire a 'beginning level' of ethical practice necessary for continuing learning in all of the four branches of nursing. This requires the nurse to demonstrate in practice:

- increasing recognition of the ethical issues and dilemmas confronting nurses in everyday practice
- a growing disposition towards striving to improve practice through reflection and clarification of values
- the use of a developing framework of nursing knowledge and theory rather than personal opinion to inform moral judgement and to guide ethical practice
- application of key ethical principles in practice to specific practice situations.

As nurses progress beyond this initial stage through the different levels of learning and practice, it is envisaged they will become aware of the gaps in their knowledge and of the need to continue, as part of professional practice, the building and updating of their knowledge and theory frameworks. In addition they will want to further develop their analytical thinking ability and critical judgement in order to participate more effectively in moral deliberation when confronting specific moral issues in practice.

Professional nurses need to be able to analyse complex arguments if they are to justify and challenge ethical decisions in health care, devise possible courses of action and evaluate them through deeper reflection (Whaite 2000, unpublished). This chapter aims to support nurses at the 'beginning stage' of this lifelong learning process of striving towards ethical practice competence.

ETHICS IS THINKING AND DOING

You will already have your own ideas about what is meant by 'nursing ethics' (Activity 3.1).

You might have come up with several ideas that reflect your understanding of the term. Your response may well include Codes of Conduct, values and beliefs, the law, human rights, justice, confidentiality, personal viewpoints, respect for persons, doing good, not doing harm, being honest and many other aspects. Nurses often find it easy to produce such lists of words, phrases and sentences, but what is not so easy is to explain what they mean. Does everyone share the same

Activity 3.1

Imagine that you are asked to explain to someone from another planet what the term 'nursing ethics' means. What would you tell them? Write down the words, phrases, sentences and examples you would use to help them understand what nursing ethics currently means to you.

meaning for a particular word or phrase? Surely, the same words can have different meanings for different people? Too often it is assumed that all parties in a debate or discussion are thinking and talking about the same phenomenon, when in reality they are not. Clarification of the meaning of the words and terms we use, and of how these are linked to each other, is needed if we are to give a meaningful explanation of nursing ethics.

A starting point in this clarification process is that nursing ethics is about what nurses *do* in practice. The emphasis and focus for the study of ethics is on action as well as knowledge – how actions are good or bad, right or wrong, and their consequences.

In giving health care, nurses and other health carers increasingly find themselves in situations where they are asking themselves what is morally the right thing to do, and how do they decide what is the right thing to do. These two questions occupy the field of study in ethics referred to as *normative ethics*.

Normative ethics implies that we are taking part in the practice of ethics itself. When we argue about the rights and wrongs of, say, not telling a patient or client the truth, we are arguing in ethics. 'Normative' refers to the standards or principles that should guide our decisions about what we ought to do. Normative ethics seeks to influence our actions and to provide answers to two fundamental questions:

1. What kinds of things are ultimately good?

And, if we know the answer to this ...

2. How do we decide what actions are right?

Another field of study in ethics, *meta-ethics*, implies that we may not be taking part in the practice of ethics itself. We are asking questions about ethics, and about the nature and basis of ethics. A fundamental question in meta-ethics is to ask whether there could be a true answer to the ethical questions raised in practice. While this chapter is primarily concerned with the field of normative ethics, the view held here is that the study of meta-ethics becomes increasingly relevant to the developing ethical practice competence of all health care professionals and, it is argued, should be included at higher levels of study.

Ethics is a complex process of enquiry

Ethics, which has been and will continue to be shaped through the ages, is a complex form of enquiry in pursuit of some standard with which to judge actions in a moral sense; a standard which can be understood through defining the meaning of moral terms 'rightness', 'wrongness', 'goodness', 'badness'. In deciding what actions are right, we can evaluate behaviour as right and wrong, good and bad, from a number of points of view, of which morality is only one (Rowson 1990). Others include those of law, social convention, professional codes, religious codes, politics and a practical approach.

An example of judging behaviour from a socially constructed viewpoint might be our opinion of the behaviour of a college lecturer who takes off his clothes when addressing the assembled students. This behaviour would be considered wrong insofar as it does not conform to the customary way of behaving in the context of such an organisation or in society itself; it defies social convention. But would it necessarily be *morally* wrong?

Is the moral point of view different from the one in this example, which is based on social convention? What is moral goodness or badness in relation to conduct? What is the standard by which to judge action in a moral sense? The answer to this may well be found in the evidence provided to support any judgement made.

A judgement of what is right or wrong in a legal sense can be supported with evidence from the statute book. A judgement of right or wrong in a social convention sense can be supported with the evidence of cultural codes, rules and etiquette. However, the evidence to support a judgement about whether or not action is right or wrong in a moral sense is not so accessible. Legal evidence, cultural codes, rules, etiquette are not in themselves sufficient evidence to support a judgement about right or wrong in the moral sense.

Although all of these points of view may provide some evidence for making a moral judgement, they are not sufficient in themselves. Different evidence for the moral truth needs to be found, based on a set of external or internal rules and principles from several sources.

What are the standards that underpin such moral action or conduct? What is the source of our moral knowledge? And what influences the choices we make about what action to take in a particular situation? Ethical enquiry is a process which requires the nurse to engage with different sources and kinds of nursing knowledge and theory in pursuit of a standard as evidence to support a moral judgement of right and wrong action or behaviour in practice. No one single source or kind of knowledge is sufficient in itself to guide action but each can help to inform a decision about what is right to do or not do in a specific situation.

Values and beliefs

A source of evidence and a major focus of study within normative ethics is the identification, critical analysis and evaluation of the value basis for practice, including moral values and beliefs – those values and beliefs, which have a moral sense of goodness, badness, rightness and wrongness. For instance, justice is associated with the moral sense of goodness, whereas injustice equates with badness and vice. Political, economic and social values, cultural values, the law and criminal justice system, organisational, professional and personal values are all brought to the practice situation and will all come under the spotlight for scrutiny within the field of normative ethics.

Moral values held by the individual are unique and personal to that individual. When a decision is to be made between competing and conflicting values about what is, morally, the right thing to do, evidence has to be provided to support the action chosen.

In summary, a precondition to reaching a beginning level stage of ethical practice competence in order to participate ultimately in the complex process of ethical enquiry requires the student to start building comprehensive knowledge and theory frameworks for practice. Study of the subject disciplines within the nursing curriculum, and bringing to conscious awareness all of the values and beliefs these frameworks are constructed around, including those considered to be unique to nursing provides a source of evidence for nurses' ethical practice.

Caring: a key value

A review of the literature (Sadler 1997) supports the view that caring is a key concept and value which underpins nursing and its development as a cognate discipline. Through the study of the concept of care and its application to nursing it is likely that students will be increasingly struck by the subjectivity of the meaning of the term 'caring'. It not only means different things to different people but is also context-dependent in that its meaning will change depending on the situation in which care is given. This can range from the acute hospital situation and care of the person who is undergoing surgery to a range of community locations and health promoting activity, for example teaching parenting skills.

The literature captures the different dimensions of caring (Morse et al 1990), for example giving physical care, or interaction with another person including feeling for, or being with and valuing, somebody (Sadler 1997). Caring involves emotions and feelings and is a moral ideal which is reflected in the UKCC Code of Professional Conduct (UKCC 1992). Nursing theory introduces students to some key concepts related to nursing and caring, including empathy (Olson & Hatchett 1997), patient/client need (Lauri et al 1997), use of self and holistic, humanistic dimensions of caring (Watson 1997). What is important is that although a great deal of literature is available to nurses, literature that is passionate about the construction of nursing around this key value, 'caring', the reality sometimes falls short of the rhetoric.

Consider Case study 3.1. Observing the practice of these nurses it would be difficult to see how such a value as 'caring' could be guiding their practice in the real world.

There would seem to be a huge gap between what the literature and professional code claim are values around which nursing is constructed and the values around which the practice of the nurses in this report may be constructed. Do you think the alleged practice of the nurses in the unit reflects a valuing of people as persons and a respect for human rights, a valuing of elderly persons and a valuing of caring? What might you assume, from observing their practice, about the values they have chosen to construct their practice around in the real world? Do they demonstrate any valuing of themselves or their work as nurses? Do you think they demonstrate that they value their relationships with patients or value patients as persons who have different needs?

Personal value choices

Another important source of knowledge to access during the process of ethical enquiry is knowledge of the self and, in particular, knowledge of self with others. This refers to personal knowing about those often hidden and extra dimensions in our lives which include personal values, beliefs and attitudes. Identifying, clarifying and choosing the values we prize and ascribe to our knowledge and thoughts is an important process in the study of nursing ethics. Morality includes reasoning about the whole area of value judgements we make in our whole lives, including those of nursing practice. This involves the nurse adopting a thoughtful and questioning approach to practice, standing back and taking stock of her practice, asking the questions 'What does what I find myself doing in practice tell me about the values and beliefs that are actually guiding my practice?' (Greenwood 1998); 'Are these the same or different compared with what I claim are my values and those which should guide my practice, including the values discussed in the literature and professional codes?'.

A classic nursing study (Stockwell 1972) showed that nurses labelled and stereotyped certain patients as 'difficult' or 'unpopular', which logically suggests the care they received was adversely affected. The criteria used for applying such labels included patients who asked questions about their care, offered an alternative view about their care, or were considered by the nurses as not belonging to the ward and therefore having no right to be there. Some of these patients were admitted or had occupied a bed long term because there was no more suitable place for them to be transferred for continuing care. It is tempting to dismiss studies that were undertaken so long ago and to conclude this could not happen in today's health care services.

Case study 3.1

A care of the elderly unit in Scotland came under internal investigation by the hospital Trust following revelations about the standards of nursing care for patients. An anonymous phone call alerted the Trust to alleged mistreatment of patients on a long-stay ward for 32 patients. After an inquiry, the following were some of the allegations revealed in the Trust report:

- Financial irregularities, such as money going missing from the ward safe; money taken from a patient's Christmas card; money left by a relative for a ward trip going missing, with half later returned.
- A patient being encouraged to drink Osmolite (which is not for oral consumption). The patient was allegedly told it was beer.
- An Asian patient, who was vegan, deliberately being given meat. The patient was said to have subsequently vomited.
- Medication being administered to a patient who was lying down. When it was pointed out that the patient was aspirating, the nurse concerned allegedly said 'Tell me when she is dead'.
- A nurse failing to get a priest for a dying Catholic patient but telling the relatives it had been done.
- Patients being forced to face the wall.

(Extracts taken from News Focus 1996.)

Go back to Case study 3.1. Is there a possibility that these nurses were not in touch with their value basis for practice? If they were to bring those values to conscious thought do you think that they might have discovered some values which would be impossible to defend as a guide to action in a moral sense? Was there perhaps some negative labelling and stereotyping going on, as described by Stockwell (1972)? Were these nurses contributing to negative labelling and stereotyping of elderly persons? If you want to explore this topic further you are advised to read Stockwell's work and more recent studies in relation to sexuality (Hayter 1996) which report the lack of emotional and interpersonal caring for gay and bisexual patients, including those diagnosed with AIDS. The problem again arises of labelling, and therefore stigmatising, patients so that they are not as valued as other patients and not treated fairly in the treatment they receive, which does not effectively meet their emotional, psychological, social and spiritual care needs.

Think about other groups within our society who also report feeling vulnerable to being stereotyped and experience being treated differently and often unfairly as a result. Do the elderly come to mind as a group who feel prone to being labelled, often based on negative stereotypes? Other groups you might have thought about include disabled persons and persons from ethnic minorities. Within health care services, as well as other public services, there is a great deal to be done in educating health carers, including nurses, to understand and value the differences between different people's cultures and religions (see Ch. 5). Essential to such education is the development of a willingness and disposition within professional nurses towards continuous striving for ethical practice competence. Nurses need to be in touch with their value base for practice and to demonstrate integrity and courage in challenging inappropriate values as a guide to practice. This means being effective in practice in contributing to enhancing patient/client health and well-being and adopting ethical practice, which prevents the exclusion of vulnerable groups from health.

Facts and values as evidence for moral decisions

As well as personal knowledge, knowledge gained by direct observation of the external world – the *empirical* or scientific way of knowing – also underpins thoughts and knowledge in nursing practice. During the process of ethical enquiry as an integral part of nursing practice, the professional nurse will engage with empirical knowledge, including nursing theory and research. This is knowledge from a different source and of a different kind, knowledge which is arrived at through observations we make about phenomena in the environment. From what we observe in a particular situation, we arrive at knowledge through the process of induction, i.e. generalising from the specific to the general. This involves the nurse in concrete thinking and empirical testing, systematically measuring directly observed phenomena to arrive at knowledge of the facts believed to be true. Clinical governance, recently introduced by the current government, places a responsibility on each practitioner for her own individual care, emphasising the importance of quality, consistency and responsiveness to patient/client need (Wilson 1998) (see also Ch. 2).

Again go back to Case study 3.1 and think about the evidence base for practice. Do you think the practice of these nurses was guided by research findings and facts claimed about the most effective nursing interventions, or particular theoretical understanding about the nature of relationships and human needs? Or was their practice based solely on personal opinions, including values – those hidden dimensions of our lives, never reflected on and which may go largely unchallenged?

A common error in reasoning is claiming facts as the sole evidence for judging what we do as right and wrong in a moral sense. Hume (1978) argued that beliefs and values are something separate from the body of empirically derived knowledge. Unlike statements of fact, beliefs and values cannot be proved or disproved using scientific methodology: the moral worth of any action can never be observed. We cannot discover empirically whether or not action is right or wrong in a moral sense, which makes statements about morality qualitatively different from statements of fact. Using the 'is/ought' distinction described by Hume (1978) can prevent us falling into the trap of confusing evidence of what *is* (fact) with evidence of what *ought* to be (evaluative evidence, based on value judgement). Hume explained that it is possible for two people to agree about all the facts observed in a particular situation and yet differ in the values that they assign to these facts, as it is humans who add moral content. Nowhere in the facts is it possible to discover rightness or badness in the moral sense. These evaluative judgements are based on one's own values of what ought to be. It is false logic to base moral truth on fact.

The 'is/ought' distinction is well recognised in the study of ethics. All statements can be divided into factual or partly factual, and evaluative or partly evaluative elements. A skill is to distinguish what is factual from what is evaluative. Value statements are often smuggled into factual statements and are stated as fact. It is very important to notice this and to challenge it when reasoning about what ought to be in a moral sense.

Hume's proposition was that one cannot reach a decision about what ought to be done in a moral sense based on the facts. It does not follow the rules of logic to look at a fact and then to say in a factual way that it is morally wrong (Box 3.1).

When we evaluate an action as wrong, right, good or bad from a moral point of view, different evidence is needed. The facts are insufficient in themselves as evidence for whether or not the action is morally right or wrong. While empirical knowledge does contribute to informing ethical decisions and practice which is effective in meeting patients'/clients' needs, it is insufficient in itself as evidence for guiding ethical judgement and practice.

In addition to the 'is/ought' distinction, there are some other common errors leading to reasoning that does not follow the rules of logic. It is useful to be aware of these errors, both in one's own thinking and reasoning and in that of others (Box 3.2).

Being aware of some of the common errors in reasoning in nursing ethics can help in developing

---

Box 3.1   Facts and values: the 'is/ought' distinction

Consider the following statement:
Jean took £10 from her grandmother's handbag.
   This is factual because it can be tested out empirically: we can observe the act.
   Now consider this statement:
Stealing from another person is morally wrong.
   This is evaluative. If, however, one were to think that this evaluative statement, smuggled in here, is fact, one could wrongly conclude as fact the following:
Jean was wrong to take £10 from her grandmother's handbag.
   Here we have a value statement that has been smuggled in without being examined. To the description of facts has been added one's own values of what ought to be, which is now passed off as fact, i.e. what is. Unbeknown to the observer, Jean's grandmother may well have instructed her to take the money!

Box 3.2   Some fallacies or errors in reasoning in ethics

• *The 'is/ought' distinction:* a skill is to identify what is factual and what is evaluative. Value statements are often smuggled into factual statements and stated as fact. It is important to notice this and challenge it when arguing in ethics.
• *Using force:* making another person accept the conclusion of an argument on the basis of force alone, without supporting evidence for your conclusion.
• *Using personal blame:* blaming another in a personal way for a decision he has taken rather than trying to understand the reasons for the decision.
• *Appeal to the majority:* the false claim that since everybody does something or thinks in some particular way, it must be right.
• *Authority versus expertise:* people within the hierarchy being invested with moral expertise they do not have, based simply on their position of power in the organisation.
• *Preaching dogma:* the refusal to allow any evidence that contradicts one's own conclusions or arguments about moral rightness or wrongness; protecting one's choices and actions against challenge and criticism; the nurse or doctor refusing to question any ethical argument or conclusion or to allow questioning of her own conclusions.

---

moral thinking and the ability to reason in the search for the truth about moral knowledge. In summary: ethical enquiry is a complex process, which is triggered when nurses, patients and clients are faced with ethical issues and dilemmas in practice. This enquiry, in pursuit of evidence to support a moral judgement of right and wrong action in practice, is enriched through nurses engaging with different sources and kinds of knowledge and nursing theory. No one single source of knowledge is sufficient as evidence in itself, but each can contribute to informing judgement and action in a specific situation.

ETHICS AND THE PRACTICE OF NURSING

Among the more general reasons for the growing interest in nursing ethics is an awareness that questions of values and moral choice are central to many developments in health care. Biomedical and technical advances have created higher expectations and increasing demands, while rationing of health care resources is inevitable. Increasingly, decisions about the allocation of health care resources at all levels of the organisation are seen to be not always in the interests of particular groups or individuals.

The context of health care and the ethics of resource distribution

Essential to the development of ethical practice competence is the need for nurses to learn about the complex and largely unpredictable global, political, economic and social environment of health care. Many of the challenges confronting patients/clients and health professionals in practice will arise from the key drivers of change emerging from the global context of health care (Warner et al 1998), including inequality, economic performance, financing of health care, integration in Europe, devolution and urbanisation. For example, there may be a mismatch between that which is possible technically and that which is possible socially and economically – some of the arguments about the rightness or wrongness of the 'morning after' pill question the rightness/wrongness of using such technology from a social and economic point of view. Will there be an increase in inequality in the UK, or a decrease? Will there be a collective intent to see equity of access to health care for all or a widespread belief that it is up to individuals to organise their own health care provision?

There are more questions than answers in attempting to predict the ethical challenges which may well confront nurses and patients/clients as a result of the impact on health and social care from the key drivers of change emerging from the global context of health care.

Demographic trends can be predicted with more certainty. In the year 2020 the elderly population will have increased, particularly the oldest old group (Kinsella 1996) who consume health and social care resources far out of proportion to their numbers (Suzman et al 1992, Ranade 1993). There is less certainty about the potential impact of a predicted rise in disability (Fries 1990, Butler 1997) and what proportions of overall life expectancy will be given to being active, disabled or institutionalised. Each possibility will make different demands on health care systems and give rise to a number of ethical challenges in the fair distribution of resource.

Society's values, beliefs and attitudes towards ageing shaped and reshaped within such a context will be significant too. These may or may not have significance in shaping the key ethical issues and health care challenges in practice of nurses in the future.

Add to any best guess scenario the political ideology of individualism which would now seem to be well entrenched within health care policy, with patients' rights, partnerships in care, consumer empowerment, patient led services, consumer led research. Who will get the lion's share of health care in the future? Will it be the group that shouts loudest? How representative of us all might this group be? Will parity and equity of information be ensured to empower patients and clients to make informed choices and avoid health exclusion of others?

The future looks uncertain and the ethical challenges facing society and health care practitioners are difficult to predict. Nevertheless, this is an important area of study for the student who is building comprehensive knowledge and theory frameworks for ethical practice competence. There can be little doubt that ethical issues and dilemmas will continue to be a recurrent feature in nursing practice and in many instances will be attributed to advances in science and technology and to the political, economic, and social environment in which health care is taking place.

In summary, many of the ethical issues arising in health care practice give rise to a broad spectrum of views from a range of sources regarding what is the right thing to do and how to decide right action in a moral sense. The professional nurse will require the knowledge and skill to: access a diverse range of opinions, views, values and beliefs from the context of health care and the different sources of nursing knowledge; to analyse the evidence and arguments, to generate options and to evaluate these so as to defend or challenge appropriately the action taken or not taken.

Take a possible scenario in health care where a question is raised about whether or not to use a particular drug to treat a group of patients/clients who are diagnosed with a particular medical condition. Through randomised control trials this drug has been found to be extremely effective, and indeed superior to any other drug available for treatment of this condition. The nurse practitioner responsible for prescribing is very much in favour of patients receiving this drug, as are several patients who have accessed information about treatments via the internet and through discussions with the nurse. The drug is much more expensive than the other, less effective drugs.

Many perspectives will be brought to such a situation. How is it to be decided who gets what in the distribution of health care resources? If the more expensive drug is given to this particular group, does it mean that other patients will lose out? Would the current market society argue that young people should take precedence over older people in the distribution of resources, given the predicted demographic trends? Is age a morally relevant property in this example? These and many more arguments brought to the situation,

representing different perspectives and viewpoints, will need to be located for scrutiny within the knowledge and theory frameworks brought to the process of ethical enquiry by the professional nurse. What are the implications for the nurse prescribing an alternative drug which is known to be less effective but which costs less, particularly when she has informed and advised patients about the more effective drug?

Ethical dimensions of care

By the very nature of their work, nurses are involved with, and intervene in, other people's lives, often at times when they are at their most vulnerable. This provides the opportunity for nurses to do a great deal of good or a great deal of harm in a moral sense. The possibility of nurses doing good or harm depends partly on factual knowledge and partly on the values underpinning their knowledge and thoughts. Factual knowledge and personal, professional and universal values must be consciously and critically evaluated for their potential to do harm or good.

Consider Case study 3.2. Imagine yourself as John's key worker. What do you feel about the failure of the doctor and nurse to provide John with information and explanations about his care and treatment, or to allow him the opportunity to talk about his feelings and express his priorities regarding his needs? In particular, what do you feel about their failure to involve John in any decision making about his care and their complete disregard of his refusal to cooperate? What would you like to say, and how would you intervene? What is the possibility of your intervention doing good or doing harm in a moral sense?

Perhaps you could identify the facts of the case. Do we know them? What are the possible value judgements that may be smuggled in and claimed as factual evidence to justify not obtaining informed consent from John? That John has a head wound that requires sutures is evident. Nowhere in the facts of the case can be found evidence that it is morally right to ignore John's basic right to give informed consent because he has a learning disability. Are there other value

Case study 3.2

John has learning disability and lives in a supported community home for people with a learning disability. He attends a local resource centre during the week and is still in touch with his family. On his way to the resource centre one day John was knocked down by a cyclist while he was standing on the edge of the pavement waiting to cross the road. He struck his head on the pavement and was bleeding profusely from a laceration to his scalp. A bystander called for an ambulance to take John to hospital. John was extremely distressed and began behaving aggressively towards the ambulance crew. He was anxious to reach the centre and to make contact with the people he knows there. On reaching the hospital John was seen by the nurse in the accident and emergency department. The doctor examined John's head, prescribed a tetanus injection and suturing of the scalp laceration. Throughout the examination John asked to make contact with the centre. He was placed on a trolley to await the nurse who would insert the sutures and administer the injection. Up to this point John's requests to see someone from the centre had gone unheeded. On the arrival of the nurse John informed her that he was not having the sutures or the injection and that he was leaving to go to the centre. The nurse, patting John's head, instructed him to lie still while his head was sutured and to take down his trousers for the injection. John verbally refused to cooperate and became increasingly distressed as the nurse proceeded to suture his scalp wound, unfasten and pull down his trousers and give the injection despite his verbal refusal and lack of cooperation.

At no point during John's stay in the accident unit were any explanations given to him about the treatment it was considered he required or whether there could be any alternatives. He was given little information beyond brief instruction by the doctor and the nurse with the expectancy that he would comply.

No attempt was made to reassure him or to contact the centre on his behalf to convey his wish for someone to attend the accident department to be with him. No attempt was made to explain to John the nature of his injury and treatment so that he could give informed consent. His consent to treatment and care was not sought by either doctor or nurse nor his permission given for the invasion of his privacy and the invasive medical treatment carried out by the nurse.

It seems John was expected to do as he was told!

judgements operating here and being claimed as fact? Could it be that these professionals erroneously believe all people with learning disability are incapable of making their own decisions and therefore have no right to do so? Do they think

that it follows that what they do in continuing treatment against John's wishes is morally good and in his best interests? Can treating John in this way be morally justified, based on the facts? It could also be argued that the knowledge base of the doctor and nurse in this case about the nature of learning disability and the facts of law concerning informed consent was very limited anyway. (Chapter 4, on the legal aspects of nursing, outlines the legal requirements for informed consent.)

Professional values in nursing practice and ethics

A code of ethics states the primary goals and values of the professional nurse. When individuals become nurses, they make a moral commitment to uphold the values and special moral obligations in such a code. The Nurses, Midwives and Health Visitors Act (1979) gave power to the United Kingdom Central Council for Nurses, Midwifery and Health Visiting (UKCC) to give guidance on standards of professional conduct. As a result, the UKCC formulated a Code of Professional Conduct in 1983, which was revised in 1984 and 1992 and is under revision again. This year will see changes to the regulatory body for nursing with the replacement of the UKCC and the national boards with the Nursing and Midwifery Council. (See Chapter 11.)

The professional nurse is expected to work within the guidelines and to embrace the values and beliefs expressed within the Code of Conduct. The code is pivotal to professional practice in placing the health and well-being of the patient/client as central to health care practice (see Ch. 11). Guidance is given about what is the right thing to do, but within the limits on decision making (how to decide what is the right action in a given situation) offered by the Code of Conduct, the professional nurse has to decide for herself what she ought to do. A key question for the nurse in anything she does is always, 'How will this benefit the patient?'. Reflective practitioners will ask whether or not what they are doing is giving their patients the best deal and, if not, how the situation can be improved.

The patient is the central focus for what nurses do

What happens if nurses lose sight of this, or do not share this professional value? Perhaps again you could reflect on the two case studies (3.1 and 3.2). Do you think the nurses and the doctor placed the patients' needs for health and well-being at the centre of their practice, or rather their own needs and those of the organisation, which might be to get the job done quickly and efficiently?

In summary: whatever the ethical challenges facing nurses, patients and clients, the health and well-being of individual patients/clients, patient and client groups, families and whole communities is the focus for what nurses do. Nursing ethics is an integral part of what nurses do in practice and is inseparable from everyday practice. It is a complex form of enquiry in search of a standard to judge and evaluate ethical practice, which is triggered in practitioners when facing ethical challenges.

The study of ethics provides some frameworks for professional nurses to use in their practice to help in clarifying thinking, logical reasoning and problem solving when determining what should be done in a moral sense. In addition to the study and use of legal frameworks in practice, values clarification, moral theory and principles are frameworks which may help nurses with the complex process of ethical enquiry. All of these can help clarify thinking and logical reasoning when analysing, justifying and/or challenging complex arguments and deciding and evaluating courses of action.

VALUES AS THE BASIS FOR MORAL THOUGHT AND ACTION

A major focus of study in nursing ethics is to identify, clarify, critically analyse and evaluate one's own and others' values and beliefs underpinning moral decisions and choice of action in practice.

Values are those assertions or statements that individuals make – through behaviour, language, choice of words or actions – that define what they think is important and for which they are willing to suffer, or even, in some cases, die. A value is a personal belief or attitude about the truth, beauty or worth of any thought, object or behaviour (Tschudin 1992).

Value choices constitute almost the whole of human freedom. We often choose to do something because of the values we hold.

FORMATION OF VALUES

Political ideology, societal and cultural values, peer group, family and community values, organisational, institutional and professional values can shape values that we ascribe to our knowledge and thoughts. Whether or not we are aware of them or have consciously chosen or assimilated them, our lives are lived by certain standards and values. These values influence what we choose to do in our own life domain with our body, life, property and privacy, and are also a basis for judging the actions of others. Activity 3.2 considers consciously chosen values.

It is possible to discover that not all values instilled in us by any of the external agencies, including parents, are necessarily our own. Rogers (1951), in his theory of personality and behaviour, considers that the child learns to respond to the environment in a way that pleases his parents and avoids their displeasure. The child learns to deny his own valuing system and is conditioned into accepting the value framework of parents and other influential people and institutions. Through this classical conditioning,

Activity 3.2

Try to bring to mind a particular value you learned from a parent or someone else you consider to have been influential in your life and which has influenced your thinking and choices of action in the way you have lived your life.

Is this value one that you still apply in your life to guide your actions?

What are your grounds for continuing to hold onto, or not continuing to hold onto, this value that those others instilled in you?

children perceive the prejudices, bias and feelings of their parents and influential others, even when they are unspoken. A parent might recoil in disgust at the sight of members of an ethnic group, which could result in the child importing strong feelings and pervasive attitudes which may, according to one view in psychology, predict future behaviour. Rather than offend influential others, we may leave unquestioned some of the values imposed upon us and which we have assimilated into our own value frameworks as our own. Values are dynamic in that, with the experience of living and exposure to others, constant questioning and search for meaning, personal values can change. They are not static (Activity 3.3).

Personal value systems

It is not always easy to identify the particular values and standards by which we live our lives. With the increasing complexity of moral issues and dilemmas confronting health care professionals has come a greater openness in discussion and debate about values. Carper (1978) identified ethical knowledge as a major element of the knowledge base of nursing. To be effective in practice, it is essential for nurses to strive to get in touch with these extra dimensions in our lives so as to begin to know the value basis for their practice in order to justify, defend or challenge decisions made and the subsequent action taken in practice.

Getting in touch with this personal value base is a crucial first step in the study of nursing ethics. Tschudin (1992) advises that values can be brought into consciousness through discovering meaning. This means not being content with superficial levels of meaning and merely responding to prevailing circumstances, but striving and searching to discover a richer level of meaning about life, its purpose, the worth of one's self, who and what we are, and ourselves with others. The source of our values is to be found through the discovery of meaning in our lives, which comes out of learning about ourselves: finding out what kind of person we are, our likes and dislikes, personality, temperament and whether we are thinking or feeling people. Through the study of theories about the formation of values from psychology and sociology, we may be helped to further our understanding of what has influenced our own personal value systems. People do not always behave in a way their expressed attitudes, beliefs and values would lead us to expect. This includes nurses. The study of social psychology may interest those nurses who wish to further discover meaning in relation to their own and others' behaviour.

Through reflecting on what we do in work, recreation and hobbies, we can discover meaning about ourselves, our purpose, our aims and what we seek to accomplish. Our values and meaning in life come out of what we do in our lives.

Frankl (1978) believes that we discover meaning in our lives through experiencing nature and culture, being open and receptive to our experiencing, and hearing nature's stories and the experience of people from different cultures within our society. From this we develop our values and meaning in life.

Frankl (1978) also believes that we discover meaning and values through the experience of our own and others' suffering. Suffering as a result of pain, disease, poverty, injustice, bereavement and disablement affects us: it shapes us, challenges us and is a source of our values (Activity 3.4).

It should be increasingly obvious that today's nurses cannot remain indifferent to the fact that nursing ethics is applied to the public and political domain as much as to the personal and clinical practice of nurse and patient. By virtue of the nurse opening herself to the patient/client

Activity 3.4

As a nurse, even if it meant a great personal cost to you, would you give up driving your car when air quality was reported as not meeting an acceptable high standard?

Is it better to keep an area of land to preserve various species of animals, plants and birds, or to build a new motorway so that more people can enjoy better access by car?

Reflect on these questions. What are your personal value choices? Discuss these with your colleagues. Do you all share the same opinions?

Pain, disease, poverty, bereavement and injustice are all associated with suffering. Have you experienced any of these or experienced observing others' suffering? Did your own or others' experience result in you changing your views and values?

Values are not static: in searching for and discovering meaning they can change. Discuss your answers to the above questions with colleagues.

interpretation of the experience of health, illness, nursing and health care, she has a professional responsibility to influence and inform decisions about: ecological and environmental issues; social and health policy; housing; health education; health promotion; research; resource allocation; and the politics of health, both nationally and internationally. Thus today's professional nurse is not solely confined to nursing ethics individualised within a caring relationship with patients but also needs to operate in the public arena through political networks.

Learning values through observation, reasoning and experience

Knowing nursing includes the area of ethical knowing. Factual knowledge, personal, professional and universal values, all must be consciously and critically evaluated for their potential to do good or harm.

Values that are based on prejudice or bias and values that are assimilated without question may result in behaviour and a choice of action that has the potential to do harm. This can occur either when giving individualised care at a local level or when developing and implementing community

policy at a national level. The tendency is for the personal value system of individuals involved to override all else. Getting in touch with meaning can lead to uncovering of such values, which are sometimes not easy to defend if they have been unconsciously assimilated or are based on prejudice. Getting in touch with such values requires courage; it may be disturbing if the values are based on prejudice, and may result in strong attitudes being expressed. Getting in touch with values can place us in a position of conflict with those we work with and with political, social and organisational values.

In a recent issue of *Nursing Standard* (News Focus 2000) it was reported that, at a conference for nurses, a nurse and a midwife whose mother had recently died after days of delayed treatment hit out at fellow professionals for being unfeeling. They talked about their own suffering and the trauma they experienced seeing their mother deteriorate and die over 5 days. They claimed that they were ignored by nurses and made to feel they were in the way. No one came to them to ask if they needed anything or even to acknowledge them with a word or a gesture. The hospital in this case is refuting the claim that nurses were unfeeling and did not help this patient and relatives who were so vulnerable. Thoughtless action, however it is intended, particularly that which is experienced as being in conflict with professional values, has greater potential to do harm than good to the whole family if it goes unchallenged. Our values and meaning in life come out of what we do. Thus, opening ourselves to the patient's and family's interpretation of meaning of their experience, reflecting on what we do in practice, enables us to learn about ourselves as people and as nurses.

Experiences in practice such as the situation described above give nurses the opportunity to get in touch with the real values which might be driving practice, bringing them to conscious awareness so that they can be confirmed and/or challenged and reviewed for their potential to do great good or great harm. In this way, if there is a mismatch between the claims being made of being concerned about the health and well-being of patients/clients and the patient's/client's experiencing of care, then this can be addressed in order to provide care that is experienced as humane and that more effectively responds to patient/client need.

Model for value clarification

Value clarification is an attempt to bring into conscious awareness the values and underlying motivations that guide one's actions. A strength of value clarification is that one expresses value preferences and priorities in an open and honest way. Questioning our value choices will help us to see how and why we make our decisions. Sometimes it is not easy to defend our choices when challenged. Choosing, prizing and acting upon our own and others' values always involves a choice, even if that choice is to follow others without question.

Raths and colleagues (1966) provided a model for value clarification (Box 3.3).

The nurse who knows her value basis has at some stage thought about it, compared it with alternatives and acted on this choice. In reality, the process may not always be so clear as the simple model outlined in Box 3.3. Getting in touch with your own personal valuing framework can help you find meaning in relation to your own and others' behaviour.

A drawback of value clarification is that one's preference does not provide justification for one's choice. No matter how carefully we have arrived at our choice, it does not mean that it is the one that is morally good and praiseworthy. A preference as a basis for action may well bring about morally bad and blameworthy action and cannot be sufficient grounds or a standard for defending moral thought and ethical practice. Value clarification, while a useful framework to help nurses in discovering what is the morally right thing to do (i.e. health care as a moral endeavour in promoting health and well-being), does not help the nurse to decide between the different claims about what actions are right in a particular situation. What is important is that nurses reflect in and on their practice in order to expose and challenge the potential for gaps between what they say and claim is good about their practice and what they actually do (Greenwood 1998), which may be experienced by patients/clients as not good, or even harmful. Nurses need to be open to the potential for the differing value systems of individual patients and clients. Several small-scale studies (which are not generalisable because of unrepresentative samples) found some mismatch between the aspects of caring valued by nurses and those valued by patients (McKenna 1993, Dyson 1996, Lauri et al 1997, Watson & Lea 1997). There is a lack of evidence that patients/clients and nurses perceive what they value about care in the same way. It would seem to be crucial that nurses do not adopt the attitude that they know what is best if the patient/client needs are to be the focus of health care and of nurses' practice.

In summary, getting in touch with social, organisational, professional and personal value frameworks, evaluating the sources of these values and their potential to do good or harm provides the nurse with a framework for ethical practice which is integral to reflective practice frameworks. Sources of values which may be based on prejudice, bias and negative stereotyping, if they go unchallenged, may result in choices of action that have the potential to do a great deal of harm and adversely affect a person's health and well-being. It is better to be in touch with these so as to take control of any behaviour or actions which may be adversely affecting the care provided for patients and clients.

Box 3.3   Value clarification

When you value something, you:

choose freely
- from alternatives
- after considering the consequences of each alternative

prize
- are proud and happy with the choice
- affirm this and tell others

act
- to act on one's value choice
- to integrate the value in the way life is lived

ETHICAL THEORY AS A BASIS FOR MORAL THOUGHT AND ACTION

PHILOSOPHICAL MEDICAL ETHICS AS A BASIS FOR NURSING ETHICS

Ethical theory, a branch of moral philosophy, offers different ways of viewing how phenomena and actions possess ethical values. The study of philosophical medical ethics based on moral theory provides the nurse with another framework for how to decide what is the right thing to do when faced with an ethical issue in practice.

Devising ethical theory

Seedhouse (1998) sees it as the work of moral philosophers to devise and refine technical ethical theory. The aim of the moral philosopher is to design a theory that is internally coherent, that contains principles that are consistent and complement each other, and that will enable a person to act morally, whatever the situation in life. The focus for technical ethics is the process of clarification and criticism when arguing in ethics. Inconsistency, contradictions, illogical arguments, assumptions, generalisations and appeals to emotion and intuition are deemed inappropriate by the traditional moral philosophers. Great value is placed on the role of reason, impartiality, detachment and the rules of logic when arguing in ethics. Access to the moral truth to guide right action is through this detached process of moral reasoning.

The bioethical model

Moral philosophers put forward two very different theories and forms of reasoning in technical ethics as a basis for judging right and wrong action in the moral sense. These are *deontology* and *utilitarianism*. Both theories offer ways of viewing how phenomena and actions possess ethical values. The study of these theories provides another framework for nurses to develop a more comprehensive understanding of the specific meanings of moral value and moral worth when applied to thinking, values and beliefs and choice of action in practice. The bioethical model is based on the two moral theories and the principles of autonomy and justice (Beauchamp & Childress 1994).

Deontology as a foundation for medical and nursing ethics

This category of moral theories is about a view of morality that prescribes a form of reason which requires sticking to moral rules or duties because they are right in themselves, and that certain duties are right acts in themselves and fundamental to the idea of morality. Deontology is not concerned with the results of actions but with motive. Without exception, the deontologist acts out of a sense of a perceived duty, whatever the consequences. The act itself is judged as a right and moral way to act. These rules may be constraints on what we do to obtain what is of ultimate value. If the deontologist accepts the rule that he should never kill another innocent human being, he can only comply with this rule or break it. Consider this question: Would you be ready to kill an innocent human being if, by doing so, you could somehow prevent the killing of several other innocent human beings? If you say 'No' then your answer is consistent with treating the non-killing of innocent human beings as a rule, as would the deontologist. By breaking the rule more lives could be saved. The deontologist, however, would keep to the rule as a right rule and standard for judging right action.

Deontological theories are justified on several grounds. One is that people have a moral duty to obey God's moral laws. A problem here is that different people understand 'God's law' to mean different things, depending on which God they recognise. Another ground for justifying such theory is the claim that natural law – the laws of nature – include moral laws that bind everyone and can be known through reason. Again the question about the source and what we mean by 'nature' and 'natural laws' arises. However, so long as the deontologist can state what the duty is, it does not seem to matter to him where the rule comes from, nor that it needs to be empirically defined. One could find in today's society evil deontologists who consider that harming people of particular race or ethnic group is a duty to purify the race. A moral deontologist follows duties as a priority, claiming that they are morally important and worth following despite the consequences. Examples of duties followed by deontologists include keeping promises, telling the truth, not killing, doing no harm and always doing good. Deontologists are concerned with the way in which people act and how they intervene in other people's lives.

A problem with this theory is that following duties without exception does not always produce the best consequences in the short term or, in some instances, the long term. A deontologist may select only one duty or, alternatively, a range of duties. Selecting only one duty is hardly a guide to acting morally; selecting a range of duties inevitably causes conflict at times between competing principles. For example, it might be that to tell the truth and to do no harm in a particular situation are in conflict: in order to do no harm, one might be compelled not to tell the truth. In this situation, the deontologist must either list a hierarchy of principles or decide which of these are of supreme importance and which are of less importance, or select a single primary duty. The deontologist will be challenged to give a good reason why he has acted in a particular way. For example, if you have promised a person confidentiality, and he tells you that he has stolen money from his mother, you will have to apply moral reasoning in order to decide which of your duties should take precedence. You may also believe that retributive justice should always be administered. Keeping your promise to the person means that it is possible that justice will not prevail in this case, whereas breaking your promise means that retributive justice may well be administered.

In this situation, you would apply the deontologist's moral reasoning in order to decide which of your duties should take precedence, not to break promises versus justice and fairness. If both rules are right rules, then how does the deontologist decide without breaking one or other of the rules? It would seem the deontologist has no way of deciding between the rules using this form of reasoning. The deontologist will have to consider factors that are not purely questions of duty and will be confronted with considering the consequences. While deontologists would consider it sensible to consider the consequences of actions, they would not overrule moral duty on the grounds of consequence in order to bring about the most favourable outcome in the short term. Deontologists would not support the weighting of the rules by appealing to the consequences. They may consider that there are certain duties that are of supreme and abiding importance. If, in the above scenario, a case is made to support the principle of justice as a supreme duty, the moral grounds for supporting the choice of action in this particular situation are that the act itself is judged as a right and moral way to act. It is the right rule in this particular situation only, and action that complies with a right rule is right action. It is purely a question of duty, rather than of consequences. Deontologists consider that it is wrong to override moral duties to bring about the most favourable consequences.

Act deontology

This is one of several types of deontology. It considers that each context, situation, person involved and judgement made in a moral sense is unique. The overriding duty in act deontology – in every situation – is that the person who is to make a moral choice and decide what ought to be done does so based on honest personal judgement. This will depend on how he sees each unique situation. It is not being true to oneself as a moral agent blindly to follow rules or do what one is told to do. Everything rests on the person who is to judge and to decide in each situation.

Within the complex world of health care and nursing, Seedhouse (1988) argues that act deontology is impracticable, as it would be well nigh impossible to base health care practice on such a philosophy that advocates individuals making their own decisions. It could be extremely confusing and chaotic if there was no consistency in moral intervention.

Seedhouse argues that some aspects of people's lives and situations have common features.

Thus it is possible to make some generalisations and to provide health care workers, including doctors and nurses, with some rules and principles of conduct to guide them in ethical practice.

Rule deontology

Instead of claiming that a person's moral choice depends on how he sees each unique situation, and on personal integrity in being honest and exercising true personal judgement as a moral agent, rule deontology asserts that a person's moral choosing should depend upon a set of rules that should be followed without exception. An advantage of this approach is that the rule deontologist's actions will be more predictable. Codes of professional practice could be described as a version of rule deontology.

Problems could again arise on occasions when it might be better to break the rule. For example, one might reason that it would be better to break a promise if new evidence had come to light since the time of making the promise.

If a set of rules is chosen, there may again be a situation in which conflicts between them are revealed. How then does the rule deontologist choose between the rules that are now in conflict? One solution offered is to rank the rules in order of worth or importance. Again, the problem with this is that a situation may arise in which it could be logically argued that it would be better to break the supreme, primary rule or duty. As already revealed, deontology does not offer sufficient guidance about how to weight the rules in a situation without having to appeal to consequences or just personal opinion, and when to do this. Arguments based solely on personal opinion about the weighting of competing duties or rules in a situation does not seem to provide good enough reason for preferring one rule and rejecting another.

Kantian ethics

The philosopher Immanuel Kant (1724–1804) proposed a rule deontology perspective. If a particular rule or duty is right in one situation, it is right in all situations; it is a general rule. The person deciding what ought to be done in those situations has a duty to obey the rules. Kant claimed that we do many things out of a sense of duty because of external influences such as the anticipation of reward or the fear of sanctions; in these situations, there is no sense of moral duty. Acting out of a sense of duty comes from the willingness to do so from within the person. There are no pressures, it is a natural inclination to act morally. Each rule or principle that is acted on out of 'a good will' is truly a morally good decision. It is a universal moral law, right in all circumstances. Such universal ethical principles are always followed, irrespective of the consequences.

In summary, the main issues for deontologists are that the source and precise nature of the principles, rules and duties by which a person judges right or wrong are open to debate and argument. In addition, what does the deontologist do when principles/rules conflict and the rule applies without exception? A deontologist can only keep or break a rule. If all rules are right rules and guide right action, then the deontologist has no way of deciding, using this form of reasoning, which is the rule that will bring about the highest level of morality. Several deontologists have offered some ways forward which the nurse may find of interest for further study.

Utilitarianism as a foundation for medical and nursing ethics

There are two main approaches to the ethics of consequences – *consequentialism* and *utilitarianism*. A consequentialist will decide how he should act by considering alternative actions and assessing the likely outcomes of proposed actions, i.e. whether the act will produce more benefits than disadvantages. The choice of the course of action to take will be based upon which action will bring about the greatest amount of benefit and the least amount of harm.

Utilitarianism was the approach proposed by Jeremy Bentham (1748–1832) and John Stuart Mill (1806–1873). The consequence thought to be beneficial was the greatest balance of good over evil, good being defined as happiness or pleasure. The utilitarians would argue that once we have formed a view about what things are good, it would follow that we could decide whether an action is right by asking if it does more to increase that good – for example happiness – than any other action that the person could do. It makes sense to maximise a value, to increase it as much as possible. If it is happiness that is valued, then the person can choose between acts that will lead to there being more or less happiness in the world. Consider again the question asked earlier: would you be ready to kill an innocent human being if, by doing so, you can somehow prevent the killing of several other innocent human beings? An affirmative answer suggests that you regard the reduction of killing of innocent human beings as a value, as would the utilitarian. Thus you would take away one life but save several more, maximising a value, the reduction of killing. The utilitarian uses the standard of maximising value to judge the rightness/wrongness, goodness/badness of actions in a moral sense – simply whether what they do will produce the best consequences – unlike the deontologist, who judges actions as right or wrong on the basis of their compliance with some right rules or principles irrespective of their consequences. Defining those values to be maximised in measurable terms is problematic, and measures of utility other than happiness are now considered. In health care, benefit is usually described in terms of health status, added life years, quality of life years, disability adjusted life years, health gain, and freedom from pain and disability. Whatever the definition of benefit, it must be measurable.

Exploring the meaning of the examples given here, and the value basis of decisions based on a calculation of outcome, raises much controversy and disagreement among health care professionals, health service managers and health economists. Defining these in measurable terms is equally problematic. In the calculation of the balance of benefit over non-benefit, all those involved are considered to be of equal importance to all others in the assessment. All persons are taken account of in the calculation of the effect of the chosen action. This impartiality and

detachment is seen as a strength of the theory, in that it is a position that challenges individual self-interest and bias.

The action taken is justified according to the outcomes achieved in terms of the best consequences. Acts are morally right only if they have utility (are useful) in bringing about the best consequences.

Act utilitarianism

The person taking this approach will look at each situation from the perspective that the context, situation, persons involved, benefits and judgement made is, in a moral sense, unique.

Seedhouse (1998) argues that, in the complex world of health care, it is unrealistic to expect people to go through new calculations each time. Much work is being done in the area of producing measurable outcomes where difficult decisions are to be made about rationing of health care resources. Much controversy surrounds this work, including the view that taking such an approach means that not all persons are valued equally nor treated fairly. Major critics of utilitarian theory claim that this approach can lead to decisions that seem to be patently unjust.

General utilitarianism

The person taking this approach will ask what the consequences would be if everyone were to pursue a particular course of action. It is a useful question to ask in that it enhances our view of reality in terms of the far-reaching consequences of actions.

Rule utilitarianism

The person taking this approach will calculate the best consequences to result from obedience to predefined rules, to which no exception is acceptable. Always to keep a certain predefined rule will be to produce the greatest good. The rule has greater utility in terms of consequences and has been established based on a process of calculation of which rules, if always followed, produce the greatest balance of good over evil.

In health care, following the theory of rule utilitarianism provides a basis for ethical practice that has been arrived at through a thorough review of past experiences. One shortcoming is that, sooner or later, the rule utilitarian will be faced with a rule to which it would be better not to adhere, in that it will not result in producing the greatest balance of good over evil. Rules are rigid; they are also created by people who may well be biased and prejudiced in some way.

Issues for utilitarians include the difficulty in defining what constitutes 'happiness' or 'the common good'. By whose definition? Does winning the lottery and having material things mean happiness? Is it happiness that gives everything value, or a life of spiritual contemplation? Or is it simply getting what we want? Who are the 'all' whose happiness is to be taken into account? Are we to extend our concern to all beings capable of pleasure and pain? How far are we to consider the interests of posterity when they seem to conflict with those of existing human beings? If a standard is adopted which applies to the majority, then what about the rights of the minority? Do they not matter equally?

Deontology and utilitarianism compared

It would seem there are problems with the philosophical basis of the theories of utilitarianism and deontology as a framework for medical and nursing ethics. Neither is sufficient in itself to provide an adequate theory for moral decision making and for justifying moral action taken in practice. Despite this, philosophical medical ethics as a basis for nursing ethics must be one area of study in any programme of nursing ethics.

Think about the two opposing theories and consider Case study 3.3.

PRINCIPLES OF BIOMEDICAL ETHICS

Traditionally, the moral principles of beneficence (to do good) and non-maleficence (to do no harm) have been the basis of the doctor–patient and

Case study 3.3

Recently the debate over the separation of the conjoined twins raged for weeks in the public arena and brought to public attention some complex legal issues and ethical dilemmas.

The key ethical issues concerned a child's right to life and right to death. Against the parents' wishes, the courts ruled that doctors should separate the girls, despite the fact it would lead to the death of one of the twins and leave the other with potential disabilities.

The parents, Catholics who came from another culture, wanted the girls to be left to live their short lives in peace without surgery until their inevitable deaths. The medical profession applied to the courts for permission to operate and separate the twins, knowing it would lead to the death of one twin in order for the other to survive.

Consider the moral theories deontology and utilitarianism as frameworks for guiding right action in an ethical sense. Can you identify with the utilitarian argument? Remember actions are judged as right actions depending on their capacity for maximising a value – in this case life itself. Who is bringing this argument to this situation? Is it right to maximise life by saving one life at the expense of another?

Can you identify with the deontological argument? Remember actions are judged according to whether they accord with a right rule or principle – in this case it is wrong to kill or instigate someone's death. Who is bringing this argument to the situation and what do you think is the source of their rule?

There are many other issues you may wish to think about in this complex and tragic case, for instance the question about the quality of life of the surviving twin and the danger the twins are being used as a means to an end in terms of medical research and progress.

(For further reading see Brykczynska 2000.)

nurse–patient relationship. The professional's duty, as an expert, was to act in the best interests of the patient, and the patient was seen as taking a relatively passive role within the relationship.

More recently, however, thinking in philosophy has moved towards the need to address patients' wishes. Respect for autonomy is a principle that is becoming central to the doctor–patient or nurse–patient relationship in health care.

It could be said that resource allocation is the 'problem' facing health care today. The care services are facing new demands as a result of changing patterns of need and the expectations of clients, and rationing of resources is inevitable.

Finding methods of rationing health care resources based on a moral principle of justice is a major challenge to all health care professionals working at all levels of the health service. The principles of autonomy and justice as fairness are pivotal to current health care practice and central to many of the arguments within medical and nursing ethics (Gillon 1994).

The principle of autonomy

The concept of autonomy has come from the philosophical work of freedom. A basic distinction to make is between negative freedom and positive freedom. Negative freedom means the absence of constraint or coercion, a person being said to be free to the extent he can choose his own goals. Berlin (1969) questions the value of this notion of freedom from interference to 'men who are half naked, illiterate, underfed and diseased'. There are situations in which individual freedom is not everyone's primary need. Thus, it is argued, personal freedom is not enough; what is needed is positive freedom – the means or power to act. Seedhouse (1998) argues that the measure of freedom a person has is the extent to which he has knowledge; he considers knowledge as another necessary condition in order to be free.

Autonomy has different meanings for different people. Gillon (1986) writes about the control a person has over his own life and choices as 'the will'; the will of the person must be respected. Seedhouse (1988) expresses concern that if autonomy of will is all there is, we could, in health care, risk neglecting opportunities to help people enhance their lives. Seedhouse argues for the notion that autonomy is a quality, a part of being human. Autonomy as a quality can exist only so far as certain conditions are present; to be able to understand one's environment, to make rational choices and to be able to act on the choices made.

Autonomy is a matter of degree. It can be considered on a continuum with 'no control' and 'total control' at the extremes. The greater the degree of autonomy, the more a person is able to do in his life. Autonomy is a quality that can be possessed to a greater or lesser degree in different areas, situations and times in our lives. Admission

to hospital can result in fear and distress and reduce a person's degree of autonomy, and thus his ability to function in that particular situation and at that particular time. Working with patients to produce the conditions necessary for autonomy is a large area of nurses' work.

A dilemma exists when it is felt that it is more important to act in the best interests of a patient than to respect his autonomy. Overriding a patient's autonomy is serious, and an action that must be justified. An area of patient/client autonomy nurses work with in practice is respecting and maintaining patient/client confidentiality, which is discussed later in the chapter.

The principle of justice

The basic point of view is that we should value people equally and treat everyone alike unless there is a difference between people that is relevant to treating them differently. In health care some differences are relevant to differences in treatment, for example someone may be very ill and very distressed and need more physical and emotional care than someone else who is more independent. Health care workers sometimes disagree over which variations between patients they consider justify differences in treatment.

There are different ways of understanding the meaning of justice. An *egalitarian* view of justice in health care is concerned with the distribution of health care resources according to individual need. Individual needs must be met by equal access to services and an adequate level of health care to meet those needs. Justice here is based on need.

A *libertarian* view of justice holds that the most important value is individual liberty and choice. Here, the best kind of state is one that protects individuals, leaves them alone and lets them enjoy the rewards of their labour. Justice relates to how hard one has worked or how well one has done – justice according to merit.

A *rights* view of justice implies that someone has a duty or obligation to the person exercising his right. Different sorts of rights are talked about, including natural rights, legal rights and moral rights (deontology). Clearly, a patient has legal rights not to suffer harm as a result of negligence on the part of any health care professional.

There are differing points of view regarding the nature of rights, so justice may be apportioned on the basis of different rights.

If we want to be just, we need to resolve the conflict between the different principles of justice, as illustrated in Activity 3.5. Justice as fairness is pivotal to nursing practice, which is based on a belief about the equality of people and a valuing of the uniqueness of each individual. Generally it is thought that we should value people equally and treat everyone alike unless there is a difference between people which is relevant to treating them differently, and this can be justified ethically. We should regard people as equally important, regardless of their race, gender, religion, culture, age, medical diagnosis, wealth and so on. We should not treat them differently or discriminate against them in any way just because they belong to these groups. (Nurses working in practice to promote equality of persons through anti-discriminatory practice are discussed again later in the chapter.)

Activity 3.5

Consider two girls. The owner of the snack bar promises each girl £5 for cleaning the kitchen. When the job is done each girl has a right to £5. This is what was agreed. This puts justice according to *right* above all else.

What if one girl does an excellent job and the other girl does a poor job? The owner of the snack bar then judges that the girl who did an excellent job deserves more reward than does the other girl, so he pays the first girl £8 and the second girl £2, thus putting justice according to *merit* above all else.

Then the snack bar owner learns that the hardworking girl comes from a well-to-do family, whereas the second girl is from a large family and is known to go hungry at times so that her small sisters can eat. The owner of the snack bar now judges that the second girl, who did a poor job, obviously needs more money, as she is going hungry in order to feed her sisters. Thus he pays both girls £5, with an extra £2 for the second girl to buy food. This puts justice according to *need* above all else.

How would you be just? Which of the principles of justice would you put first? Defend your position.

CARING AS THE BASIS FOR MORAL THOUGHT AND ACTION

There has been a backlash against modern moral philosophy, mainly by those who would wish to promote a return to virtue ethics. This includes some feminist moral philosophers whose values are reflected in the writings of nurse theorists who would seek to promote the concept 'caring' as a guide to ethical nursing practice. The concept of caring has occupied a prominent position in the nursing literature and has been presented as the essence of nursing practice by many nurse theorists and writers (including Leininger 1981, 1984, Gilligan 1982, Noddings 1984, Benner & Wrubel 1989, Tschudin 1992, Watson 1997).

Benner & Wrubel (1989) claim that inherent in nursing practice is the moral sense of caring. Caring as a basis for nursing ethics is a central value that underpins a special way of being and doing within the nurse–patient relationship that can promote good and enhance patients' and nurses' lives. Many of the writers above refer to the implicit moral sense of caring, a universal value that guides practice.

Writers from the caring movement strongly oppose importing into nursing theories from other disciplines, including moral philosophy. There is concern that the moral sense in nursing practice that relates to day-to-day choices and their potential to do good or harm will be lost.

A major criticism is that modern philosophy is misguided because it rests on the incoherent notion of a law without a lawgiver. More importantly, theories that emphasise right action seem incomplete because they neglect the question of character. They concentrate instead on rational calculation or the application of highly abstract universal principles by which rational beings should be guided.

Both deontology and utilitarian theories share an admiration for the rules of reason to be appealed to in a moral context to support right action. The modern moral philosophers who would decontextualise reasoning about particular issues/dilemmas, usually of a dramatic nature, using rules and principles, prize being detached and impartial during this process. They would denigrate any appeal to feelings and emotion. Feminist moral philosophers (Held 1990) and some nurse theorists (Noddings 1984) claim ethical decisions cannot be made in this detached mechanical way. In addition, they raise a major challenge for the modern philosophers in the form of the question of whether reason motivates action. They argue that theories of ethics that emphasise right action will never satisfactorily provide an account of what is actually done in practice. It is one thing to contemplate through reason the weighting of moral principles and to undertake rational calculation when deciding what is the right thing to do. But does it follow on from deciding what it is right to do using moral theory frameworks that you are motivated to act? The argument is that this will depend on the character of the person contemplating the act.

Knowing the right thing to do does not necessarily mean that the nurse is motivated to take what is judged to be right action. The taking of action will depend on the particular qualities, virtues and vices of the nurse's character. Those who would revive virtue ethics, including feminist moral philosophers and those of the caring ethic movement in nursing, suggest we should stop thinking about obligation and duty and concentrate on asking 'what would a human being look like who lacked the virtues?'. The central questions are about character. To understand ethics, nursing ethics, we must understand what makes a good person, one who is motivated to act ethically. The claim is that a good person is a person of virtuous character and so virtues become the subject matter of ethics. A recent survey (Plunkett 1999) of over 200 nurses in the USA reported that the most disturbing ethical dilemma confronting them in their practice was having to work with colleagues they described as being unethical and impaired. They described their colleagues, who were sometimes observed seeming to condone unethical practice through their inaction, as not being motivated to enhance the health and well-being of their patients/clients.

Seedhouse (1988, 1998) refers to 'ethics in the general sense'. The person who deliberates in a general sense of ethics realises that *all* thought and action can and should produce moral reflection; all action has potential for good or harm. Too often, nurses confine themselves in ethics to the kind of dramatic ethical dilemmas well deliberated in the public arena, but these are only the tip of the iceberg. So much of ethics in everyday practice goes unnoticed, without reflection; this is the bulk of the iceberg that remains out of sight.

The writers from the caring movement highlight particular features of the caring relationship, including ways of relating, the existence of particular conditions within the relationship, specific aims for interacting and the presence of particular caring qualities or characteristics of the caregiver (Noddings 1984, Watson 1985, 1997, Leininger 1988, Hall 1989, Koldjeski 1990, Marck 1990, Morse et al 1990, Brown et al 1992, Boykin & Schoenhofer 1993).

Gilligan (1982) found in her studies that there was an emphasis on empathy and concern for the well-being of the other within the caring relationship. In one study, nurses and patients described a sense of fulfilment as a direct result of nursing care delivered out of a moral sense.

Noddings (1984) wrote about some of the virtuous caring qualities, being non-judgemental and accepting of the patient, empathy and person-to-person relating, as particular conditions existing in a caring relationship. In order to create these conditions, the caregiver needs to develop self-awareness and empathy both as qualities and as skills. This means not only trying to step in and out of the patient's inner private world to glean meaning, but also developing the skill to convey to the patient the ascertained meaning of his inner private world.

Several writers describe certain virtuous caring qualities and characteristics of the caregiver. Roach (1987) identifies compassion, competence, confidence, conscience and commitment. Leininger (1981) refers to 27 differing caring constructs, including compassion, concern, empathy, love, nurturance, presence, support and trust. Other writers have identified knowledge, patience, honesty, trust, humility, hope and courage. Total caring requires one to be free of self-centredness. Through self-actualisation and the development of these qualities and characteristics, the nurse will strive for the good of the self and others, and good in general. Character is the source of ethical nursing practice, both for deciding what is the right thing to do and the motivation to act.

All of the values and claims expressed by those of the caring movement are also open to serious challenge, and none enjoys the status of demonstrable truth. There is a danger in nursing of the unquestioning wholesale adoption of the humanistic existential ethic, which could lead to subtle indoctrination of that ethic (Barker et al 1995). Also there is a predicament in nursing in adopting this ethic which is linked to gender (Davies 1995, Rafael 1996,). This comes from a traditional view of caring as 'women's work' (Morse et al 1990), that it comes naturally and requires no particular knowledge or skills. Those who manage nursing resources may well, if they hold this view, undermine the value nurses themselves place on the work they do through not providing them with sufficient resources to ensure the incorporation of caring activities within nursing workloads.

Foot (1978) questions adopting an ethic of caring that is so dependent upon putting others interests before one's own. She challenges this in the light of a society that would seem to refuse to value caring, placing instead greater value and emphasis on individualism and egoism, and having little regard for selflessness and concern for the well-being of others.

The caring model as a basis for nursing ethics would seem to be orientated by the values of the agapistic or altruistic models developed by ancient and mediaeval philosophers such as Aristotle and St Thomas Aquinas. One source of appeal might well have been the emphasis on the development of natural virtues, including providence, wisdom, temperance, courage and justice. Ethics is about virtues of character that are acquired through man's rational thought, desire and action. To develop a virtue is to express one's essence as a rational responsible agent, so, to that extent, the cultivation of virtues must be part of a rational agent's good.

A virtue is a trait of character that is manifested in habitual actions. Actions spring from a firm and unchangeable virtuous character. For instance an honest person is truthful as a matter of principle, not just occasionally or when it is to his advantage. We distinguish between virtues and vices in that virtues are good to have and are possessed by the sorts of persons we prefer, while other sorts of persons, those with vices, we prefer to avoid. Thus a virtue is a trait of character that is manifest in habitual actions that it is good for a person to have. According to Aristotle, a virtue is a mean state with reference to two vices between excess and deficiency of action and feeling, and ethical action is about responding appropriately. This is determined by the reason of the wise (i.e. rational) person. Being generous is part way between being extravagant and being miserly, and courage is a mean between foolhardiness and cowardice. Each of the virtues has its own distinctive features and raises its own problems.

VIRTUE ETHICS: A REVIVAL

Several philosophers (MacIntyre 1993, Rachels 1998), increasingly frustrated by the impersonal form of the dominant moral theories of utilitarianism and deontology, have begun to revive virtue theory. The question of what one ought to do in any given situation is not concerned with calculating the consequences, balancing interests or resolving conflicts of rights. It is about what kind of person is making the decision. Virtue theory seeks to describe the types of character we might find admirable and praiseworthy, raising questions about what a good person would do in a particular situation.

The argument put forward in support of the revival of virtue ethics is that notions of moral duty and obligation are no longer compatible with today's worldviews. It is felt that modern societies have inherited fragments of conflicting ethical traditions and that people are feeling confused. A claim for a return to virtue ethics is that the virtues are needed to conduct our lives well. We are rational social beings who want and need the company of others. We live in communities, among friends, family and fellow citizens. Such virtues as courage, loyalty, generosity, honesty are needed for living with all of these people successfully, whatever the culture or race. The virtues all have the same general sort of value – they are qualities needed for successful living.

Questions need to be asked about whether or not we can resurrect in modern life the virtues of Aristotle and the code of an 18th-century aristocrat, which has its origins in a time when societies were not democracies. Stressing the perfection of the individual and the future of man, how does this fit with the view that all men are equal? Does a man who does not measure up to this perfectionist ideal of character have less worth? Is this view compatible with moral equality and justice?

Many would argue that it is not possible for an ethical theory which is based entirely on a virtuous character to do all the work of ethics. The idea of a core of all virtues suggests there is only one good way to live and one good way for society to develop, whereas there are many different ways to live and many possible different worlds in the future, each requiring different systems and practices, and people with different kinds of virtue, for its development. However, there is a view we all have a great deal in common despite our differences: for example, everyone needs courage and generosity because in all situations there will be property to be managed, goods to be distributed, and some people will be worse off than others; honesty is needed because no society can exist without communication between its members; and loyalty is needed because everyone needs friends, and to have friends one must be a friend, so everyone needs loyalty.

It would seem that the supporters of virtue ethics as a framework to guide ethical nursing practice consider it to be a profound fault of non-virtue theories that so little attention is paid to the major areas of life that form character. In nursing, more needs to be learned about the impact of 'caring' as a virtue guiding decisions and action in practice. What are the character traits of the virtuous and the non-virtuous nurse? Virtue ethics is appealing because it provides a natural and attractive account of moral motivation, whereas other moral theories are deficient in this, emphasising only right action, which does not necessarily motivate action.

There is a connection between virtue ethics and some of the concerns voiced by feminist moral philosophers (Held 1990). These writers would argue that modern moral philosophy incorporates a male bias with its appeal to impartiality and reason, where relationships are impersonal, contractual and often adversarial. They argue that women's experience of moral problems leads them to be especially concerned with actual relationships between persons: they are inclined to attend to the particularities of the context within which a moral problem arises, rather than remain distant and unattached. Women often pay attention to feelings of empathy and caring to guide their action rather than relying on abstract rules of reason. Emotion is respected by feminist moral philosophers in the process of gaining understanding.

Virtue ethics makes the question of character its main concern. It is an incomplete theory in that while it provides understanding about moral character and motivation to do the right thing, it does not provide a guide to deciding on the right action. Adding this theory to traditional moral theory of right action provides an account of virtues and the motivation for taking the right action. While nurses may be able to reason when arguing in ethics and reflect deeply on their values, they may not reach a point where strongly held beliefs are challenged. They may not be motivated to do so!

MAKING MORAL DECISIONS IN NURSING PRACTICE

Few studies of nurses' experiences of ethical decision making and ethical behaviour in practice are to be found in the literature.

STUDIES IN MORAL DEVELOPMENT

Studies in moral development are based on the cognitive theory of moral development proposed by Kohlberg (1984). This work advanced and extended the work of Piaget on the moral development of children. The theory holds that the underlying cognitive structures or principles that an individual uses to resolve moral dilemmas develop through a series of six sequential stages, each embodying a qualitatively different kind of moral reasoning and representing a form of thinking about morality. In the initial stages, where rudimentary levels of decision are made, anticipation and fear of punishment and obedience have a major impact on decisions. Moving up the scale, conventional acceptance of society's values and rules has a major impact on decisions made. At the top end of the scale, moral decisions are made on the basis of universally valid ethical principles. Stages five and six are the highest stages of cognitive development, which not everyone achieves.

Accepting this theory, it could be assumed that a cross-section of society, including doctors and nurses, will reveal a sizeable number at many of the moral stages. At each succeeding stage there is greater appreciation of the welfare of others and a greater desire to resolve moral dilemmas in a fair and equitable way.

An implicit assumption is that those who have reached a higher stage of moral reasoning are more likely to act morally than are those at the lower stages. However, there is no empirical evidence to support this assumption. The cognitive theory itself is criticised by those who support caring and feminist ethics (Gilligan 1982) and social learning theory (Bandura 1997) as providing a dominant male view with respect to the staged process and moral development and reasoning being a purely cognitive process. Hoffman (1979) demonstrated a tendency of children as young as 2 years old to empathise with others and express this in a rudimentary way.

Studies examining nurses' reasoning ability (Rest 1990, McAlpine et al 1997) have been based on Kohlberg's work and assumptions that a relationship exists between hypothetical reasoning, practical reasoning and actual behaviour in the real, lived, experienced world of nursing practice. A significant pattern in these studies is that measuring instruments ask subjects to rank lists of issues in responding to hypothetical situations. This says little about the subject's own thinking about the issues or whether or not they would recognise for themselves the moral issues involved. Such lists may prompt thinking which would not otherwise have occurred. These studies in the literature have asked nurses to say what they ought to do and what they would do in response to a particular hypothetical situation, but none has investigated what nurses actually do in practice.

Although of limited value due to study inaccuracies and instrument misuse, these studies raised important issues. Factors other than the ability to reason were reported by the researchers as having the potential to determine moral action in practice. Influence could be from the environment, the work setting, the personal characteristics of the nurse, the perception of the role and role relationships, differing values and beliefs among professionals (Joudrey 1999), conflicting loyalties, organisational values, supportive and unsupportive environments, power and power relationships and forms of power sharing.

INFLUENCES ON THE ETHICAL DECISION-MAKING PROCESS

Erlen & Frost (1992) described a common experience of nurses in relationship with doctors, 'perceived powerlessness', which led to nurses describing themselves as ineffective in influencing moral decisions. Nurses perceived themselves as 'victims' of the system and the many constraints to ethical practice arising in the system (McAlpine et al 1997). On the other hand, Udén and colleagues (1992), when comparing the experiences of doctors and nurses, found that doctors reported feeling isolated, lacking support and feeling insecure in their work because they were criticised by nurses. Doctors described nurses as not being willing to explore problems deeply.

As yet, the experience of nurses in practice is a little-known phenomenon. There are other factors, besides the ability to reason at a high-principled level and follow rules of logic, that may well have an influence on moral reasoning and the practice of nursing. One probability is that new entrants to nursing are still exposed to the strong and rapid socialisation into a traditional mindset (Aroskar 1982, Stein et al 1990, May 1993, Fitzpatrick et al 1993) of the nurse as obedient and unquestioning 'handmaiden'. This is a rich and challenging field for nursing research (see Ch. 11).

THE NATURE AND ISSUES OF POWER WITHIN RELATIONSHIPS

The study of power and politics goes hand in hand with ethics. To be a professional nurse means that one exercises a public role. The professional nurse is dealing with different power relationships and the use of that power, both within her work – in clinical practice, research, management education and politics – and outside the nurse–patient relationship – with colleagues, other disciplines, managers, the organisation, professional bodies, pressure groups, unions and politicians at local, national and sometimes international levels.

The practice of ethics in all of these relationships is intimately tied up with the power issues of control, compliance, conformity, manipulation, coercion, facilitation, enabling, negotiation, domination and the use of authority. Study of sociology and psychology within the nursing curriculum offers the nurse access to further exploration of the concept of power, related concepts and their application to nursing practice, particularly within relationships.

Whatever the philosophical basis for nursing ethics in practice, political knowledge and ability is essential for informing decisions and choice of action. Ethical decisions so often come into conflict with the realities of power between professionals, different influential groups, persons at different clinical and management levels, and individuals and communities.

The nurse with a public role has a responsibility to try to use her political influence actively to shape health policy and influence public opinion on health matters. Nurses have a responsibility to the wider community and to society. Working with people every day can give nurses first-hand experience and information about whole communities, their health status, inequalities and health care needs.

CONFIDENTIALITY

As discussed earlier, autonomy is a complex moral principle which is even more complex when applied in practice. Working with autonomy in practice involves nurses demonstrating respect for patient/client autonomy and/or working to promote patient/client autonomy in many areas of care. One such area is respecting confidences through protecting what is private and personal. Clause 9 of the Professional Code of Conduct (UKCC 1992) states that each registered nurse should:

respect confidential information obtained in the course of professional practice and refrain from disclosing such information without the consent of the patient/client or a person entitled to act on his/her behalf, except where disclosure is required by law or by the order of a court or is necessary in the public interest.

All nurses, including students of nursing, are expected to abide by the code.

What is confidential information?

Working with the moral principle of autonomy in protecting what is private and personal, the nurse would clearly need to understand exactly what 'confidential information' is, and also what would constitute a breach of confidentiality. By virtue of their role, nurses have access to information about patients/clients that has not necessarily been given in the strictest confidence, but nevertheless may be private and personal. For example, a person might be unable to give confidential information, in the sense that he can understand what confidential information is, because he has dementia, severe learning disabilities, is unconscious, or confused. Another instance may be the nurse on a community visit in a person's own home who comes across information which is not necessarily information 'given in confidence' but which is nevertheless private and personal.

What counts as confidential information and what does not must never be assumed. To break confidentiality is a serious matter and strong evidence is required to support the reasoning behind a decision to share information about patients and clients. The dominant view within nursing is that *all* information about patients and clients should be regarded as confidential (Cain 1999). This is the benchmark for professional ethical practice.

Breaching confidentiality and informed consent

Any sharing of information, even among health or social care professionals, is a breach of confidentiality. The sharing of information about a client's/patient's health is only made possible within health care teams directly involved in the patient's/client's care where the patient/client has given informed consent to the sharing of information. By giving permission, the patient/client (not the health or social care professional) has extended the boundary to include those persons with whom information is shared. A breach occurs when information is shared without the patient's/client's informed consent.

Consider the scenarios in Case study 3.4. Decide whether there has been a breach of patient/client confidentiality. Give reasons for your answers.

You may have considered that the nurses who were overheard talking did not identify the patients by name, that the assignment was not read by anybody, that the cleaner did not look into the patient records, the community nurse's partner did not share the information with the authorities.

However, in each of these cases it would not be too difficult to identify the particular patient/client the information relates to. For instance, the dining room at the hospital is used by staff and visitors who can locate the patient/client by virtue of which ward or unit the nurses are working on. Some nurses may know the unit and the patient/client by virtue of having worked there themselves. It could also be possible that any member of hospital staff or a visitor knows of the patient and can identify him/her from information that is being discussed, e.g. particular characteristic, occupation, where they live, friends and acquaintances, etc. The point here is that the nurses failed in every case to protect personal and private information. That the cleaner did not access the records or the student assignment remained unopened and the patients/clients may not have been identified is irrelevant. It is enough to fail to protect private and personal information for a breach of confidence to have taken place. In

Case study 3.4 Five scenarios

First scenario
Two student nurses are having lunch in the hospital dining room and are overheard by another nurse from a different ward, discussing the care they had provided for a patient that morning. They are discussing how difficult it was to communicate with this patient, whom they describe as being rather 'miserable and smelly'. At no time do they mention the patient's name or the name of the ward.

Second scenario
A staff nurse undertaking a specialist nursing course has brought her assignment to discuss with other nurses on the ward. It contains some extracts from several patient care plans.
  Leaving in a rush that evening after a busy day she forgets the assignment and leaves it in the changing room. On her return the next day she finds the assignment where she left it. It is unopened.

Third scenario
After a busy day, a health visitor forgets to lock her cabinet at the health centre. It contains records and confidential information about one of her client families. The cabinet is closed and the office is locked. The evening domestic unlocks and enters the office to empty the bins. The health visitor returns the next day. The records are intact.

Fourth scenario
You are working on a very busy ward caring for patients when the care worker shouts down the ward that she needs some help with Mrs Tingle who has soiled her bed for the fourth time that morning. All the patients in your vicinity look up and smile.

Fifth scenario
While visiting a patient at home, a community nurse and a student nurse witness the patient's married daughter emptying the contents of her shopping on the table. There are many expensive items and the mother questions her daughter about where she got the money to pay for them. The daughter informs her mother that her friend has stolen them from the supermarket and that this is a regular occurrence. The community nurse mentions this to her husband in conversation at home that evening.

each and every case there is a serious breach of confidence, even if that breach does not result in a person being identified. Even if no information is disclosed the risk of a breach lies in the possibility the person the information relates to could be traced. In failing to protect private and personal information there is a breach, just as there is a breach when information is disclosed.

SOME ETHICAL ISSUES

Working with the principle of autonomy requires nurses to work with clients/patients in caring relationships where there is respect and trust. From the outset, clarifying and deciding through obtaining informed consent about what information is shared between the client/patient and nurse and what is to be kept confidential helps in building that trust.

What counts as confidential must never be assumed.

Grounds for breaking confidentiality are that the patient/client has given informed consent to the sharing of information. An ethical issue arises where a patient/client is unable to give informed consent. Sharing of information, even within the health care team, would be a breach of confidentiality. Arguing in ethics, a strong justification could be made for breaching confidentiality in that the professionals directly involved in care have a moral and legal duty to care for the patient/client. To neglect the patient's/client's needs, which are the reason health care professionals have access to the information in the first place, would not be defensible. The benchmark still applies that sharing of personal and private information would only be with the team directly involved in the patient's care and the boundaries would not be extended to others.

Sometimes a claim is made to justify breaking confidentiality on the grounds it is in the interests of the individual, group of individuals or the rest of society. A calculation is made of the aggregate of benefit for all those affected and the utilitarian standard used to justify breaking confidentiality. However, this needs to be balanced against the rights of the individual to give informed consent.

A complex example of this may be in the case of a child who is dying from a condition that is currently incurable and has requested that no further treatment is given. The parents ask that the child be given some treatment that is still at an early stage of development and not tried and tested, but that this information is not given to the child, who might refuse. To keep such a confidence may be colluding with others, denying the child's autonomy to make an informed choice and the child's right to know the truth. Withholding information from the child and sharing information with others, including parents, without the child's consent is a breach of confidentiality. The grounds for such breaches of confidentiality are often claimed as being in the best public interests, which include individuals, groups and society. The parents in this case may be acting out of a motive of self-interest in that they are desperate for the child to survive. This may well blind them to the rights of the child. The question would be whether or not these are good enough grounds for such breaches of confidence. Resolving issues like this, which can arise in practice, requires the participation of nurses who have achieved high-level ethical practice competence. There are many ethical challenges arising from this situation in addition to the notion of confidentiality which will require resolution. By virtue of their roles, all nurses have access to information about patients and clients that is not necessarily given in strictest confidence yet may be private and personal. For this reason, what counts as confidential information must never be assumed by the nurse.

In practice, all information about clients and patients should be regarded as confidential. To break confidentiality is a serious matter and requires strong evidence to support an argument in ethics for sharing information about patients/clients with others, including health and social care professionals, in the absence of the patient's informed consent.

Fair and antidiscriminatory practice

Fair and antidiscriminatory nursing practice, recognising and respecting alternative cultures and beliefs, is constructed around the valuing of the individual as a person with rights (Clause 5, UKKC 1992). It includes a positive acceptance of differentness, for example arising from ethnic origin, cultural beliefs, personal attributes, social status, property, birth, health problems, political and personal opinions or any other factor (Clause 7, UKCC, 1992).

The health service (DoH 1998, 1999) is underpinned by values of equity and fairness and holds that health services should strive to provide care which is based on the best possible evidence and guided by patients' needs and expectations. *All patients, without exception, should have equal access to a high standard of care, regardless of where they live, their ethnic and social origin, race, colour, cultural beliefs, personal attributes, health problems or any other factors.*

As already discussed, the moral principle of justice is highly complex in terms of its meaning and application in practice. Taking the notion of justice according to rights, an understanding of what constitutes an individual's rights is a vital goal for nurses if they are to strive to promote and uphold the rights of patients/clients to fair and equitable care.

Violating the rights of patients/clients in their care is one of the worst offences that nurses or health professionals can be found guilty of.

What are rights?

Organisations such as the United Nations (UN) try to determine through universal agreement what human rights are and how they can be upheld in countries throughout the world. The UN defines rights and makes declarations which it expects member nations to sign and abide by. The Universal Declaration of Human Rights (UN 1948) has 30 articles and states that 'everyone is entitled to all rights and freedoms within the declaration without distinction of any kind such as race, colour, language, religion, political/other opinion, natural or social origin, property, birth or other status. Some of the most important articles are listed in Box 3.4.

Upholding rights

In trying to uphold human rights for all people, special attention has to be paid to those groups who are at most risk of having their rights violated. Think of the human rights abuses throughout the world today. There are many examples in the world of oppression, dispossession, cultural and geographical dislocation. You might have brought to mind the torture of political dissidents in some countries, including those nurses who

---

Box 3.4 The Universal Declaration of Human Rights (UN 1948)

The declaration has 30 articles. These are some of the most important:

- All human beings are born free and equal in rights
- Everyone is entitled to all rights and freedoms set forth in the declaration without distinction of any kind, such as race, colour, sex, language, religion, political or other opinion, national or social origin, property, birth or other status
- Everyone has the right to life, liberty and security of person
- No one shall be held in slavery or servitude
- No one shall be subjected to torture or to cruelty, inhuman or degrading treatment or punishment
- Everyone has the right to recognition everywhere as a person before the law
- No one shall be subjected to arbitrary arrest, detention or exile
- Everyone charged with a penal offence has the right to be presumed innocent until proved guilty according to the law in a public trial at which he has had all the guarantees necessary for his defence
- No one shall be subjected to arbitrary interference with his privacy, family, home or correspondence, nor attacks upon his honour and reputation
- Everyone has the right to seek and to enjoy in other countries asylum from persecution.

In 1950, the UK and a number of other European states became signatories to the Convention for the Protection of Human Rights (the European Convention on Human Rights) which came into force in 1953. By the convention, the European Court of Human Rights was set up to adjudicate upon complaints of breaches of Human Rights by individuals within the territories of the signatories to the convention, collectively known as the Council of Europe. By being a signatory to the convention, the UK government guaranteed its citizens the protection of the rights afforded by the convention. However, those rights were not incorporated into UK domestic law until October 2000. Before this date, a citizen who believed that the rights afforded to him by the convention had been breached had to bring an application before the European Court Of Human Rights. UK citizens can now rely on those rights in an action in the domestic courts.

---

have tried to influence health and social care policy to bring about improvements in health and social services in order to enhance the health and well-being of whole communities.

There are cases where these nurses advocating for patients have been systematically tortured and imprisoned without trial. You might like to bring to mind the rights you enjoy as a citizen in the society you live in. Is the society that you live in an equal society? Do all of its citizens enjoy full and equal rights? Discuss your views with colleagues. Your own and colleagues' views will be influenced by your political beliefs and by your experiences as a member of that society. As a woman in Britain you may identify continued discrimination in working practice employment through restrictive child care services. If you have a disability you may find that discrimination against you persists through the lack of safe access to particular public places. The chapter on law (Ch. 4) will provide additional information for the reader about a number of parliamentary Acts seeking to give full and equal rights to different persons in society. The development of human rights legislation in Western society is one with a short and slow history over the past 100 years. Currently under consideration is the proposal to introduce legislation to promote and protect the rights of older persons. The necessity for such legislation would seem to confirm that despite human rights declarations and codes, not all citizens enjoy the same human and civil rights as every other member of the society to which they belong. Particular groups of people report experience of finding their basic human rights violated. Some of these groups include black and ethnic minority people, the elderly, those dependent on care due to medical and physical conditions, persons diagnosed as mentally ill. Recently there have been high profile cases and inquiries into alleged violation of the human rights of persons involving some of the public services in England.

The patient as citizen has rights

A right is a justification or fair claim; being entitled to a privilege or authority to act a person may legally (agreed through national and international laws) or morally (universal agreement through declarations and codes) claim. Rights may also be negotiated by individuals in reaching an agreement on how to relate to each other, for example a contract of employment or a learning contract between student and clinical assessor.

The patient/client as a citizen has rights which impose an obligation or duty on health care staff who provide care. Incomprehensibly, it could at best be assumed, this seems to have been forgotten by the nurses and doctor referred to in Case studies 3.1 and 3.2. Nurses who accept that patients/clients admitted to an institutional setting still enjoy the same human and civil rights as every other member of society to which they belong also accept they have an obligation to respect and promote those rights. It is part of acting as an advocate and a partner in the patient's/client's care.

One way in which patients/clients may experience their human or civil rights being violated is that others begin to make decisions on their behalf. A recent case reported in the media was of a doctor who wrote in a 67-year-old patient's notes that the patient was inappropriate for resuscitation. The patient learned about the decision through requesting access to her patient record several months after her recovery from an infection. The decision had been taken by a doctor who had never met the patient nor sought her view. Campaigners said the case highlighted the way older people are being discriminated against by 'ageist' health care staff. The patient, who described herself as fit, agile, alert and articulate, with a quality of life and a few good years left, felt written off by the hospital and treated as if her life was not worth living. Her right to equitable and fair treatment and care had, she felt, been violated.

A recent development in Western society has been the formalising of the rights of various groups in society in citizens' charters.

Understanding difference

Arising out of a valuing of the individual as a person with human and civil rights is a positive acceptance of difference. Acceptance alone, however, is not sufficient. The nurse needs to explore differences between patient/client and nurse in an attempt to better understand what it means, for instance, to be black and live in a predominantly white culture; what the patient/client interprets from his own and others' experience; what the nurse understands about the patient's/client's interpretation and its match with her own. A lack of a shared understanding, even if difference is accepted, would seem likely to adversely affect the care given. The experience of racial and cultural prejudice, discrimination and disadvantage is widespread, for instance the experience of racial discrimination and the impact of stereotyping on mental health and mental health care in relation to Afro-Caribbean culture (Fannon 1993, Boyce 1998). A common experience described is the pressure on the individual to 'fit in' to a system that is informed largely by stereotypical perceptions of black people as 'non compliant, irrational, aggressive, emotional, and non verbal'.

Acceptance of difference means that patients are encouraged to assert their difference and the way of life they share with others of a particular race or ethnic group.

Look at Case study 3.5. Do you think the health care professionals concerned accepted the differences between the culture of the patient/client and their own culture? If you think they did, how well do you think they understood the patient's interpretation of her experience and what effect do you think this may have had on the patient's care. Reflecting on this case afterwards, one of the nurses involved raised several important issues for discussion with colleagues. This nurse had felt uneasy about Mary's detention and was relieved when the Section was rescinded. The nurse described how it had felt like being 'sucked in' to a situation where Mary was being treated within a system that did not seem to take account of her individual needs. The nurse recalled from cultural studies that culture influences the way in which distress is conceptualised, communicated and resolved with others. If a person feels stressed in an alien culture, it is unlikely he will find it easy to use the ways of the dominant culture to articulate and express distress and to obtain help. What is more likely is that the person under stress utilises the ways that come more naturally to him, the ways of his own culture. Were Mary's race, gender, culture and social circumstances sufficiently acknowledged and understood, together with their impact on her distress and ways of coping with this? Mary was

Case study 3.5

Mary is an Afro-Caribbean woman who came to live in England in 1995. By her first husband she has two children in their teens. She married her second husband shortly before coming to England.

Mary has an uneasy relationship with her husband and has always felt convinced that he is intent on doing her harm through his practice of voodoo. Expressing her fear and distress to her general practitioner 2 years ago resulted in Mary's referral to a psychiatrist who diagnosed 'paranoid delusion' and prescribed antipsychotic drugs.

Mary now lives separately from her husband but still has contact and believes he has the power to do her harm – including physical harm – even from a distance.

At a recent visit to the day hospital Mary told one of the nurses that she had a knife in her bag with which her husband intended to kill her. The nurse immediately spoke to the psychiatrist who instructed Mary should be admitted for a period of assessment and review of medication. Mary did not agree to this and became very agitated in response to the nurse's continued insistence that she should agree to admission. Mary refused and was admitted under Section 2 of the Mental Health Act. On attempting to leave, Mary was prevented by the nursing staff, whom she then began to attack physically. Security were called and Mary was restrained and taken to the secure unit.

Mary appealed against the Section. It was rescinded by the hospital 3 days later and she went home.

This situation left the nurse feeling uneasy and triggered her to engage in the process of enquiry, getting in touch with the value base for practice and finding a standard for judging the actions of the professionals involved, in terms of the rightness/wrongness, goodness/badness of their intervention in a moral sense.

well known to the services, yet no one demonstrated that they were trying to understand the practices Mary's husband was participating in and what this might mean for Mary living in two cultures – participating in the dominant white culture in which she lived, worked, accessed and used mental health services, while at the same time participating in those ways of life, including religion, customs and spiritual practices, which are shared with others of one's own race or culture, the minority culture in this situation. The nurse considered that there had been a complete breakdown in communication. Mary had not been given a chance to explain what was going on for her, or about her fear of the power she believed her husband had over her; that he had been able to control her to the extent that he had willed her to carry a knife with which she believed he would kill her. Had the sight of the knife been sufficient to trigger fear among the nurses and an instant gut reaction resulting from the assumption that black equals violent? Did this override the trigger that could have motivated the nurse in this situation to construct an ethical enquiry around the judgements that were being made and the choices of ways of intervening in Mary's life?

An ethical challenge arising in practice for mental health nurses is the nature of mental illness itself. Is Mary suffering from some biological dysfunction in the brain which can be treated with medication or is her distress a result of the frustration and distress arising out of trying to cope with the tensions of living in two very different cultures? Locating Mary's care within a medical framework, with a seemingly vague diagnosis, may result in ignoring a crucial aspect of her problem. Was Mary's behaviour irrational, was she lacking insight, or was this no more than a response to being treated unfairly, her voice unheard? Was Mary's physical attack on the nurses merely self-defence and physical resistance to what appeared to involve solely the exercise of power by the professionals to detain her? Detaining her in this way just served to frustrate and anger her and to increase the powerlessness she felt in her relationship with the doctor and nurses.

One argument in defence of this intervention could be if there is therapeutic benefit for the patient. Mary was detained for several days only and did not receive any treatment or therapy during this time. She experienced it as punitive and degrading and a betrayal by the nurses she had known for some time. It was felt that racist fears and assumptions had been triggered by the sight of the knife.

Challenging one's own and others' practice in this way requires courage, energy, vigilance and confidence as the experience can be subtle, leaving the nurse unsure about what may be happening. The nurse in this case demonstrated integrity and a striving to achieve practice that is fair and antidiscriminatory through examining the value basis for practice, acknowledging the professional's obligation to respect and uphold the human and civil rights of every individual, and seeking to change practice. Nurses in particular have an obligation to support patients and clients in a system that may well have difficulty interpreting and understanding difference. Being vigilant helps nurses avoid contributing to the unfair and unjust treatment of patients and clients. This may not always be easy, particularly for students who find themselves in dependent relationships with qualified nurses. However, in many practice situations students will have the opportunity and privilege to reflect with practitioners such as the nurse in Case study 3.5.

Ethics is not about being saintly or omnipotent. It is about accepting our humanity and recognising our strengths and failings and their impact on others when we are intervening in their lives. We must be motivated to strive towards being with others in a way that enhances health and wellbeing and be prepared to face up to, and change, our practices when we discover they diminish rather than enhance the lives of others. Developing a beginning stage ethical practice competence requires nurses who are willing to question their own and others' practice, to get in touch with their own and others' values and to challenge bias, prejudice and stereotyping which can adversely affect the care particular patients or groups receive. In addition, they should be willing to build the theory and knowledge frameworks with which to scrutinise some of their ideas and findings in practice – practice informed by knowledge frameworks versus practice solely based in personal opinion which is rarely reflected on or exposed to challenge.

PRESCRIPTION FOR ETHICAL REASONING, DECISION MAKING AND ACTION

The focus in this chapter has been on the individual making a judgement about what is morally right or wrong to do in a particular set of circumstances. To assist individuals in this process, several different prescriptions are offered as frameworks and guiding principles for nurses in their decision making, when making moral choices and when taking action in nursing practice.

Ethics is not a subject with a shallow end in which you can paddle around the edges; you need to jump in at the deep end. Tschudin (1992) quotes Joseph Conrad: 'it is not the clear sighted who lead the world. Great achievements are accomplished in a blessed, warm mental fog.' Ethics is a complex process of enquiry, which, ideally, is triggered in the nurse through the recognition of ethical issues and dilemmas arising in the nurse's practice situation. This enquiry requires the nurse to engage with a comprehensive knowledge and theory base using different kinds of discourses and perspectives versus personal opinion as evidence to support judgements and a standard to guide action in practice. The search for meaning is never easy, but there is a way through the fog, given commitment and determination. The key is not to get overwhelmed at this initial study stage. Nursing ethics is integral to all nursing practice and demands of the nurse a lifelong process of striving towards high-level ethical practice competence. Professional nurses are required to analyse complex arguments in order to justify and challenge ethical decisions in health care, to advise and to evaluate possible courses of action.

Getting in touch with one's personal value base is a crucial first step in the study of nursing ethics. Keeping in touch thereafter is equally important. Questioning their value choices will help nurses to see how and why they make the choices they do and expose any mismatch between what they claim is good to do and what they actually do in practice.

All of the values expressed by the caring movement are open to serious challenge. There is still a need for nurses to examine the appropriateness of caring as a basis for nursing ethics in practice. Thus it must continue to be an area of study in any programme of nursing ethics.

Linked to caring as a basis for nursing ethics is the attempt at a revival of virtue ethics, which holds that certain characteristics and virtues are an alternative basis for guiding moral thought and action. Much is still to be learned through empirical research about the many areas of life in which character is formed.

The research basis for a prescriptive theory in nursing ethics is sparse. A review of the literature indicates there is an urgent need to explore the relationship between hypothetical reasoning, practical reasoning and actual behaviour in the real lived world of practice, and to explore, through empirical research, all the factors that would seem to be influencing moral choices made in practice.

Finally, the professional nurse, in her work in clinical practice, research, management, education and politics, is dealing with the issues of power and politics in all relationships at all levels. Ethical choice decision making and choosing courses of action so often create tensions and come into conflict with the realities of power and politics in any of these relationships as in particular situations. There is a need for the study of power and politics to go hand in hand with the study of nursing ethics: one cannot practise nursing ethics without political knowledge and ability in today's complex health care system.

Through the use of narrative, nurses must tell their stories about their experiences in the practice of nursing ethics. A framework for building a case study file can be used to reflect on and record significant events and situations where there are moral issues or problems (Box 3.5). This can help nurses to tell their own stories and to learn more about their own and others' moral values and choices, emphasising the importance of the individual.

The description of ethics in practice is still awaited. It would seem that the prescriptions offered as frameworks in this chapter to guide practice are insufficient in themselves to provide an adequate theory upon which to decide moral decisions, justify and motivate moral action. However, all are essential areas of study in nursing ethics. This body of knowledge and understanding can then be taken into practice, so that the student and the professional nurse can learn about and begin to articulate the moral sense of

---

Box 3.5   A framework for building a case study file of ethical issues and dilemmas

Build a case study file of the ethical issues and dilemmas that you or others have found challenging in practice. You might find the following questions useful to guide your reflection on your documented case studies. Remember your obligation to protect confidentiality. Do not place information in your file that can directly identify any persons (e.g. do not use names, addresses, locations). Remember that it is a breach of confidentiality to fail to protect private and personal information, even if that information is not shared or a person identified. The questions are constructed to guide nurses' reflection and beginning analysis in developing a beginning level ethics practice competence:

1. *Identify the ethical issue*
   - What is the dilemma?

2. *Examine the issue*
   - What are the values and beliefs (your own and others) being brought to the situation? Are there conflicts? Whose? Why?
   - Nursing and the organisation. Are there conflicts? Whose? Why?
   - Are there rights and duties involved? Whose? Why?
   - Are there disputed facts about the evidence base for care?
   - Is there any research? Is it valid and reliable?
   - What are the ethical principles involved? (e.g. autonomy, justice, beneficence, non-maleficence)
   - What does the law say?
   - What does the profession have to say? (e.g. codes of practice)

- What do other professionals have to say? (e.g. codes of practice, contracts)
- What does the organization have to say? (e.g. policies, procedures, protocols)
- Who is deciding? Why?
- What are the choices of action?
- What are the arguments for choosing between the possible choices of action? Use moral theory and nursing as caring to formulate these. Which are weak arguments? Which are strong? Why?

3. *Propose a course of action*
   - Am I confident to propose a course of action and to act on it? Why?
   - How would I justify choosing or not choosing? Acting or not acting?
   - What have I learned from this experience?
   - What still needs to be learned?
   - How will this experience affect my developing practice?
   - What might I do differently next time?
   - What do I need to do next?

Further stages of questioning (not included here) are designed to take the nurse engaged in higher-level study and practice into deeper reflection, analysis and challenge of some of the arguments, logical reasoning, making judgements, deciding, justifying and evaluating different courses of action.

---

nursing practice, thus contributing to the development of nursing's ethical knowledge base.

Achieving a beginning level ethical practice competence requires the nurse to:

- build and begin to use comprehensive knowledge and theory frameworks within which to consider ethical issues and dilemmas and to defend and challenge action in practice
- recognise the gaps in nursing knowledge and seek to resolve these
- move away from making decisions and acting solely out of one's own personal values and opinions, unreflective right and wrong judgements
- further develop knowledge and understanding about self with others and behaviour through getting in touch with those extra dimensions in one's own and

others' lives which include values, beliefs and attitudes
- increase ability to recognise ethical issues in practice through creating and maintaining a case study file.

REFERENCES

Allmark P 1995 Uncertainties in the teaching of ethics to students of nursing. Journal of Advanced Nursing 22(2): 374–378

Aroskar M 1982 Are nurses' minds set compatible with ethical practice? Topics in Clinical Nursing 4(1): 22–32

Bandura A 1997 Social learning theory. Prentice Hall, New Jersey

Barker P J, Reynolds W, Word T 1995 The proper focus of nursing: a critique of the 'caring' ideology. International Journal of Nursing Studies 32(4): 386–397

Beauchamp T L, Childress J E 1994 Principles of biomedical ethics, 4th edn. Oxford University Press, Oxford

Benner P, Wrubel J 1989 The primacy of caring: stress and coping in health and disease. Addison Wesley, California

Berlin I 1969 Four essays on liberty. Oxford University Press, Oxford

Boyce K 1998 Asserting difference: psychiatric care in black and white. In: Barker P, Davidson B (eds) Psychiatric nursing: ethical strife. Arnold, London, ch 11, pp 157–170

Boykin A, Schoenhofer S 1993 Nursing as caring. National League for Nursing Press, New York

Brown J, Kitson A, McKnight T 1992 Challenges in caring. Chapman and Hall, London

Butler R 1997 Ageing beyond the millennium. Nuffield Trust and Age Concern, Cymru/Wales

Brykczynska G 2000 Not quite the judgement of Solomon. Paediatric Nursing 12(9): 6–8

Cain P 1999 Respecting and breaking confidences: conceptual, ethical and educational issues. Nurse Education Today 19: 175–181

Carper B 1978 Fundamental patterns of knowing in nursing. Advances in Nursing Science 1: 13–24

Davies C 1995 Gender and the professional predicament of nursing. Open University Press, Buckingham

Department of Health 1992 The patients' charter. HMSO, London

Department of Health 1998 A first class service: improving quality in the NHS. Stationery Office, London

Department of Health 1999 Making a difference: strengthening the nursing, midwifery and health visiting contribution to health and health care. Stationery Office, London

Dyson J 1996 Nurses', conceptualisations of caring attitudes and behaviours. Journal of Advanced Nursing 23(6): 1263–1269

Erlen J, Frost B 1992 Nurses' perceptions of powerlessness in influencing ethical decisions. Western Journal of Nursing Research 13(3): 397–407

Fannon F 1993 Black skin, white masks. Pluto Classic, London

Fitzpatrick J, White A, Roberts J 1993 The relationship between nursing and higher education. Journal of Advanced Nursing 18: 1488–1497

Foot P 1978 Virtues and vices. Basil Blackwell, Oxford

Frankl V 1978 Man's search for meaning. Hodder and Stoughton, London

Fries J F 1990 The compression of morbidity: near or far? Millbank Q 67: 208–232

Gallagher V, Boyd K 1991 Teaching and learning nursing ethics. Scutari Press, London

Gilligan C 1982 In a different voice: psychological theory and women's development. Harvard University Press, Cambridge

Gillon R 1986 Philosophical medical ethics. John Wiley, Chichester

Gillon R (ed) 1994 Principles of health care ethics. John Wiley, Chichester

Greenwood J 1998 The role of reflection in single and double loop learning. Journal of Advanced Nursing 27: 1048–1053

Hall J 1989 Towards a psychology of caring. British Journal of Clinical Psychology 29: 129–144

Hayter M 1996 Is non-judgemental care possible in the context of nurses' attitudes to patients' sexuality? Journal of Advanced Nursing 24: 662–666

Held V 1990 Feminist transformations of moral theory. Philosophy and Phenomenological Research 50: 321–344

Hoffman M 1979 The development of moral thought, feeling and behaviour. American Psychologist 34: 958–966

Hume D 1978 A treatise of human nature, ed. P Nidditch, 2nd edn. Oxford University Press, Oxford

Joudrey R 1999 Caring and curing revisited: student nurses' perceptions of nurses' and physicians' ethical stances. Journal of Advanced Nursing 29: 1154–1162

Kinsella K 1996 Demographic aspects. In: Ebrihim S, Kalache A (eds) Epidemiology of old age. British Medical Journal in collaboration with the World Health Organization, London

Kohlberg L 1984 Essays in moral development. Vol. 11: The psychology of moral development. Harper and Row, New York

Koldjeski D 1990 Towards a theory of professional nursing caring: a unifying perspective. In: Leininger M, Watson J (eds) The caring imperative in education. National League for Nursing, New York, pp 45–57

Lauri S, Lepisto M, Kappeli S 1997 Patients' needs in hospital: nurses' and patients' views. Journal of Advanced Nursing 25: 339–346

Leininger M (ed) 1981 Caring: an essential human need. Proceedings of Three National Conferences. Charles Slack, New Jersey

Leininger M 1984 Care: the essence of nursing and health. Charles Slack, New Jersey

Leininger M 1988 Caring: a central focus of nursing and health care services. In: Leininger M (ed) Care: the essence of nursing and health. University Press, New York, pp 45–59

MacIntyre A 1993 After virtue: a study in moral theory. Duckworth, London

Marck P 1990 Therapeutic reciprocity: a caring phenomenon. Advances in Nursing Science 13(1): 45–59

May T 1993 The nurse under physician authority. Journal of Medical Ethics 19: 223–227

McAlpine H, Kristjanson L, Poroch D 1997 Development and testing of the ethical reasoning tool (ERT): an instrument to measure ethical reasoning of nurses. Journal of Advanced Nursing 25: 1151–1161

McKenna G 1993 Caring is the essence of nursing. British Journal of Nursing 2(1): 72–75

Morse J, Solberg S, Neander W, Bottorff J, Johnson J 1990 Concepts of caring and caring as a concept. Advances in Nursing Science 13(1): 1–14

News Focus 1996 Nursing Times 92(40): 16–17

News Focus 2000 Nursing Standard 15(10): 8

Noddings N 1984 Caring: a feminine approach to ethics and moral education. University of California Press, London

Olson J, Hanchett E 1997 Nurse expressed empathy, patient outcomes and development of middle-range theory. Image: Journal of Nursing Scholarship 29(1): 71–79

Plunkett P 1999 New Hampshire nurses: what are our concerns, resources and education in ethics? Nursing News 49(3): 3

Rachels J 1998 The ethics of virtue and the ethics of right action. In: Cahn S M, Markie P Ethics history theory and contemporary issues. Oxford University Press, New York, ch 35, pp 669–681

Rafael A 1996 Power and caring: a dialectic in nursing. Advances in Nursing Science 19(1): 3–17

Ranade W 1993 A future for the NHS? Care in the 1990s. Longman, London

Raths L, Harmin M, Simon S 1966 Values and teaching. Merrill, Columbus, Ohio

Rest J 1990 Guide for the defining issues test. University of Minnesota, Minneapolis

Roach M 1987 The human act of caring. Canadian Hospital Association, Ottawa

Rogers C 1951 Client centred therapy. Constable, London

Rowson R H 1990 An introduction to ethics for nurses. Scutari Press, London

Sadler J 1997 Defining professional nurse caring: a triangulation study. International Journal of Human Caring 1(3): 12–21

Seedhouse D 1988 Ethics: the heart of health care. Wiley, Chichester

Seedhouse D 1998 Ethics: the heart of health care, 2nd edn. Wiley, Chichester

Stein L, Watts D, Howell T 1990 The doctor nurse game revisited. New England Journal of Medicine 322(8): 546–549

Stockwell F 1972 The unpopular patient. Royal College of Nursing, London

Suzman R M, Willis D P, Manton K G (eds) 1992 The oldest old. OUP, New York

Tschudin V 1992 Values: a primer for nurses. Workbook. Baillière Tindall, London

Udén G, Norberg A, Lindseth A, Marhanga V 1992 Ethical reasoning in nurses' and physicians' stories about care episodes. Journal of Advanced Nursing 17: 1028–1034

United Kingdom Central Council for Nursing, Midwifery and Health Visiting 1992 Code of professional conduct. UKCC, London

United Kingdom Central Council for Nursing, Midwifery and Health Visiting Commission for Education 1999 Fitness for practice. UKCC, London

United Nations 1948 Universal declaration of human rights. UN, Geneva

Warner M, Lonley M, Gould E, Pice K A 1998 Health care futures 2010. Welsh Institute for Health and Social Care, University, Glamorgan

Watson J 1985 Nursing: the philosophy and science of caring. University Press of Colorado, Colorado

Watson J 1997 The theory of human caring: retrospective and prospective. Nursing Science Quarterly 10(1): 49–52

Watson R, Lea A 1997 The caring dimensions inventory (CD1) content validity, reliability and scaling. Journal of Advanced Nursing 25: 87–94

Wilson J 1998 Clinical governance. British Journal of Nursing 7(16): 985–986

FURTHER READING

During your studies all of your reading about nursing theory and nursing research will contribute to your learning about nursing ethics and achieving a beginning level ethics practice competence. The more comprehensive your nursing knowledge and theory base, the richer the process of ethical enquiry can be. This means you can bring all of your learning in the curriculum to your study and practice of ethics. It is important nurses access the literature manually and electronically on a regular basis to read and keep up to date about nursing, health, health and social policy and politics.

The following are some key texts for the nurse who wishes to read more fully about some of the moral theories introduced in this chapter:

Cahn S M, Markie P (eds) 1998 Ethics history, theory and contemporary issues. Oxford University Press, New York

Singer P (ed) 1994 Ethics. Oxford University Press, Oxford

The following are some useful texts for the nurse who wishes to read further about some of the current challenges for nursing and caring:

Norman I, Cowley S (eds) 1999 The changing nature of nursing. Blackwell, Oxford

Seedhouse D 2000 Practical nursing philosophy: the universal ethical code. Wiley, Chichester

Walsh M 2000 Nursing frontiers, accountability and the boundaries of care. Butterworth-Heinemann, Oxford

The following is one of several useful texts for the nurse who wishes to read further about reflective practice:

Johns C, Freshwater D (eds) 1998 Transforming nursing through reflective practice. Blackwell, Oxford

The following is one of several useful texts for the nurse who wishes to read further about power and nursing practice from a sociological perspective:

Wilkinson G, Miers M 1999 Power and nursing practice. Macmillan, London

4

Legal issues

Helen Caulfield

CHAPTER CONTENTS

Importance of the law   113

Sources of law   114
Legislation   114
Common law   115
Differences between the law and the
   nursing professional body   115

Legal forums   115
   Courts   116
   Employment tribunals   116
   Inquests   116
   Public inquiries   116
   Lawyers   116

Criminal law   116
Criminal law affecting nursing   117
   Abortion   117
   Death and dying   118
   Assault   119

Civil law   119
Civil law affecting nursing   119
   Consent   119
   Negligence   123
   Confidentiality   125

Documentation   126
   Data Protection Acts 1984 and 1998   127
   Access to Medical Reports Act 1988   127
   Access to Health Records Act 1990   127
   Wills   127
   Accident and incident reports   127

References   127

Further reading   128

A good foundation in legal principles for nursing will increase each nurse's confidence in practising nursing skills, and an enhanced ability to identify potential legal problems will enable nurses to become the advocates of their patients and clients. This chapter on the legal aspects of nursing aims to:

- consider the importance of the law to nursing
- describe sources of the law and the system by which the legal process works
- explore criminal and civil law with respect to various aspects of nursing practice and different client groups
- outline the legal requirements for particular types of health care documentation.

IMPORTANCE OF THE LAW

Nurses face increasing dilemmas in their practice which require an assessment of the professional, ethical and legal aspects of many situations. Some may be obvious: for example what is the nurse's role when the police arrive at an accident and emergency department and ask for details about a patient's condition? Some, however, are more subtle: what about the patient with AIDS who is in great pain and requests the nurse to increase pain-relieving medication to an extent that both know will result in the patient's death? How do nurses in the community respond to a patient who assaults them – do they have to continue providing nursing care or does the law also allow a measure of self-defence? When a nurse wishes to provide care to a child who flatly refuses to receive any treatment, how does the nurse respond, and what is the legal position of the child's refusal?

Many nurses faced with these and other situations will look to their professional Code of Conduct for guidance, or they may ask managers for assistance. Knowledge of the legal principles involved will also be important to help nurses recognise the lawful boundaries applicable to these health care situations. Employers and other members of the health care team will also know that they are required to act within the law and that failure to do so could mean a potential action in civil or criminal law.

The role of nursing is becoming more independent in some areas, and it is increasingly important that nurses working in these fields are aware, on an individual basis, of the legal principles that apply to their work. Such knowledge leads to greater confidence on the part of the nurse.

Patients and their families have an increased awareness of their rights and appear to be more willing than in the past to challenge health care decisions. Publications such as the Patient's Charter increase patients' confidence to demand better standards of care and treatment. There is a perception that litigation will play an increasing part in the provision of health care services, and more people are turning to the courts for assistance on the extent and degree of health care that should be provided.

Legislation is now playing a fundamental role in determining boundaries for the provision of health care. Along with legislation providing for NHS Trusts and extended community care, other Acts of Parliament deal with, for example, access to health records, transplantation, abortion, provision of mental health care and childcare.

It is becoming more important for nurses to be aware of these developments in the law, and just as important for nurses to ensure that their own practice is reflected in future legislation. The nurse who acts as the patient's advocate will influence social policy-making by demanding high standards of health care provision, and a

working knowledge of legal principles in this field will enrich the nurse's own approach to her work.

SOURCES OF LAW

LEGISLATION

A statute is an Act of Parliament that sets out the law in a formal document. Examples of statutes are the Children Act 1989, the Human Embryology and Fertilisation Act 1990, the Data Protection Act 1998 and the Health Act 1999. Each Act follows a formal and detailed procedure of debate and voting in the House of Commons and the House of Lords. Statutes form a body of law that set out in detail how individuals must act. If someone fails to act in accordance with any part of a statute, a criminal penalty may be imposed. For example, there are criminal penalties in the Medicines Act 1968 which set out the level of fine that can be imposed on a nurse who prescribes without authority.

Secondary legislation is a process by which quicker legislation can be passed with minimal debating time in the House of Commons. The Nursing, Midwives and Health Visitors Act 1997 creates a legal duty for the United Kingdom Central Council for Nursing, Midwifery and Health Visiting (UKCC) to hold professional conduct hearings into allegations of improper conduct on the part of a nurse. The rules that govern the conduct hearing itself are provided in a statutory instrument (Nurses, Midwives and Health Visitors Rules 1993). The effect of this statutory instrument is to oblige the UKCC to follow a certain procedure in its investigation and hearings of these matters.

A further source of legislation comes from Europe, which requires member states to implement Community law through their own Acts of Parliament. European legislation, which is also known as European Directives, encompasses a variety of issues, including the 1990 European Directive (90/269/EEC) on the manual handling of loads and Directive 92/85/EEC on the protection of the rights of pregnant workers.

COMMON LAW

Where no legislation exists to determine the law on a particular subject, common law will be used.

Common law is made by judges who sit in court and determine how a legal dispute between two or more parties is to be resolved. The law relating to negligence, for example, is not defined in a statute but has evolved over time through various court decisions. These decisions form a body of law. Patients who allege that negligent treatment has led to injury will have their disputes heard in court, and the legal principles that apply will be those of the common law of negligence.

In many health care situations, an application can be made to the court for guidance on legal issues where no legislation exists. In 1993, the legal issues surrounding the withdrawal of treatment from a patient in a persistent vegetative state were discussed in court in the case of *Airedale NHS Trust* v. *Bland* [1993]. Among the arguments raised were questions of whether it was lawful to withdraw artificial hydration and nutrition from the patient, knowing that it would lead to his death. This was the first time this situation had been raised, and no other legislation existed to clarify the issues involved. Such cases become legal precedent, so that future decisions can refer back to the judicial reasoning that took place in earlier cases. The principles laid down by the court in Bland's case have already been followed in at least one other situation (*Frenchay Healthcare NHS Trust* v. *S* [1994]).

DIFFERENCES BETWEEN THE LAW AND THE NURSING PROFESSIONAL BODY

The UKCC is the regulatory body of the nursing, midwifery and health visiting professions, and was set up by an Act of Parliament, the Nurses, Midwives and Health Visitors Act 1979, later amended by two further Acts (Nurses, Midwives and Health Visitors Acts of 1992 and 1997). The UKCC is charged with acting as Parliament's representative in regulating the profession. The UKCC has drawn up a Code of Conduct (revised in June 1992) which sets out the extent of the professional duty required of a nurse, midwife or health visitor. It is a requirement of the UKCC that the professions adhere to the Code of Conduct, and failure to do so will potentially lead to a nurse, midwife or health visitor being disciplined or even removed from the Register.

The UKCC determines professional duty, which may differ from the nurse's legal duty. A nurse's legal duty can be defined by looking at relevant statutes and common law. There is, for example, no legal duty for a nurse to promote the interests of a patient, but there is a professional duty to do so under the Code of Conduct, paragraph 1. A nurse who appears in court for any reason may be found liable in negligence, or guilty of a criminal offence, and while the courts have power to order a nurse to pay compensation or to impose a criminal sentence, they do not have power to order that a nurse be prohibited from working as a nurse. The UKCC alone holds the power to determine whether or not the nurse has behaved in a professional manner.

The UKCC will not require a nurse to behave in a manner that is unlawful, and the principles behind each section of the Code of Conduct are based on the common law (see Ch. 11).

The result of this is that a nurse has a professional duty to the UKCC that may be different from the legal duty owed to clients, colleagues and employers (Wright & Caulfield 1994).

LEGAL FORUMS

Disputes that need to be resolved within the legal system will be heard in public. It is rare for a legal case to be resolved by a judge in private, although in cases where a vulnerable person is involved, such as in child abuse or mental health cases, it is common for the person to be referred to by their initials so that their full identity is protected. It is always open to the parties involved in the dispute to reach an agreement before the public hearing. This avoids any resultant publicity and helps to keep legal costs down. There are several types of legal forum, each governed by its own procedures.

Courts

There are civil courts and criminal courts, ranging from magistrates courts to high courts, each of which has its own system of resolving particular cases. Courts are considered in more detail below.

Employment tribunals

Employment tribunals deal with disputes relating to employment, including discrimination and redundancy. Each party is required to pay its own costs at the end of a case. The tribunal has power to hear employment cases and make rulings, which include the power to order reinstatement or a payment of compensation if a finding of unfair dismissal or discrimination is made. The Arbitration and Conciliation Advisory Service (ACAS) will attempt to arbitrate between both sides to assist in reaching a settlement before the hearing.

Inquests

The purpose of an inquest is to investigate the circumstances of a death that may not have been natural or expected. A coroner directs the hearing and can put questions directly to a witness. A jury sits and listens to the evidence and return a verdict in relation to the circumstances of the death. Any nurse who is required to attend an inquest should notify her manager to ask for guidance. Most employers should provide legal assistance to any nurse in this situation. Where it seems that there may be a conflict, the nurse should contact her professional body or trade union.

Public inquiries

A matter of national concern can be handled by a public inquiry, set up and funded by the government, in which witnesses are asked to give evidence in a formal setting. Nurses who are requested to give evidence should seek assistance in handling both the hearing and any consequent publicity. A report is published after the inquiry has ended and recommendations will be made to remedy the problems leading to the crisis. For example, the Kennedy Report in 2001 looked into the background of the deaths of children at Bristol Royal Infirmary and published recommendations that have to be considered by the government, which is then required to say which recommendations will be accepted.

Lawyers

The people who work within the legal system are called lawyers and may be solicitors, barristers, judges or legal executives. Solicitors are able to advise clients directly about the legal position on a case and are based in offices accessible to the public. They can represent clients in some courts and generally advise on a wide range of issues from conveyancing to divorce. Barristers are self-employed lawyers instructed by solicitors who may require detailed research into the law or may need to use the specialised advocacy skills of a barrister in court. The general public cannot approach a barrister directly and must go through a solicitor. After 10 years, a barrister may wish to become a Queen's Counsel (QC) and then take on more complex cases. Murder trials must be presented by a QC.

Judges are generally barristers, although more solicitors are being encouraged to apply for such positions. The role of the judge is to direct the hearing in a civil or criminal trial and ensure that the correct rules of law and procedure are applied. In a criminal case, the judge will determine the sentence if the defendant has been found guilty. In civil cases, the judge will decide the level of compensation to be awarded to a successful claimant.

Legal executives work in solicitors' offices, and although they are not as highly qualified as solicitors, they can deal with their own cases and see clients. Lawyers or doctors can apply to become coroners and preside over inquests; they are subject to their own rules of procedure and conduct.

CRIMINAL LAW

The criminal law is found in statutes. Anyone breaking the rules in a particular Act of Parliament could be guilty of a crime. For example, if a nurse steals sheets from the linen cupboard of a hospital and is discovered, she could be guilty of theft under the provisions contained in the Theft Act 1969. The police have powers to investigate a suspected crime. If the police believe that there is a criminal case, papers are sent to the Crown Prosecution Service, where an independent assessment takes place to decide whether or not prosecution should take place. If it should, the case is initially heard in the magistrates court.

Every town has a magistrates court. Magistrates (who are not lawyers) are drawn from the community and have power to decide a person's guilt or innocence and to pass sentence. When a case comes before the magistrates court that is beyond the legal powers of the magistrates to deal with, for example a charge of murder or rape, the magistrates refer the case to the crown court. In the crown court, barristers represent both the defendant and the prosecution. A judge directs the hearing before a jury of 12 people, again non-lawyers chosen from the community. It is the task of the jury to decide *beyond reasonable doubt* whether or not the defendant is guilty, and they carry out their deliberations in secret. If a finding of guilt is made, the judge can hear evidence from the defendant (a plea in mitigation) before deciding on an appropriate sentence.

The function of criminal law is to determine the boundaries of behaviour acceptable to society and within which members of society are allowed to act freely. The criminal law system is designed to allow the defendant to dispute the allegations before a representative section of society.

CRIMINAL LAW AFFECTING NURSING

A crime occurs when the legal provisions in a statute are broken. It must be shown beyond reasonable doubt that a crime has been committed, to the satisfaction of a jury, before the person charged can be convicted. While it is unlikely that nurses will face the prospect of prosecution for a criminal offence in their professional careers, the advances of clinical care are constantly being

tested against provisions that make up the criminal law. For example, it is an offence under the Suicide Act 1961 to assist a person to commit suicide, and there are difficulties for health professionals in interpreting this, particularly where a patient may be requesting extra medication to cope with a painful illness, which may be sufficient to end his life.

Most of the problems in assessing whether clinical treatment may or may not be criminal occur at the beginning or the end of life, and the law has gone some way in assessing the extent of the nurse's legal role in these areas.

Abortion

The criminal law relating to abortion is found in the Abortion Act 1967, with amendments subsequently made in s.37 Human Fertilisation and Embryology Act 1990.

It is an offence under the Abortion Act to procure an abortion unless certain conditions have been fulfilled. Where two doctors have formed an opinion in good faith that the pregnancy would involve a risk of injury to the physical or mental health of the pregnant woman or to any of her other children, and as long as the pregnancy has not progressed beyond its 24th week, a termination of the pregnancy may be lawfully carried out by a doctor. It is possible to terminate a pregnancy after the 24th week if a risk exists of grave permanent injury to the pregnant woman, including a risk to her life, or where there is a substantial risk that the child might be born with severe physical or mental handicap.

Abortion is therefore unlawful unless the criteria set out in the statute are fulfilled. The moral and ethical debate surrounding the termination of pregnancy will continue to influence any future legislation, and much debate centres on the rights of the fetus and the point at which the fetus becomes a person. The law gives full legal status to an infant born alive. A stillborn delivery has no legal standing, as the law does not give any legal rights to an embryo or fetus until it is capable of being born alive.

The Abortion Act 1967 allows a person with a conscientious objection under s.4 of the Act to

Case example 4.1

In the case of *R. v. Salford Health Authority ex p. Janaway* in 1988, a doctor's receptionist refused to type the letter referring a patient for a termination. She justified her refusal by claiming conscientious objection under section 4 of the Abortion Act 1967. The court found that the receptionist was so removed from the actual treatment that s.4 did not apply to her. This test of proximity is a difficult one to assess in relation to nurses, particularly where they may be expected to move around a hospital in a far more flexible manner than a doctor, who may be assigned to a particular ward.

withdraw from participating in treatment connected with a termination, except where treatment is needed to save the life of the woman or prevent grave permanent injury to her health.

The role of nurses in abortion is problematic and possibly not fully recognised by the legislation or subsequent judicial cases. While it is clear that a nurse may rely on s.4 conscientiously to object to participating in the treatment connected with an abortion, this would seem to apply only to the abortion itself. It is less clear whether or not a nurse could refuse to care for a woman who was transferred to a general medical ward following an operation. Case example 4.1 considers how far this legislation extends.

Death and dying

Allowing the patient to die can be complex in law. There is a legal difference between letting something happen and active intervention to ensure that it occurs. The law accepts that each person has the legal right to determine what will happen to his body, and interference by a third party may be unlawful.

There is no legislation that allows euthanasia, and the intentional killing of another person is murder. Where a health care practitioner wishes to assist a patient to die through some form of intervention, a charge of manslaughter may be brought if the intervention was unlawful. This will be the case even where the patient requests assistance, for example by an increased level of

medication in order to cause death. In *R. v. Cox* [1992], a doctor was convicted of attempted murder after he gave an injection of potassium chloride to a patient with an incurable illness, knowing that she would die almost immediately.

It is lawful to provide treatment to relieve pain and suffering even where this may have the unintended effect of hastening death, and treatment for these purposes will not constitute manslaughter. In the Cox case, the injection of potassium chloride was intended to cause death rather than to relieve pain and suffering, and was, as such, a criminal offence.

Where the patient is unable to be involved in the decision-making process, the legal concept of 'best interests' has been used to decide the most effective care that should be provided. This has arisen in relation to the selective non-treatment of severely handicapped neonates. When a child is born with severe physical and mental handicaps, the choice is to provide intensive therapy, usually involving surgery, to alleviate symptoms and prolong life, or to make a decision to provide only pain-relieving medication when there is a possibility that the child will die. When such cases come to court, the argument of best interests is used to determine which treatment programme should be followed. In *Re C* [1989], the court directed that a hydrocephalic child should be treated in such a way that she would end her life peacefully. It was considered to be in the best interests of the child that she be given non-invasive treatment.

In the Bland case cited above, a different situation was presented to the court. The patient had been in a persistent vegetative state for over 3 years following injuries sustained at Hillsborough Football Stadium. He was on a ventilator, and was receiving artificial hydration and nutrition. The court was asked to consider whether the withdrawal of artificial hydration and nutrition would be lawful. Legal argument took place in the High Court, the Court of Appeal and the House of Lords, where it was agreed that there was no prospect of recovery from this condition and that the withdrawal of the treatment would be in the patient's best interests. It was accepted that, by removing this treatment the patient would die, and that it was lawful for the doctors to proceed in this manner as continuation of the treatment would be futile. In the absence of any subsequent legislation, it will be for the court to decide the criteria to be used in assessing the legal definition of a patient's best interests when deciding whether treatment should be given or withdrawn.

Assault

It is a reflection of the changing nature of relationships that there is an increasing number of recorded assaults by patients on nurses. These occur most commonly in community, psychiatric and accident and emergency nursing. Most employers have a policy that means the assailant is not reported to the police, and no prosecution takes place. Very often, the attack may be the manifestation of the illness that is being treated.

Where a prosecution does take place, it will be heard in the magistrates court, and the nurse attacked will be required to give evidence. If the assailant is found guilty, the magistrates have powers to order that an amount of compensation be paid to the nurse by the assailant.

If the injuries sustained are serious and result in the nurse taking time off work to recover physically or psychologically, it is possible to make an application to the Criminal Injuries Compensation Authority, which can make a separate award of compensation for injuries received as a result of a violent attack without the necessity for a criminal prosecution.

Nurses are legally entitled to use a measure of self-protection if they fear an attack from a patient. The measure of self-defence must be in proportion to the threat or attack itself: it would be reasonable for a nurse to push a patient who was threatening to strangle her, but it would not be reasonable for a nurse to do this if the patient were shouting abuse. Most hospitals have introduced control and restraint courses, from which nurses can learn non-violent means of deflecting perceived or actual attacks. When any attack takes place, even if there is no injury, it is imperative that it is reported immediately so that appropriate steps for the safety of the nurse and the patient can be taken.

CIVIL LAW

Civil law is designed to resolve differences between individuals. As a consequence, civil law encompasses a wider range of issues than does criminal law, including negligence, employment, divorce, childcare, libel, defamation and any other matter that is not criminal in nature.

Because civil law is concerned with disputes between parties, court hearings do not require the use of magistrates or a jury (with the historic exception of libel hearings, which need to be heard before a jury). Matters that involve smaller value claims are heard in the county court and more complex or higher value claims are heard in the high court.

CIVIL LAW AFFECTING NURSING

The majority of health care situations that need legal involvement will be civil matters. It will be far more common for a nurse to be affected by civil law than criminal law decisions. Some of the most important areas of civil law are assessed here. The development of health law is constantly reshaping nursing practice, although the basic principles set out below should remain unchanged.

Consent

It is an established part of law that no treatment can be given to a person without consent – this is a fundamental foundation of the law. Any clinical professional who touches a patient or client without consent commits a battery that is both a civil and a criminal offence. It is extremely rare for a health care professional to be prosecuted under the criminal law for battery, but civil actions brought by patients for an unlawful touching are more common (*Devi* v. *West Midlands RHA* [1981]; *Marshall* v. *Curry* [1993]). If a nurse gives an injection to a patient who has not consented to being touched, the nurse will have acted unlawfully and will have committed a battery (see Ch. 14).

It is important that the consent itself must be obtained in a way that does not render it invalid.

If a nurse tries to persuade a patient to agree to invasive treatment by, for example, threatening the patient, it will automatically mean that any agreement given by the patient becomes invalid, as the consent was not obtained voluntarily. In this situation, even where the patient says yes and signs a consent form, the consent will have been obtained in an unlawful manner and any subsequent treatment will also be unlawful.

In order for a consent to be valid it must consist of three elements:

- The person giving consent must have the capacity to do so.
- The consent given must be informed.
- The consent must be given in a voluntary manner.

1. The person giving consent must have the capacity to do so. It is vital that a person giving consent has the capacity to understand what is involved in the proposed treatment. It is accepted that adults over the age of 18 automatically have the relevant capacity to understand and make their own decisions about medical and nursing treatment.

2. The consent given must be informed. Informed consent has caused much discussion among health care professionals. Just how much information needs to be given to a person before he has enough on which to make a decision? The most famous case on this point is that of *Sidaway v. Board of Governors of Bethlem Royal Hospital* [1985] (Case example 4.2).

There is no duty imposed by law on a health care professional to inform the patient of all the likely risks or advantages in the proposed treatment, and the courts have held that the extent of what to tell the patient lies within the doctor's discretion. If the patient asks questions, these should be answered truthfully, but again the doctor can use discretion on the amount of information that should be volunteered, and can withhold information for good reason (although this may require later justification if the case ever comes to court).

How does an individual nurse decide what information should be given and what could be held back? The test for this was formulated in the

Case example 4.2

Amy Sidaway agreed to an operation. She was not told that there was a very small risk that her spinal cord might be damaged. In the operation the risk materialised, and she suffered partial paralysis. She argued that she would not have consented to the procedure had she been told of the risk, and her claim in court was that her whole consent was invalid as she had not received sufficient information to make an informed consent. This argument was rejected by the House of Lords, who found that the doctor had fulfilled his duties in relation to informed consent by telling the patient of the material risks, alternatives to the treatment and the nature and consequences of the proposed treatment. In addition, there is a duty on the doctor to assess whether the particular patient requires any further information.

case of *Bolam* v. *Friern Hospital Management Committee* [1957], in which the court decided that the standard of care required of a nurse is to act in accordance with a recognised body of nursing opinion and practice. The standard is therefore determined by the nursing profession itself and not by reference to an individual patient. This standard of care has been criticised for failing to give sufficient weight to the patient's own circumstances, and it has been suggested that a nurse or doctor should provide the patient with all the information in her possession in order to enable the patient to make an informed decision. This has been largely rejected by the courts as being impractical and overburdensome on the health care professional.

3. The consent must be given in a voluntary manner. Consent must be freely given and no threats or implied threats used. Threats such as the use of a compulsory section under the Mental Health Act 1984 if treatment is not accepted nullify the consent. Whether treatment is voluntary will depend on what information is given to the patient and how this is presented. Coercion or manipulation of the patient would tend to imply that the consent has not been obtained voluntarily.

Once these three criteria have been established, a valid consent can be given to treatment or care. Most hospitals require patients to sign a consent form before agreeing to invasive treatment, and some health professionals have mistakenly placed too much emphasis on such a signature being obtained. A signed consent form does not prove that the consent is valid, but it is usually good evidence that a discussion on consent has taken place. In this context, a consent form is important evidence, but it should never be considered the sole factor needed to be taken into account in establishing proper consent with patients.

Particular aspects of consent in relation to different sections of society need separate consideration, and are dealt with below.

Young people

Those over the age of 18 years are allowed to make their own decisions about treatment and care. Between the ages of 16 and 18 years, adolescents can consent to treatment under the provisions of the Family Law Reform Act s.8 (1). The more problematic area concerns adolescents under the age of 16. The legal position is established in *Gillick* v. *West Norfolk and Norwich AHA* [1985], which allows adolescents under 16 years to consent to treatment provided they have sufficient understanding and intelligence to enable them to understand fully what is proposed. Adolescents of sufficient understanding to make an informed decision have the right to consent to examination and treatment. They also have the right to refuse the treatment or care. The question of deciding whether or not an adolescent is capable of understanding is determined by the doctor, although it is likely that nurses, for example, would be able to give treatment to children when they have made a professional assessment that the child has the understanding to know what is proposed and involved in the nursing treatment.

Where the child is not capable of giving consent, the guardian of a child under the age of 16 years may give valid consent on behalf of the child.

The court has, however, indicated that such a child does not have the final say in refusing treatment, and has held that any refusal of treatment by a child is not conclusive (*Re W* [1992]). It is open to the parents or guardians to override that refusal and to consent to the treatment proposed by the health professional. Where a nurse is confronted with a strong difference of opinion between a child and a parent or guardian over proposed treatment, the nurse should always seek advice to ensure the correct weight is given to the child's wishes. In some situations, it may be necessary to ask the court to decide between the conflicting wishes. For example, if a 14-year-old girl involved in a road accident refuses any blood transfusions because of her religious beliefs, her parents may want to override her refusal so that treatment can proceed. It may be difficult for the doctor or nurse to determine how far the child's wishes should be taken into account. In this type of situation, a court would be able to hear the evidence and make a decision to be followed by all parties.

Adults

In contrast to the rights of a child to refuse treatment, the court of appeal upheld a case in 1992 that affirmed in strong terms an adult patient's right to refuse medical treatment (*Re T* [1992]). In this case, a woman aged 22 years was involved in a car accident and, while in hospital, told medical staff both orally and in writing that she did not want a blood transfusion should one become necessary. Her condition deteriorated and she was placed on a ventilator. When it became apparent that a blood transfusion would be required, she was unable to give specific consent or refusal. The court of appeal upheld the view that a competent adult patient has a right to refuse medical treatment even if the outcome will be that the patient will die. Any health care professional who ignores a valid refusal and carries out treatment will commit a battery. The impact of this case means that a terminally ill patient can refuse to receive any further treatment, and the doctor or nurse who accords with these wishes will not be held responsible for committing the crime of aiding and abetting a suicide.

What about the patient who is admitted in a state of unconsciousness who is clearly unable to provide consent to any proposed emergency treatment? It would be difficult to support a view that any subsequent touching or treatment would constitute battery in the absence of consent, because it is simply not possible to obtain this from the patient. The law accepts that treatment should be given where it is in the best interests of the patient to save life or preserve health, and that, in these circumstances, there is no necessity to obtain consent. It is, however, not possible for non-urgent medical or nursing treatment to be given to such a patient and in these circumstances, it would be unlawful to proceed with that treatment. It is necessary in those situations to wait for the patient to regain consciousness and then obtain consent.

There may be an issue of conflict between a mother and her unborn child where the mother's refusal of treatment puts the life of the child at risk. The court of appeal was asked to consider this issue (*St George's Healthcare NHS Trust* v. *S* [1998]). A woman with pre-eclampsia refused a caesarean operation. The NHS Trust asked the high court for a declaration that the operation would be lawful, despite its being against the mother's wishes. They argued that the operation was necessary to save the life of the child. The court granted this declaration and ordered that the caesarean operation proceed, on the basis that it was in the interests of both mother and child to have the operation as, without this intervention, it was likely that both would die. This ruling was overturned by the court of appeal which has now issued guidelines that all Trusts and health authorities need to follow. The court of appeal confirmed that where the mother is competent, her decision not to have treatment must be respected. Where she refuses treatment that is recommended, that must be recorded in her notes. It is only where the mother is not competent that treatment can be given in her best interests.

Elderly care

Nursing older people brings its own complications when assessing consent, particularly where there is dementia. It could well be that capacity based on understanding will vary within the same person. The older person suffering from dementia may have periods of complete lucidity in which he can determine exactly what he wants in terms of medical or nursing care. On other occasions, this may not be possible. In these situations, it will be necessary for the nurse to assess the patient's ability to understand the proposed treatment or care before each procedure takes place. Dementia may be a situation in which medical technology will allow a clearer assessment of these periods of fluctuating capacity, but, in the meantime, it remains one of the hardest areas to resolve in terms of capacity and consent.

This particular difficulty is highlighted in a situation in which a patient refuses to have a particular type of treatment or care. Some difficulty may exist for nurses who are motivated to act in the best interests of the patient. When the older person's choice accords with nursing practice, the level of competence of that person is rarely assessed. Since the older person agrees with the treatment that is being proposed, many nurses automatically assume that the patient has capacity to consent. Because the treatment being proposed will always be in the patient's own interests, it is assumed that a patient who consents to that treatment is showing the necessary capacity to understand what is involved. Difficulties arise when a patient refuses certain treatment. In such a situation, it seems that nurses demand a much higher level of understanding in order to satisfy themselves that the patient has capacity, even though he is now actively choosing a course not deemed to be in his best interests.

The importance of a refusal from an older person seems to be that it triggers a fresh evaluation of understanding, but it does not mean that because the person refuses to agree with the nurse's proposals that he has necessarily lost the understanding that is crucial to give consent. There have been no cases dealing with this problem yet that would provide legal guidance.

Mental health

Adults who are incapable of giving consent because of mental illness can receive treatment under the provisions of the Mental Health Act 1984 for that disorder. However, there may be some situations in which a person with a mental disorder may require medical treatment for some

Case example 4.3

In September 1993, doctors at Broadmoor Hospital discovered gangrene in a patient's foot and informed him that unless the foot and part of the leg were amputated, he faced imminent death. The patient, who suffered from chronic paranoid schizophrenia, was transferred to the local hospital. He refused to consent to the amputation. He applied to the court for an injunction restraining the hospital and the surgeons from amputating his leg, both then and in the future, unless he gave his express, written, valid consent. The judge was satisfied that the patient understood the proposed treatment and believed what he had been told about it, and that the patient was capable of balancing the risks. Although his general capacity was impaired, the judge found that it was not established that the patient did not understand the nature, purpose and effects of the treatment he refused (*Re C* [1994]). The ruling in that case gives clear authority for the legal binding status of advance directives, which has importance particularly for mental health patients who may wish to give an advance directive about their future treatment. A patient who suffers from psychotic states of mind may have rational and lucid periods, in which he has sufficient capacity to make a decision to decide on future mental, medical and nursing treatment.

other condition. The dilemma here is that the person has no capacity to consent on his own behalf, and, because he has reached adult status, there can be no guardian to make the decision for him. In such circumstances, there will be a hearing before a judge to determine whether or not the proposed treatment is in that person's best interests. Cases that have involved a proposal to sterilise mentally incapable male and female adults throw this issue of consent into sharp focus. The court of appeal has found that the patient has the right, if he is unable himself to choose, not to have invasive surgery unless and until it has been demonstrated that it is in the patient's best interests (*Re A (male sterilisation)* [2000]).

The court has held that some patients with mental disorder can refuse treatment for a condition unrelated to that disorder (Case example 4.3).

Negligence

The possibility of an action in negligence is one that is feared by more nurses than any other

area of law. When a procedure goes wrong and involves injury to a person, the possibility of an action in negligence must always be considered. The same applies equally if a nurse is herself injured in the course of employment, and it is open to the nurse to consider bringing a claim of negligence against the employer. The law on negligence has been determined through common law, and the following principles emerge that need to be established before a claim in negligence can be successful:

1. There must be a duty of care owed by one person to another. This principle was established in the case of *Donohoe v. Stevenson* [1932]. In that case, a woman in a tea shop drank a bottle of ginger beer and discovered the remains of a decomposed snail at the bottom. She was ill as a result. The court held that the manufacturer of the ginger beer owed a duty of care to its ultimate consumers to provide them with a beverage free from impurity. The principle of the duty of care applies in a nurse–patient relationship as well as an employer–nurse relationship, and a duty of care exists between these parties that could give rise to an action in negligence.

The extent to which one person may owe a duty of care to another has been discussed in relation to nervous shock suffered by a person who witnesses an accident. While anyone may suffer nervous shock by witnessing injuries occurring to another person, the courts have held that in order to justify a claim that the person causing the accident owed a duty of care to prevent nervous shock, it is necessary to show a family relationship with the injured person.

2. The duty of care is broken when one person fails to do what a 'reasonable' person would or would not do in the circumstances. The test to determine whether or not a person has acted as a reasonable person is judged by an objective test called the Bolam test (from *Bolam v. Friern Hospital Management Committee* [1957]). The standard of care required of a nurse in establishing whether or not a duty of care has been broken is to assess what a reasonable nurse would or would not have done in the circumstances according to a recognised body of nursing opinion. If a patient on a 24-bedded ward falls out of bed and breaks a leg, it is open to the patient to claim that the staff owed a duty of care to ensure his safety and well-being. In order to prove that the duty of care has been broken, it will be necessary for the patient to demonstrate that reasonable steps could have been taken to prevent him falling out of bed.

3. The injury caused must arise directly from the duty of care that has been broken. This is best illustrated by the case of *Barnet* v. *Chelsea & Kensington HMC* [1969] (Case example 4.4).

It is worthwhile considering at this point the different standards that might be applied to nursing practice by the law and by the nursing professional body. In Case example 4.4, it is shown that the law requires all three elements of

Case example 4.4

Three night watchmen presented at a casualty department complaining of vomiting. The nurse on duty took their details and telephoned the casualty officer, who listened to the nurse's report and gave telephone advice that the men should go home and seek GP treatment. The nurse accurately relayed this information to the night watchmen. Shortly afterwards, one night watchman died, and the post mortem revealed that all three had been subject to arsenic poisoning after someone had laced their flasks of tea, which they had drunk earlier that night. The widow sued the hospital in negligence.

The court held that both the nurse and the casualty doctor owed a duty of care to the night watchmen. It was found that the nurse had behaved as a reasonable nurse, according to the Bolam test, in taking advice from the casualty officer and relaying this to the night watchmen. It was therefore ascertained that the nurse had not broken her duty of care, and therefore any claim in negligence against her failed at that point.

The casualty officer's decision not to come and investigate the night watchmen was held to be sufficient to break the duty of care, as it was demonstrated that a reasonable casualty officer would have examined the men. However, independent medical evidence showed that the night watchman would have died in any event because of the arsenic poisoning, and the lack of intervention on the part of the casualty officer was not a material cause of death. It could not be demonstrated therefore that the death was directly attributable to the negligent omission of the casualty officer. In these circumstances, the action in negligence failed.

negligence to be proved before an action can succeed. In this case, therefore, even if the nurse had broken her duty of care, the law would not have made a finding of negligence against her, because the death was not connected with her action. It is interesting to note that the UKCC does not require that the third legal element of negligence be proved before they can investigate whether a nurse has been guilty of misconduct, and the UKCC may indeed investigate the actions of a nurse without reference to any legal position in a finding of negligence.

In an action for negligence, there is a time limit of 3 years from the date the injury occurs or the person becomes aware of the injury to the date on which the court must be notified that a claim is being brought. No claim in negligence for personal injury can be made outside this 3-year period. Where children have been injured potentially as a result of negligence, they are allowed to reach adult status before the 3-year period runs. Therefore if a 6-year-old is involved in a road traffic accident in which somebody else was responsible, that child is allowed to reach the age of majority (i.e. 18) and then have a further 3 years (i.e. until the age of 21) before notifying the court of an intention to sue for negligence.

In most nursing practice, the principle of vicarious liability will mean that any omission or error made by a nurse that may result in an action for negligence will not be brought directly against that nurse but against the nurse's employer. The principle of vicarious liability means that the employer is responsible for all the actions of its employees that are carried out in the course of employment. However, the fact that a nurse may not be named on the court documents does not mean that she will not be very closely involved in any subsequent proceedings, and that nurse will generally be required to give evidence in court.

In an emergency situation, it may not be possible to assess how a reasonable nurse should act in the circumstances. Where a patient is involved in a road traffic accident and a nurse comes across the scene outside the course of her employment, there is no positive duty on the nurse to become involved in helping the injured victims. If the nurse chooses to become involved and apply what first aid knowledge she has that may help the situation, no action in negligence can be brought against that nurse if the steps taken make the condition of the patient worse. Although the general public may mistakenly assume that any nurse is also a qualified first aider to deal with accident situations, this is not always the case.

Confidentiality

Confidentiality is a fundamental part of the nurse–patient relationship. Information given to a nurse in the context of a nurse–patient relationship must be protected. The law on confidentiality also applies to other professionals who are in a professional relationship, and covers lawyers and their clients as well as, for example, banks and their customers. The law will uphold and protect confidentiality in situations where a relationship is established in which one person agrees to give information about themselves to another in the trust that it will be kept confidential.

Any information given to a nurse should not be passed on to a third party without consent. It is accepted that the nurse may be required to pass some patient information to other members of the health care team if it is necessary for the team to know of the patient's condition to provide effective health care. In this situation, it is implied that the patient gives consent for the nurse to pass on the relevant information.

If a nurse passes information about the patient to a third party outside the health care team, a breach of confidentiality will have occurred. It is possible for the patient to bring a civil action against the individual nurse and to sue the nurse for breach of confidentiality. Equally, it is open to a patient who is told that information is about to be passed to a third party to bring a civil action and seek an injunction, in which the court will be asked to make an order preventing the information being passed to a third party (Case example 4.5).

Where a breach of confidentiality has occurred that is successfully pursued in court, it will result in a payment of compensation to the aggrieved patient.

No breach of confidentiality will occur when a court order requires specific disclosure of patient

Case example 4.5

In 1988, a journalist discovered details of two hospital doctors who had been diagnosed as having AIDS. The journalist intended to publish details about the doctors. The hospital employing the doctors sought an injunction to prevent publication. In court, the journalist argued that such disclosure was justified on the grounds that it affected the public interest, but this argument was rejected by the court, which ordered an injunction to prevent publication of the article (*X* v. *Y* [1988]).

information. A court order demanding disclosure overrides the duty of confidentiality, and nurses are under a legal duty to comply fully with the terms of any court order. No breach of confidentiality occurs in these circumstances.

Equally, where a patient consents to information being passed to a third party, no breach of confidentiality occurs. Consent is the key issue, and the law requires that no disclosure to a third party is made without this consent.

The only defence allowed to a breach of confidentiality is that it is justified in the public interest. The burden falls on the person breaking the confidence to prove that his actions were so justified.

The UKCC Code of Conduct follows these legal principles, and the UKCC has published further guidance dealing with this subject (UKCC 1996). (See also Chapter 11.)

The prime difficulty for nurses in the area of confidentiality is in determining whether or not information can indeed be passed to a third party if the patient specifically declines to give consent. Individual nurses will need to assess whether or not there is sufficient public interest arising in any case to determine whether a breach of confidentiality would be justified. Even where a nurse makes this assessment, a court may take a different view of the justification and rule that a breach of confidentiality had occurred that was not justified.

The justification for a breach of confidentiality in the public interest has evolved through civil cases in which confidentiality has been a key issue. The courts have, in the past, held that such breaches are justified where a person had been involved in criminal activity or behaved so disgracefully that it was judged in the public interest to expose that behaviour. In these cases, no breach of confidentiality has occurred. These cases have generally involved confidentiality connected with banking practice.

There are also circumstances in which there may be no wrongdoing on the part of an individual but where it is considered vital to make confidential information known on a public basis. An example of this would be a significant breakthrough in medical technology, such as the first successful heart and lung transplant.

There have been no legal cases that deal with a nurse's proposed or actual breach of confidentiality. In *W* v. *Edgell* [1990], the case concerned a doctor's breach of confidentiality. In this case, the patient sued Dr Edgell for disclosing a psychiatric report to the medical director of a special hospital. The report indicated that the patient was unfit to be considered for discharge. The patient had specifically refused to give consent for this report to be disclosed to the medical director, and when Dr Edgell took this step, the patient sued for breach of confidence. It was not disputed in the court that the report had been disclosed to the medical director against the specific wishes of the patient. The doctor argued that this breach of confidence was allowed on the grounds that disclosure was justified in the public interest. He maintained that there was a fear of real risk to public safety were the patient discharged. The court of appeal accepted this defence and made no order of compensation. They commented that only the most compelling circumstances would justify a doctor acting in this way, and that the defence of disclosure in the public interest should only be used in the strictest circumstances possible. The court felt that, in every case, the doctor should seek to obtain the patient's consent before breaching confidentiality.

The UKCC takes a similarly guarded approach to breaches of confidentiality in dealing with the public interest element. It considers that disclosure in the public interest could be justified if the nurse became aware of issues affecting society in

which criminal activity of a serious nature, such as child abuse or drug trafficking, was involved.

Some contracts of employment include a clause requiring the nurse to keep confidential all information learned about the work environment, and in some cases, the nurse is required to respect this confidence even after the employment contract has terminated and the nurse is working elsewhere. In addition, many hospitals now have policies for staff to follow when police or journalists make enquires about a patient. The decision of whether or not to provide such people with information about a patient is not one that any member of staff should make without assessing the employer's policy on this issue. There is no requirement to pass information to police making enquiries, even when they are investigating criminal activity, unless the nurse in charge feels that such criminal activity falls within the boundaries provided by the UKCC in defining the public interest. In addition, that nurse should also be able to justify her own actions at any later stage should the patient make a claim that a breach of confidentiality has occurred.

DOCUMENTATION

Should patients be allowed to keep their own medical and nursing notes and read what is written on them? In the past, patient records have been kept secret even from patients, and disclosure was generally only allowed with a court order. Recent legislation allows the patient to have greater access to the information written in certain circumstances, which is viewed as increasing patient autonomy.

The Secretary of State for Health assigns by delegation to the health authority or NHS Trust the duty to keep records on patients. The paperwork on which these records are completed belongs to the health authority or NHS Trust; it does not belong to the patient, and the patient has no right of automatic access to the records that are kept.

Legislation allows the patient to have access to the information kept in certain circumstances, as outlined below.

Data Protection Acts 1984 and 1998

These Acts and the subsequent Order allow the patient to have access to electronically stored data by giving sufficient notice in a required form. The Acts do not apply to manually kept records.

Access to Medical Reports Act 1988

This Act only applies to reports made for insurance or employment purposes, and does not cover any notes made about a patient's condition. A patient has a right to see a medical report compiled by a doctor with responsibility for his clinical care if this is then to be sent to an insurance company or employer.

Access to Health Records Act 1990

This Act provides a right of access by patients to records kept about them that were created on or after 1 November 1991. A request can be made in writing, enclosing the set fee plus reasonable photocopying charges, and the patient can then receive copies of these notes. No fee can be charged for records that are less than 40 days old. This Act only applies to manual records. It means that there is no right to access manually kept information created before 1 November 1991.

It is open to the holder of the manually or electronically stored records to refuse disclosure if, in the opinion of the holder, it is decided that disclosure would cause serious harm to the physical or mental health of the patient. The Act does not require the holder of information to justify such a decision.

Wills

Adults of sound mind can sign their own will, and it is open to anyone to write out the will for themselves, although it is always better if a solicitor drafts the will to avoid any possible misinterpretation or confusion about the wishes of the person making the will. Anyone can witness a will being signed, although they lose their entitlement to benefit from the will if this happens. If a patient wants to leave a gift to a nurse in a will, the nurse should check her employer's policy and seek professional advice to avoid the possible implication of fraud. A nurse who is receiving a benefit from the will should not witness it.

The rules for signing a will need to be complied with exactly for the will to be valid. The person making the will is called the testator. The testator needs to sign the will in the presence of two independent witnesses, who then need to sign their own names on the will in the presence of the other witness and the testator. It is not sufficient for two people to attend as witnesses and sign the will at separate times; if this happens, the whole will becomes invalid.

Accident and incident reports

It is important that all incidents involving a nurse are recorded on the appropriate accident or incident report, even where no injury has been sustained by the nurse. Accident reports are necessary in assessing risk that may arise in the place of work, and the available statistics may need the employer to take some steps to reduce the occurrence of incidents that lead to injury.

REFERENCES

Airedale NHS Trust v. Bland [1993] 1 All ER 821
Barnet v. Chelsea and Kensington HMC [1969] 1 QB 428
Bolam v. Friern Hospital Management Committee [1957] 2 All ER 118
Devi v. West Midlands RHA [1981] CA 491
Donohoe v. Stevenson [1932] AC 562
Frenchay Healthcare NHS Trust v. S (1994) The Times, 19 January 1994
Gillick v. West Norfolk and Norwich AHA [1985] 3 All ER 402
Marshall v. Curry [1993] 3 DLR 260
Nurses, midwives and health visitors (professional conduct) rules 1993. SI 1993 No. 893. HMSO, London
R. v. Cox (1992) 12 BMLR 38
Re A (male sterilisation) [2000] 1 FLR 549
Re C (a minor) (wardship: medical treatment) [1989] 2 All ER 782
Re C (adult: refusal of medical treatment) [1994] 1 All ER 819
Re S (adult: refusal of medical treatment) [1992] 4 All ER 671

Re T (adult) (refusal of medical treatment) [1992] 4 All
    ER 649
Re W (a minor) (medical treatment) [1992] 4 All ER 627
St George's Healthcare NHS Trust v. S [1998] 2 FLR 728
Sidaway v. Board of Governors of Bethlem Royal Hospital
    [1985] 1 All ER 643
United Kingdom Central Council for Nursing, Midwifery
    and Health Visiting 1996 Guidelines for professional
    practice. UKCC, London
W v. Edgell [1990] 1 All ER 835
Wright S, Caulfield H 1994 Defining nurses' and doctors'
    duty of care. Nursing Standard 9(12–14): 31
X v. Y [1988] 2 All ER 648

FURTHER READING

There are relatively few books and articles available on the application of the law to nursing practice. The majority still cover medical practice. The following suggestions deal with nursing issues:

Mason J K, McCall Smith R A 1994 Law and medical ethics,
    4th edn. Butterworths, London
Brazier M 1992 Medicine, patients and the law, 2nd edn.
    Penguin, London
Montgomery J 1989 Nursing and the law. Macmillan,
    London
Dimond B 1995 Legal aspects of nursing, 2nd edn. Prentice
    Hall, London

5 Managing cultural diversity in care

Alison Spires

CHAPTER CONTENTS

Introduction   129

What is culture?   130
Culture and health care   131
Culture and nursing care   132

Transcultural care   132
Making transcultural care a reality   135
Is there a problem with transcultural care?   138

Providing culture sensitive care   138
An example from nursing practice: pain   138
Does this model work in practice?   139

Good practice in transcultural care   141
Patient assessment   141
Patients' explanatory models   142
Spiritual needs   142
Communication and interpretation   143
Eating and drinking   143
Personal hygiene and washing   144

Conclusion   144

References   145

Further reading   146

After reading this chapter you will be able to:

- provide a simple definition of culture and discuss culture in the general context of health care
- apply the concept of culture to nursing care
- describe the concept of transcultural nursing care and discuss ways in which transcultural nursing care can be made a reality
- identify some problems with the concept of transcultural care
- discuss how culture influences pain perception and the management of pain
- describe how good nursing practice in the area of transcultural care can be achieved.

INTRODUCTION

There is no doubt that, in this third millennium, the UK is already a multicultural society. The islands which make up the UK have within their borders many different groups of people who see themselves as culturally distinct from their neighbours. People are proud of their Scottish, Irish, Welsh or English ancestry, and of the cultural dimension of that ancestry. They are also just as proud of the fact that they are highland or lowland Scot, mountain or valley Welsh, Londoner, Liverpudlian or Bristolian English, rural or urban dweller. But it is not only in the 'traditional' UK groupings that culture is important and distinctive. History tells us that over the years the UK has become a host country to many waves of immigrants. People have come to these shores from many countries: for economic reasons, as invited workers, as political refugees or to escape persecution because of their beliefs. It can be argued that even within one single society many different cultures exist – men and women, boys and girls, old and young, ill and healthy, all these groups in any society are expected to behave in ways that their culture feels is appropriate for them.

Cultures are also divided into subcultures. The National Health Service (NHS) can be said to be a subculture of British society and, within the NHS, nursing, medicine and physiotherapy, for example, can be identified as further subcultures. Each subculture has its own clear and distinctive set of implicit guidelines for behaviour. New entrants to health care professions are often referred to as needing to be 'socialised' into their professions. It is clear that health professionals do form a separate cultural group within society, but can the same be said for patients? Is there a 'patient' culture? Helman (1994) states that society does indeed divide up its members according to their health status as 'healthy' or 'ill'. However, this may be a label applied by a health professional to a person rather than by the person to himself.

There are other ways of dividing society up into categories of subcultures. An important category is to do with race and ethnicity. Balarjajan & Raleigh (1993) inform us that about 6% of the population define themselves as being from an ethnic origin other than white Caucasian. This percentage is likely to have increased in the years between the 1991 and the 2001 censuses. The 1991 census was the first to elicit information about ethnic origins of the population of the UK. The percentage of minority ethnic groups is not currently high, but according to James (1995) this is likely to double over the next 40 to 50 years. Without doubt each different cultural and minority ethnic group adds value to the diversity and complexity of UK society. Valuing the cultural background of each and every client and patient is crucial in the provision of culturally aware and culturally sensitive nursing care. Cultural diversity in caring is an important and fundamental issue for nursing.

WHAT IS CULTURE?

In order to explore the concept of cultural diversity in caring, culture itself must be defined. Culture has many meanings. Some people when they talk of culture are referring to art, opera, and music. To others, culture can mean the distinguishing characteristics of a workplace (for example we often talk of the culture of the National Health Service, the culture of the armed forces or of the civil service). From an anthropological perspective, culture is taken as meaning the set of guidelines which individuals use which tells them how to behave in their own particular part of society. Helman (1994) uses the analogy of a 'lens' through which an individual perceives and understands his own world. Anthropology theory suggests that people's behaviour is partly governed by the specific society in which they grow up and in which they live. Culture provides the guide for determining values, practices and beliefs within any given society. It determines how people accommodate themselves within their own culture because it is related to the way that people live. Culture relates to morality, beliefs, social norms and accepted behaviour. Individuals in any culture are expected to adopt and comply with that culture's rules. What is acceptable in one culture may not be acceptable in another. For example, female circumcision (also known as female genital mutilation) is an accepted and deep-rooted practice in a number of African countries. Ng (1999) states that some 50% of Kenyan girls are still being circumcised. In the UK, however, there is legislation in place which prohibits the practice, and the World Health Organization does not support it.

Culture determines how nurses and patients react and respond to the actions of nursing interventions. 'Transcultural' nursing, as the term implies, means that the provision of nursing care is to do with a meeting of two or more cultures – the culture of the nursing profession, the nurse's own cultural background and the cultural background of the patient, and maybe even male–female culture, age–youth culture. Transcultural care thus focuses on issues to do with the way each cultural group understands what health is and the causes of illness, what treatment is intended to achieve and what contribution nursing care makes to the total picture. Our behaviours as people in all our roles in life are learned from observing others in our immediate society, and in comparing what we do with what others do we alter our own behaviour to fit in. This is a useful way of describing culture from a health care point of view since it allows us to look at our own nursing culture, and also be concerned with the cultural background of the individuals who become patients and clients of the health care services.

CULTURE AND HEALTH CARE

The National Health Service was set up in 1948 to cater for the needs of a fairly homogenous 'British' culture. Mares and colleagues, writing in 1985, felt that the service had not really begun to take into account the composition of the population in the provision of care. They felt that NHS service provision and staff training were still geared to the way of life, family patterns, dietary norms, religious beliefs, attitudes, priorities and expectations of the majority population. In 1994 Thomas & Dines felt that initiatives by the NHS to meet the health care needs of ethnic minority groups appeared inadequate, and that there was little evidence of what might constitute good practice in this area. Papadopoulos, writing in 1999 about Greek Cypriots living in London, felt that their health care needs had not yet been fully recognised. Vydelingum's research (2000) indicated that patients of South Asian origin felt a general dissatisfaction with their health care in hospital settings. Despite a number of reports from the Department of Health in the 1990s (DoH 1992, for example) which highlighted the particular needs of minority ethnic groups, it seems that such ideas have not yet been translated fully into action in the NHS. One of the reasons for this, and a problem for the NHS, is the blanket terminology used, for example the term 'ethnic

Case example 5.1 Unintentional racism

An example of unintentional racism from my own experience of living in London in the 1980s concerns an all-female GP practice. While sitting in the waiting room prior to an appointment with my GP, I observed a young woman of apparently South Asian origin, who did not appear to speak English, hand over an NHS card to the receptionist. I interpreted this as her wish to join the practice list, as did the receptionist. The receptionist shook her head and told the lady very slowly and very loudly to go down the road to another doctor 'because he speaks your language'. What the receptionist did not know, of course, was what language the lady actually spoke, what her ethnic origin was, or her reasons for wanting to register with an all-female practice. The woman may well have been directed by the receptionist to a doctor who spoke a different language from her and may have come from a different ethnic group. She may not have wanted to register with a male doctor. She was given no choice, and we can interpret the receptionist's actions as being a racist, stereotypical response – grouping all Asian people together in one homogenous whole and failing to realise the differences between the various South Asian ethnic groups.

minority' seems to be used to cover everyone who is not of the white indigenous population (Case example 5.1).

Whatever we might like to think, there are still numerous examples of racism and prejudice in the NHS; some might term this 'institutional racism'. These examples range from not providing interpreter services and using patients' own young children as interpreters, to not providing appropriate food or calling it 'special' food, failing to provide services for particular medical conditions common in specific ethnic groups, and failing to adapt patient records to reflect particular naming systems. Yet numerous examples of good practice can also be found. These include health promotion literature in different languages, the provision in some areas of interpreter services for patients, the provision of education for health professionals in the areas of culture and race, the provision of literature for health professionals to consult, for example, the *Multicultural Information File* (MCRIC 1994) and *Organ Donation: Religious and Cultural Issues* (UK Transplant Co-ordinators Association, undated).

James (1995) spelt out for us the health disadvantages that encumber the black and ethnic minority populations of the UK. The rates of ill health and mortality in minority ethnic groups differ from those of the white population and differ between minority ethnic groups themselves. Black and ethnic minority communities face additional disadvantages to those of the white population in that they are more likely to be concentrated in lower paid occupations, are more likely to be unemployed, are more likely to live in poor housing and have access only to schools which are poorly equipped. In terms of health (Balarjajan & Raleigh 1993) the following have been identified:

- higher perinatal mortality among African, Caribbean and Asian babies
- higher rates of congenital abnormality among Asian infants
- higher mortality from coronary heart disease in people from the Indian subcontinent and African Commonwealth countries
- higher prevalence of hypertension, cerebral vascular accident and diabetes among people from the Caribbean, Indian subcontinent and African Commonwealth countries
- higher rates of diagnosis of schizophrenia in Asian, African and Caribbean men.

James (1995) identified some major influences on health and illness in these particular cultural groups. More research is needed to determine the aetiology of illness in these groups. It is not sufficient simply to say that differences result from 'cultural differences'.

With these issues in mind there is much that nursing can do to provide culturally sensitive and culturally aware care, and to acknowledge cultural diversity in health care. The rest of this chapter therefore seeks to explore the issue of transcultural care, and concludes with some ideas for good nursing practice in the area of culture sensitive care.

CULTURE AND NURSING CARE

McGee (1992) tells us that it was Florence Nightingale who first articulated the need for nursing care to take into account the cultural dimension of a society. Nightingale asserted that women who worked in India must know the language, religions, superstitions and customs of the women they cared for. However it is only in the last few years that this cultural dimension to nursing care has begun to be addressed in nursing textbooks and nurse education programmes. For many practitioners this still represents a gap in their knowledge and unfortunately many nurses continue to think that it is enough to provide care that is 'individualised'. It is simply not enough to say 'I treat everyone equally', or 'I treat everyone as an individual' because this may imply that a nurse has not thought through the implications that a person's cultural background has for his care. It may also imply that the nurse has not thought through the implications that her own cultural background has for the nursing care that is offered.

The United Kingdom Central Council for Nursing, Midwifery and Health Visiting (UKCC) Code of Professional Conduct (UKCC 1992) urges nurses to take note of the background of patients in making decisions about their care. The Code of the International Council of Nurses (ICN 1974) states that the need for nursing is universal. Inherent in nursing is respect for life, dignity and the rights of man. It is unrestricted by considerations of nationality, race, creed, colour, age, sex, politics or social status.

TRANSCULTURAL CARE

It was Madeleine Leininger (1991) who first put forward a model for cultural aspects of caring. She coined the phrases 'transcultural' and 'cross-cultural' care in referring to the fusion of nursing and anthropology. She felt that anthropology had a significant contribution to make to modern nursing. She argued that just as patients' culture influences their beliefs about health and illness, so the cultural background of health professionals will influence their beliefs and value systems about illness states and how they are managed, and about health and how it is maintained.

Transcultural care has been in existence for as long as nursing has. Anyone who gives care to another person does so in the context of the cultures from which they both come. Sometimes that may be the same culture; sometimes it may be different cultures. In any nurse–patient interaction there can be misunderstanding as well as understanding; some misunderstandings may be based on cultural issues. What has happened in recent years is that cultural issues in health care have become more clearly articulated. The need for increased cultural awareness and understanding, awareness of racial and ethnic group issues and race discrimination have become important items on the modern health care agenda.

Andrews & Boyle (1995) represent transcultural care as a synthesis of nursing concepts and other borrowed concepts, suggesting the following:

- caring exists in all cultures
- the way in which caring is carried out is culture specific
- the meaning of caring varies cross-culturally
- what constitutes care varies cross-culturally
- where care matches client expectations, the more accepted it will be.

They suggest that caring in a transcultural sense is concerned with shared meanings and the degree to which carer and client agree or disagree on the cultural symbols of health, illness, disease and caring. These meanings are said to influence all carer–client interactions.

For effective transcultural care a nurse needs basic knowledge of how different cultural groups define and treat illness, promote and maintain health, prevent illness and structure their health care systems. Many authors have articulated their own beliefs about what constitutes transcultural care. Andrews & Boyle (1995) see transcultural care as a fundamental element of all care, not just care given to minority ethnic groups and foreign populations. The nurse skilled in transcultural care techniques will possess sophisticated assessment and analytic skills, will plan care with sensitivity to an individual's culture and will implement interventions that are culturally

relevant and acceptable. Such a person as a 'transcultural nurse' should not exist; instead all nurses and all health professionals should be culturally aware and skilled in delivering culture sensitive care. The existence of 'transcultural nurse' emphasises difference, and suggests that the nurse should be 'consulted' when a patient from a different cultural group to that of the health professional is being cared for. It must not be just about how white people look after black people, and it is not just about the care of ethnic minority groups.

Leininger's (1991) view that 'every nurse comes from a particular group ... and we cannot come to a care situation free from our religious, social and cultural influences' is important in understanding our own communication processes in a health care context. People are not always aware of the extent to which these influences operate in their daily lives, and see themselves as possessing 'normal' thoughts and behaviours. This can lead to the 'pathologising of culture', which is when cultural expression itself is seen as abnormal in a health context.

Abdullah (1995) agrees with this view, stating that caring involves the intellectual analytical ability of the nurse to relate relevant and culturally appropriate knowledge in the delivery of effective care. Providing quality individualised patient care cannot be achieved without considering the context of the client as a whole person and factors associated with the client's personal being such as culture, belief and tradition. This means that each nurse has to think about her interactions with patients from all kinds of cultures and backgrounds, and has a responsibility to learn about a patient's culture.

Herberg (1989) states that transcultural care is concerned with the provision of care in a manner that is sensitive to the needs of individuals, families and groups who represent diverse cultural populations within a society. Developing cultural sensitivity is something that comes with the experience of meeting people from diverse backgrounds and acknowledging that there is a need to learn, and then to use that learning in an appropriate way. Nurses and other health professionals therefore need to understand the variables in people's behaviours – such as differences in values, religion, dietary belief and practices, social hierarchical structure, family patterns, beliefs and practices related to health and illness – if they are to begin the process of offering culturally sensitive care.

DeSantis (1994) goes further and suggests that nurses need more than cultural sensitivity. They need competence in the use of culture.

Transcultural care therefore is the integration of the concept of culture into all aspects of nursing and the provision of health care. In terms of nursing care it is the ability to step out of, or suspend, one's own cultural traditions (values, beliefs and practices) in order to try and perceive the situation as others do. DeSantis suggests the following components of transcultural care:

Nurse–patient negotiation. There is no room in any nurse–patient interaction for the nurse to make all the decisions about care. If the nurse does this then everything is viewed from the nurse's own cultural perspective, and it may not be appropriate care for that patient. Many patients, particularly older people, may be content for the nurse to make a large number of decisions about care on their behalf. Even if this is the case, the nurse and patient will have agreed that this should be.

Simultaneous dual ethnocentrism. What do we understand by this term and why is it important? Culture always operates, is always present and always influences what patients and nurses do in any health care encounter. We all make judgements according to our own belief systems, which in turn are culturally determined. The concept of dual ethnocentrism makes nurses aware that everybody operates under the influence of their own specific culture. Nurses can then begin to appreciate the culture of the 'other', and can then attempt to use aspects of the patient's belief system in mutually acceptable care interventions.

Multiple cultural contexts and clinical realities exist in the nurse–patient encounter. Each nursing care encounter is the interaction of three cultures:

- the nurse's professional culture
- the patient's interpretation of the health care system based upon his own culture

- the context in which the nurse–patient encounter takes place (institution, home, surgery).

This allows us to understand that there are multiple realities operating simultaneously in all health care situations.

Patients are cultural informants. Nurses can help patients to explore the meaning of the health care situation for them during, for example, the assessment process. Part of this is for the health professional to assess things such as patients' explanatory models. Differing cultures may have different ways of explaining the same signs and symptoms; each culture puts its own meaning on health and illness events. The patient is the authority on his own culture, and the nurse must take what the patient says about it as the truth for that patient. Individuals can be viewed as unique products of their own culture, with a unique perception of their own health and illness experiences, and this uniqueness is incorporated into the health care encounter.

The cultural dimension is fundamental to the nature of nursing. If culture is not seen as something separate to be assessed, the cultural dimension of care can be incorporated into the nursing process in a more routine way. The use of a separate cultural assessment tool may make it seem that culture is associated only with ethnic/racial/cultural/religious aspects of an individual, rather than something that affects every single individual in everything that they do.

Nurses who are competent in the use of culture will therefore be:

- aware of the limitations that their own cultural values, beliefs and practices impose upon them
- open to cultural difference
- have a patient/client-orientated focus
- use cultural knowledge and resources to address health care problems.

It is important to recognise one's own cultural perspective, especially if one is part of a dominant or majority culture. The realisation that life may be different for others may be slow in its impact on some nurses. It is possible to suggest that the transcultural nurse is one who has studied other cultures in depth. This is a view that suggests 'other' cultures are glamorous and exotic and emphasises the differences between cultures. It is not necessarily helpful to view other cultures and societies as exotic as it 'dresses-up' culture in a false and stereotypical fashion.

Nurses may function as 'cultural brokers', who strive to perceive the situation from the patient's perspective, compare it to their own and mediate between the two to produce interventions that are mutually agreed and appropriate to the care situation. Nurses must always scrutinise their own beliefs and practices in relation to those of their patients. In this way nurses' own cultural beliefs are brought further into their consciousness.

MAKING TRANSCULTURAL CARE A REALITY

Tripp-Reimer and colleagues (1984) suggest that 'cultural brokerage' provides the way for nurses and other health professionals to carry out transcultural care. This includes the following ideas, and could form the basis of a cultural dimension to the assessment and planning stages of the nursing process:

• An assessment of how the patient and family understand the current health care problem and intended treatment.
• Comparison of both the nurse's and the patient's perspectives. The nurse can explain and interpret medical diagnosis and treatment and explain nursing care to the patient, yet is able to take into account the patient's own explanatory model.
• The result of this is an effective working partnership, with both the nurse and the patient understanding each other's perspective.
• There may be occasions when nurse and patient cannot find mutually acceptable understanding, and nursing interventions are not possible.
• If neither is able to find solutions the nurse has the responsibility to compromise, but such problems should be referred to appropriate sources of help. No nurse need feel that she is without peer or manager support in difficult situations.

• Each party must abide by the solutions and monitor progress.
• If no compromise is possible the patient has the right absolutely to decide on what health care measures to take, although there may be legal and ethical reasons why this may not be appropriate in specific incidences.
• Onward referral must be used when no compromise is possible or when the nurse feels unable to accept the patient's decision. This is the nurse's responsibility. The patient also has the right to seek assistance elsewhere.

There are problems with this kind of open, non-judgemental approach to care and much of this has to do with ethical issues. For example, members of some faiths, notably Jehovah's Witnesses, may object to a blood transfusion, yet it is hard for nurses to see a patient exsanguinate before their eyes when a blood transfusion would save the person's life. If the patient is a child, it is harder still. Much transcultural care literature seems to imply that nursing and caring must be value free and non-judgemental; but this dehumanises nurses and other health professionals – no one individual can be forced to be all-accepting. In such cases nurses and doctors may feel more comfortable with the decisions about care and treatment being taken by a court of law. But nurses can allow themselves to intervene directly in other situations. For example, if a parent hits a child in hospital (even if physical chastisement is part of the family or group culture) a nurse can remonstrate with the parent. In the UK, nurses can register a conscientious objection to abortion, and not take part in such a procedure, even though it may be allowed legally.

DeSantis (1994) suggests that brokerage has three forms: first, it focuses on patients to help them cope with the health care situation; second, it focuses on practitioners to assist them to provide care in a culturally acceptable and appropriate way; and third, it provides for a mediation between patients and practitioners who have different health care orientations. The end point of brokerage may be simply an understanding of another person's point of view.

Nursing therefore needs to incorporate cultural assessment devices into nursing assessment. There are some examples of specific cultural assessment devices around, but these are often unwieldy and, while being comprehensive, are perhaps of little value clinically. They also tend to be separate from other assessment tools, and may just be providing one more form to be filed away in a patient's notes.

Nursing also needs theory and concepts related to the issue of culture and care. No longer is it enough merely to exhort nurses to be culturally aware and give culturally sensitive care, nor to present inventories of cultural practices, which promote a recipe approach to care. Such theories and concepts include understanding of the differences between culture and ethnicity. Culture is the observable factors such as food, dress, language, values and beliefs. Ethnicity refers to a subjective perspective of one's own heritage and to a sense of belonging to a group that identifies itself and is identified by others as distinguishable from other groups. Culture therefore includes those things about the ethnicity of the person. There needs to be a balance between knowledge that is ethnospecific and the introduction of concepts which are useful in an understanding of people across cultures. We need to understand how cultural bias may make interventions less effective as well as to understand approaches that can be used to make health care interventions more effective.

A goal for transcultural nursing care could thus be described in this way:

To provide care that is relevant and culturally acceptable to patients.

But it is also important that care is culturally acceptable to the nurse as well as to the client.

Most nursing models and theories mention the importance of understanding a patient's social background; we could take this to mean their cultural background. Roper and colleagues' (1996) model – a model of nursing based on a model of living – recognises that there is a social element to each of the activities of living. The activities which are socially based (working and communication for example) have more overt emphasis, but it is nevertheless important to recognise that physiological activities of living (such as breathing, eliminating, eating and drinking) also have clear-cut sociocultural elements. A disadvantage of this approach is that it makes it easy to slip into a reductionist approach, whereby we ask questions such as 'What do different cultures eat?'. We may end up with statements such as 'Jews don't eat pork'. Although this is a necessary aspect of understanding a culture, it does compartmentalise the approach. Transcultural nursing is not about intra-ethnic or intracultural variation. This lends itself to stereotyping and means that descriptions of cultural norms are not always helpful when it comes to offering culturally sensitive care.

Leininger's 'Sunrise' model (1991) (Fig. 5.1) attempts to depict her theory of cultural care universality and diversity, and offers perhaps a wider perspective than models such as that of Roper and colleagues. However, models such as this look very complex, so that we tend to lose sight of their intention, and may have difficulty in understanding exactly what it is they are meant to depict and convey.

It may be a useful exercise for nurses to look at a number of different models and try to tease out the cultural element in each of them (see Ch. 13). Most have something to say about 'social' influences. Human societies are clearly complex structures, but we need a simple model that puts culture into an appropriate context and shows how it affects the nurse–patient relationship.

A simple model (Fig. 5.2) for examining culture and its relationship to nursing care takes on board all the necessary factors. This model offers a concept on transcultural care where we see that the nurse–patient relationship is at the core of nursing care, the assessment component of the nursing process is a key factor, and both patient and nurse bring their own personal cultural experiences to their encounter. This model can apply for any 'health' or 'illness' event.

Littlewood (1989), in discussing the link between nursing and anthropology, said that anthropology might be more useful in terms of nurses' understanding of patients' subjective worlds than, for example, knowing about physiology. Western systems of healing place primacy on a biological understanding of disorders.

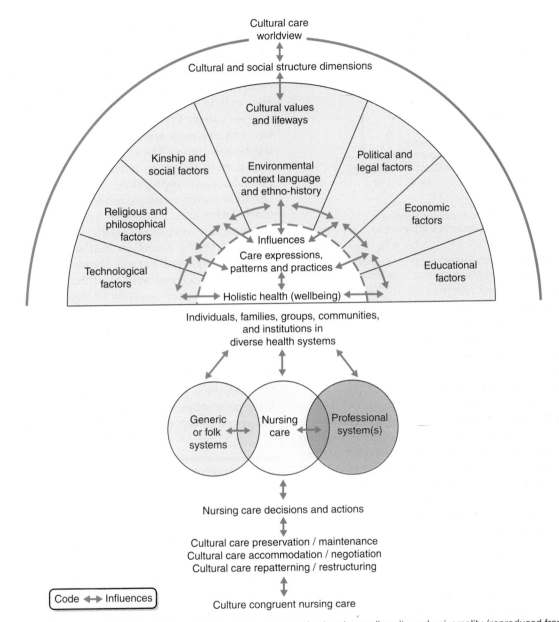

Figure 5.1 Leininger's 'Sunrise' model to depict her theory of cultural care diversity and universality (reproduced from Leininger 1991).

Nursing could be a very powerful force and try to supplement this understanding by seeing things more from the patient viewpoint, recognising that illness is both physically and socially disruptive. This suggests that nurses could begin to incorporate the patient's explanatory models of illness into their own assessment of the patient.

Rather than just ask the patient for their understanding (which may or may not fit into the nurse's preconceived notions) the nurse could ask the patient 'How will you know when you are healed (or better)?'. Models of illness (even simple things such as coughs and colds) are in general culturally determined.

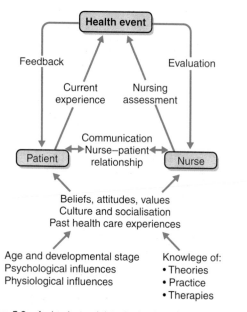

Figure 5.2 A simple model to depict the influence of culture on the nurse–patient relationship for any health event.

IS THERE A PROBLEM WITH TRANSCULTURAL CARE?

There is a real danger that ethno-specific or culture specific care can result in over-generalisation and lead us into making assumptions about individuals' health practices that can lead to cultural stereotyping. There is some fear therefore that transcultural care may well reinforce the very problem of paternalism and ethnocentric care that it seeks to address. Some nurses may feel that if they offer 'individualised' care, they offer culture sensitive care. These 'transcultural nurses' may be so bound up with their own beliefs and values in offering such care that they cease to be sensitive to anything other than their own belief and value system. Some nurses may project their own cultural expectations as they attempt to offer culture sensitive care, making it difficult, if not impossible, for patients to express their own ways of thinking and behave as they would do normally.

Culture is not a static but a dynamic process, and within any one culture the experience of the individual varies and changes with time. There may be a danger in providing culture specific care as it may divert attention away from the uniqueness of the individual.

Mason, in her 1990 research, compared mothers in Jamaica and Northern Ireland and found no causal relationship between cultural background and maternal behaviour. Differences between women's experiences of motherhood within the two cultures were just as great as those between the two cultures. There is an argument therefore that to draw up a list of culture specific practices is not appropriate, because of the huge variation within a culture as well as between cultures. There may actually be very little that we can recognise as culture specific.

Mason (1990) warns us that we should not make gross generalisations about people based on our preconceived notions of their 'culture'. If we do this we may be guilty of stereotyping and ignoring individual specific needs. Nurses may then run into the trap of further dividing cultures, and the usefulness of this is questionable. People are certainly 'cultural' beings, but it is not helpful always to view patients in this way; for example a person in pain may simply need their pain relieved rather than have their pain behaviour interpreted as culturally determined.

PROVIDING CULTURE SENSITIVE CARE

AN EXAMPLE FROM NURSING PRACTICE: PAIN

Pain is the most commonly occurring universal symptom of disease, illness and injury, and is the most frequent and compelling reason for seeking health care. Pain as a problem has exercised the minds of philosophers and medical men down the centuries, and it still poses a problem for modern health care. It is a primary danger signal that all is not well with the body, and is a central perception, not merely a primary sensory modality – that is, pain is felt with the whole being, and affects the way a person thinks, feels and behaves. It forces individuals to take note that something is amiss.

From what we know of pain, the physiological mechanism does not vary widely from person to person or from culture to culture. What does vary considerably is the psycho-cultural component of pain, and this gives rise to many different pain behaviours across cultures. This makes pain a very difficult symptom for health professionals to deal with. Definitions of pain are culturally influenced and its expectation, manifestations and management are all embedded in cultural contexts. So not only should health professionals consider how they might conceptualise the importance of pain relief (based on physiology), they might also consider how they might understand the whole meaning of the pain experience for an individual based on that individual's psychosocial make-up.

Pain behaviour is the result of a complex physiological, psychological, social and cultural interaction, a concept put forward by Melzack & Wall (1989) as the gate control theory of pain. In building upon Melzack & Wall's work, Bates (1987) suggests that pain behaviours are learned though two powerful psychosocial processes: that of social learning (Bandura 1977, cited in Bates 1987) and that of social comparison (Festinger 1954, cited in Bates 1987).

Social learning theory suggests that our behaviours in relation to entities such as pain are learned as we grow up in the social world by imitating the behaviours of others and by appropriate reinforcement of behaviour. For example it is common in the UK for families to reinforce 'brave' pain behaviour in children, and this is likely to lead to stoic 'stiff upper lip' responses as adults.

Social comparison theory suggests that people are continually evaluating themselves and trying to present themselves to others in the best way that they can. When a person is in pain, he will wish to behave in a way that is congruent with the rest of the social group. Thus the behaviours related to pain in any one cultural group become the socially desirable behaviours.

These theories lend support to the notion that we learn our pain behaviour as part of social learning, beginning in very early childhood, and by mechanisms of social comparison. That is, we continually compare our own behaviours in all sorts of situations to the behaviour that we

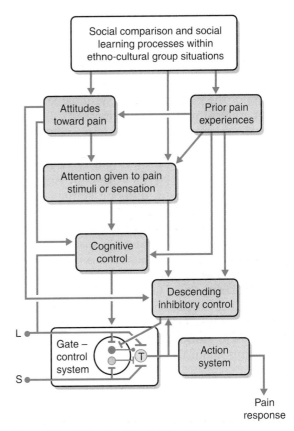

Figure 5.3 A biocultural model of pain perception (reproduced from Bates 1987).

observe in others, and our pain behaviours will become the socially desired behaviours of our specific cultural group. Bates suggests that it is likely that the cultural group experience influences the psycho-physiological processes responsible for pain thresholds (when a stimulus is reported as causing a pain sensation) perception of pain severity and pain response (Fig. 5.3).

DOES THIS MODEL WORK IN PRACTICE?

There have been numerous studies on pain behaviours and responses in different cultural groups over the last 50 years, but such studies are only of value if we use the results to make a difference in the understanding and management of pain. Knowledge of cross-cultural variations in pain behaviours only helps if such knowledge is used by health professionals in their assessment and treatment of pain. This kind of knowledge can be dangerous – it can lead to the stereotyping of people and their response to pain, and this in turn can distract us from an individualised plan of care for the person in pain. We must learn to accept intracultural variation as well as inter-cultural variation in all behaviours related to health and illness.

Some of the first cross-cultural research into pain was conducted by Zborowski in 1952. He looked at Americans of differing cultural back-grounds who were in hospital for a variety of health problems (herniated intervertebral discs, neurological disorders and other disorders). He found differences in pain behaviours between the cultural groups, but also similarities. Where there were similarities there were often different mean-ings ascribed to pain by the differing cultures. Two important features arise from Zborowski's study. First, those patients who made more complaints about their pain were often labelled 'problem' patients (Jewish and Italian people) and, second, those who tended to express their pain with minimal expression and were with-drawn were often labelled 'model' patients (people of Irish, Anglo-Saxon and German ori-gin). This demonstrates how culture can be dam-aging if nurses stereotype.

Just as patients have their own culturally determined pain behaviours, so too will nurses come to a patient encounter with their own cul-turally determined attitudes to people in pain. There is vast potential for culture clash here, with the result that pain can go unrelieved because the pain behaviour of a person from one culture is not recognised as such by the carer from another culture. More recent cross-cultural research into pain has looked into this concept. Davitz and col-leagues (1976) conducted research on 554 nurses in six different countries to test their attitudes towards pain and suffering. They demonstrated that there were marked cross-cultural differences in the way nurses from different countries rated pain and distress, based on patient vignettes. For example, Japanese and Korean nurses indicated that they believed the patients in the vignettes suffered higher degrees of pain than did American

and Puerto Rican nurses. American nurses scored the lowest ratings of patients' pain. Clearly the implication here for nursing practice is that pain may go unrecognised and therefore unrelieved. The Royal College of Surgeons report on pain after surgery (1990) states that for pain to be unre-lieved is bordering on professional negligence. We need therefore to construct pain assess-ment tools that can somehow take the cultural-behavioural element of pain into account, and make the nurse's assessment more objective and free from her own cultural influences. This is not likely to be an easy task. Calvillo & Flaskerud (1993) compared Mexican and Anglo-Saxon American women's responses to cholecystec-tomy pain, and found that there was a huge gap between what patients said about their pain and what their nurses said. Nurses evaluated *all* pain as being less than the patients' evaluations of their own pain. This presents a powerful argument for changing current pain management regimens to put pain control into patients' hands. Pain is such an intensely personal experience and it is simply not possible to experience another person's pain. Pain assessment is therefore very difficult.

Differing cultural backgrounds, as we have seen, are likely to produce differing pain behav-iours; however, there is as much intracultural variation as there is intercultural variation. The cultural background of carers is an important determinant of inferences of pain and distress, and this in turn suggests that there is a need to assess pain and evaluate responses to pain thera-pies in relation to the ethnic and cultural back-ground of the patient. There is a need to address methods of pain management for different cul-tural and ethnic groups, and nurses need to understand that differing cultures attach very different meanings to pain.

In recent years much work has been done in trying to explore different methods of pain relief, and some of this has been based on cross-cultural research. For example, acupuncture, a traditional Chinese approach to pain management, was for many years considered 'fringe' medicine. How-ever, since the 1970s there has been a gradual acceptance of the efficacy of pain relief from acupuncture and it has now become a popular and effective method in the mainstream of modern medicine. Other methods from other cultures may well become accepted into Western medical thought.

Few studies on cross-cultural aspects of pain have been done in the UK (an example is Thomas & Rose 1991) and the area is ripe for research. We need to understand much more about the way cultural factors influence pain experiences. Bates (1987) argues that we must pay attention to how people learn to think about pain, which she suggests is culturally determined. She also suggests that we need to pay attention to a whole host of other variables which will vary cross-culturally, such as attitudes, values and experiences, and look at how these influence psychological, verbal and behavioural responses to pain. Culture thus appears to be inextricably intertwined with all the other aspects of an individual, and it cannot be ignored in offering care. The model in Figure 5.2 can also be represented as a model for understanding the cultural influence in pain (Fig. 5.4) and this simple model can hold true for many other health and illness events.

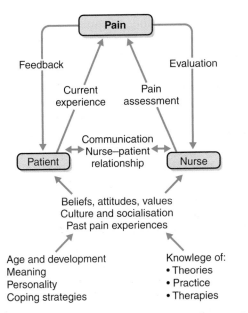

Figure 5.4 Figure 5.2 adapted to depict the influence of culture on the nurse–patient relationship when the patient is in pain.

It must be possible to determine what good practice in transcultural care should be. It should be based upon the key elements of knowing and understanding each patient's cultural background, the nurse's understanding of his or her own background, effective patient assessment, appropriate evaluation of care, the patient's own experience, and good communication within an effective nurse–patient relationship.

GOOD PRACTICE IN TRANSCULTURAL CARE

This section is not intended to be an all-encompassing summary of what differing minority ethnic and cultural groups do in their everyday lives, nor will it provide all the answers for the nurse. There are many other texts that can do that. It is merely intended to give some examples of areas in which the nurse can make a difference in the provision of care that is culturally sensitive. (Further reading suggestions are given at the end of the chapter.)

Patient assessment

Nursing care plans will usually contain some kind of assessment tool which helps the nurse take a nursing history from the patient and identify problems which can be managed by nursing intervention. Such assessment tools could incorporate a cultural element, but the nurse has to be careful not to make the questions asked seem unusual in any way. Cultural enquiry perhaps should become part of the norm for assessment. It is usual practice for a patient to be asked his religion; this may open the way for a nurse to enquire if that means anything specific in terms of, for example, food preferences and personal hygiene practices. Once the information is obtained it must be used. Vydelingum (2000) quotes South Asian patients in his study who felt that questions were asked only for the sake of the form being completed rather than seeking real information that could be used in the construction of a care plan.

Patients' explanatory models

Everyone views their health situation from their own cultural background and experience. Nurses are uniquely placed to bridge the gap between the medical viewpoint and that of the patient. By placing emphasis on the patient's understanding of the illness, anxieties and possible misunderstandings can be minimised. Patients are usually asked their personal understanding of their medical condition or for their explanation of the operation they are having, and this will be faithfully documented. Littlewood (1989) suggests that it is the nurse more than most health professionals who has the possibility of exploring the person's understanding of illness, and who can negotiate between the goals of the doctor and the goals of the patient. Herberg (1995) suggests that nurses' attitudes are influenced by a value system of rational, analytic and biomedical practices. Therefore nurses must be careful not to allow their own attitudes to stand in the way of accepting ideas, beliefs and practices about health care which are incongruent with their own. Put simply, the nurse must believe in the patient's viewpoint.

Spiritual needs

As mentioned above, patients normally will be asked their religious beliefs as part of the admission/assessment procedure. It is important to be aware that a professed religion does not necessarily mean that a person is active in that religion; or that agnostic, atheist or humanist perspectives mean that a patient does not have any kind of spiritual life. Nurses should be willing to engage in communication with patients about their spirituality, and indeed can do this without necessarily having the same beliefs. Religious beliefs should be documented carefully. Terms such as Christian, Hindu, Moslem, Jew all need further definition, lest the person the nurse identifies to help the patient is from the 'wrong' sect. This could cause great offence. Neuberger (1987) suggests that religious labels are partly anthropological – they provide guidelines for the way people live, group themselves in particular communities, mark life-cycle events and keep distance from other groups. For example, Eisenbruch (1984) argued that, although death itself is universal, the response to death is not and each cultural group will have its own appropriate responses. In the UK, the most generally acknowledged way of dealing with loss, as with pain, is the 'stiff upper lip'; a response of stoicism that is alleged to have its roots in Victorian values. Grief is viewed as essentially a private emotion and great emphasis is put on a rapid return to normality. However, the death of Diana, Princess of Wales, demonstrated that such stoic reactions may be changing. The public outpouring of grief seemed an uncharacteristic British response, and led to much comment in the press.

Murray-Parkes, Laungani and Young (1997) note that there have been few crosscultural studies on grief and mourning, suggesting that one reason for this is the reluctance of anthropological researchers to interpret their observations of grief and mourning in other cultures. Series in the nursing press and books by authors such as Green (1991) and Neuberger (1997) have gone a long way in assisting nurses in their understanding of the customs and rituals associated with death and dying in different cultural groups. Neuberger gives the example of how Jewish people deal with death. She asserts that Jews are very much in the 'here and now', with a deep and strong hold on life, and a belief in an after-life and a physical resurrection. Such an emphasis on life, Neuberger argues, makes Jews 'less than good' at dealing with a dying family member and this may be interpreted by nurses as callousness. A body is not left alone after death, and the custom of having 'watchers' who stay with the body day and night after death and recite psalms is still continued by many Jews. Clearly this may pose a problem for nurses, so the provision of a side room may be helpful to both the family and to nurses in dealing with the numbers of people involved.

It is important to acknowledge that it may be difficult for patients to adhere to the traditions and rituals of their religion while in hospital. At the very least, privacy can be offered, and nurses do have some obligation to know and understand something of their patients' belief systems if they are to offer appropriate care.

Communication and interpretation

Where interpreters are used to assist patients to communicate with health care professionals, it should be appropriate for the situation. Many women would not want a male interpreter, especially if problems of a highly intimate nature are being discussed, and indeed vice versa. Richardson (1994) suggests that interpreters must understand the issues involved and be able to help the patient (and family) understand. It is preferable to use professional interpreters and many hospitals keep a register, and also provide leaflets for patients informing them how to access the service. (See, for example, the leaflet produced by Chelsea and Westminster Hospital in eight different languages (Chelsea and Westminster Health Care, undated). Despite this, an English-speaking friend or relative is still required to make the initial approach to the hospital.) Professional services are preferable to the use of family members or volunteers from hospital staff because a professional interpreter will ensure that information is presented as given and will not edit it, which may render it inaccurate. This will also help to ensure that the patient and health carer talk to each other and not to the interpreter. Members of staff are often used as volunteers to interpret for patients, but such use can take them away from their own jobs. Extreme caution should be taken if children are to be used as interpreters for family members. They may speak English well, but will have a very limited medical vocabulary, are not able to grasp the concepts involved, and certainly should not be expected to cope with the responsibility. It would be devastating if, for example, a child were asked to interpret news of cancer, or other serious illness.

Eating and drinking

Eating and drinking are part of what we all do every single day of our lives. The more common dietary preferences are generally catered for in the provision of food and fluids in hospital. Most hospital menus will give a choice so that people who are vegetarian, or wish to eat, for example, a low fat diet or a high fibre diet, can eat their preferred food. Many people do not mind what sort of food they eat or how it is prepared. However, for some people such aspects of eating and drinking are very important manifestations of their religion or culture. Although all cultures have a shared need of food, ethnocentric thoughtlessness can result (Gerrish et al 1996). People should not be expected to suspend their beliefs or their food preferences because they are ill. Families may wish to overcome deficiencies in hospital catering by bringing in food prepared at home; but while this may solve a problem for one individual, it does nothing to address the issue in general terms (Case example 5.2).

A situation such as the one in Case example 5.2 is unlikely in the year 2000, as most people now understand so much more about all kinds of foods. However the South Asian community continues to have a much higher than average risk of coronary heart disease and diabetes. For various reasons Asian families may be unaware of current Department of Health guidelines on healthy eating. Local health promotion initiatives on food preparation can assist women from minority ethnic groups in this respect. Asian cookery clubs set up in south Bedfordshire helped women to

Case example 5.2

In 1977 an elderly man of Ugandan Asian origin, with newly diagnosed diabetes, was admitted to a medical ward. His family brought him his main meals. On one occasion the consultant physician happened to be in the ward at dinner time and, observing the gentleman eating chapattis, turned to the ward sister and wagged his finger, ordering 'no chapattis, sister!'. Following on from this, the ward sister consulted with the hospital dietician who arranged to talk to the family through an interpreter and advised them on the correct balance of carbohydrate and fat in the patient's diet. The ward sister was then able to inform the physician that she was satisfied the patient was eating an appropriate diet for his diabetes.

adapt their traditional cooking in line with dietary recommendations. Evaluation of these clubs demonstrated that this model of helping individuals to follow healthier diets was effective in facilitating dietary change (Snowdon 1999).

In the 1970s it was unusual for a hospital to provide Asian menus. Today, hospitals should provide menus to cater for a wide variety of different food preferences. The nurse has a responsibility to make such menus available for all patients who need them, and to assist each patient to make appropriate choices from that menu. However, Vydelingum (2000) cites a number of authors who have found that there is still poor provision of nutritional services to meet religious needs. Thomas & Dines (1994) have suggested that where Asian meals are provided, they are rather limited, usually being vegetarian, and that provision for Afro-Caribbean meals is virtually non-existent. The Multicultural Information File (MCRIC 1994) is an example of how appropriate information can be given to nurses and other health professionals. It sets out clearly a food and health policy, stating that it will require extension to take into account the more specific needs of the many cultural groups resident in south Glamorgan. For example, the policy states that religious or cultural laws governing food preparation should be adhered to and respected.

Personal hygiene and washing

Attention to these aspects of personal care occupies much nursing time, and ensuring the comfort and cleanliness of patients is a core activity of nursing. A patient of white British origin may be entirely happy to wash in the bath, or under a shower, or from a bowl of water put by the bed. He may not like removing underwear for surgical procedures, but will comply with such a request from a nurse. However, a patient of Asian origin, for example a Hindu, may find such practices as washing from a bowl of water unacceptable because running water is considered essential for cleanliness. Nurses must learn to adapt their practices in this respect to allow the patient to feel clean and comfortable. Patients of Muslim origin distinguish between the 'clean' right hand

Case example 5.3

In the operating theatre, it is the responsibility of the whole operating team to ensure that the *kaccha* is kept in place. An incident was described by a theatre nurse who was studying a course in transcultural care. The patient had kept the *kaccha* on during the journey to the operating theatre and while being anaesthetised. After the patient was moved onto the operating table, a member of the theatre staff had started to remove the garment. The theatre nurse prevented this from happening and advised that the *kaccha* should be wrapped loosely around one ankle. She reminded the theatre staff that in much the same way, many Christian people and those to whom the symbolic meaning is important, do not like to have a wedding band removed. It is a small but significant task for the nurse to tape it to the finger to guard against loss or damage, and the same principle should apply to the symbols of other faiths.

and the 'dirty' left hand. The siting of intravenous infusions is therefore important. Sikhs wear five identifying symbols, including the *kara*, a steel bangle which should never be removed, and *kaccha* (undershorts), which are intended to reinforce notions of sexual morality and modesty. *Kaccha* are never removed totally; the wearer changes *kaccha* by removing one leg from the old pair and putting it into the leg of a new pair before removing the old pair from the other leg. This garment is also worn when showering (Case example 5.3).

CONCLUSION

It can be argued that a transcultural view of caring will assist the nursing profession to see all patients as empowered human beings. To move nurses into culturally informed clinical practice, the concept of culture must be viewed as basic to the nature of caring, and responsible for shaping human responses to health, illness and other life situations.

Modern nurses in the 21st century must attempt to provide health care within the context of understanding the effects of culture on patients and on themselves. In a multicultural and multi-racial society this simply cannot be ignored. When nurses and other health professionals develop competence in culture and begin to operate from a transcultural position, the field of transcultural nursing will cease to exist, because transcultural nursing is nursing!

REFERENCES

Abdullah S N 1995 Towards an individualised client's care: implications for education. The transcultural approach. Journal of Advanced Nursing 22: 715–720

Andrews M M, Boyle J S 1995 Transcultural concepts in nursing care. Lippincott, Philadelphia

Balarjajan R, Raleigh V S 1993 The health of the nation: ethnicity and health: a guide for the NHS. Department of Health, London

Bates M 1987 Ethnicity and pain: a bio-cultural model. Social Science and Medicine 24(1): 47–50

Calvillo E R, Flaskerud J H 1993 Evaluation of the pain response by Mexican American women and their nurses. Journal of Advanced Nursing 18: 451–459

Chelsea and Westminster Health Care (undated) Interpreting service. Chelsea and Westminster Health Care Trust, London

Davitz L L, Sameshima Y, Davitz J R 1976 Suffering as viewed in six different cultures. American Journal of Nursing 76(8): 1296–1297

Department of Health 1992 Health of the nation: a strategy for health in England. HMSO, London

DeSantis L 1994 Making anthropology clinically relevant to nursing care. Journal of Advanced Nursing 20: 707–715

Eisenbruch M 1984 Cross-cultural aspects of bereavement. 1: A conceptual framework for comparative analysis. Culture, Medicine and Psychiatry 8: 283–309

Gerrish K, Husband C, MacKenzie J 1996 Nursing for a multi-ethnic society. Open University Press, Buckingham

Green J 1991 Death with dignity: meeting the needs of patients in a multi-cultural society. Nursing Times Book Service, London

Helman C 1994 Culture, health and illness, 3rd edn. Butterworth-Heinemann, Oxford

Herberg P 1989 Theoretical foundations of transcultural nursing. In: Andrews M M, Boyle J S Transcultural concepts in nursing care, 2nd edn. Lippincott, Philadelphia

International Council of Nurses 1974 Code for nurses: ethical concepts applied to nursing. International Nursing Review 21(3–4): 103–104

James J 1995 Ethnicity and transcultural care. In: Basford L, Slevin O (eds) Theory and practice of nursing. Camion Press, London

Lea A 1994 Nursing in today's multicultural society: a transcultural perspective. Journal of Advanced Nursing 20: 307–313

Leininger M M (ed) 1991 Culture care, diversity and universality: a theory of nursing. National League for Nursing Press, New York

Littlewood J 1989 A model for nursing using anthropological literature. International Journal of Nursing Studies 26(3): 221–229

McGee P 1992 Teaching transcultural care: a guide for teachers of nursing and health care. Chapman Hall, London

Mares P, Henley A, Baxter C 1985 Health care in multiracial Britain. Health Education Council/National Extension College, Cambridge

Mason C 1990 Women as mothers in Northern Ireland and Jamaica: a critique of the transcultural nursing movement. International Journal of Nursing Studies 27(4): 367–374

Melzack R, Wall P D 1989 The challenge of pain. Penguin Books, Harmondsworth

Minority Cultures Resource and Information Centre 1994 The multicultural information file. MCRIC and Cardiff Community Health Care and South Glamorgan Health Authority, Cardiff

Murray-Parkes C, Laungani P, Young B (eds) 1997 Death and bereavement across cultures. Routledge, London

Neuberger J 1987 Caring for dying people of different faiths. Lisa Sainsbury Foundation Series. Austen Cornish, London

Ng F 2000 Female genital mutilation: its implications for reproductive health. An overview. British Journal of Family Planning 26(1): 47–51

Papadopoulos I 1999 Health and illness beliefs of Greek Cypriots living in London. Journal of Advanced Nursing 29(5): 1097–1104

Richardson J 1994 Cultural issues in critical care nursing. In: Millar B, Burnard P Critical care nursing: caring for the critically ill adult. Baillière Tindall, London

Roper N, Logan W, Tierney A 1996 The elements of nursing: a model for nursing based on a model for living, 4th edn. Churchill Livingstone, London

Royal College of Surgeons 1990 Report of the working party on pain after surgery. Royal College of Surgeons, London

Snowdon W D 1999 Asian cookery clubs: a community health promotion intervention. International Journal of Health Promotion and Education 37(4): 135–136

Thomas V J, Rose F D 1991 Ethnic differences in the experience of pain. Social Science and Medicine 32(9): 1063–1066

Thomas V J, Dines A 1994 The health care needs of ethnic minority groups: are nurses playing their part? Journal of Advanced Nursing 20: 802–808

Tripp-Reimer T, Brink P J, Saunders J M 1984 Cultural assessment: content and process. Nursing Outlook 32(2): 78–82

United Kingdom Central Council For Nursing Midwifery And Health Visiting 1992 Code of professional conduct. UKCC, London

UK Transplant Co-ordinators Association (undated) Organ donation: religious and cultural issues

Vydelingum V 2000 South Asian patients' lived experience of acute care in an English hospital: a phenomenological study. Journal of Advanced Nursing 32(1): 100–107

Zborowski M 1952 Cultural components in responses to pain. In: Conrad P, Kerns R (eds) The sociology of health and illness. St Martin's Press, New York

FURTHER READING

Burr J A, Chapman T 1998 Some reflections on cultural and social considerations in mental health nursing. Journal of Psychiatric and Mental Health Nursing 5(6): 431–437
Students intending to undertake branch studies in mental health will find this article aids their understanding of cultural issues in mental health.

Chappiti U, Jean-Marie S, Chan W 2000 Cultural and religious influences on adult nutrition in the UK. Nursing Standard 14(29): 47–51
This article gives a more detailed account of dietary needs for selected religious and cultural groups.

Farrington A 1993 Transcultural psychiatry, ethnic minorities and marginalisation. British Journal of Nursing 2(16): 805–809
Students undertaking branch studies in mental health nursing will find this article will aid their understanding of cultural issues in mental health.

Kelleher D, Hillier S 1996 Researching cultural differences in health. Routledge, London
This book is a useful resource on research into cultural differences in health and provides good background information.

Mwasandube P 2000 Mixing cultures: the challenges for nursing. Nursing Management 7(2): 21–25
This article highlights cultural problems facing the NHS from both a nursing care and a patient perspective.

Radley A (ed) 1995 Worlds of illness: biographical and cultural perspectives on health and disease. Routledge, London
This book reviews finding from medical sociology, health psychology and medical anthropology; and in relating these findings to specific disease processes helps to answer some of the questions about cultural aspects of disease.

The Transcultural Nursing and Health Care Association was set up in 1998. There are plans for a journal. Internet access: http://www.fons.org/network/tcnha

2 Theory supporting nursing care

SECTION CONTENTS

6. The physiological basis of nursing   149

7. The psychological basis of nursing   197

8. The sociological basis of nursing   225

Theory supporting
nursing care

6

The physiological basis of nursing

Gillian Snowley

CHAPTER CONTENTS

Recurring principles of physiology   150

The cell   151
The cell and nuclear membranes   151
Transport across membranes   152
The nucleus and genetic material   152
Cell division   154
Mitosis   154
Meiosis   154
Inheritance   155
Human hereditary disorders   156
The Human Genome Project   160
Genetic modification   162

The sustenance of life   163
Energy from cellular respiration   163
The importance of enzymes in
cell chemistry   164
Factors affecting enzyme action   164

Homeostasis and the body systems   167
Regulation mechanisms in
homeostasis   167
The skin and homeostasis   169
The cardiovascular system and
homeostasis   172
Blood   172
The heart   176
The arterial system   176
Capillaries   176
The venous system   178
The lymphatic system   178
The respiratory system and
homeostasis   179
The mechanisms of lung ventilation   180
The digestive system and homeostasis   181

Ingestion   181
Obtaining food   181
Digestion   181
Motility of the alimentary canal   182
Gastrointestinal secretions   183
Absorption   184
Defecation   185
The renal system and homeostasis   185
Formation of urine   186
Excretory function of the kidneys   187
The importance of healthy kidneys   188
Micturition   188
The nervous system and homeostasis   188
The processes of nervous regulation   190
The endocrine system and
homeostasis   190
Hormones   191
The immune system and homeostasis   191
How the immune system works   192
Immunity and immunisation   193

References   195

Further reading   195

In a single chapter, it is impossible to convey more than a few of the basic principles and objectives for understanding the physiological self. This chapter attempts to lead the reader towards the underlying purpose of body function, namely the constant endeavour by the body to remain physically and chemically 'balanced' or homeostatic. In doing this, the text aims to:

- introduce the basic physiology of the cell
- outline, with specific examples, the principles of cell division and inheritance
- describe the production of energy in the cell
- explore homeostasis, focusing on specific body systems and using examples relevant to nursing practice to explain both how problems may arise and the role of health professionals in re-establishing the balance.

Much of physiology is an account, largely in terms of physics and chemistry, of *what* happens *where* in the body. In the past, detailed information about the minute structure of the cell was considered to be of academic interest only, but it is now evident that cytology (the study of the cell) is of major significance to physiology and pathology (the study of disease) and hence to health care. The other main area of physiology deals with the coordination of the individual parts of an organism to form an efficiently functioning whole: how the whole is greater than the sum of its parts, and how the parts behave as if they know of the existence of each other and of the whole.

RECURRING PRINCIPLES OF PHYSIOLOGY

To attempt to cover completely the depth and the mysteries of the physiological self in one chapter is not only an impossibility but also a belittling of the subject and of those who have studied it

and made their knowledge available to others. However, certain principles or themes recur throughout the study of physiology, and may be summarised as follows:

- *Function is based on structure.* Human movement, for example, depends on the structure of muscles, bones and nerves, and on their anatomical interrelationship. The dependence becomes even more evident when microscopic and more intricate structures are studied. One of the most intensively studied tissues is skeletal muscle, whose ultrastructure is revealed by electron microscopy and provides an explanation of muscular contraction.

The principle that function depends on structure applies also to biochemical events. For example, changing the shape of an enzyme molecule by heating it to above 40°C may render it biologically non-functional.

- *Genetics determines biological function.* It is generally agreed that the information content of a DNA (deoxyribonucleic acid) molecule is responsible for the structure, function, behaviour and survival of a species. DNA carries the genetic code, and every part of body structure and function is determined by this code. Every detail of structure and function, every second of chemical activity, is ultimately subservient to the transmission of the genetic code to the germline (reproductive cells) for the survival of the species. Physiology is the discipline whose study reveals how this is achieved.

- *Homeostasis ensures survival.* All organisms survive, in their lifetime, because of their ability to maintain a constant environment for their cells and tissues. In human beings, this environment is the fluid that surrounds the body cells (tissue fluid). The content of this fluid must be regulated to provide adequate nutrients to the cells (and to remove toxic waste) at the correct rate and temperature and within a narrow range of acidity/alkalinity. Much of the study of physiology is the study of how systems work to produce homeostasis.

These principles are explored further in this chapter. It has not been possible to provide an explanation of basic biochemical principles, nor is basic anatomy of tissues, organs and systems dealt with in any detail, but the microstructure of cells and molecules is outlined where this is essential to an understanding of physiology. (See the Further reading list at the end of this chapter for helpful texts.)

The cell, its boundaries and its DNA are described in the first section of the chapter. This enables the reader to move on to a brief exploration of heredity and genetics. The second section introduces some aspects of basic biochemistry, as well as factors that affect the sustenance of life at cellular and whole-body levels. The third section is devoted to the concept of homeostasis and how all the major body systems function towards its achievement. Throughout the chapter, examples are given of the relevance of physiology to nursing, health, and disorders of health. The following quotation (from Wright 1965) explains why all nurses should have some knowledge of physiology:

When a physiological response is observed, one generally proceeds to ask the questions 'How' and 'Why'? The first is a physiological one; it means: 'what are the mechanisms responsible for the change; what is the sequence of events between the stimulus and the response?' The second question is not really physiological at all; it is an appeal to the idea of purpose ... but can be very useful. Most people asking 'Why?' mean 'In what way does the response help to preserve the integrity and the efficiency of the organism, or to protect it from changes in the environment, either external or internal?'

We reasonably take it for granted that unless an organism were equipped to make such responses it would never have survived. (Wright 1965)

THE CELL

The structure of a typical cell is shown in Figure 6.1.

Our bodies are made up of cells, but, as befits a sophisticated animal such as a human being, there is a high degree of differentiation whereby these cells perform a variety of specialised functions. With the exception of red blood cells, all human cells contain at least one nucleus surrounded by a mass of cytoplasm, which may contain a variety of cellular sub-units or organelles. Probably of greatest importance in appreciating the place of the cell in the overall physiology of the body is an understanding of the nature and purpose of the cell membranes, the nucleus and its genetic importance, and the biochemical cycle of events that produces energy.

THE CELL AND NUCLEAR MEMBRANES

The limiting boundary of the cell is the plasma membrane (cytoplasmic membrane or cell membrane). The plasma membrane acts as a

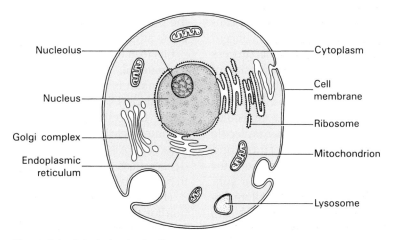

Figure 6.1 A typical animal cell.

permeability barrier that regulates the entry and exit of materials. It is composed of a double layer of phospholipids (fats) with protein molecules floating in a 'fatty' sea. Thus, the membrane structure is far from rigid, and the protein molecules are believed to be mobile within it, some extending all the way through it (protein bridges or channels). No holes or pores have been identified in the plasma membrane, and it is believed that the protein bridges allow fat-insoluble substances, for example glucose, to cross the membrane. Fat-soluble substances such as alcohol can, obviously, pass through the lipid layer.

Transport across membranes

There are several mechanisms by which substances gain entry to or leave a cell:

- diffusion
- osmosis
- facilitated diffusion
- active transport
- phagocytosis and pinocytosis.

Diffusion is the passive movement of a substance from an area of high concentration to an area of low concentration of that substance. The substance may be water or a solute such as glucose or sodium (Na^+). Diffusion requires no energy expenditure by the cell. Only small molecules make the transfer in this way.

Osmosis is the flow of a solvent (water, in the body) across a semipermeable membrane (the cell membrane) from a weaker to a more concentrated solution, i.e. from a high water concentration to a low water concentration. This process will continue until the solutions on either side of the membrane are of equal concentration.

Facilitated diffusion is the method by which molecules become attached to carrier molecules within the membrane itself. The carrier molecule is specific for the transported substance, and there must still be a concentration gradient for facilitated diffusion to occur. Glucose is a substance transported across a muscle cell membrane in this way. No cell energy is expended to achieve such transport. The limiting factor for transport is the number of free carrier molecules.

Active transport is the process by which substances transfer across the plasma membrane when there is no concentration gradient, or against the gradient, i.e. from an area of low concentration to an area of high concentration. Cell energy is expended for this to occur. Active transport is an essential mechanism for the maintenance of constant cell composition within a changing extracellular environment (see 'Homeostasis and the body systems', p. 167).

Phagocytosis and pinocytosis. Some substances or larger particles may enter cells by becoming engulfed (phagocytosis for particles, pinocytosis for water). The plasma membrane enfolds them, and they become enclosed in a fluid-filled vesicle. This method is regularly used by the mobile white blood cells that engulf bacteria. Once inside the cell, the engulfed substance undergoes chemical breakdown by intracellular enzymes. The soluble end products then diffuse into the cytoplasm while indigestible remains are released into the surrounding environment by the reversal of phagocytosis.

THE NUCLEUS AND GENETIC MATERIAL

The most prominent feature of a cell, when viewed under the microscope, is the nucleus. It is separated from the cytoplasm by a double membrane. Transport mechanisms through the nuclear membrane are not as well understood as are those of the cytoplasmic membrane, and during the process of cell division the membrane disappears altogether, to re-form later.

Electron micrography reveals irregular masses of material, called chromatin, in the nucleus. Chromatin is a mixture of protein, deoxyribonucleic acid (DNA) and ribonucleic acid (RNA). When the cell reproduces itself, the chromatin becomes clearly visible in threads known as chromosomes. Also within the nucleus are one or two denser areas known as nucleoli. These are known to be rich in RNA.

The chromosomes contain the genetic information for the whole body, but, in any one cell, not all of this information will be active all of the time. The key molecule that carries the 'genetic

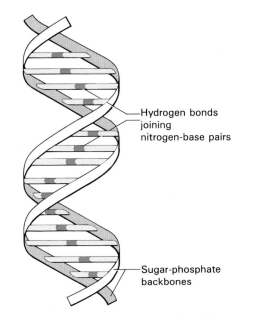

Hydrogen bonds joining nitrogen-base pairs

Sugar-phosphate backbones

Figure 6.2　The Watson and Crick model for DNA.

code' is the DNA molecule (Fig. 6.2). Genetic information (genes) determines all parts of our make-up, from the colour of our eyes to the way we walk. The particular sequencing of bases within the DNA molecule determines the synthesis of a particular protein within a cell and thus controls cellular function. RNA, found within the nucleus and the cytoplasm, is a molecule that is able to transmit the genetic information from gene to ribosomes, which is where proteins are made (Box 6.1).

With the exception of the germ cells in the ovaries and testes (i.e. ova and spermatozoa), all the nucleated cells of the human body contain 46 chromosomes, in 23 homologous pairs. Of each pair, one chromosome is derived from the person's mother and the other from the father. There are now known to be approximately 75 000 genes carried on these 46 chromosomes. The chromosomes of a homologous pair are alike in size and shape and can line up together as exactly as the two halves of a zip. There is one exception to this ruling, which is the pair of sex chromosomes. Of this pair, one is the X chromosome and the other may be the different Y chromosome, whose presence means that the person will be genetically male. An appreciation of the processes of cell

---

Box 6.1　DNA and the genetic code

DNA is a massive molecule (molecular weight in the millions) whose now well-known structure was identified by Watson and Crick in the 1950s.

It is composed of two molecular chains, which are intertwined in a helical configuration. The 'backbone' of each chain is made of sugars and phosphates. Protruding at regular intervals along the chain is one of four nitrogen base materials. Each chain of the double helix links with the other by a 'loose' chemical combination of the opposing nitrogen base (see Fig. 6.2).

It is the particular order of the bases in the two chains that determines the genetic information encoded in the DNA. It is important to remember that the base on one chain can only ever combine with one other base on the opposite chain. The four bases are:

- **adenosine**, which always links with **thymine**
- **guanine**, which always links with **cytosine**.

It is the sequencing of the nitrogen bases on one strand of the DNA double helix which conveys the genetic code. A DNA molecule is capable of reproducing itself exactly, according to the sequencing of bases on each strand. This is what happens during mitosis: as the chromosomes replicate, so does the DNA. In meiosis, as the chromosomes' strands become intertwined and partially exchanged, so do the strands of DNA, leading to genetic variation in the gametes and, therefore, the offspring.

The actual genetic code is now known to be a triplet code. A sequence of three bases on a DNA strand recognises one amino acid, so successive triplets specify amino acid sequence and hence protein structure. The codes for all 20 known amino acids are now well understood. Since proteins are made of amino acids, sometimes many thousands of triplet codings are necessary for the 'blueprint' of a single protein.

---

division is the first step to understanding how characteristics are inherited.

Factors affecting sex determination

In human beings, the female has 22 pairs of ordinary chromosomes (known as autosomes) and one pair of similar sex chromosomes (two X chromosomes, one from the mother and one from the father). The male also has 22 pairs of autosomes but has a pair of dissimilar sex chromosomes (one X chromosome from the mother, and one Y chromosome from the father). Sex inheritance is illustrated in Figure 6.3.

The possibility of having a male or a female child is equal according to this normal, chromosomal

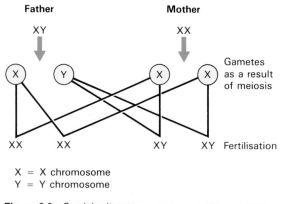

X = X chromosome
Y = Y chromosome

Figure 6.3 Sex inheritance.

inheritance. However, the sex of an individual is subject to other possible variables, despite the person's sex chromosome. All human embryos will develop as females, irrespective of whether the sex chromosome construction is XX or YY, unless male hormones are produced and function at early stages of embryonic development (usually about 6 weeks after fertilisation). It has been thought that a gene controlling male development exists and is located on the Y chromosome, but this has yet to be confirmed. The role of the Y chromosome in determining maleness is not well understood.

CELL DIVISION

Mitosis

Humans consist of approximately 10^{16} cells, but each individual is developed from a single cell. Not only must the 10^{16} cells be formed as the body grows and matures, but they must also be replaced in regeneration and repair. The type of cell division that provides for this growth and repair is mitosis. The special significance of mitosis is that it ensures a continuous succession of cells with 46 chromosomes and the same genetic endowment.

During mitosis, the nucleus of the parent cell divides into two identical nuclei, after which the cytoplasm of the cell divides. In the early stage of mitosis each chromosome is duplicated so that the nucleus contains two identical complete sets

of genes on identical pairs of chromosomes. Each chromosome is connected to its duplicate at one point called the centromere. Each identical portion of chromosome is known as a chromatid. The stages of mitosis are shown in Figure 6.4.

Although the process of mitosis produces millions of cells carrying identical sets of genes, it is important to remember that the resultant cells undergo specialisation by using only part of their inherent genetic code; for example, some cells in the pancreas produce insulin, while nerve cells conduct electrical impulses. However, this feature of specialised cells doing specialised things is, itself, coded for in the DNA.

Meiosis

Some cells become specialised to form the reproductive cells or gametes. The female gamete is the ovum, and the male gamete is the sperm. Meiosis is the cell division that produces gametes. If gametes were produced by mitosis, the human egg and sperm would each contain 46 chromosomes. The fertilised egg, formed by their union, would then contain 92 chromosomes, as would the gametes produced by the resultant adult. Thus, with each new generation, the chromosome number would double. Meiosis prevents this from happening. The two most significant outcomes of meiosis are that:

- 23 single chromosomes occur in the gamete
- genes may have switched between paired chromosomes prior to their separation at actual cell division.

The process of meiosis is illustrated in Figure 6.5. (It should be noted that genetic switching occurs in the first division stage.) The resulting cells contain a mixture of maternal and paternal chromosomes because their segregation at anaphase is entirely random. Further randomness of gene inheritance in the gametes is produced by the 'crossing-over' of genetic material between chromatids. Since the resultant cells contribute through fertilisation to the next generation, sexual reproduction ensures the production of individuals who are different from their parents and from each other. (The exception here is identical

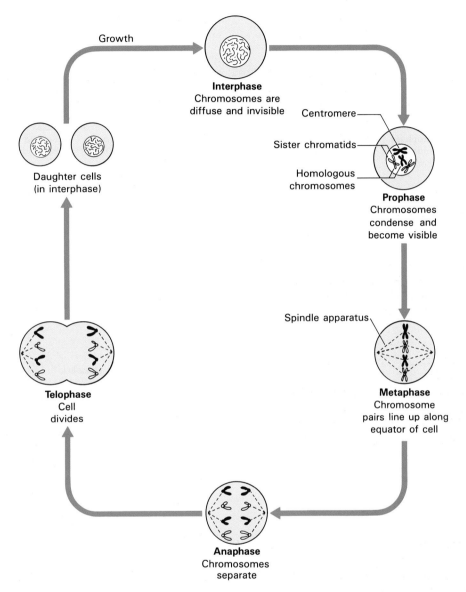

Figure 6.4   The stages of mitosis.

twins, who are formed by a mitosis of the fertilised egg.)

INHERITANCE

Meiosis provides a general picture of how the basic physiological process of inheritance works. It is the process whereby genetic material passes from one generation to the next. The foundations for the study and development of genetics and inheritance were laid by an Austrian monk, Gregor Mendel, in 1866. Mendel's work was brilliant and classical, and is still highly regarded as the first fundamental study of inheritance. The fact that he knew nothing of chromosomes and DNA, let alone cell structure, mitosis and meiosis, makes his work all the more remarkable. The modern study of genetics, however, has shown that human inheritance is infinitely more complex than is laid out in Mendel's laws. Crick and

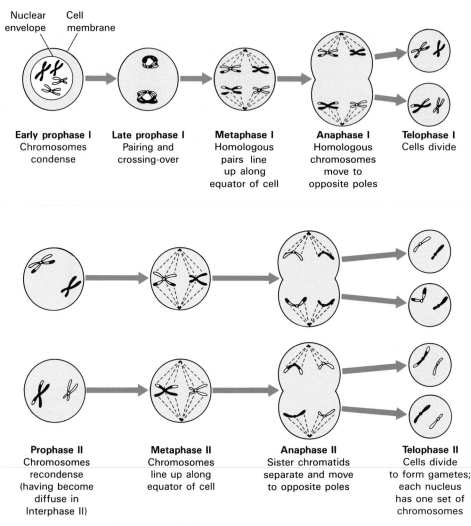

Figure 6.5 The stages of meiosis.

Watson's discovery of the structure of DNA in the 1950s heralded the beginning of modern genetics which has become an increasingly precise science and one which it is believed will dominate medicine in the 21st century. Perhaps one of the most important research projects of the late 20th century has been the Human Genome Project whose goal has been to construct a physical map of all 3.3 billion nitrogen base pairs in the haploid human genome. (A genome is the array of genes carried by an individual). At the time of writing, this international project has just been completed and further developments are eagerly awaited.

Human hereditary disorders

Human hereditary disorders are known as congenital disorders. There are three main ways in which such disorders can be inherited:

1. A *single gene* may be the cause, where the structure of the gene has been altered, i.e. the order of the nitrogen bases has been changed.
2. There may be *chromosomal abnormalities*.
3. A *genetic predisposition* may be inherited which, together with other factors within the individual or his environment, will result in a particular condition.

(See Table 6.1 for examples of human hereditary disorders.)

Mutations

By understanding what a gene is and how genes specify the formation of proteins, it is not difficult to appreciate how an alteration to gene coding, for whatever reason, alters the functioning of a cell. Indeed, it is remarkable that this happens so infrequently. Changes in genes are known as mutations and may be responsible for altered function, disease or disability, which may or may not be inherited.

If mutations occur during the production of gametes (germinal mutations), the mutant gene or genes will be inherited. Mutations may also occur in other body cells, and these mutant genes will not be inherited (somatic mutations: e.g. skin cancer due to ultraviolet radiation).

Causes of mutations are always the subject of research investigations, but known causes include environmental, physical and chemical factors. Possibly the best known of these is ionising radiation, the subject of extensive studies in relation to nuclear power plants and childhood leukaemia.

Single gene disorders

At each position, or locus, on opposing homologous chromosomes is a pair of genes specific to a certain characteristic, for example hair colour, eye colour or perhaps a disorder of some kind. If one of the pair becomes altered by mutation, the individual may exhibit altered characteristics. When the altered gene is on an autosome, it is said to be an autosomal inheritance. Autosomally inherited characteristics can be passed on to the next generation either as a dominant characteristic or as a recessive characteristic. In the dominant mode of inheritance, one of the parents will show the features of the condition and there is always a 50% chance that each pregnancy will result in an affected child. In a recessive disorder, it is possible that neither parent is affected by the condition, but if two people who are carrying the recessive gene have children, there is a 25% (1 in 4) chance that a child may have the disorder. The risk is the same for every pregnancy. See Boxes 6.2 and 6.3 for examples of these autosomal inheritance patterns, which follow the straightforward Mendelian pattern.

When the altered gene is on one of the sex chromosomes, the condition is said to be sex-linked.

Sex-linked inheritance

This is inheritance of a mutant gene, which is carried on a sex chromosome. Almost all sex-linked inherited conditions are carried on the X chromosome and thus their pattern of inheritance is said

Table 6.1	Some well-known human hereditary disorders and diseases and their consequences
Disease	**Major consequence**
Chromosome abnormalities	
Down's syndrome	Mental retardation
Klinefelter's syndrome	Sterility, occasional mental retardation
Turner's syndrome	Sterility, lack of sexual development
Autosomal dominant mutations	
Achondroplasia	Dwarfism
Retinoblastoma	Blindness
Porphyria	Abdominal pain, psychosis
Huntington's chorea	Nervous system degeneration
Neurofibromatosis	Growths in nervous system and skin
Polydactyly	Extra fingers and toes
Autosomal recessive mutations	
Cystic fibrosis	Respiratory disorders
Xeroderma pigmentosum	Skin cancers
Albinism	Lack of pigment in skin and eyes
Phenylketonuria	Mental retardation
Homocystinuria	Mental retardation
Sickle-cell disease	Anaemia
X chromosome mutations	
Haemophilia	Failure of blood to clot, bleeding
Duchenne muscular dystrophy	Progressive muscular weakness
Agammaglobulinaemia	Defective immune system, infections
Testicular feminising syndrome	Sterility, lack of male organs

Box 6.2 **Autosomal dominant inheritance**

The family tree below, through three generations, is an example of how a dominant autosomal condition is inherited. Examples of such conditions are Huntington's chorea, achondroplasia, neurofibromatosis. Both males and females can be equally affected by this kind of inheritance.

▼

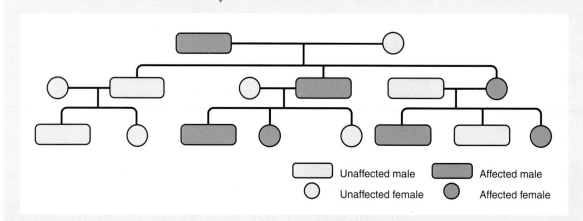

What is actually happening in the inheritance of genes is shown below. **A** represents the dominant gene for the condition and **a** is the recessive gene for the normal state. Any individual with **A** will show the characteristics of the condition. The 50% chance of inheritance may be seen in this case, even when only one parent has the condition.

The severity of these conditions can vary widely within members of the same family. A disease such as Huntington's chorea does not manifest itself until midlife, so children can be born before the parents are aware that such a condition is part of their genetic make-up.

▼

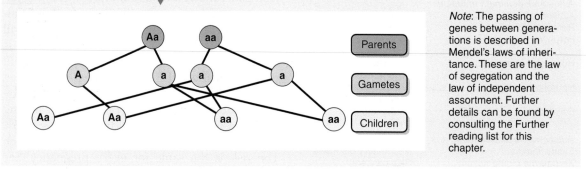

Note: The passing of genes between generations is described in Mendel's laws of inheritance. These are the law of segregation and the law of independent assortment. Further details can be found by consulting the Further reading list for this chapter.

to be X-linked. This is because the opposing Y chromosome does not carry any genes to complement those carried on the X, so a male needs to inherit only one, possibly recessive, gene to exhibit the characteristic. If the gene happens to be a disease-causing one, the male then has the disease. X-linked inheritance, therefore, usually affects only males. This pattern of inheritance means that each daughter has a 50% chance of being a *carrier* of the inherited condition (Box 6.4).

Chromosomal abnormalities

These may be either numerical or structural. Numerical abnormalities are the result of too many or too few chromosomes being present in the ovum or sperm prior to fertilisation. The embryo produced will then have an abnormal number of chromosomes, which may or may not be compatible with life. The most common cause of chromosomal abnormality is failure of

Box 6.3   Autosomal recessive inheritance

The family tree below is a typical example for an autosomal recessive disorder, shown through three generations. Both males and females can be equally affected by this mode of inheritance.

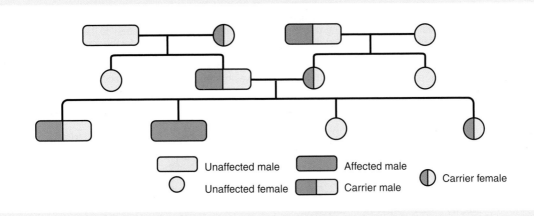

There is a 25% chance, in the third generation above, of a child being born with the condition, a 50% chance of the child being a carrier for the condition, and a 25% chance of a child being unaffected. The inheritance of the genes is shown below.

In this situation, **b** is the recessive gene for the condition and **B** is the dominant gene for the normal state. An individual with **bb** as their genetic make-up (*genotype*) will have the condition, those with **Bb** are carriers but not affected by the disorder, and those with **BB** will be unaffected.

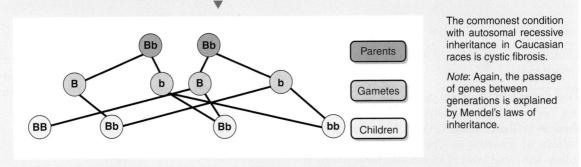

The commonest condition with autosomal recessive inheritance in Caucasian races is cystic fibrosis.

Note: Again, the passage of genes between generations is explained by Mendel's laws of inheritance.

chromosome segregation in meiosis. (See Boxes 6.5 and 6.6, which illustrate normal and abnormal gametogenesis). The commonest chromosomal congenital disorder is Down's syndrome where there is an extra chromosome present at pair 21. Structural abnormalities can involve any chromosome and one of the commonest problems is a deletion of part of a chromosome, as in fragile X syndrome, where the X chromosome looks as though it is about to become detached. In structural abnormalities, pieces of chromosome may *translocate* to a different chromosome and give rise to a congenital disorder. Chromosomal abnormalities occur in about 0.6% of live births; these small differences in genetic make-up can result in profound difficulties for affected individuals and their families and some are incompatible with life beyond the womb. Antenatal diagnosis of chromosomal abnormalities is possible at about 10 weeks of pregnancy and expectant parents are now able to make decisions about possible termination of pregnancy if a severe abnormality is found.

Box 6.4   Haemophilia as an example of sex-linked inheritance

Genes that are located on the X chromosome are said to be sex-linked because usually only the male is affected by them. A female can also have a sex-linked characteristic, providing that both her X chromosomes carry the recessive gene. Probably the most well-known and serious sex-linked inherited disorder is the blood-clotting disorder haemophilia. It has been famous as an inherited disorder in Queen Victoria's family, and, with intermarriage with European royals, the disorder has been inherited in these families. The disease has not been transmitted to living descendants of the British royal family.

Because of the different structures of X and Y chromosomes, a male (XY) will have haemophilia even if he carries only one recessive gene on his X chromosome. There is no opposing or complementary gene on the Y chromosome. A female must carry two recessive genes (one on each X chromosome) to have haemophilia. A female who is heterozygous for the condition is said to be a *carrier* although she will not have haemophilia.

When a carrier female (X*X) and a normal male (XY) have children, the following hereditary pattern is possible.

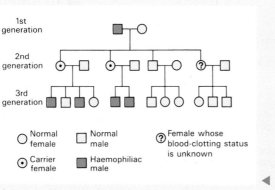

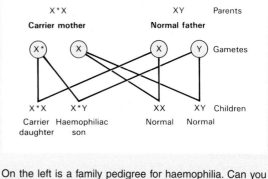

On the left is a family pedigree for haemophilia. Can you determine why the blood-clotting status of one of the women in the second generation is unknown?

Genetic predisposition (or multifactorial inheritance)

This is the largest group of genetic factors causing abnormality. In many common disorders there is evidence for genetic factors but no clear pattern of inheritance. These conditions do not follow the usual laws of Mendelian inheritance. It is now generally accepted that multifactorial inheritance involves the interaction of adverse environmental factors (either internal or external to the individual) with an underlying susceptibility which is determined by the additive effect of many genes. Unlike single gene inheritance, firm scientific evidence for multifactorial inheritance is harder to determine. Such conditions are known to involve the inheritance being the result of many genes at different loci with each gene contributing a small additive effect, i.e. no one gene is dominant or recessive to another. Examples of disorders which are multifactorial include diabetes, the tendency to particular types of cancer, coronary heart disease and schizophrenia. Much research is being carried out to determine the genetic cause of these disorders.

The Human Genome Project

For the past few decades, geneticists have been dealing with the question of exactly how genes are organised within the chromosomes of organisms. The answer is being found through the attempts to analyse the complete *genome*, or the entire haploid set of chromosomes which form the genetic material of a variety of diverse organisms from bacteria to humans. As this chapter is being prepared, classification of the complete human genome has just been completed. This international project got under way in 1990. The sequence of each gene in the human genome is now known.

Box 6.5   Gametogenesis

The production of gametes is distinctly different in men and women and this results in different clinical consequences if errors of cell division occur. The two processes are illustrated below.

Oogenesis

The most significant feature here is that the meiotic process which produces the ovum can take 50 years or more to complete. This is because the first cell division is 'suspended' (a phase known as dictyotene) from before birth of the little girl until sexual maturity of the young woman is reached and ovulation occurs. This very lengthy interval between the onset of meiosis and its completion accounts for the increase in chromosome abnormalities in the offspring of older mothers. An example is Down's syndrome, where the affected child has one too many chromosomes. (See Box 6.6 for further explanation.)

Spermatogenesis

The development of sperm is a relatively rapid process which takes about 60 days. At puberty the second meiotic division takes place to produce mature spermatozoa in abundance, about 100–200 million in each ejaculate. Spermatogenesis then becomes a continuous process which involves many mitotic cell divisions in the testes, as many as 25 per year, prior to the final meiotic divisions which produce the sperm. There is no similar paternal age effect on congenital abnormalities through chromosome number defects, although a few disorders do occur which are largely paternal in origin. Examples include Turner's syndrome (where an X or Y chromosome is missing) and Klinefelter's syndrome (where there is an additional X chromosome). Older men may produce sperm which carry mutations due to DNA copy errors during the many mitotic cell divisions which precede spermatogenesis.

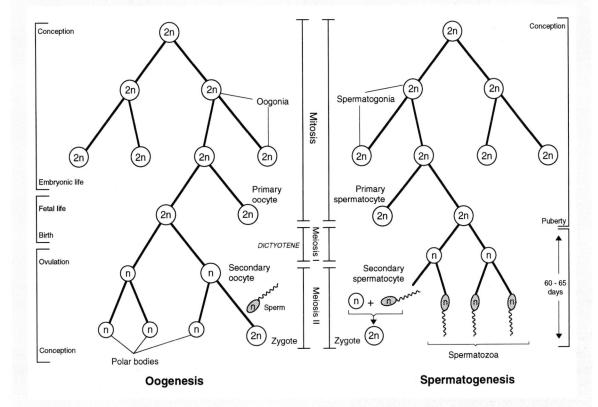

Oogenesis   **Spermatogenesis**

Undoubtedly, medicine will change as a result of this knowledge. At the moment, knowing the sequencing of genes does not mean that the function of all the genes is yet known and work continues on this. However, it is expected that within 20 years disease susceptibility will be predicted when all of the several thousand genes that cause illness have been identified. Treatment

Box 6.6   Non-disjunction and numerical abnormalities of chromosomes

Numerical abnormalities involve the gain or loss of one or more chromosomes, known as aneuploidy, or the addition of one or more complete sets of chromosomes, polyploidy. The cause of such numerical changes is the failure of normal separation of homologous chromosomes during the first meiotic division of gametogenesis, or failure of sister chromatids to separate during the second meiotic division. The diagrams below illustrate normal meiosis and the effects of the two different types of non-disjunction. They show how non-disjunction can lead to the formation of gametes with too few or too many chromosomes. If these gametes are subsequently fertilised, the resultant embryo will have an abnormal number of chromosomes. Non-disjunction occurs much more commonly in oogenesis (in the older woman) than in spermatogenesis. It is well known to

be the cause of trisomy 21 (an additional number 21 chromosome), also known as Down's syndrome. In the diagram, the gametes that will give rise to trisomy are shaded.

There are other less well known autosomal trisomies which are compatible with life, for example Patau's syndrome (trisomy 13) and Edwards's syndrome (trisomy 18). The presence of an extra X or Y chromosome causes well documented syndromes such as Klinefelter's syndrome (47 XXY), XXX females and XYY males.

The diagrams also show how a gamete with too few chromosomes may occur. Subsequent fertilisation here causes monosomy, meaning absence of a single chromosome, and this is usually incompatible with life. An exception is Turner's syndrome which is caused by a missing X or Y chromosome.

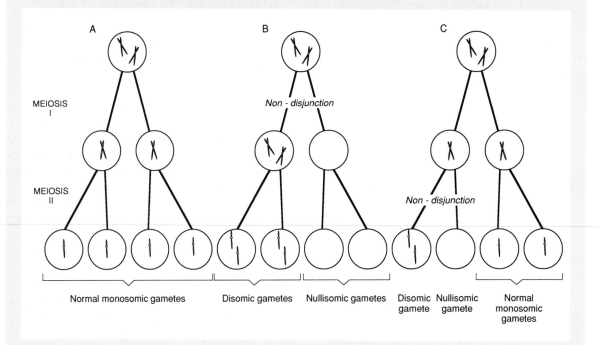

for the disease may be tailor-made for each individual according to genotype. The next decades mark the beginning of remarkable changes in the understanding of health and illness, through the development of genetics knowledge. The new knowledge also brings more questions relating to the ethical, legal and social consequences of genomic research as more information leads to difficult decisions about treatment availability, cost, privacy, to treat or not to treat and many

other issues. Detailed explanation about this most important work is beyond the capacity of this chapter, but the Further reading section will provide useful pointers.

Genetic modification

The study of genetics and its role in the cause of human disease, and how it may be treated, is widely recognised as being at the forefront of medical research. But these pioneering studies are also now applied to a thriving industry which is able to develop disease resistant crops and genetically engineered animals. Improved knowledge in the field of genetics has extremely attractive commercial applications in agriculture but there is alarm among many people that this has serious attendant risks of altering the earth's ecosystems irretrievably.

THE SUSTENANCE OF LIFE

If human physiology is a study of *what* happens *where* in the body, there needs to be an understanding of the processes by which everything keeps going. This means that some appreciation of energy in the body is necessary. The cells of the body require energy for:

1. the synthesis of large molecules, such as proteins, from smaller ones (which happens in growth)
2. the electrical activity of the nerves
3. the activation of the contractile machinery of muscle cells to produce contraction and movement
4. active transport (see 'Transport across membranes', p. 152)
5. heat production.

These five functions, the result of complex and meticulously ordered and controlled chemical reactions at cell level, support the whole range of body activities. All are energy-requiring reactions, the energy being supplied by energy-releasing reactions, of which cellular respiration is the most significant. Cellular respiration makes a sixth function, which is the result of complex and controlled intracellular chemistry, and completes the list of life-sustaining processes. However, without it, none of the other five would ever happen at all; thus cellular respiration merits consideration at this early stage.

ENERGY FROM CELLULAR RESPIRATION

Cellular respiration is the production of energy as a result of the oxidation of food material such as glucose. Since the production of energy does not necessarily correspond with the body's needs at any given moment, the body requires a mechanism for storing energy. Stored energy is the outcome of cellular respiration. The unit of stored energy is known as adenosine triphosphate (ATP). This molecule is able to release energy, when required, and it then changes into adenosine diphosphate (ADP), having lost a phosphate group.

Cellular respiration is the process by which energy-laden molecules of ATP are made. The basic ingredients for cellular respiration are food material (such as glucose) and oxygen. A large number of reactions is involved in the full breakdown of glucose to produce energy. Every stage requires the presence of its own specific enzyme, and oxygen is required for the final stage of this chain reaction. This makes cellular respiration an aerobic reaction (requiring the presence of oxygen), although, if the oxygen supply is limited, a less efficient form of cellular respiration occurs. This process, known as anaerobic respiration, produces less energy. (A by-product of anaerobic respiration is lactic acid, which produces the well-known symptom of 'cramp' in the muscles of weary athletes.)

The way in which cellular energy production is expressed is in units of ATP, the unit of stored energy. Cells can manage with a limited supply of oxygen, but their ability to carry out the full range of energy-requiring chemical activities is much diminished by a reduction in oxygen, and they cannot function for more than a few minutes if the oxygen supply is completely blocked for any reason. Nervous tissue is particularly sensitive to oxygen deficit and will not maintain its function after a maximum of about 3 minutes of anoxia (lack of oxygen).

Although glucose is the major food molecule used in cellular respiration, almost all cells, with the exception of nervous tissue, are able to use fats for energy production. Fats, when oxidised in cellular respiration, produce large numbers of ATP molecules, but unfortunate by-products are also produced. These are acidic substances, which, if produced unchecked because of a shortage of glucose, can cause highly acidic body fluids, a situation that eventually leads to death. Fats are metabolised only if there is a shortage of glucose or if glucose use is impaired, as in diabetes. Similarly, proteins can be used to produce energy, but the output is small. Proteins are used for energy production only in cases of extreme lack of glucose (such as during starvation), and, if this happens, the main protein stores (muscles) are much reduced and severe weight loss ensues.

Most of the reactions of cellular respiration occur in the mitochondria of the cells. Enzymes coat the inner, folded lining of the mitochondria. The number and inner complexity of the mitochondria increase markedly in a cell that is highly active in producing energy. Cells in the most metabolically active organ in the body, the liver, have large numbers of complex mitochondria.

It may not be necessary for the reader to know any greater detail than this about the chemistry of energy production. Much more specific detail is known, and there is a great deal of information available for the interested student. In the early stages of nursing studies, however, it will not normally be necessary to take this topic any further.

THE IMPORTANCE OF ENZYMES IN CELL CHEMISTRY

To be alive means to be producing energy by the oxidation of carbon compounds, such as glucose. Without this basic cell chemistry, nothing else will happen. Although glucose (or some other food molecule) and oxygen are primary requirements for energy production, of equal significance are the enzyme molecules that must be present for even the simplest of the oxidation reactions to take place. All enzymes are proteins, and they themselves have to be made and replaced. This, too, requires energy. Enzymes, like all proteins, are highly sensitive to changes in their environment, so that minute changes in temperature, acidity/alkalinity and concentrations of components of the cellular fluid around them may reduce or stop altogether the chemical reactions they initiate and control. Their physical molecular structure is a highly significant factor in their ability to function at all, because of the required physical linkage between the enzyme and the molecule undergoing the chemical reaction (the substrate). This means that even if the basic ingredients for energy production are present, unless the intracellular environment is perfect, cell chemistry will not proceed normally, and life will cease if imperfections persist.

Factors affecting enzyme action

Each cell contains many different enzymes, each catalysing a specific chemical reaction. Without exception, each species of enzyme molecule is a protein of very specific amino acid composition and sequence. The work of geneticists has demonstrated that proteins, including enzymes, are the primary gene products. Enzymes regulate all the synthesising and metabolising activities of the cell, but they will function only when the following conditions are fulfilled:

1. Enzymes normally function within a very narrow range of pH, although the optimum pH will be different for different enzymes.

2. Enzymes function within a very narrow temperature range. As temperatures rise, enzymes may break down chemically and be permanently denatured. At low temperatures they become inactive but are restored to activity when normal temperature is restored.

3. Frequently, the action of enzymes depends upon the presence of cofactors. Minerals (such as iron, sodium, potassium) and vitamins are cofactors in enzyme function (Table 6.2).

4. Enzymes are very specific in action – each enzyme will catalyse reactions for only chemically related substrates – and act by forming a complex, but temporary, bonding with one of the reacting molecules.

5. Enzymes are swiftly inhibited by the presence of foreign substances. (Minute quantities of some poisons can have a devastating effect by stopping enzyme activity.)

6. Some enzymes have to be stored in inactive form – a protein-digesting enzyme, for example, would otherwise destroy the organ in which it is stored.

Table 6.2 The vitamins: their actions, sources and results of deficiency (reproduced from Wilson 1990)

Vitamin	Chemical name	Source	Stability	Functions	Deficiency diseases	Dietary reference values (Department of Health 1991)
*Fat-soluble vitamins**						
A	Retinol (carotene provitamin in plants)	Milk, butter, cheese, egg yolk, fish liver oils, green and yellow vegetables	Some loss at high temperatures and long exposure to light and air	Maintains healthy epithelial tissues and cornea Formation of visual purple	Keratinisation Xerophthalmia Stunted growth Night blindness	1–2 mg
D	Calciferol	Fish liver oils, milk, cheese, egg yolk, irradiated 7-dehydro-cholesterol in human skin	Very stable	Facilitates the absorption and utilisation of calcium and phosphorus = healthy bones and teeth	Rickets Osteomalacia	2–10 μg
E	Tocopherols	Egg yolk, milk, butter, green vegetables, nuts	Destroyed by rancid fat and iron salts	Prevents catabolism of polyunsaturated fats	Anaemia Ataxia Cystic fibrosis Scotomas	15 mg
K	Phylloquinone	Leafy vegetables, fish liver, fruit	Destroyed by light, strong acids and alkalis	Formation of prothrombin and Factors VII, IX and X in the liver	Slow blood clotting Haemorrhages in the newborn	2–10 μg
Water-soluble vitamins						
B₁	Thiamin	Yeast, liver, germ of cereals, nuts, pulses, rice polishings, egg yolk, liver, legumes	Destroyed by heat	Metabolism of carbohydrates and nutrition of nerve cells	General fatigue and loss of muscle tone Ultimately leads to beriberi Stunted growth	1–1.5 mg
B₂	Riboflavin	Liver, yeast, milk, eggs, green vegetables, kidney, fish roe	Destroyed by light and alkalis	Carbohydrate and protein metabolism Healthy skin and eyes	Angular stomatitis Cheilosis Dermatitis Eye lesions	1.5–2 mg
B₆	Pyridoxine	Meat, liver, vegetables, bran of cereals, egg yolk, beans, soya beans	Stable	Protein metabolism Production of antibodies	Very rare	1.5–2.5 mg

(Cont'd)

Table 6.2 (*Continued*)

Vitamin	Chemical name	Source	Stability	Functions	Deficiency diseases	Dietary reference values (Department of Health 1991)
B_{12}	Cobalamine	Liver, milk, moulds, fermenting liquors, egg	Destroyed by heat	Maturation of RBCs	Pernicious anaemia Degeneration of nerve fibres of the spinal cord	1–2 µg
B	Folic acid	Dark green vegetables, liver, kidney, eggs Synthesised in colon	Destroyed by heat and moisture	Formation of RBCs	Anaemia	100–200 µg
B	Niacin (nicotinic acid)	Yeast offal, fish, pulses, wholemeal cereals Synthesised in the body from tryptophan	Fairly stable	Necessary for tissue oxidation Inhibits production of cholesterol	Prolonged deficiency causes pellagra, i.e. dermatitis, diarrhoea and dementia	15–20 mg
B	Pantothenic acid	Liver, yeast, egg yolk, fresh vegetables	Destroyed by excessive heat and freezing	Associated with amino acid metabolism	Unknown	Unknown
B	Biotin	Yeasts, liver, kidney, pulses, nuts	Stable	Carbohydrates and fat metabolism Growth of bacteria	Dermatitis Conjunctivitis Hypercholesterolaemia	100 µg
C	Ascorbic acid	Citrus fruits, currants, berries, green vegetables, potatoes, liver and glandular tissue in animals	Destroyed by heat, ageing, acids, alkalis, chopping, salting and drying	Formation of inter-cellular matrix Maturation of RBCs	Multiple haemorrhages Slow wound healing Anaemia Gross deficiency causes scurvy	30–60 mg

* Bile is necessary for the absorption of these vitamins. Mineral oils interfere with absorption.

Because of these demanding requirements to sustain enzyme activity, upon which the life of cells depends, the whole of the rest of human structure and function works to maintain the constancy of the environment for the sake of the enzymes, those fussy proteins that DNA produces. Maintenance of a constant internal environment is called *homeostasis*.

HOMEOSTASIS AND THE BODY SYSTEMS

Homeostasis is the tendency of the body to maintain the stability of the internal environment in the face of environmental changes and changing internal demands. It enables, for example, the individual to adapt slowly to living at high altitude or to rapidly flee from danger. Two points about homeostasis should be borne in mind throughout the following discussion:

1. Homeostasis is a dynamic process, sometimes referred to as 'dynamic equilibrium'. Everything that happens in the body is monitored constantly, with small adjustments being made. Even during sleep, a great deal happens; for example, sugar levels, blood oxygen levels and body temperature are constantly monitored and adjusted. The body never rests completely, even during sleep.

2. When homeostatic balance is not maintained, the health of the person is threatened, and disease or even death may be the result. Nursing and medical intervention is an attempt to prevent imbalance occurring or to restore homeostasis.

Maintenance of intracellular chemistry, by maintaining a balanced intra- and extracellular environment, is essential to life. The regulation of osmolarity, pH, temperature and the balance of the ions in body fluids is critical for maintaining cell function. Every system in the body has maintenance of this constant internal environment as its ultimate purpose. (The possible exception is the reproductive system, whose sole function is the long-term survival of the species rather than the short-term survival of the individual – although

homeostatic mechanisms will, themselves, ensure correct functioning of this system!)

The body systems, in homeostatic terms, are as follows:

1. *Suppliers, waste disposers and transporters.* These are systems that communicate with the external environment. They supply nutrients, water and oxygen to the tissues, and remove waste. They are the respiratory, gastrointestinal, renal and cardiovascular systems.

2. *Detectors.* These are usually nervous (sensory) receptors, which can detect internal changes of pressure, changes in muscular tone or external dangers, such as heat, cold and physical trauma. Some detectors may be chemical in nature, such as the oxygen- and carbon dioxide-sensitive cells in the brain, which detect abnormally high or low blood gas levels. Some glands also act as detectors, as seen, for example, in the pancreatic β-cells, which monitor blood glucose levels.

3. *Effectors.* These are usually muscular structures (such as in the heart, as well as muscles for breathing, shivering and major body movement) and glands. Muscles and glands act to make changes.

4. *Regulators.* These systems make sure that the detector–effector mechanism is continued, so that timing, strength and duration of response are appropriate. These systems are the nervous system and the endocrine system.

In any further study about the physiological functioning of the person, the reader should strive to discover how these individual systems contribute to the homeostatic balance of the whole body.

REGULATION MECHANISMS IN HOMEOSTASIS

The regulatory processes depend in many instances on the principle of feedback. A man-made physical system, such as a computer, can be made so accurate that it will produce a predictable result under normal and predictable conditions. Living systems, however, must be able to function to produce a balanced system within narrow limits despite large and unexpected external variations; for example, they must maintain a normal glucose supply to cells during a period of fasting. The means by which the body achieves regulation is feedback.

Most control systems in the body act by negative feedback; Figure 6.6 shows an example of such a system, the maintenance of balanced blood sugar levels. A disturbance, such as the absorption of high levels of glucose into the blood following a meal, 'signals' the sensor in the control system (in this case, cells in the pancreas). The pancreas also acts as the effector by releasing the hormone insulin. Insulin then acts on several body tissues, for example muscle and fat cells, and reduces the blood glucose level by facilitating their uptake of glucose from the blood. The response by the body has been in a negative or opposite direction to the disturbance, to compensate for the abnormality. Such mechanisms are self-regulating and automatic. There is no voluntary control over them, which is just as well because it would be impossible to manage, voluntarily, all the thousands of controlling mechanisms that operate simultaneously within the body. Such feedback mechanisms occur in every compartment of human physiology, including endocrine function, blood circulation, breathing and body temperature. Positive feedback

mechanisms are much less frequent. As the name suggests, they act in the direction of the disturbance, thus compounding the situation.

Positive feedback is generally used to produce an explosive or successively catalytic effect. Examples of useful positive feedback mechanisms include uterine contractions at birth (whereby one contraction induces further contractions and so on until the baby is expelled from the uterus) and the less obviously energetic blood-clotting mechanism (Box 6.7). Most positive feedback mechanisms are harmful, even fatal, the most well-known of these probably being progressive shock (Box 6.8).

Although homeostatic regulating mechanisms are automatic, they are not always rapid. This is because they often act via chemical messengers in the blood (hormones) or via slow-acting nerve fibres. There is often a time lapse between stimulus (abnormality) and response (restoration). Therefore, there may be too great a build-up of stimulus, or too great a production of restorative, and perfect balance may take some time to be achieved. This is what leads to fluctuations around the normal value, although these are usually within narrow limits. If the fluctuations increase and remain unrestored, homeostasis is lost, and it is at this stage that medical or nursing intervention may prevent disaster or speed

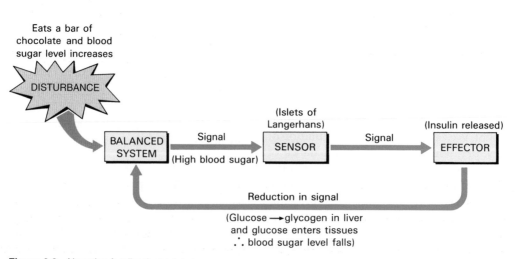

Figure 6.6 Negative feedback mechanism.

Box 6.7 Blood clotting

Blood clots (or *coagulates*) when the soluble plasma protein *fibrinogen* changes into insoluble *fibrin*. Fibrin forms a webby network of long strands, in which blood cells become trapped. The strands are sticky, so that the clot adheres to surrounding tissues, which plugs any gap and prevents leakage of blood. If exposed to the air, as at an external wound, the clot dries and hardens. Clotting (the formation of fibrin) concerns the plasma. Plasma without cells will clot: cells play an entirely passive role in being trapped in fibrin strands.

Fibrinogen is a natural constituent of plasma, but it changes into fibrin only when *thrombin* is present. Thrombin is not normally present in plasma, existing only as the precursor substance, *prothrombin*, which is another plasma protein. The conversion of prothrombin to thrombin takes place when activator substances are released from damaged tissues and platelets (*extrinsic factors*) and in the presence of certain other essential substances in the plasma (*intrinsic factors*).

The coagulation mechanism is a 'biological amplifier' (positive feedback), sometimes called a 'cascade' of enzyme-controlled reactions, whereby one substance is activated and, in turn, triggers another action and so on. Thirteen main coagulation factors have now been named. Absence of one or more of them will cause failure (or reduced speed) of clotting.

The full mechanism can be represented thus: ▶

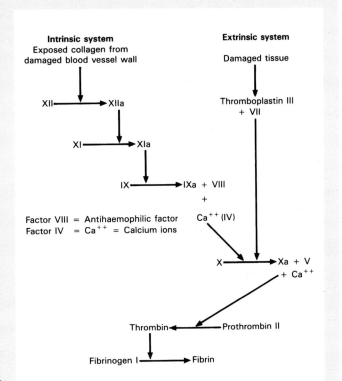

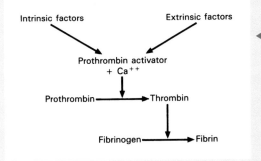

The intrinsic and extrinsic systems join in the final common pathway, which converts prothrombin to thrombin. It will not be necessary to know all of the factors and reactions, but the following simplified version should be learned.

The entire clotting sequence takes about 4–8 minutes (the clotting time). However, once Factor X is activated, the rest takes just a few seconds.

It is important to realise that blood must contain regulators or natural inhibitors of clotting to prevent the clotting mechanism spreading from the point of injury or damage to the entire system. Some of these have been identified, but the whole process is not well understood at the present time.

---

recovery. This is why it is important for nurses to know something about normal levels (and acceptable fluctuations around the normal) of the measurable components of homeostatic mechanisms in human physiology. Of equal importance is the ability to observe and detect any of these dangerous fluctuations. Probably the most obvious measurement a nurse may undertake is the person's body temperature, but the range of disturbances of homeostatic control is as vast as the numbers of chemical reactions and controlling mechanisms that support them.

Box 6.8 Shock

'Shock' means a decrease in circulating blood volume, caused by the loss of blood (*haemorrhagic or hypovolaemic shock*), poor cardiac activity (*cardiogenic shock*) or severe distress (*neurogenic shock*). Whatever the cause, the loss of circulating blood volume causes the following sequence of events to occur (at this stage, the reader may not be familiar with all of the terms used, but the important thing is the overall pattern).

Non-progressive shock

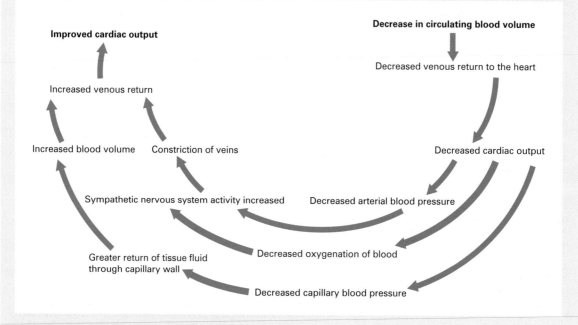

In the illustration above, negative feedback mechanisms, acting through the sympathetic nervous system, produce an increase in the circulating blood volume to improve cardiac output and so restore equilibrium.

Signs and symptoms of shock

Under conditions of shock, the circulation of blood to the vital organs (brain and heart) has priority, with the result that blood supply to the skin, gut, kidneys and skeletal muscle is reduced. Because of this, and taking account of the cycle illustrated above, it is easy to understand the common signs and symptoms observed in a shocked patient:

- pallor – owing to constriction of peripheral capillaries
- rapid pulse – owing to sympathetic nervous stimulation
- sweating – (as rapid pulse) owing to sympathetic nervous stimulation
- weak pulse – owing to low blood volume and reduced cardiac output
- oligaemia – owing to reduced kidney function
- low blood pressure – owing to reduced cardiac output.

Progressive shock

Here, the cause is so severe (usually severe haemorrhage, extensive fluid loss through burns, or cardiac failure) that the usual negative feedback mechanisms cannot compensate. Thus the following cycle occurs:

Box 6.8 *(Continued)*

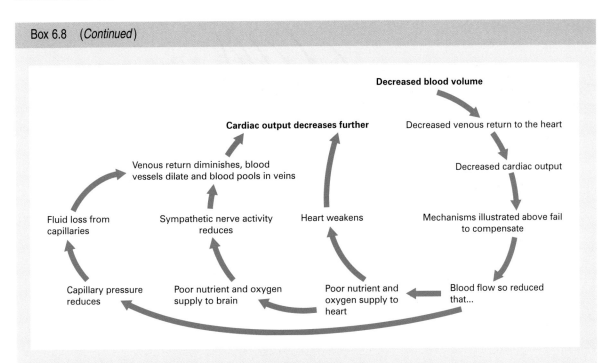

The problem is increasing, reinforcing and compounding itself: blood flow keeps reducing, which reduces cardiac output, which further reduces the flow, which weakens the heart further, etc., etc.

Treatment of shock

The priority is to improve the circulating blood volume by giving intravenous fluids, such as plasma, whole blood or normal saline solutions. Where the cause of shock is severe, in blood loss and burns (hypovolaemic) or in cardiac arrest/failure (cardiogenic), intravenous fluids are always given. In neurogenic shock (pain, bad news or other emotional shock), the shock is rarely progressive, and recovery does not normally require fluid replacement, although other care may be required, such as pain relief, reassurance and rest.

THE SKIN AND HOMEOSTASIS

The skin is one of the largest organs of the body (Fig. 6.7). In adults, it covers an area of about 2 square metres and weighs 4–5 kg. It is not just a simple thin covering that keeps the body intact and provides protection; it also fulfils several important functions:

- *Regulation of body temperature* through sweat evaporation to reduce high body temperature and diminished sweat production to conserve heat. Changes in blood flow in the skin also help regulate temperature.

- *Protection*, by providing a physical barrier against abrasion to underlying tissues, bacterial invasion, and dehydration. Hair and nails, which are extensions of the epidermis, also provide protection.
- *Sensation* as a result of abundant nerve endings and receptors that detect touch, pressure, pain and temperature.
- *Excretion* where sweat is the vehicle for removal of unwanted water and some salts and organic compounds.
- *Immunity* from certain cells in the epidermis which fend off invading organisms.

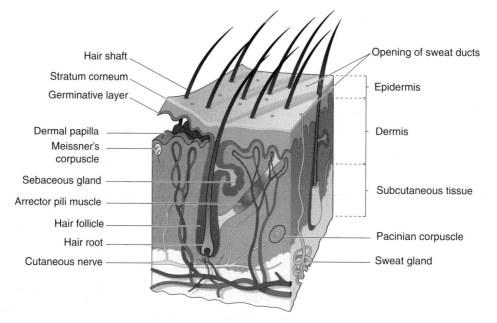

Hair shaft
Stratum corneum
Germinative layer
Dermal papilla
Meissner's corpuscle
Sebaceous gland
Arrector pili muscle
Hair follicle
Hair root
Cutaneous nerve

Opening of sweat ducts
Epidermis
Dermis
Subcutaneous tissue
Pacinian corpuscle
Sweat gland

Figure 6.7 The skin.

- *Blood reservoir* in the extensive network of blood vessels in the dermis. These may constrict to assist in redistribution of blood to more essential areas of the body (for example muscles during strenuous exercise), or they may dilate to increase heat loss from the body surface.
- *Synthesis of vitamin D* when the skin is exposed to sunlight.

Two major homeostatic activities of the skin are wound healing and temperature regulation, described in Boxes 6.9 and 6.10.

THE CARDIOVASCULAR SYSTEM AND HOMEOSTASIS

The cardiovascular system – i.e. the heart, the blood and the vessels along which the blood moves – has evolved to transport materials to and from all regions of the body. In simple organisms such as yeast cells or amoebae such a system is unnecessary because the functioning units (the cells) are in direct contact with both their nutrient and oxygen supply and their means of waste removal – normally the solution in which they live.

In the human body, the cardiovascular system transports respiratory gases, nutrients, waste products, hormones, antibodies and salts to and from all cells. Blood is a complex tissue and contains many cell types. It acts as a vehicle for many homeostatic agents and is, in fact, one itself.

Apart from the blood itself, the cardiovascular system consists of:

- the main propulsive organ, the *heart*, which forces blood around the body
- an *arterial system*, which assists in propelling the blood and smoothing the blood flow to the periphery
- *capillaries*, across the walls of which transfer of materials between blood and tissues occurs
- the *venous system*, which acts as a blood reservoir and as a system for returning blood to the heart.

Blood

Blood is the medium in which all materials are transported around the body. In its passage through the capillaries, its composition changes as components are exchanged across the capillary

Box 6.9 Skin, the effects of pressure and wound healing

The process of wound healing differs according to whether the skin damage is superficial and restricted to the epidermis or a deeper wound where injury, which could be a surgical incision, extends into the dermis. An important goal in nursing is to prevent the damage that can occur when patients are exposed to prolonged pressure on the skin – pressure sores. This has been a subject of considerable research and it is possible to prevent even the most immobile person from developing pressure sores. The status of the skin and the likelihood of developing pressure sores should form part of the initial assessment of patients in general acute nursing care. Special pressure relieving surfaces and mattresses are widely available, but the vigilance of the nurse in inspecting skin, carrying out gentle passive exercise and ensuring adequate nutrition must always be there for the vulnerable person. For those patients who are susceptible to pressure sores, the most important thing to keep off the skin is the weight of the patient! (See Chapter 14.)

Epidermal wound healing is normally rapid because the basal (continuously dividing) layer of the epidermis has remained intact. In response to injury, the basement cells enlarge and 'migrate' across the wound until they meet. Continued migration occurs right across the wound and stops when the surface is covered with new growth. Simultaneous with the migration of cells is the rapid division

of some of the remaining basal cells to replace them and thicken the new epidermis. Epidermal wound healing occurs within 24 to 48 hours after injury, assuming the wound is clean and the skin is otherwise healthy.

Deep wound healing occurs when an injury extends to the tissues of the dermis. The first phase of healing here is the inflammatory phase (see Box 6.15). After this, the blood clot which has united the edges of the wound, becomes a scab and epithelial cells beneath the scab migrate and multiply to bridge the wound. Beneath this, granulation tissue is formed where collagen fibres and damaged blood vessels from the dermis regrow. The epidermal cells continue to divide to form a strong new outer layer. This phase, known as the proliferative phase, may take many days depending on the extent of the wound; the strength of the repair is very weak at this stage so that the skin can break down again easily with any further force. During the next maturation phase, which may last for up to 80 days, more collagen fibres are deposited within the dermis, blood vessels are restored to normal, the scab sloughs off and the skin's normal strength returns.

For surgical wounds, healing into the proliferative phase up to suture removal is about 10–12 days. Where wounds are deep, wide and infected – as in severe pressure sores – healing takes a great deal longer, and this takes no account of the pain and distress to the patient.

Box 6.10 Control of body temperature

A balance has to be maintained between heat gain (body metabolism which produces heat and environmental temperature) and heat loss (largely through the skin and due to environmental temperature). Maintenance of a constant body temperature, which is essential to life, is under the control of the central nervous system and its effect on the skin and skeletal muscles. The temperature regulating centre in the hypothalamus of the brain is sensitive to the temperature of circulating blood and this centre affects body temperature by its actions on the sweat glands on the skin. The vasomotor centre, in the medulla oblongata of the brain, controls the diameters of the small arteries and arterioles in the body, including those in the dermis of the skin.

When body temperature is increased, the arterioles and capillaries in the dermis are dilated, in response to neurological stimulation, so that the extra blood near the surface increases heat loss by radiation, conduction and convection. The individual looks flushed and is aware of feeling hot. In addition, the sweat glands are stimulated to secrete sweat which is conveyed to the surface of the skin by sweat ducts. The body is cooled by the loss of heat used to evaporate the water in sweat. When the external temperature and humidity are high, or the individual is generating excess heat, sweat droplets appear on the skin. Insensible

water loss also causes heat loss by evaporation, even though the sweat glands are not active. Water diffuses from the deeper layers of the skin to the surface and evaporates into the air. Under normal conditions, this is a continuous process.

When body temperature falls, for whatever reason (low external temperature, reduced metabolism), vasoconstriction occurs in the dermis arterioles as a result of neurological stimulation because of reduced blood temperature. This reduces blood flow near the body surface and conserves heat. Other compensatory mechanisms also occur such as shivering (which is increased activity of skeletal muscles in an attempt to generate heat) and pilo-erection, which is contraction of the muscle fibres attached to the skin hairs and which makes the hairs stand erect, thus creating 'goose flesh'. This latter process generates heat and also helps to provide some insulation by trapping a thicker layer of air next to the skin.

Maintaining a constant body temperature is a fundamental aspect of homeostasis and basic nursing care will always include an assessment of body temperature and measures to maintain it at a normal level. These measures may include tepid sponging to reduce body temperature in fever, sunstroke, etc. or careful rewarming to increase core body temperature in cases of hypothermia.

walls with those of tissue fluid. Thus continuous exchange functions to maintain an optimum internal environment for cell and tissue function, and without it homeostasis would not exist.

Plasma

The fluid component of blood, plasma, is the transporting agent for nutrients, hormones, salts (electrolytes) and carbon dioxide. Of special significance in homeostasis at tissue fluid level is the plasma protein content of plasma, which exerts a significant osmotic pressure within blood and assists in the osmotic recovery of water from body tissues. Another particular homeostatic component of plasma is the protein fibrinogen and the other clotting factors, whose cascading interactions cause the formation of blood clots, a protective mechanism of singular significance (see Box 6.7). Many other plasma proteins have the specific function of giving protection against invading foreign proteins, and are known collectively as antibodies.

The cellular components of blood

The cellular components of the blood (Fig. 6.8) are:

- erythrocytes (red blood cells)
- leucocytes (white blood cells)
- thrombocytes (platelets).

Erythrocytes

These should be considered, in homeostatic terms, for two major reasons:

1. The major constituent of a red blood cell is haemoglobin. This protein molecule, with its constituent iron-containing portion, has a structure that enables it to form a rapid but reversible combination with oxygen. As oxyhaemoglobin, life-sustaining oxygen is collected in the lung tissues and transported to all body cells. The affinity of haemoglobin for oxygen keeps increasing as more oxygen is bound and delivered; this is a positive feedback mechanism that is due to

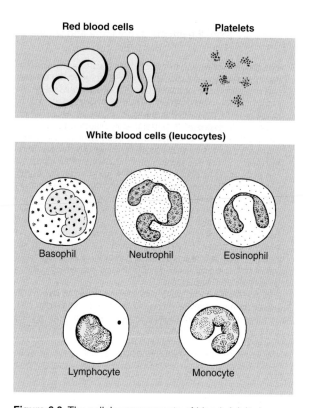

Figure 6.8 The cellular components of blood. Adults have close to 30 trillion red blood cells. *Note 1*: There are about 5×10^9 red blood cells and 7.5×10^6 white blood cells in each litre of blood. *Note 2*: Basophils, neutrophils, eosinophils and lymphocytes are sometimes known collectively as polymorphs because of their irregular shape and many-lobed nuclei.

successive minor changes in the configuration of the globin part of the molecule.

Some genetic abnormalities exist that affect the structure of the haemoglobin molecule, thereby affecting its ability to transport oxygen. The best-known of these disorders is sickle-cell anaemia, which is anaemia (lack of circulating blood oxygen) caused by a mutant kind of haemoglobin.

2. Red blood cells also carry the proteins that are responsible for blood grouping. The blood grouping proteins are known as antigens as they will stimulate antibody production (as would any other foreign protein) if introduced into the blood of a person whose grouping is different. There are a great many antigens carried on the

Box 6.11   Blood groups

About 12 different blood grouping systems have been identified, the most important of which are the ABO and Rhesus systems. Blood grouping is the result of particular *antigens* carried on the surface of red blood cells. An antigen is any substance that causes the stimulation of an antibody. Blood groups are genetically determined.

If plasma containing Antibody A comes into contact with red blood cells containing Antigen A, the cells clump together and are eventually destroyed. The clumping (*agglutination*) can cause serious blockage in small blood vessels, and red cell destruction causes anaemia and jaundice. Small concentrations of antibody do not cause seriously damaging agglutination. While exactly matched blood is normally provided for transfusion, certain transfusions are possible in emergencies, as in the following:

If donor blood contains unfavourable plasma (with antibodies) this is rapidly diluted on entering the recipient, and stands little chance of causing agglutination. However, if donor blood contains unfavourable red blood cells (with antigens), these will be immediately 'attacked' by the large volume of recipient plasma.

Unlike in the ABO system, there are *no naturally occurring Rhesus antibodies*. However, Antibody D will be built up in the plasma of a Rhesus negative (Rh⁻) person who receives Rhesus positive (Rh⁺) blood. A first Rh⁺ transfusion will not normally cause agglutination, but Antibody D remains in the plasma. A second Rh⁺ transfusion is, therefore, dangerous and to be avoided at all costs.

This principle is at work when a Rh⁻ woman carries a Rh⁺ child. Any leakage of fetal cells into the maternal bloodstream stimulates the production of Antibody D in the mother's plasma. A subsequent Rh⁺ fetus is in danger from maternal Antibody D, which may transfer through the placenta into the fetal circulation. Modern preventative medicine includes immediate postnatal Antibody D injections to Rh⁻ mothers. The Antibody D rapidly destroys any escaped positive cells and no build up of Antibody D occurs. The injected Antibody D is too small a dose to have any lasting effect on a future pregnancy.

The ABO system

Group	Antigens present on red blood cells	Antibodies naturally present in plasma
A	A	Antibody B
B	B	Antibody A
AB	A and B	None
O	Neither	Antibody A and antibody B

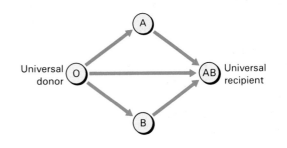

Universal donor — O ... AB Universal recipient (A, B)

The Rhesus system

Group	Antigens present on red blood cells	Antibodies in plasma
Rhesus positive	Rhesus antigen (D)	None
Rhesus negative	None	None

surface of red blood cells, but the most important to understand are those concerned with the ABO and Rhesus systems: this is because of their potentially devastating effects during blood transfusions. The actual physiological importance of these proteins to the person whose blood cells carry them is unknown: they are significant only when they cause problems, which, fortunately, is rare (Box 6.11).

Leucocytes

The homeostatic significance of leucocytes is discussed in the section entitled 'The immune system and homeostasis', below.

Thrombocytes

Often known as platelets, these are the smallest cellular components of blood. Their major function is in the arrest of bleeding, by adhesion to the endothelium of a damaged blood vessel. They form a platelet plug, which can stop blood flow (see Box 6.7). In a situation of vessel damage, platelets also produce an activator chemical, which assists in the blood-clotting mechanism. Thrombocytes are significant homeostatic regulators.

The heart

The mammalian heart has evolved to become a sophisticated muscular pump, capable of sustained and untiring activity and able to respond to the changing homeostatic needs of the body. A detailed consideration of the structure of cardiac muscle shows that the tissue has similarities to ordinary skeletal muscle, but that its cells are electrically coupled. Cardiac muscle is capable of spontaneous contraction, even if removed from the body and kept in a warm, nutrient- and oxygen-rich solution. Within the body, the muscle is coordinated to contract rhythmically and strongly by the nervous stimulation of the tissue.

The electrical stimulation of the heart is initiated in the pacemaking region, and electrical activity spreads over the heart from one cell to another because of electrical coupling. As the wave of excitation spreads, so the cardiac cells are stimulated to contract. Any interference with this electrical transmission, such as may occur with cardiac tissue death (usually due to a disrupted blood supply to the tissue and called myocardial infarction), can stop the coordinated pumping action of the heart.

The mechanical pumping action of the heart, once initiated by the pacemaker, is a controlled system of fluid flowing through chambers, sustained by the action of valves that prevent backflow and disturbance (Fig. 6.9). Wear and tear, or disease of the valves can affect this smooth flow and lead to mechanical stress on the cardiac muscle, with resultant loss of vigour, accompanied by heart enlargement.

These mechanical activities may be the subject of careful investigation for sounds of abnormal valve closure or abnormal blood flow sounds in the heart.

The arterial system

This consists of a series of branching vessels whose walls are thick, elastic and muscular. Arteries serve four main functions:

1. to act as a conduit for blood between the heart and capillaries
2. to act as a pressure reservoir for forcing blood into the small-diameter arterioles
3. to dampen oscillations in pressure and flow generated by the heart and produce a more even flow to the capillaries
4. to control the flow of blood to different capillary networks via selective constriction of branches of the arterial tree (e.g. if there is serious blood loss, capillaries to the brain, heart and kidneys may be kept open, while those to the gut and/or extremities may be shut down).

Arterial blood pressure is controlled, largely because of the proportion of muscle and elastic tissue in arterial walls. The arteries alter their control within quite large ranges of pressure, which may be augmented by increased heart rate and strength or by restriction in capillary flow, or decreased by the opposite phenomena. The muscle and elastic layers alter in proportion the further away from the heart the artery is. Those nearest the heart require great elasticity to dampen the surges of blood, while those nearer the periphery need more rigidity to sustain supply to the tissues. Blood pressure is altered by heart activity and changes in peripheral resistance, but remains remarkably constant (in the short term) within one individual, largely due to the action of arteries.

Capillaries

These microscopic vessels are the end-point of all that happens in the physics of the cardiovascular system. It is through their walls that materials are exchanged with the tissues, and this activity is the essence of homeostasis (Fig. 6.10).

Under normal conditions, the volume of the plasma and the volume of tissue fluid that it is supplying change very little, despite massive

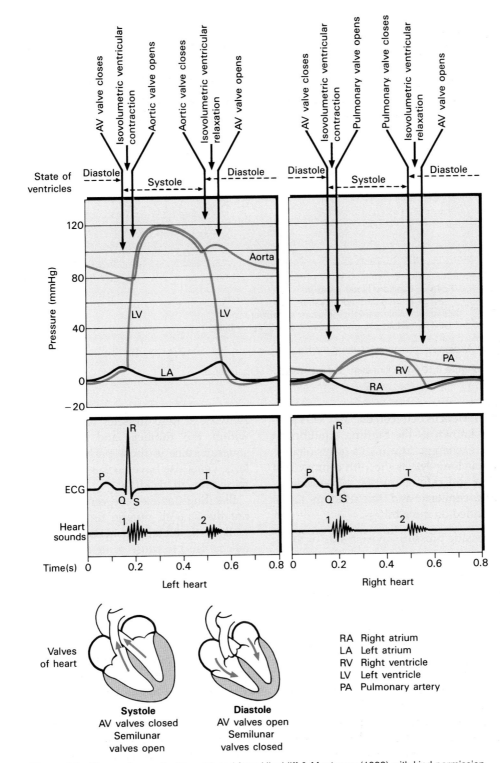

Figure 6.9 The cardiac cycle. (Reproduced from Hinchliff & Montague (1988) with kind permission from Baillière Tindall.)

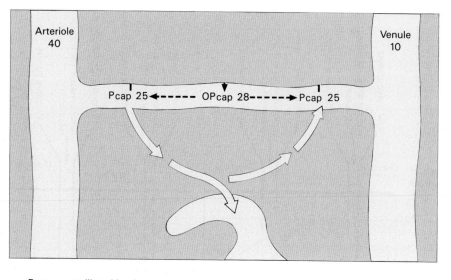

Pcap = capillary blood pressure
Pif = interstitial fluid pressure
OPcap = colloid osmotic pressure in capillary
OPif = colloid osmotic pressure in interstitial fluid

All figures refer to pressure in mmHg

Figure 6.10   The formation and reabsorption of tissue fluid.

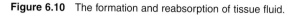

transfer of substances between the two. This phenomenon is known as the Starling equilibrium of capillary exchange. Starling, a physiologist, pointed out as long ago as the 19th century that the direction and rate of transfer of substances between the capillary and the fluid in tissue spaces depended on three things:

1. the hydrostatic pressure on each side of the capillary wall
2. the osmotic pressure of protein in the plasma and in the tissue fluid
3. the properties of the capillary wall (its semipermeability).

The venous system

This is a large-volume, low-pressure system with vessels of large internal diameter. It acts as a storage reservoir for blood, which is returned steadily to the heart for redistribution.

Blood flow in veins is affected by a number of factors other than contraction of the heart. Activity of limb muscles and pressure exerted within the thoracic and abdominal cavities squeeze veins in those parts of the body. Long, large veins also have pocket valves in their walls; these prevent backflow.

Bleeding depletes the venous blood reservoir, but the smooth muscle tissue in the arteriolar walls is stimulated into action (negative feedback mechanism) to cause some reduction in outflow to the skin and gut and thus help to maintain venous blood pressure.

The lymphatic system

Any consideration of the cardiovascular system would be incomplete without reference to the lymphatic system. This system is a drainage system additional to the veins. Most of the tissue fluid returns to the blood capillaries, but a little remains to be drained by the lymphatic capillaries, which originate as blind-ending, microscopic tubules within the tissues. As well as returning excess fluid to the cardiovascular system (which the lymph vessels join in the large veins of the neck), any leaked plasma proteins readily enter the lymph vessels, whose hydrostatic pressure is very low. Lymphatic capillaries are also important in the absorption of fat from the intestine. The lymphatic system also includes lymph glands, which filter debris and are the main centres of lymphocyte production (see p. 191, 'The immune system and homeostasis').

THE RESPIRATORY SYSTEM AND HOMEOSTASIS

Oxygen, combined with carbon compounds, is used to produce energy in tissue respiration, as previously described; during this process carbon dioxide is produced as a waste product. The body must, therefore, have a mechanism for transferring oxygen to and removing carbon dioxide from the tissues as quickly and efficiently as possible. Transportation of these materials is carried out by the cardiovascular system, as already described, but the actual exchange of these gases between the external world and the individual is the function of the respiratory system.

In more primitive animals, the gases are exchanged by passive diffusion across the body surface (cf. the moist skin of a frog or earthworm, or the cell membrane of an amoeba). The human gas exchange surface is provided by the microscopic alveoli of the lungs. These provide the following requirements for gaseous exchange:

- The surface area of the exchange membrane is large in comparison with the body volume to be supplied (human alveoli would fill a tennis court if spread out).
- The exchange surface is thin, and permeable (alveoli have walls one cell thick).
- The surface is moist to facilitate diffusion (the lining of alveoli is always moist).
- Stagnation of the medium close to the surface of the epithelium is avoided by:
  - movement of air across it by ventilation of the lungs, and
  - removal of diffused materials by circulating blood at the surface of the alveoli: capillary blood supply to the alveoli is rich and intimate (very close and intertwined).

Box 6.12 Smoking and lung damage

Disorders such as asthma, bronchitis and emphysema have in common some degree of obstruction of the air passages. The term 'chronic obstructive airways disease' (COAD) is used to refer to them. Airflow obstruction causes cough, wheezing and laboured breathing (dyspnoea). Cigarette smoking is the leading cause of bronchitis, emphysema and lung cancer and can trigger an asthmatic attack or exacerbate the condition.

The effect of smoking on the lungs is to produce constant irritation to the bronchial epithelium, with subsequent enlargement of the glands and mucous secreting goblet cells lining the bronchial airways. This leads to the secretion of an excessive amount of mucus which stimulates coughing; the typical symptom of **chronic bronchitis** is the regular expectoration of thick greenish yellow sputum. Constant irritation of the bronchial lining from persistent smoking can lead to **emphysema** which is the result of alveolar wall disintegration, with subsequent reduction in the surface area for gaseous exchange in the lungs. Emphysema leads to reduced blood oxygen levels and even very mild exercise leaves the person breathless. Continued alveolar destruction causes air to be trapped in the lungs so that the person has to work to exhale, a key symptom of the disorder. **Bronchogenic carcinoma** (the commonest form of lung cancer) occurs when the bronchial epithelium has become so damaged by the irritation of smoking (or other substance such as asbestos) that its basal cells divide rapidly and break through the basement membrane. At this stage goblet cells disappear and may be replaced with malignant cancer cells. If this happens, the new growth spreads throughout the lung and may block a bronchial tube resulting in breathlessness. People who have not apparently been exposed to tobacco smoke do occasionally develop bronchogenic carcinoma but its occurrence is 20 times higher in smokers than it is in non-smokers.

The rate of gas transfer across this respiratory surface depends on the rate of lung ventilation *and* on the blood flow to the surface; these factors, in turn, depend on total ventilation volume and cardiac output. So, lung function and cardiovascular function are here interrelated. Disturbance to the exchange of gases across the alveolar surface, such as occurs in inflammation of the bronchial passages for whatever reason, creates homeostatic imbalance for the individual. The consequences of this can be very serious (Box 6.12 describes smoking and lung damage).

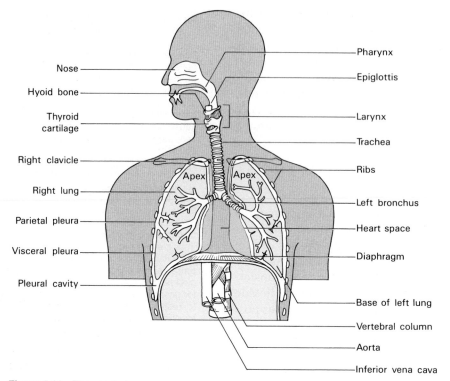

Figure 6.11 The respiratory organs.

The mechanisms of lung ventilation

The lungs are elastic, multichambered bags that are suspended within an airtight pleural cavity and open to the exterior via a single tube to the trachea (Fig. 6.11). The space between the lungs and the wall of the thoracic cage is lined with a pleural membrane and filled with a thin layer of pleural fluid. This thin cavity provides a flexible, lubricated connection between lung and thoracic wall. When the thoracic cage changes volume, the gas-filled lungs do so also.

During normal breathing, the thoracic cage is expanded and contracted by the action of the muscles in the diaphragm and between the ribs (intercostal muscles). When the diaphragm and intercostal muscles contract, the thoracic cavity enlarges, the lungs expand (because of the pleural membrane attachments) and air is drawn in via the trachea. Expiration is the opposite of this and happens when the respiratory muscles relax. Thus inspiration is *active* and expiration is *passive* (Fig. 6.12).

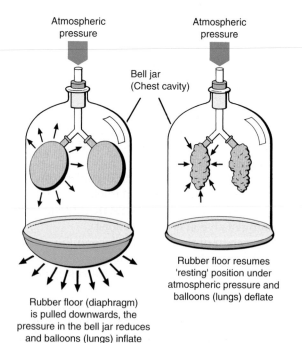

Figure 6.12 A model to illustrate the process of inspiration and expiration.

If the airtightness of the thoracic cavity is damaged by injury or puncture of the pleural membrane, air enters the pleural cavity and the lung(s) collapse. This is a state known as pneumothorax, and, except in very severe cases, it can be cured by slowly allowing the air to move out of the pleural cavity through a secondary, airtight drainage system.

Contractions of the respiratory muscles are controlled by specialised receptor neurones (central chemoreceptors) in the respiratory centre of the brainstem. These neurones respond to changes in carbon dioxide (CO_2) and oxygen (O_2) levels in the blood, and they control the rhythmic nature of breathing. There are also extremely sensitive stretch receptors in the lungs themselves, which prevent over-expansion of the lungs. The neuronal mechanisms causing rhythmic breathing are complex and poorly understood at present.

In addition to these neural mechanisms – which produce normal, rhythmic, quiet breathing – chemoreceptors in the carotid and aortic bodies (on the carotid and aortic arteries) respond to changes in O_2 and CO_2 levels in arterial blood. It is always the CO_2 increase that causes a response before a lowered O_2 level does. Since an increase in CO_2 causes increased acidity of the blood, it is possible that the response is due to the reduced pH rather than the CO_2 itself.

Whatever the combination of mechanisms, the rate and depth of breathing alter unconsciously according to O_2, CO_2, pH, emotions and sleep. Control can be voluntary, too, as in the fine changes needed for the complex human activities of singing, whistling and just talking. The limitations of voluntary control over normal ventilation can be seen, however, in breath-holding, which is always overcome by the eventual need to breathe!

THE DIGESTIVE SYSTEM AND HOMEOSTASIS

Ingestion

All living organisms depend on external sources for the raw materials and energy needed for their growth, normal functioning and repair. Food, which provides energy as well as material for the production of new tissue, is obtained from a variety of plant, animal and inorganic sources. The chemical energy for fuelling all processes in the animal body comes ultimately from a single source, the sun. Solar energy is not available directly to animals. Only autotrophic (or self-nourishing) organisms – i.e. chlorophyll-containing plants – can harness light energy to produce biochemical molecules for growth and energy conservation.

All animals are heterotrophic: they derive all their energy-yielding and body-building carbon compounds from ingested foodstuffs, which are, ultimately, derived from autotrophic organisms (Fig. 6.13).

Obtaining food

Before food can be used for tissue chemistry, growth and repair, it must first be obtained. Obtaining nutritional essentials is, clearly, a key to the survival of any species. Much of human enterprise is an effort towards finding enough to eat, although in comparison with other animals we have become less in need of the natural mechanisms to 'catch' or gather food, or to prevent ourselves from becoming a meal for predators. However, the complexities of the nervous system, sensory organs and muscular system have, in fact, evolved in part to ensure survival by obtaining sufficient food.

Digestion

Once food is obtained, it must be digested before any of it can be used by body tissues for energy production and body-building. Digestion is a chemical process in which special digestive enzymes catalyse the breakdown of large foodstuff molecules into simpler compounds that are small enough to diffuse or be transported across cell membranes for incorporation into cell chemistry.

The digestive system itself is a tube, or canal, with a receiving end (the mouth) and a discharging end (the anus). Its structure is varied to suit the function of its components (Fig. 6.14). For propelling material along the tube in the stomach and intestine, its walls are muscular. For carrying out enzymatic digestion in the stomach and small

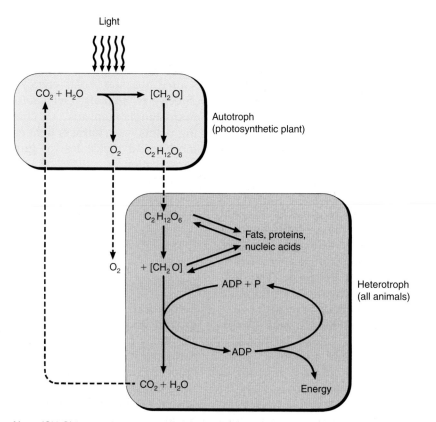

Note: (CH₂O) is an abbreviation formula for carbohydrate

Figure 6.13 Flow of chemical energy in the living world. In plants, high-energy sugars ($C_6H_{12}O_6$) are made, using light energy, from the raw materials of carbon dioxide and water. In the heterotroph, which eats ready-made high-energy compounds, the sugars and other foodstuffs yield energy when oxidised in the tissues.

intestine, the lining contains enzyme-secreting cells; supplementary digestive glands open into the gut. Where digested nutrients are transferred into the bloodstream, the lining is deeply folded to increase the absorptive area. Of significant importance in digestion are two functions: the motility of the gut and the secretion of gastrointestinal enzymes.

Motility of the alimentary canal

The muscles in the wall of the gut are arranged in a layer of circular muscle and a layer of longitudinal muscle. All gut muscle is smooth, involuntary muscle. The coordinated contractions of these muscles produce peristaltic waves of constriction, which propel the contents down the length of the tube. Movement of the contents within the tube is caused by a different sequencing of contractions (circular muscles contract in bands along the gut, causing intermittent segment formation, which squeezes and churns the food). Swallowing involves integrated movements of the tongue and pharynx, as well as peristaltic movements of the oesophagus. These actions move food out of the mouth and down the stomach without the person choking. Once in the stomach, food is mixed and squeezed vigorously by peristaltic activity and is retained in the stomach by closed cardiac and pyloric sphincter muscles at each end of the stomach. Like heart muscle, gastrointestinal muscle is capable of spontaneous

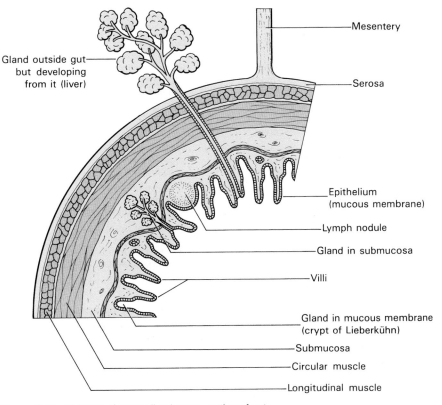

Figure 6.14 Diagram of generalised cross-section of gut.

contraction, but, in the gut, the automatic contractions are much slower. They are coordinated by a range of influences, including nerve control and hormonal mechanisms, and by the actual presence of food in the stomach and intestine.

Gastrointestinal secretions

The alimentary canal produces both endocrine and exocrine secretions.

Endocrine secretions

Endocrine glands are ductless glands that release their secretions (hormones) directly into the bloodstream for distribution to the target tissues (see 'The endocrine system and homeostasis', p. 186). Some hormones important in the digestive process are also released from special tissues within the gut itself (Table 6.3).

Exocrine secretions

Exocrine glands are very important in the gut. The output of an exocrine gland flows through a duct into a body cavity, such as the mouth, gut, or urinary tract. In the alimentary canal, these secretions are a mixture of water, salts, mucus and digestive enzymes. Their timing and duration of activity is controlled and coordinated by nervous and hormonal collaboration. The main initiating stimulus for the secretion of digestive juices is the presence of food within that portion of the tract. For example, saliva is secreted freely when food is in the mouth; it is impossible to prevent such secretion by volition, and this applies elsewhere in the alimentary tract.

With the exception of bile, all digestive juices contain enzymes that successively break down large food molecules into their smallest and simplest form, ready for absorption into the bloodstream (Table 6.4). Bile contains no enzymes, but

Table 6.3   The gastrointestinal hormones (adapted from Eckert 1988)

Hormone	Tissue of origin	Target tissue	Primary action	Stimulus to secretion
Gastrin	Stomach and duodenum	Secretory cells and muscles of the stomach	HCl production and secretion; stimulation of gastric motility	Vagus nerve activity; peptides and proteins in stomach
Cholecystokinin–pancreozymin (CCK–PZ)	Upper small intestine	Gall bladder Pancreas	Contraction of gall bladder Pancreatic juice secretion	Fatty acids and amino acids in duodenum
Secretin	Duodenum	Pancreas; secretory cells and muscles of stomach	Water and $NaHCO_3$ secretion; inhibition of gastric motility	Food and strong acid in stomach and small intestine
Gastric inhibitory peptide (GIP)	Upper small intestine	Gastric mucosa and musculature	Inhibition of gastric secretion and motility; stimulation of Brunner's glands	Monosaccharides and fats in duodenum
Vasoactive intestinal peptide (VIP)	Duodenum		Increase of blood flow; secretion of thin pancreatic fluid; inhibition of gastric secretion	Fats in duodenum

Table 6.4   The digestive enzymes (adapted from Eckert 1988)

Enzyme	Site of secretion	Site of action	Substrate acted upon	Products of action
Salivary α-amylase	Mouth	Mouth	Starch	Disaccharides (few)
Pepsinogen [→] pepsin	Stomach	Stomach	Proteins	Large peptides
Pancreatic α-amylase	Pancreas	Small intestine	Starch	Disaccharides
Trypsinogen [→] trypsin	Pancreas	Small intestine	Proteins	Large peptides
Chymotrypsin	Pancreas	Small intestine	Proteins	Large peptides
Peptidases	Pancreas	Small intestine	Large peptides	Small peptides (oligopeptides)
Lipase	Pancreas	Small intestine	Triglycerides	Monoglycerides, fatty acids, glycerol
Enterokinase	Small intestine	Small intestine	Trypsinogen	Trypsin
Disaccharidases	Small intestine	Small intestine	Disaccharides	Monosaccharides
Peptidases	Small intestine	Small intestine	Oligopeptides	Amino acids

it does contain alkaline bile salts that physically break up and disperse fats for their easy digestion by enzymes.

Absorption

Two products of digestion must find their way into all the tissues and cells of the body. The first stage in this process is by transport through the cells that line the gut. Transport is by a mixture of diffusion, facilitated diffusion and active transport. Most nutrients are absorbed across the lining of the small intestine, but a few will be absorbed from the stomach if, for example like alcohol, they are simple and soluble enough. Once they have left the gut, nutrients move into the blood and lymphatic capillaries with which the gut wall is richly endowed. Digested fats enter the lymphatic capillaries and are then transferred to the venous system (see 'Lymphatic system', above), while sugars, amino acids and water more readily enter the blood capillaries.

Box 6.13 The liver

The liver is the largest and probably the most metabolically active organ in the body. It does not belong to any one system as such, yet it is intimately involved in the biochemistry of the whole body. Its cells have abundant mitochondria (always a sign of fiercely active cells), and the liver tissues are heavily supplied with blood. It appears that all liver cells are capable of carrying out all the chemical functions of the liver. These can be summarised as follows:

Functions concerned with blood. The liver plays an important part in the production of erythrocytes in fetal life. It is also the place where old erythrocytes are broken down and their haemoglobin converted to bilirubin, which is excreted within the bile. The liver also manufactures all plasma proteins, except for the immune gammaglobulins. This protein manufacture includes the clotting factors prothrombin and fibrinogen.

Functions concerned with food. The liver stores carbohydrate in the form of glycogen. Under the control of hormones, liver glycogen is the main source of blood glucose, whose maintenance is vital to life. Carbohydrate can be manufactured in the liver from non-carbohydrate sources such as fats and proteins. This is an important function in times of fasting and starvation.

Of great importance with foodstuffs is the liver's function in detoxifying excess *protein* products (amino acids). In the liver, amino acids are broken down into ammonia and other compounds. The ammonia, which would be toxic if left to accumulate, is converted to relatively harmless urea, which is then excreted via the kidneys.

The role of the liver with regard to fats is equally significant. It produces bile salts, which are stored in the gall bladder and then released onto food in the small intestine. These salts assist in the physical breakdown (emulsification) of fats in food. They act as detergents. Fat-soluble vitamins (A, D, E and K) are stored in the liver. The liver also stores some fats as fatty acids and these can be metabolised in a variety of ways to produce energy and heat. This metabolism is particularly important in conditions of starvation or when insufficient carbohydrate (glucose) is being absorbed by the tissues. The latter state is the case in diabetes mellitus, in which alternatives to carbohydrate have to be metabolised to maintain life. The breakdown of fats in this case produces waste products called ketones, which can cause acidosis. Fortunately, this condition can now be reversed rapidly providing that medical and nursing care is sought.

Functions concerned with detoxification. The liver is the most important organ in the metabolism of drugs and alcohol. Most of these substances, if taken in moderation, are modified by the liver, excreted and eventually cleared completely from the body. A few cause lasting damage to the liver cells, which, of course, are then less efficient in their detoxification activity. In particular, high doses of paracetamol, Distalgesic and alcohol are known to cause severe liver damage, which can provoke liver failure.

The biochemistry of drugs and poisons and their metabolism within the liver is the subject matter of pharmacology textbooks. It is not essential to know these complexities, but the principles of assessing potential dangers and therapeutic doses in association with liver functions must always be applied when drugs are prescribed and administered.

Defecation

Most food absorption is complete by the time the gut contents reach the colon. Into the colon move the indigestible remains and water from the food itself and from the digestive juices. Water is gradually absorbed as the contents are moved along the colon, so that what remains for egestion, or defecation, is a semi-solid mass of largely cellulose material (roughage) and dead bacteria, with some water and bile pigments.

The muscular coordination of defecation is initiated by an involuntary nervous sensation (often termed 'the call to stool'), which is then usually accompanied by some measure of voluntary effort. Where nervous control is not yet matured (in babies) or has been damaged (e.g. by stroke, or by cerebral or spinal cord trauma), defecation is not voluntarily controlled; in the latter case, this can cause severe distress to sufferers and to carers.

THE RENAL SYSTEM AND HOMEOSTASIS

Regulation of a constant internal environment demands that the levels of water and intra- and extracellular solutes are constantly monitored and altered, as necessary, to restore balance. This process is known as osmoregulation. Also, the cellular environment must be freed of potentially toxic wastes that accumulate as a by-product of metabolism. This process is known as excretion. The renal system is the major excretor and osmoregulator in the body. (See Box 6.13 for detail about the production of nitrogenous waste.)

Although there may be hourly and daily variations in fluid (osmotic balance) within the tissues, the healthy body is generally in an osmotically steady state over the long term. Water enters the body with food and drink, and leaves in the urine, faeces, sweat and expired air. The 'fluid balance' (i.e. water in = water out) is relatively straightforward, but osmoregulation also has to maintain a favourable solute (e.g. sodium, potassium, chloride and acid/base) balance within the intra- and extracellular fluids. This balance is required during periods of feeding, fasting, exposure to extreme temperatures, exercising and so on (see Ch. 14).

All of these activities will also alter the rate at which excretory products (urea, carbon dioxide and water) are manufactured. The renal system is able to regulate body fluids for all these changes. At least one adequately functioning kidney is vital to life. The gross anatomy of the kidney is shown in Figure 6.15. There are normally two kidneys, lying one on each side against the dorsal inner surface of the lower back. They are small (about 1% of total body weight) but receive a remarkably large amount of blood (about 20–25% of the total cardiac output).

The functional unit of the kidney is the nephron (Fig. 6.16). This is closed at one end (Bowman's capsule), and opens at the other into the collecting duct system at the renal pelvis. Associated with the Bowman's capsule is a bunch of arterial capillaries known as the glomerulus. This close anatomical association of blood capillary and actual tubule is responsible for the first step in urine formation. The blood is filtered at the glomerulus, and the filtrate begins its journey along the nephron. Of particular significance to the osmoregulatory function of the kidney is the loop of Henle and its associated blood capillary supply, which also follows a looping structure.

Formation of urine

There are four processes that contribute to the ultimate composition of urine:

1. glomerular filtration
2. tubular reabsorption
3. tubular synthesis
4. tubular secretion.

Glomerular filtration. The blood is, effectively, 'sieved', and the factors determining which substances leave the blood and enter the nephron are molecular size, electrical charge and blood pressure. In healthy people, the only substances that do not enter the nephron are blood cells and plasma proteins. Water, Na^+, potassium (K^+), chloride (Cl^-), glucose and urea are all passed into the nephron.

Tubular reabsorption. The original filtrate composition is rapidly modified, so that about 75% of the water is reabsorbed before it gets to the loop of Henle. Glucose, in healthy people, is reabsorbed completely along the nephron, and water and other solutes are selectively reabsorbed according to their varying concentrations in the blood plasma. Urea is about 50% reabsorbed, and Na^+, Cl^- and H_2O reabsorption levels are critical in maintaining homeostasis. Water and Na^+ reabsorption are controlled by antidiuretic hormone

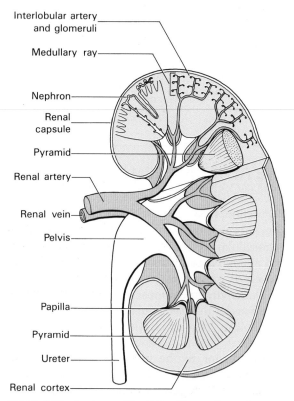

Interlobular artery and glomeruli

Medullary ray

Nephron

Renal capsule

Pyramid

Renal artery

Renal vein

Pelvis

Papilla

Pyramid

Ureter

Renal cortex

Figure 6.15 Anatomy of the kidney. The nephrons lie parallel to one another, with their collecting ducts opening through the papillae into a central cavity (the renal pelvis). The urine passes from the pelvis into the ureter, and from there to the urinary bladder.

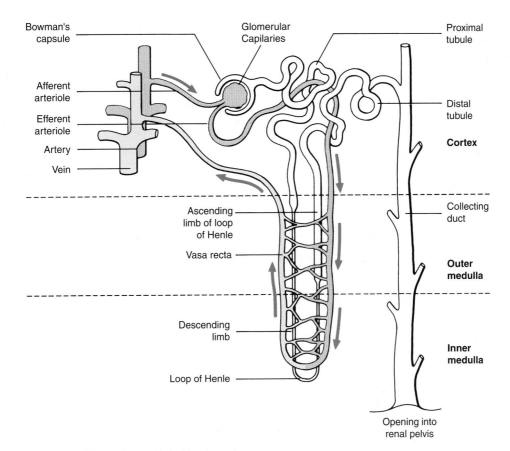

Figure 6.16 The nephron with its blood supply.

(ADH) and aldosterone respectively. The structure of the loop of Henle and related blood vessels is critical in allowing for the formation of a highly concentrated urine, if necessary, well above the concentration of blood plasma.

Tubular synthesis. Some excretory substances, mainly nitrogenous waste materials that are derived from escaped amino acids in the glomerular filtrate, are produced in the tubule and added to the urine.

Tubular secretion. As urine passes down the renal tubule, exchange of materials between urine and plasma can occur. There is sometimes a need for substances to be secreted from the blood into the urine (the opposite of reabsortion). By secretion, acidic ions (H^+), uric acid and potassium are removed from the blood for excretion.

All terrestrial animals, including humans, are faced with the risk of dehydration. Indeed, for humans this becomes a stark reality in desert-like conditions or during periods of water starvation of over 24 hours. The structure of the kidney, with its loop of Henle, is specific to birds and mammals, which are the only animals able to produce a urine that is more concentrated than blood.

Excretory function of the kidneys

In addition to the vital function of the kidneys in osmoregulation, their excretory function is also life-saving. Nitrogenous waste products, such as ammonia, from the breakdown of proteins are highly toxic if allowed to accumulate. If proteins are eaten to excess (eating too much meat is common in Western society), they cannot be stored, so are converted, by the liver, to urea (see Box 6.13). Urea is excreted via the urine, and although coincidental to the osmoregulatory activity of kidneys, the process is vital none the less. Urea excretion by the kidneys is a straightforward passive process of filtration and normal diffusion. Excretion of urea is interrupted if the liver or kidneys are damaged or diseased.

The importance of healthy kidneys

Apart from the acutely life-threatening dangers of cardiovascular or cerebral disorders, the most dangerous diseases are those that affect the kidneys. It is well understood that acute failure of the heart or brain can deprive tissues of oxygen, and that death can result within a few minutes, but renal failure, while not usually the cause of immediate death, can produce severe and lasting deviations from normal tissue function because of interruptions to homeostasis. This is equally life-threatening if left untreated, and may require intervention in the form of renal dialysis, in which unwanted substances are removed from the blood, or renal transplant surgery.

The kidneys are also vital for some non-excretory functions. For example, they are believed to produce the hormone erythropoietin in response to a low blood oxygen level (hypoxia) in the renal arteries. Erythropoietin stimulates the production of red blood cells (erythropoiesis) in the bone marrow and other sites (for further information, see Hinchliff & Montague 1988).

Micturition

The pelvis of the kidney gives rise to the ureter, which empties into the urinary bladder. The formation of urine is complete as it reaches the renal pelvis, and below the kidney the renal system can be considered as mere plumbing. Fortunately, this plumbing allows for the storage of urine in the bladder, with occasional release. This release is under neural control, which responds to stretching of the bladder wall by relaxing the bladder sphincter muscle: urine is then expelled (micturition). As in defecation, emptying of the bladder is not voluntarily controlled if the nervous system is immature or damaged.

THE NERVOUS SYSTEM AND HOMEOSTASIS

Nervous systems are undoubtedly the most intricately organised structures to have evolved on earth. The human nervous system contains anything up to 10^9 cells, which, during development in the fetus, become arranged into the neural circuits that make up the system. No part of the body – no system, organ or tissue – is without its own neural circuit. In spite of the complexity of organisation within the nervous system, the large number of nerve cells that comprise it are not accompanied by an equally large number of methods of working.

The function of the nervous system depends almost entirely on the same repertoire of electrical signals produced by the same physical and chemical changes across nerve cell membranes. The sophistication of the nervous system lies in the complexity of its organisation, which results in an immeasurable number of connections.

Neurones

The rapidity of neural communication is due to the structure and function of the individual nerve cells or neurones. Neurones are known as 'excitable' cells because they respond readily to physical or chemical changes in their environment and convert these responses into nerve impulses. Impulses can be transmitted at speeds of up to 120 m/s, and may travel along neurones that are, themselves, up to 1 m long (Fig. 6.17). The axons of most neurones are surrounded by a multilayered lipid and protein covering called the myelin sheath. This fatty sheath electrically insulates the axon and increases the speed of nerve impulse conduction. If this sheath becomes damaged, as, for example, in the demyelinating disease multiple sclerosis, the speed of nervous transmission may be much reduced.

Transmission of impulses

The physiological behaviour of a neurone depends upon its anatomical form and on the properties of its membranes. For example, the long axon (as in Fig. 6.17) has the ability for rapid

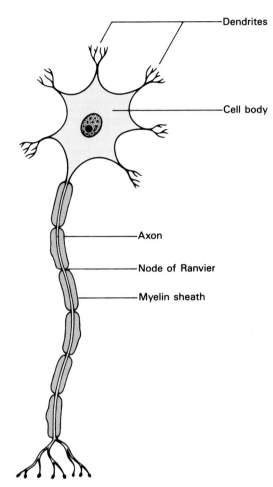

Figure 6.17   Structure of a neurone.

Labels: Dendrites, Cell body, Axon, Node of Ranvier, Myelin sheath

---

Box 6.14   Transmission at synapse

Before the development of electron microscopy in the 1940s, it was uncertain whether the nervous system was a continuous web of tissue, or whether there were distinct 'gaps' between neurones. The latter is now known to be the case and these gaps are called synapses. This discovery means that electrical excitation must be transmissible across a gap to another neurone, and/or to the cell of an organ which is being stimulated to act (e.g. a muscle). This transmission may be either electrical or chemical.

Electrical transmission. In this type of transmission, electrical current simply transfers from the pre-synaptic cell membrane to the post-synaptic cell membrane. This permits very rapid transmission and is known to occur within cardiac muscle and smooth muscle cells. It is well suited to rapid transmission in a group of nerve cells or across a series of cell–cell junctions such as are found in those tissues.

Chemical transmission. The vast majority of synaptic transmissions involve chemical transmitters. The pre-synaptic neurone liberates a transmitter substance that interacts with receptor molecules on the post-synaptic membrane. The post-synaptic cell is usually 'triggered' into action, which may be further transmission of electrical potential towards the next cell, or a different kind of excitation that results in muscular contraction if the next cell is a muscle fibre. Many transmitter chemicals are now identified and research still continues. Both excitatory and inhibitory transmitters are known to exist. The best known neurotransmitters are acetylcholine and noradrenaline, both of which are released in the autonomic nervous system.

---

conduction of electrical impulses from the cell body to the target structure, which is usually a muscle. The membranes of neurone terminals are specialised for the secretion of transmitter substances into the extracellular fluid between it and the target organ (e.g. muscle) cells, or for electrical transmission to another neurone (Box 6. 14).

This highly simplified version of nervous transmission within nervous tissue itself and between neurones and target organs gives an indication of how fully and rapidly the regulating mechanism can operate. To understand how nervous tissue makes and transmits impulses, it is necessary to know about the electrical and biochemical activity of cells. That is beyond the capacity of this chapter but it can be followed up by consulting one of the texts from the Further reading list.

Components of the nervous system

Anatomically, the nervous system has the following components:

- the central nervous system (CNS), consisting of the brain and spinal cord
- the peripheral nervous system, consisting of cranial nerves, spinal nerves and autonomic nerve fibres.

Although not part of the nervous system as such, special sense organs (eyes, ears, tongue, nose and skin) are richly supplied with specialised receptors and, via these, have direct links with the nervous system.

The processes of nervous regulation

The main sequence of events in nervous regulation is shown in Figure 6.18. A stimulus is anything that excites a neurone. Internally, it may be, for example, raised hydrostatic pressure within tissue fluid, an excess of CO_2 in the blood, or raised body temperature. Externally, it may be sound waves stimulating the nerve endings in the ear, a feather tickling the skin, or acid in a lemon affecting the taste buds. There are many different structural types of sensory receptor, responsive to many different kinds of stimulation, but their overall function is to raise awareness in the CNS of a change of circumstances. The excitability of the sensory receptor is translated into electrical impulses transmitted along sensory nerve fibres to the CNS (so-called afferent nerves). Specialised groups of cells in the brain and spinal cord interpret the received sensory information and, if necessary, initiate a homeostatic response via another kind of nerve cell whose fibres (efferent nerves) terminate in muscles or glands that are required to produce a response (of contraction or secretion). Not all sensory stimulation reaches consciousness. This is because it is interpreted either within the spinal cord with no cerebral (brain) interaction, or because the part of the brain used for interpretation of the signal is not within the consciousness area.

Unconscious nervous homeostasis includes control of breathing, heart rate and force of heart contraction, digestive tract activity, sweating, and vasodilatation in body temperature control. These are all activities controlled by the nervous system and of which we are normally unaware (except for sweating or 'glowing' when hot). Conscious sensations involve vision, hearing, taste, smell and touch, which special sense organs are responsible for initiating. While, for much of the time, such sensations do not provoke a homeostatic response, there may be occasions when they do, and these are related to basic survival needs to flee from or face danger (the 'flight or fight' response). Their role is considered to be much more significant in more primitive animals.

It will be helpful to know more about the nervous system and its application to nursing (see the Further reading section, below). Its significance in maintaining homeostasis should always be an important consideration, but the nervous system is responsible for many of the less well understood higher-order activities, such as speech and perception, in humans.

THE ENDOCRINE SYSTEM AND HOMEOSTASIS

Just as the muscular activity of the body would be impossible without the coordination and

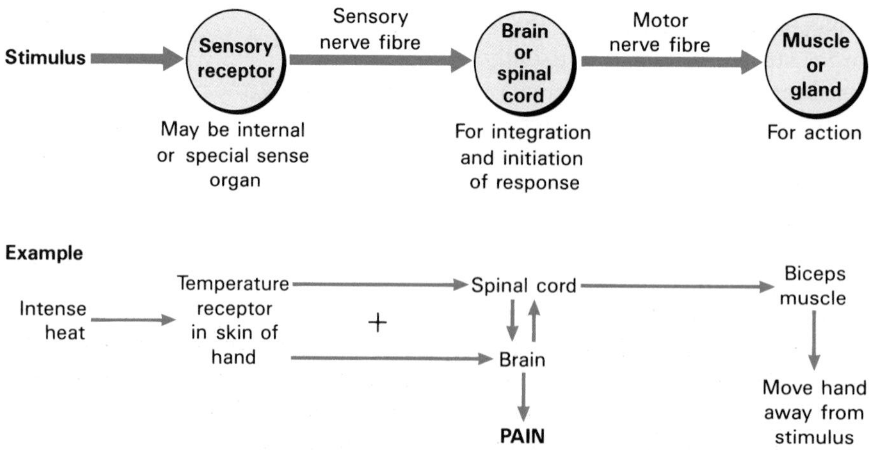

Figure 6.18　The sequencing of nervous regulation.

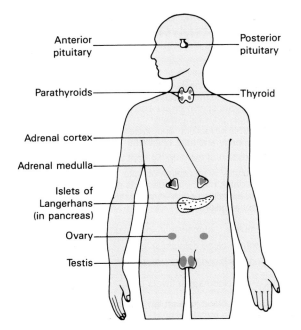

Figure 6.19 The major endocrine glands.

control exerted by means of the electrical signals of the nervous system, so also would the metabolic activities of the body (such as growth, maintenance and reproduction) be impossible without the coordination and control exerted by chemical agents. These chemical messengers are known as hormones and are secreted from a number of organs, the major endocrine glands being shown in Figure 6.19. The activity of a number of endocrine glands is regulated through the activity of the hypothalamus in the brain.

Hormones

A hormone is a chemical released directly into the bloodstream to be carried in the circulation to a distant target tissue. In addition to the hormones secreted by the endocrine glands, other groups of hormones are released into the bloodstream from nervous tissue. The hypothalamic hormones are neurohormones. There is also a group of hormones known as local hormones; these are secreted from various tissues to act on nearby targets, and include histamine and some of the intestinal hormones (Table 6.5).

The term hormone comes from the Greek for 'arouse to activity'. It is known that the hormone molecules react with specific receptor molecules on the surface of their target cells. By an interaction of the hormone molecule with the receptor molecule, a series of cascade-type, enzyme-mediated reactions is initiated within the cell. Although hormone molecules come into contact with all the tissues in the body, only cells that contain the receptors specific for the hormone are affected by that hormone.

The amount of hormone produced by an endocrine gland is very small. Blood concentrations are low and target cells are extraordinarily sensitive to their hormone. The typical blood plasma level of a hormone would be similar to the concentration achieved by dissolving a pinch of sugar in a large swimming pool full of water.

The secretion and circulation of hormones both take place relatively slowly, unlike the rapid reaction times experienced in nervous control activities. Thus the endocrine system is well suited for regulation that is sustained for minutes, hours or days. Such long-term control is required for regulating blood osmolarity (water/salts balance), blood sugar levels, growth and metabolic rate. The reproductive cycle in women also requires cyclical and sustained hormonal control. The quick-acting nervous system and the slower, sustained activity of the endocrine system complement one another in the overall regulation of physiological activity (Table 6.5).

Homeostatic control may be lost if hormones are under- or over-secreted. The normal mechanism for controlling secretion level is by negative feedback, as described earlier. Malfunctioning endocrine glands (causes for this not being completely known but including congenital abnormality, heredity and viral infection) upset homeostatic regulation most severely.

THE IMMUNE SYSTEM AND HOMEOSTASIS

The immune system defends the body against a variety of foreign substances, including microorganisms (which cause infection), transplanted cells, tissues or organs, and irritants such as pollen. The mechanisms involved enable the individual

Table 6.5 The major hormones and their functions

Gland	Hormone	Functions
Anterior pituitary (adenohypophysis)	Thyroid stimulating hormone (TSH)	Controls the activity of the thyroid gland
	Adrenocorticotrophic hormone (ACTH)	Controls the activity of the adrenal cortex
	Follicle stimulating hormone (FSH)	Controls the menstrual cycle in females
	Luteinising hormone (LH)	Stimulates sperm production in males
	Growth hormone	Controls physical growth
	Luteotrophic hormone	Controls production and secretion of milk during pregnancy and after childbirth
Middle lobe of pituitary	Melanocyte stimulating hormone	Deposition of melanin pigment in melanocyes in skin
Posterior pituitary (neurohypophysis)	Antidiuretic hormone (ADH)	Regulates reabsorption of water from renal tubules
	Oxytocin	Stimulates uterine contractions during childbirth
		Causes milk ejection from breasts during infant suckling
Thyroid	Tri-iodothyronine (T_3) Thyroxine (T_4)	Stimulate metabolism in the tissues generally
	Calcitonin	Controls blood calcium levels
Parathyroid	Parathyroid hormone	Controls blood calcium levels
Pancreas (islets of Langerhans)	Insulin Glucagen	Control blood sugar levels
Adrenal cortex	Aldosterone	Controls blood sodium ion (Na^+) levels
	Cortisol	Regulates metabolism of carbohydrates, fats and proteins
		Complex involvement in stress responses
	Sex hormones (androgens and oestrogens)	Control sexual development
Adrenal medulla	Adrenaline Noradrenaline	Prepare body for action: 'fight or flight' response
Ovaries	Oestrogen Progesterone	Produce female secondary sexual characteristics
		Act on uterine lining during each menstrual cycle
Testes	Testosterone	Produces male secondary sexual characteristics
		Stimulates growth of seminiferous tubules
Placenta	Human chorionic gonadotrophin (HCG)	Maintains oestrogen and progesterone production in early pregnancy

to recognise and respond to the 'foreignness' of a wide range of biological substances that are potentially harmful if present in the body.

There are several important defences that prevent foreign substances from entering the body. The most obvious is the skin, but others include the mucous linings of the respiratory and digestive tracts, which trap foreign particles or stimulate their expulsion by coughing and sneezing. In addition, some body secretions, such as gastric juices, are acidic and therefore destroy disease-producing bacteria.

However, foreign materials can enter the body via damage to the skin, by ingestion or inhalation of pathogens, by deliberate introduction of 'foreign bodies' via transplants or blood transfusions, or by the development of abnormal tissues within the body (e.g. cancerous growths). In every case, the presence of foreign material is likely to provoke an automatic series of responses designed to destroy or contain its damaging effects. Unfortunately, the response mechanisms do not distinguish between harmful 'foreigners' (infections) and potentially life-saving ones (transplants): the nature of the response is geared to neutralise foreign substances that have the potential to interfere with the delicate balance of homeostasis.

How the immune system works

The immune system works in two main ways:

1. direct physical attack
2. antibody production.

Direct physical attack

When foreign matter penetrates the defences of the skin and mucous membranes to enter the superficial tissues (such as in a spot or boil) or the bloodstream, it encounters special white blood cells known as polymorphs and monocytes. These cells engulf particles, including infectious agents, and destroy them. This is phagocytosis (referred to in 'Transport across membranes', above). These phagocytic cells can carry out their function within the bloodstream, or they can migrate out of the blood vessels into affected tissues in response to a chemical stimulus from the foreign materials.

Tissues that have been damaged or which contain foreign substances evoke an inflammatory response (Box 6.15).

Antibody production

A vascular immune response occurs when the phagocytic cells are unable to recognise (chemically) the invading agent, or are unable to engulf foreign particles because they lack the appropriate chemical receptors to do so. In this case, a more subtle and sophisticated type of germ warfare may be engaged, or may occur simultaneously. This is the production of antibodies, i.e. proteins manufactured specifically to attend to and neutralise invading or foreign substances. Substances that stimulate the production of antibodies are known collectively as antigens. The hallmark of the immune system is the specificity of an antibody for a particular antigen.

Antibodies are manufactured by cells called lymphocytes, some of which circulate in the blood and some of which exist in lymphatic tissues within the body. Antibodies act by directly attacking the foreign cells and neutralising them by locking on to their surface, but the special feature of lymphocytes is that they carry genetic information to cope with an almost infinite variety of antigens, i.e. they can produce a protein antibody for any antigen. Once a lymphocyte has been processed to 'recognise' and interact with a particular antigen, it remains in the blood or lymphatic tissue, able to recognise it again should a further invasion occur. The specificity of the antibody/antigen relationship is what makes this recognition possible. A second infection will thus be 'neutralised' rapidly, preventing widespread damage. This is immunity in its simplest explanation. Its discovery led to the development of artificial immunisation against severe infections, whereby a reduced dose is introduced to the individual in order to stimulate production of antibodies against a further attack.

Immunity and immunisation

Immunity has been achieved when an individual is no longer susceptible, or has a reduced susceptibility, to one or more antigens. Gaining immunity to infectious diseases (or other antigens) is an important factor in health care programmes, and nurses need to be familiar with the processes by which immunity may be acquired.

Passive immunity

This occurs when individuals have not produced their own antibodies. The simplest example of such immunity is the natural transfer of antibodies from mother to baby, both prenatally, via placental exchange, and postnatally, through breastfeeding. This 'transfer' of antibody is mostly extremely beneficial, and confers to the child the ability to fight off early infections until it is able to produce its own antibodies.

Artificial passive immunity is provided when people receive specific antibody injections against infectious diseases. The effect is immediate but shortlived, lasting only until the antibodies are destroyed in the recipient's body. Passive immunisation is reserved for situations where a person is at risk from a dangerous disease but has had no previous opportunity to develop a personal active immunity (i.e. has had no previous contact with the disease). An important example of passive artificial immunisation is in the prevention of Rhesus incompatibility in pregnancy (see Box 6.11).

Active immunity

This occurs when individuals produce their own antibodies in response to the presence of the

Box 6.15 Inflammation explained

Inflammation is the protective response of the body to irritation or injury. The word 'inflame' means, literally, 'to set afire', and the suffix 'itis' denotes an inflammatory response, as, for example, in appendicitis and arthritis.

Common causes of inflammation

- mechanical – caused by direct trauma
- chemical – corrosion of tissues by direct contact, for example acid burns to the skin or acid reflux from the stomach to the oesophagus
- allergenic – for example pollen in hayfever, contact objects causing dermatitis, some foods, insect bites and stings
- infective – either external (topical) or systemic
- thermal – excessive heat or cold, which causes tissue damage.

Physiology of the inflammatory response

The blood vessels local to the damaged area dilate, increasing blood supply to the area. The dilated vessels become more permeable, and fluid escapes into the surrounding tissues. The escaped fluid, or exudate, contains fibrinogen and immunoglobulins. Polymorphonucleocytes are attracted to the area where they destroy damaged tissue and invading microbes by phagocytosis. Histamine is released from local tissues.

The local signs of inflammation

These commonly include:

- redness – due to vasodilatation
- heat
- swelling – due to accumulation of tissue fluid
- pain – due to increased activity, through disturbance, of local pain receptors
- loss of function – due to pain, swelling and protective 'guarding' by adjacent muscles.

The systemic responses to inflammation

These may include:

- a rise in body temperature
- general malaise with poor appetite
- changes in blood electrolyte levels
- changes in plasma protein levels, owing to immune responses
- an increase of white blood cell levels
- increased activity of lymphatic tissue ('swollen glands').

Managing inflammation

Local and simple inflammation requires the relief of pain and management of the swelling. Wherever possible, foreign bodies and pus should be removed. Systemic responses to inflammation, such as with infections, surgery or other internal causes, require more extensive intervention to reduce the stimulus, for example by using antibiotics for infection.

In all cases, the need to achieve restoration of homeostasis is the key component, but the patient may be distressed and will need management of this, alongside attention to physical and social needs.

Anaphylactic shock

In extreme cases, a localised cause of inflammation, such as a bee sting, may cause a rapid and extreme systemic response, leading to a case of allergenic shock, or anaphylactic shock. This is very rare but life-threatening, and requires urgent medical intervention with intravenous adrenaline and life-sustaining measures such as cardiopulmonary resuscitation.

Anaphylaxis is, fortunately, rare, but it is a clear example of a case where the internal homeostatic mechanisms are unable to meet the unusual demands of an external disruption to a stable internal environment (see Box 6.8).

---

specific antigen. Immunity may have been acquired naturally, where the immune system has responded by producing antibodies to fight the antigens of a naturally occurring infection. These antibodies then remain, often for many years, so that a further invasion of the antigen is immediately attacked, and no further disease occurs. A common example of active natural immunity is that which occurs for chickenpox.

Active immunity can also be artificially stimulated. A small, safe dose of the disease-producing organism, or some of its components or products, is given to an individual. Routes of administration vary, according to the disease and vaccine, but many more are now oral preparations rather than injections. The recipient's immune system responds by producing antibodies that provide protection from the serious disease. This kind of immunity (active artificial) is now widely used in health care programmes. Common illnesses now almost completely preventable by this method include diphtheria, whooping cough, poliomyelitis, tuberculosis, measles and rubella (German measles), because the antibodies are long-lived. Artificial immunity for influenza is less certain, because the influenza virus repeatedly changes its protein specificity, so needs repeatedly different antibodies for its destruction.

All nurses need to be familiar with the development of natural immunity and its exploitation in programmes of immunisation for children and for any individuals at risk of infection.

Immunological mechanisms are essential for survival, and have formed the basis for significant research in the past few years. With the increasing ability of surgeons and medical engineers to undertake transplants, a major problem of tissue rejection (of foreign protein material) has required massive investigation.

A number of illnesses arise because of autoimmunity, when immune reactions are directed against an individual's own cells. Examples include rheumatoid arthritis, some cases of diabetes mellitus and ulcerative colitis. Probably the greatest challenge at the time of writing is the problem of AIDS (acquired immune deficiency syndrome), whose name explains the condition in terms of immunity.

REFERENCES

Eckert R 1988 Animal physiology, 3rd edn. W H Freeman, Oxford
Wright S 1965 Applied physiology, 11th edn. Oxford University Press, London
Hinchliff S, Montague S 1988 Physiology for nursing practice. Baillière Tindall, London
Mueller R F, Young I D 1998 Emery's Elements of medical genetics, 10th edn. Churchill Livingstone, Edinburgh
Wilson K J W 1990 Ross and Wilson's Anatomy and physiology in health and illness, 7th edn. Churchill Livingstone, Edinburgh

FURTHER READING

Cree L, Rischmiller S 1991 Science in nursing, 2nd edn. W B Saunders/Baillière Tindall, Sydney
Helpful for readers who wish to understand more about basic physical sciences and their place in physiology for nurses. Full of nursing examples that illustrate underlying physical principles.

Hinchliff S, Montague S 1988 Physiology for nursing practice. Baillière Tindall, London
Provides extensive description of physiology of all the systems.

Mueller R F, Young I D 1998 Emery's Elements of medical genetics, 10th edn. Churchill Livingstone, Edinburgh
A classical text which has been through 10 editions in 30 years and so has followed the development of genetics through exciting times. This is a very helpful reference for both the newcomer to genetics and to the student who wishes to go beyond the basics.

Scott Hawley R, Mori Catherine A 1999. The human genome: a user's guide. Academic Press, San Diego
An entertaining text which gives all the science of genetics from Mendel to the genome project, but written in a manner to engage every reader, whatever their background. Intended to 'put genetics in the middle of people's lives'.

Tortora G J, Grabowski S R 1993 Principles of anatomy and physiology, 7th edn. Harper Collins, New York
A huge book, but designed as an introductory text for students and assumes no prior knowledge of the subject. It is geared to students entering the health care professions and includes clinical applications wherever relevant. Beautifully illustrated with great clarity.

Wilson K J W 1990 Ross and Wilson's Anatomy and physiology in health and illness, 7th edn. Churchill Livingstone, Edinburgh
Covers anatomy in good detail. Well illustrated. A good support to any student of physiology.

7

The psychological basis of nursing

John Wilkinson

CHAPTER CONTENTS

The contribution of psychology to nursing 199
What is psychology? 199
An introduction to psychological themes 200
Absolute and negotiated knowledge 200
Commonalities and differences between people 201
Autonomy and constraining factors 201
Consciousness and the unconscious 202
Why is psychology relevant to nursing? 202

Nature, nurture and human behaviour 203
Predetermined and contextual components of human nature 203
The psychodynamic perspective 203
The behaviourist perspective 205
The cognitive perspective 207
The humanistic perspective 209

Acknowledging people as individuals 210
Diversity of health beliefs 210
The self-concept 210
Self-concept and self-esteem 211
Health locus of control 212

Making assessments 213
Attention 213
Perception 214
Person perception 214
Attribution theory 215

Using memory effectively 216
Memory registration 216
Memory storage 217
Memory retrieval 217

Problem solving 218
Problem solving and evidence-based decision making 218
Expertise and problem solving 219
Developing problem-solving expertise 220

Stress 221
An environmental approach to stress 221
A physiological approach to stress 221
An interactional approach to stress 222
A composite explanation of stress 223

Conclusion 223

References 223

Further reading 224

Psychology is a social science which seeks to understand and explain human mental processes and behaviour. An understanding of the subject offers insights into how and why people are sometimes very different and sometimes very similar. Exploring the relationships of individuals with their social context has the potential to enhance the quality of health care provision in a range of settings. As a social science and academic discipline, psychology is underpinned by research, the main focuses of enquiry being approaches which seek to interpret and to understand the subjective nature of human experience and those which seek objectively to measure relationships between variables in order to demonstrate causality. These research aims are congruent with modern health care where there is increasing recognition of the contribution that each person makes to his or her own experience of health and illness and an emphasis upon practice which is directed by research and other evidence. Through an exploration of psychology, health care professionals are better informed to understand health and illness behaviour, the management of health care and therapeutic relationships between the provider and recipient of care within a health care context.

This chapter gives the reader a selective overview of a number of aspects of human mental processes and behaviour which are relevant to nursing. It refers to some helpful further reading from both health care and psychological literature and illustrates the relevance of the issues raised through the use of examples of application drawn from clinical practice.

Space is limited within an introductory chapter such as this one, and readers who wish to explore psychology in more detail are recommended to consult an introductory psychology source such as Gross (1996), which is an excellent text in terms of clarity of expression and comprehensiveness of the material included. However, due to its general

nature, the specific links to health care applications are limited. There are a number of specialist psychology texts written for a health professional readership such as Payne & Walker (1996) or Niven (2000) which also merit looking at if you wish to follow up in more detail the topics raised in this chapter.

It must be noted that psychological theory which is relevant to nursing should not be regarded as being separate from other aspects of professional practice. This chapter should therefore be considered in the context of the rest of the book, particularly Chapter 9 ('The nurse as communicator'), which highlights the application of appropriate aspects of the psychology of human interaction, and Chapter 10 ('The nurse as health promoter'), which highlights the application of appropriate aspects of the psychology of social cognition.

This chapter:

- introduces psychology in order to argue its relevance to inform professional nursing practice
- considers nature and nurture perspectives to highlight the predetermined and contextual components of human nature
- considers psychodynamic, behaviourist, cognitive and humanistic perspectives as different ways of explaining human development, thinking and behaviour
- acknowledges the diversity of lay and professional health conceptualisations and the need to individualise health care in response to this variance
- examines the self-concept in relation to self-awareness, self-esteem and locus of control
- illustrates how both empirical and interpretive types of data collection are relevant to nursing assessments
- gives an explanation of how, given that the processes of attention and expectation influence the way in which the world is perceived selectively, nursing assessments need to be conscious rather than automatic
- outlines person perception and attribution theory to caution against bias and other

errors of judgement which may compromise the accuracy of nursing assessments

- **considers registration, storage and retrieval processes to suggest ways in which memory function may be enhanced to improve the retention of information which is important to health care**
- **discusses problem solving in relation to evidence-based decision making in the context of contemporary health policy**
- **explores domain-specific expertise in order to suggest ways to develop improved problem solving strategies**
- **represents stress using environmental, physiological and transactional approaches and highlights reactive (i.e. using defence mechanisms) and proactive (i.e. using cognitive techniques) coping strategies.**

THE CONTRIBUTION OF PSYCHOLOGY TO NURSING

WHAT IS PSYCHOLOGY?

Psychology is the study of the mind and mental processes in order to seek to understand and explain human experience. The subject matter of psychology thus includes how human beings think, behave and experience the world. It could, therefore, be argued that everyone is an expert in psychology because the subject is merely a formalisation of the common sense understanding of ourselves and others which is built up through life experience. To a certain extent this is true. Common sense, professional nursing and psychology all attempt to explain mental processes such as thinking, understanding and experiencing emotions. However, whether you have studied psychology or not, even our own mental processes are not directly accessible to interpretation (Activity 7.1).

It is doubtful whether anyone experiences life in a totally predictable and ordered way. The complexities of life are a serious challenge to an expectation that it is possible to introspect in a way that takes account of all the countless factors which have the potential to influence the way the human brain functions. Of course, even if introspection were an effective key to understanding ourselves, personal insights are only part of human experience. It is difficult to conceive of a field of nursing that does not involve substantial interaction with other people, both as individuals and in groups. Accepting that one's own mental processes are not directly accessible to comprehensive interpretation, those of others are even more elusive (Activity 7.2).

As already discussed, it is likely that one person will think about a given incident quite differently to others. It would be quite surprising if two individuals interpreted the behaviour of a third person in the same way, but even if similar responses are reported, this may be because there is a degree of mutual influence. Consider whether someone else, for example a parent or personal tutor, would make the same interpretation as yourself: the point is, of course, no one knows; nor do they have a direct way of knowing!

 Activity 7.1 Personal introspection

Think about what you were doing earlier today. Focus upon all the thoughts, emotions and behaviour that were going on as you went about your normal business. (Psychologists call this accessing of mental processes 'introspection'.) How easy would it be to offer a rational account of why you behaved the way you did and not in any other way? If you think you are able to explain in detail the causes of your feelings and behaviour, how can you be sure that your interpretations of your introspection are complete and accurate?

 Activity 7.2 Comparing and contrasting introspections

Get together with a friend and experience a short interaction with a third person, perhaps in a café or shop. Discuss with your friend your introspections about what was going on. How do your thoughts compare and contrast with those of your friend? Now focus upon your interpretations of the behaviour you observed acted out by the third party. Do you and your friend agree or differ in the conclusions you have drawn about the third person?

Despite the complexity of human thought and behaviour, and its inaccessibility, making sense of one's own and other people's mental processes and behaviour is fundamental to human interaction. Without an understanding of ourselves and others, human interaction has the potential to be reduced to simple rule-based relationships. It would be inappropriate for nurses to relate to everyone with whom they had professional contact in the same way without any regard for individual needs. An important contribution of psychology to understanding human experience is that it offers a wider range of alternative explanations of personal introspections and interpretations of observations of others' behaviour beyond those which are generally available as common sense explanations. The reason why psychology is able to expand, and sometimes challenge, common sense explanations is that psychology is structured around explanations which are informed by theories which in turn have been developed through research. An understanding of psychological theory provides opportunities to support or challenge common sense interpretations of the mental processes of oneself and others.

AN INTRODUCTION TO PSYCHOLOGICAL THEMES

Within the psychological literature are found a number of themes which represent different ways of interpreting mental processing and behaviour. These themes are outlined below (and summarised in Table 7.1) and will be referred to

when they arise at relevant points within the chapter.

Absolute and negotiated knowledge

One view of the world is the 'positivist' one. This is underpinned by an assumption that there are absolute truths which cannot be falsified despite attempts to do so using evidence collected in research. Positivist research data are empirical, i.e. can be experienced and measured by one or more of the senses. Numerous examples of a positivist assumption of absolute truth are found in the medical model of illness. A traditional medical model assumption is that illness is attributable to disease which has predictable pathology and which can be detected and treated with predictable outcomes. Cognitive psychologists in the positivist tradition study how human beings process information and have developed causal relationship representations of how these processes might occur within all human beings; for example variations in human memory can be explained by assuming that everyone's memory works in the same way, variation in memory function being explained by some people being better than others at using and applying memory processing.

In recent years the absolute assumptions of the medical model have increasingly been challenged (Gabe et al 1994). An alternative perspective is that of knowledge being negotiated. This means that human beings define and interpret their experiences depending on innumerable factors which do not easily lend themselves to

Table 7.1 Psychological themes

Theme	Examples of areas of psychological study	Examples of relevance to clinical practice
Absolute and negotiated knowledge	Positivist and interpretive research	Evidence-based practice and reflective practice
Commonalities and differences between people	Idiographic and nomothetic ways of exploring human similarities and individuality	National Service Frameworks (to standardise clinical practice) and individualised assessment to inform holistic care planning
Autonomy and constraining factors	Theories to explain stress and coping	Responding to, and coping with, stressful situations
Consciousness and unconsciousness	Theories to explain memory	Making clinical assessments based on patient histories

identification and measurement. For example, in discussing evidence-based practice in the context of clinical governance, Ferlie (1999) reports that midwives argue that current positivist research on the clinical assessment of women is not sufficiently broad to encompass their individual views and preferences. Psychological theory and investigation is frequently concerned with interpretation of the interplay of such diverse factors. Humanistic psychologists value highly the idiosyncratic nature of human experience and put subjective interpretations at the heart of their research.

Commonalities and differences between people

The study of psychology embraces assumptions that people are similar in how they think and experience the world. There are parallels here within a traditional medical model view of health and disease. The established medical model understanding of disease is that it is predictable in that all who contract a particular illness are affected in the same way and should respond in a similar way to the same form of treatment. This is the thinking behind standardised approaches to care as represented in recently disseminated National Service Frameworks (e.g. for heart disease, diabetes mellitus and mental health). If it is assumed that human beings are generally more similar than they are different, then it is good practice to develop ways of measuring those aspects of similarity. For example, in physical care it is sometimes useful to measure physiological

factors such as blood pressure; and in social care the measurement of social factors such as income can be appropriate. However, as has already been identified, psychological factors such as emotional response to disease are not easily measured directly. Hence indirect approaches, using techniques such as stress or personality questionnaires, are sometimes used clinically and in research. The technical term for the measurement of criteria on a predetermined scale is *nomothetic* enquiry.

A contrasting view of humankind is that every person is uniquely individual with respect to his mental processes, and this is frequently thrown into relief when a person becomes unwell. Such a view is prominent in aspects of health care where the emphasis is upon the nursing process: individualised assessment, planning, implementation and evaluation of care with a view to deliver holistic practice (Leddy & Pepper 1993). Central to the assumption of individual differences is that clinical assessment must be comprehensive, person-centred and without pre-judgements setting up expectations. The technical term for the assessment of an individual without any predetermined criteria is *idiographic* enquiry.

Table 7.2 compares nomothetic and idiographic enquiry.

Autonomy and constraining factors

Autonomy is associated with having the free will to select and act according to one's inclinations with independent thought and control over choice (Wilkinson 1997a). In psychology, autonomy is

Table 7.2 Idiographic and nomothetic enquiry (adapted from Ellis 1996)

Idiographic	Nomothetic
Focuses on the inner world of personal experience	Focuses on the outer world of observable behaviour
Subjective experience important	Objective measurement important
Uses a single or a few in-depth individuals or case studies	Uses large numbers of subjects to yield a representative sample
Values individual interpretation and intuition	Values the demonstration or falsification of causal relationships between isolated variables
Generalisations to larger populations are not appropriate	Aims to generalise to larger populations
Emphasises the uniqueness of individuals	Emphasises statistically significant commonalities and differences between people

recognised through acknowledging that people are idiosyncratic and do not always express the opinions nor exhibit the patterns of behaviour that might be expected. For example, some people feel more in control in stressful situations than others and this may facilitate either a sense of empowerment to cope or a sense of responsibility which leads to panic.

However, the concept of autonomy may be illusory: 'to believe that man is the author of his destiny is not to deny that he may be tragically limited by his circumstances' (Kelly 1979). What is being suggested by the psychologist George Kelly is that an understanding of autonomy must acknowledge that choice is always influenced by constraining factors. People who are under-confident may feel that they are avoiding a stressful situation through choice, but this choice may be better informed if it is made with some insight into influencing factors such as coping strategies.

Consciousness and the unconscious

Consciousness refers to our sense of awareness of our own thoughts and to events occurring around us. Consciousness includes an immediate sense of 'here and now' – i.e. everything that is going on around an individual at any particular moment in time. It also includes everything which is readily available for retrieval from memory, which then moves from preconsciousness storage into conscious awareness. When taking a history from a patient as part of a clinical assessment, a nurse is asking the patient to report what they are experiencing (consciousness) and this is expanded by questioning which draws additional information from their preconscious.

However, much of human functioning occurs unconsciously. A good example of unconscious processing is something which is done frequently, such as driving a particular journey. When asked to comment upon a regular driving experience, many people are unable to report accurately what happened the last time they made such a journey. For many people, getting to a familiar destination is so unremarkable that they have very little recollection of the process – it

has become automatic, and because there was little conscious attention paid it is said to have occurred unconsciously (not the same as the unconsciousness associated with a general anaesthetic, but with a similar effect upon diminishing the richness of the experience). Poor conscious awareness can compromise patients' accounts when taking a history and so nurses need to be aware of strategies to enhance patients' perception and memory to add accuracy and richness to their accounts.

WHY IS PSYCHOLOGY RELEVANT TO NURSING?

Current UK health policy (DoH 1998) is increasingly recognising the contributions that individuals and social groups make to experiences of health and illness. The contribution of nurses to facilitating health is now recognised as an essential component of their practice in addition to their traditional role in the management of illness (National Health Service Executive 1998). One of the key challenges to nurses is to work with individuals and social groups to promote a sense of personal responsibility and control over their lifestyles in relation to health (Fatchett 1998). However, patients (and indeed health care professionals, including nurses) may hold health beliefs which are highly idiosyncratic and difficult to understand, particularly when viewed out of context (Wilkinson 1999). Despite the development of policy and the considerable professional interest in patients' involvement in their own health, the nurse adviser to the Health Service Ombudsman reports that communication deficits are the major cause of complaints about health care (Martin 1997). Great emphasis is placed upon nurses engaging in good quality communication which is based upon shared meanings with patients (UKCC 1996). To be able to do this, nurses need to recognise that people think and behave in very different ways.

It has already been argued that psychology seeks to explain human mental processing and behaviour. A better insight into some of the commonalities and differences between people is fundamental to understanding the relationship of the individual's health and illness experiences within his social context and engagement in the health care system. Such insights are important to help nurses to understand those with whom they work in order to inform enhanced assessment, planning, implementation and evaluation of care strategies tailored to individual needs. Throughout this chapter a range of examples will be offered which demonstrate how psychological theory offers nurses credible options to a diverse range of challenges that are encountered in clinical practice.

NATURE, NURTURE AND HUMAN BEHAVIOUR

PREDETERMINED AND CONTEXTUAL COMPONENTS OF HUMAN NATURE

There is a longstanding debate concerning the interplay between nature, nurture and human development. The issue is perhaps best summarised by Pervin (1978) with the phrase 'Am I me or am I the situation?', which is questioning the relative strengths of internal and external influences upon the way in which a person develops psychologically. 'Nature' refers to the assumption that an individual's psychological self is the way it is because it is internally determined by genetic make-up in the same way that physical self is biologically determined. Hence factors such as level of intelligence, degree of extroversion/introversion or emotional stability are predestined by genes in the same way as physical characteristics. However, while some physical attributes are generally fixed (e.g. sex, eye colour, skin colour), others are subject to some limited change within a range of parameters, for example there is the potential to grow a little taller (or fatter) depending upon diet and exercise. In health care there is presently much interest in the genetic determinants of disease. This is reflected in the strategy for nursing and midwifery education (UKCC 1999).

An acceptance of potential for change is associated with the externally mediated 'nurture' assumption of psychological self. This view is in many ways a much more optimistic stance than an assumption of fixed or very limited change because it recognises the potential for psychological growth and development over which each individual has some control – an acceptance of the influence of external factors recognises the importance of parenting, education and learning from experience, for example. In health care, therapy is often influenced by nurture assumptions, e.g. communities for people with special learning needs are designed to foster development through learning from therapeutic experience. In contrast, where there is less acknowledgement of possibilities for change, such people are more likely to be provided with a care environment which is more custodial than therapeutic.

There are four prominent theories which seek to explain human psychological development, each of which is linked to predetermined and contextual components of human nature:

1. the psychodynamic perspective
2. the behaviourist perspective
3. the cognitive perspective
4. the humanistic perspective.

Although there are limitations to each approach as a comprehensive approach to explaining human behaviour, all have important implications for nursing practice. A challenge to nurses is to think about ways in which aspects of each perspective can be combined to inform a way of working which reflects a suitable balance for the care setting and user population.

The psychodynamic perspective

The psychodynamic perspective is associated with Sigmund Freud (1856–1939), a medical practitioner, physiologist and psychotherapist who lived and worked in Vienna and subsequently in London. With a background in biological science it is not surprising that the origins of the psychodynamic approach attach importance to the influences of nature. However, as a psychiatrist, Freud was interested in how and why people suffered mental tension and he was concerned with therapy to effect change, which suggests acceptance of the effects of nurture as well.

Freud's early studies were concerned with using different idiographic methods of accessing the unconscious in order to explain how it influenced the behaviour and experience of his patients. The theory was developed from case studies of patients who sought help for neuroses such as anxiety states and depression. However, most of Freud's patients were middle class Jewish women and hence the theory is based upon a population which is not generally representative of humankind. Techniques Freud employed were hypnosis, interpretation of dreams and free association whereby he listened to his patients as they related their feelings and experiences while they reposed on the famous couch in his consulting room. Through analysis of the psyche (i.e. psychoanalysis) of his patients, Freud was able to make detailed assessments and from these developed

his psychodynamic theory of human development. The theory is centred around a homeostatic notion of balance in a similar way to the physiological balance of hormones within the endocrine system. Psychological energy, argues Freud, is mainly related to powerful energy instincts which tend to be freely expressed by animals, but which have to be mentally controlled by humans to comply with acceptable social behaviour. According to the psychodynamic perspective, healthy human development is dependent upon ways of thinking and/or behaving which enable psychological energy to be released in formats which are socially acceptable. These drives therefore need to have a means of controlled release – termed 'catharsis' by Freud – in order to prevent tension and neuroses. These cathartic expressions – termed 'mental defence mechanisms' – are considered to be a

Table 7.3 Commonly used mental defence mechanisms (from Stevens 1983 and Wilkinson 1997b)

Defence mechanism	Example in practice*
Repression is the exclusion of distressing drives from conscious awareness (failing to acknowledge an issue)	Denial of bad news, such as not accepting the implications of being told about having a terminal illness
Suppression is not responding to conscious awareness of distressing drives (ignoring something in the hope that it will go away)	Not responding to a symptom such as deteriorating hearing because of wishing to avoid being labelled as having a disability
Regression is a retreat to a previous stage of development (seeking psychological comfort in a state which is considered to be more safe)	Not exercising a right to informed consent through avoiding making decisions about treatment options – expecting health care professionals to take complete control
Displacement is the redirection of a drive from one focus to an alternative target (seeking out a perceived easier option)	Relatives who unconsciously direct their anger at nurses when they are perhaps angry with the patient or themselves
Sublimation is the channelling of drives into socially acceptable outlets	A patient who is very angry about disfiguring surgery may direct their aggression into working tirelessly for a self-help group
Projection is claiming that others are exhibiting one's own repressed drives	A nurse who has not come to terms with her own sexuality may express homophobic prejudices against gay patients
Reaction formation occurs when a repressed drive is counterbalanced by exaggerating an opposite tendency	An elderly patient who has been discharged from hospital and who is lonely, frightened and has poor confidence constantly expresses how pleased he is to be home
Rationalisation is where a distressing experience is reinterpreted as being a positive opportunity	A child who is isolated from his normal family, school and social routine due to illness uses the opportunity to become an expert at a particular area of interest
Isolation is when a drive becomes detached from the emotions which are commonly associated with a particular situation	A nurse working in an emotionally challenging speciality such as palliative care appears to be unaffected by working with the dying and their relatives

* Please note that the examples given are just that, and that the presence of the situations depicted are not necessarily indicative of a mental defence mechanism being employed.

normal part of mental development; they come into existence in childhood and are continued throughout adulthood. Psychological harmony is maintained if mental defence mechanisms are used as coping strategies to respond to anxiety-provoking experiences, but they should not be overly relied upon to the detriment of tackling stressors directly when this is appropriate.

A nurse who understands mental defence mechanisms will have enhanced self-awareness into her own use of such mechanisms, and will also be sensitive to the use of them by patients and colleagues. Table 7.3 summarises common mental defence mechanisms.

Nurses are workers for whom emotional engagement with others is part of their primary task and, as such, have been described as 'emotional labourers' (Falconer 1999). Menzies (1961) has argued that to be able to cope with the distress of working closely and continuously within an emotionally draining environment, the context in which nursing is practised has developed a system of defence mechanisms. Like the defence mechanisms that are used by individuals, these are frequently unconscious. The difference lies in what Menzies describes as collusive agreements within the social system of the institution itself. Examples of social defence mechanisms are summarised in Box 7.1.

Box 7.1 Menzies' social defence mechanisms in nursing (from Barber 1993)

1. Splitting up the nurse–patient relationship
2. Depersonalisation, categorisation and denial of the significance of the individual
3. Detachment and denial of feelings
4. The attempt to eliminate decisions by ritual task performance
5. Reducing the weight of responsibility in decision making by checks and counter-checks
6. Collusive social redistribution of responsibility and irresponsibility
7. Purposeful obscurity in the formal distribution of responsibility
8. The reduction of the impact of responsibility by delegation to superiors
9. Idealisation and underestimation of development possibilities
10. Avoidance of change

It is reasonable to question whether the social defence processes identified by Menzies over 40 years ago still exist in contemporary practice, given the emphasis upon nurses being knowledgeable doers rather than practising in a routine, automatic and unthinking fashion. Paul Barber, a nurse himself, reports the persistence of these social defences from his own experiences as a patient (Barber 1997). Barber's experiences offer insights for carers which reveal that the world of the providers of health care may be very distant from the world of those who receive health care. This is regrettable in itself, but particularly so if one considers the argument that there are forces present which seek to perpetuate the status quo.

The psychodynamic perspective has a number of strengths. In addition to describing human behaviour, it seeks to explain this within a theoretical framework based upon the widely accepted biological principle of homeostasis. Many people find the theory plausible, so much so that concepts such as 'the unconscious' and 'denial' have been absorbed into our culture.

There are, however, also a number of challenges that can be levelled. Freud's approach is idiographic, using very few cases of people who had come to him for therapy, and as such his small and selective research sample is not generalisable to a wider and more diverse population as a whole. Although the behaviour of people is observable, we have already established that the reasons behind their behaviour are not directly accessible. A positivist critique of the psychodynamic perspective is that it is unfalsifiable and therefore impossible to test and disprove, and hence is not proven.

The behaviourist perspective

The behaviourist perspective arose in part as a reaction against problems that the psychodynamic perspective poses for positivist scientific study. Where Freud's theory is a classic example of an idiographic approach to human development, behaviourism (so called because of an emphasis upon observing behaviour) is characteristically nomothetic in its approach. As long ago as the late 1600s, a philosopher John Locke offered the suggestion that human beings are born as *tabula rasa* (meaning a blank slate), and thus everything a person becomes is as a result of what he learns through behaviour. The origins of behaviourism are thus firmly linked to the nurture interpretation of human development.

It was not until the late 19th century that behaviourism developed theoretically as a consequence of experimental research when the famous Nobel prize winning researcher Ivan Pavlov first reported the phenomenon of classical conditioning. Pavlov demonstrated that dogs are able to learn to express established behaviour (salivation) in novel circumstances (the sounding of a bell) if appropriate stimuli (the bell and food) are paired together, and that this is sustained over time (the dogs salivated in response to the bell in the absence of food being available). The process was subsequently replicated in humans by John Watson, using a white rabbit and a loud noise to induce fear in a child in response to the rabbit alone (ethically questionable these days, but presumably not considered so in the 1920s when Watson did his research).

The implications of classical conditioning are important for nurses. For example, consider a person who is mentally ill and who is presenting with challenging behaviour. If a nurse responds to this situation by threatening to give an injection as a punishment for such threatening behaviour, then the patient may pair punishment and medication rather than pairing medication and therapy. The same nurse (or indeed all nurses) may then be associated with threat rather than help, a situation sometimes referred to as 'white coat syndrome'. It is important for nurses to recognise that they may be responded to for what they represent, rather than as the person they are as an individual.

Another well-known psychologist, B. F. Skinner, in the 1950s and 1960s developed the concept of operant conditioning. This differs from classical conditioning in the important respect that whereas in classical conditioning the behaviour is established (e.g. salivating) but introduced in novel circumstances (in response to a bell), in operant conditioning both the circumstances of the behaviour and the behaviour itself are novel.

Skinner demonstrated experimentally with animals such as rats and pigeons, and also with humans, that if a particular pattern of behaviour leads to a desirable outcome, then the pattern of behaviour is more likely to be repeated because the desirable outcome is rewarding and has the effect of positively reinforcing the behaviour.

The implications of operant conditioning are important for nurses. For example, consider a person who is recovering from a stroke and whose care plan is centred around rehabilitation. Using the operant conditioning technique of shaping, the nurse can encourage the patient to take increasing responsibility for feeding himself. In positive reinforcement it is important to ascertain that the stimulus, such as increased independence in eating, is perceived as desirable by the recipient of the reinforcement. If patients are being reinforced simply by the presence of the nurse giving praise, then they may become demotivated and uncompliant in their progress with the rehabilitation since they may fear that increasing independence will eventually reduce their contact with the nurse at mealtimes.

An important strength of the behaviourist approach to explaining human behaviour is that it is based upon rigorous observation and experimentation which yield replicable empirical data (i.e. behaviourist approaches such as classical and operant conditioning are able to predict and influence behaviour). The nomothetic approach to behaviourist perspective research has given confidence in generalising the findings widely and consequently behaviourist principles have strongly influenced educational policy through reward systems, from the use of house points in schools to the award of degrees in universities for desirable work. Nurses are often faced with problems in their practice which require practical solutions: clarification of the relationships between factors which can be paired through positive reinforcement offer simple and easily applied strategies to direct practice.

A major limitation, however, lies in the overly simplistic view of human behaviour which neglects to take into account that people are able to think, make idiosyncratic choices and are frequently unpredictable. For example, despite pairing cigarette smoking with disease and attaching value to being a non-smoker, many adolescents choose to take up the habit. Perhaps this is because a stronger pairing is between smoking and being accepted by peers, or because smoking is a way of exercising control which is part of adult independence. Clearly, linking behaviour to simple paired associations or reinforcement is not as simple in real life as it might be in a psychology laboratory. Behaviourism can be criticised as being reductionist as it does not acknowledge the complexities of human experience.

The cognitive perspective

The cognitive perspective, like the behaviourist approach, is underpinned by an assumption that behaviour is shaped by the environment. An important difference, however, is a central focus upon thinking processes as an integral part of determining behaviour. Cognition involves the integration of thought processes in response to two factors. Concept driven processing includes our human nature, the nurture influences of previous experiences and the learning that has occurred as a consequence. Data-driven processing refers to the information which comes to conscious attention through our sensory organs of sight, hearing, smell, touch and taste. This relationship is represented in Box 7.2. It suggests that although a number of individuals may experience the same event, the effect of this upon their mental processes and behaviour may be very different. For example a qualified nurse and a student nurse may assess the same patient but draw different conclusions because they interacted in different ways. This is because each individual may notice and interpret different aspects of the way the patient presents himself and come to different conclusions as a consequence.

A prominent psychologist in the development of the cognitive perspective was Jean Piaget (1896–1980), working in Europe in the middle part of the 20th century. Piaget conducted research based upon observations of children involved in the normal activities of play and acquiring language skills. He tested his theories by setting problem solving challenges to see if he could learn

Box 7.2   **Representation of cognitive processing**

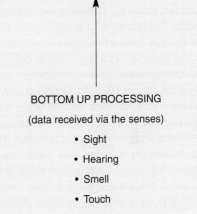

TOP DOWN PROCESSING

(individual mental concepts derived from previous personal experience)

- Memories
- Attitudes (beliefs and values)
- Self-awareness
- Personality characteristics

COGNITIVE PROCESSING

(behaviour determined by an interaction between top down and bottom up processing)

BOTTOM UP PROCESSING

(data received via the senses)

- Sight
- Hearing
- Smell
- Touch
- Taste

from, and predict, human behaviour. Piaget's theory of cognitive development links mental processing and behaviour with four key concepts:

Schema. A schema is a mental representation which is developed through experience and action. A student nurse will have a schema of nursing which will be developed as a consequence of experiencing and learning about nursing. Schemas are not fixed, being subject to changes which result from learning from experience. Schemas are useful ways of communicating with others because a shared schema enables insight into another person's mental processing and behaviour. However, it is important to be aware that schemas can differ markedly between individuals. A nurse who values patient empowerment will have a different schema to that of a patient who feels that nurses are there to do everything for those who are sick, rather than to facilitate independence as part of a health model. Such a patient will expect nursing behaviour to enable patient passivity and be alarmed if nurses are working in a way which promotes patient activity. It is therefore important for nurses to understand their own schemas and those of the colleagues and patients with whom they are working. Otherwise a notion of working in partnership with other health care professionals and patients to achieve common goals will be seriously compromised.

Assimilation is concerned with fitting new experiences into existing schemas so that there is the maintenance of consistency with mental processing. For example, a patient who wishes to be passive may interpret a more facilitative style of nursing as one particular nurse being uncaring and unrepresentative of what he considers most nurses to be like. In holding this belief, the patient's schema will not change and he is likely to remain passive and continue to expect nurses to take responsibility for his care. The challenge to nurses here is to work with the patient to explain why their own active contribution to health care is important so that they are able to accommodate their schema to effect change.

Accommodation is concerned with altering an existing schema to take account of new experiences and understanding because the existing schema is no longer a useful representation of experience and behaviour. For example, patients who receive an explanation and rationale for why their active involvement in their own care is central to promoting independence and recovery may alter their schemas about the role of nurses. In doing so, they are likely to accept that nurses are sometimes most effective when in a facilitative rather than interventionist mode and alter their behaviour to respond to this positively.

Equilibrium. Piaget argued that understanding develops as a function of disequilibrium between an existing level of adaptation and the challenge of new situations. When a new experience or new information cannot be comfortably assimilated into an existing schema, then accommodation occurs to generate a new or adapted schema, a process termed 'discovery learning' or learning from experience. It is important for nurses to appreciate the considerable adjustment that is required to return to a state of equilibrium when disequilibrium has occurred as a consequence of illness or hospitalisation. Change is often perceived as being distressing and this may be responded to through the use of mental defence mechanisms (see Table 7.3) or in a stress response.

As in the behaviourist perspective, an important strength of the cognitive approach to explaining human behaviour is that it is based upon rigorous observation and experimentation. Development of the cognitive approach in this way yields replicable empirical data and these enable theories to be applied and tested. Nurses who are aware of the notion of schema development are better able to understand why people act in the way they do in particular situations. Health psychologists have developed social cognition models which seek to represent how people process information and are used to predict health related behaviour (Conner & Norman 1996). The nomothetic approach to cognitive research has given confidence in generalising the findings widely and consequently cognitive principles have strongly influenced education policy through learning based upon the creation of structures which motivate problem solving, finding out for oneself and learning from doing. In nursing education these principles have been used to develop curricula based upon enquiry-based learning (UKCC 1999).

A limitation of the cognitive approach lies in the assumption of inherent human motivation to learn from experience and to subsequently change as a consequence. It is not uncommon to encounter people who have a great deal of experience of doing something badly, but who do not seem to be able to learn from this and change accordingly. Contemporary research into cognitive processing is concerned with artificial intelligence which is modelling human reasoning on a computer, yet it is questionable whether human beings are as rational as the cognitive perspective suggests. In addition to considering the rational side of human thinking and behaviour, it is also necessary to explore an approach which has the acknowledgement of human feelings and emotions at its heart.

The humanistic perspective

The humanistic perspective shares an idiographic approach with the psychodynamic perspective. A central difference is that while the latter lays emphasis upon the constraining influences of drives and the achievement of homeostasis, the former has strong assumptions about the liberating potential of human autonomy. The humanistic approach emerged in the USA in the 1960s as a reaction to criticisms that the cognitive perspective is overly technical and fails to recognise that human beings are highly individual, and that the very nature of being human is to exercise one's right to choose to express individuality, whether this is the same as or different to anyone else. A key message for nurses to take from the humanistic perspective is to be tolerant of, and indeed to celebrate, human differences.

Carl Rogers (1974) suggests that each person is at the centre of his own continually changing world of experiences and each person behaves in a way which reflects this unique view of the world based upon subjective experience. To understand oneself is the first step in understanding others, because it is through recognising our own internal frames of reference that we will be able to put these to one side to understand someone else through their particular reference system. For example, a person who is concerned with his own body image is likely to adopt a value system and behaviour patterns in relation to appearance and diet. It is important to be self-aware about behaviour and the reasons for this in order to accept that there are alternative viewpoints before being able to understand someone who is seeking professional help with an eating disorder.

Psychologists working within the humanistic approach have a generally optimistic perspective on human behaviour and mental processing. It is assumed that human beings have a natural inclination to want to achieve their personal goals and will actively make efforts to do so. Hence it is claimed that each person has a high degree of autonomy over personal destiny. A useful analogy here is to use a nurturing horticultural parallel. Like seeds in a packet, every person is different and has a different potential to grow and develop. Seeds which are planted in fertile soil and which receive nutrition, protection and attention will tend to maximise their potential while those which are scattered on barren earth and left to their own devices are less likely to develop optimally, and some will perish. All seeds will try to grow, but those that are understood, have an interest taken in them and are appropriately cared for are more likely to grow best within their natural potential. In nursing it has already been commented that the nature of the work is sometimes emotionally draining. The humanistic approach directs nurses to be in touch with their own feelings and to be aware of the emotions which influence behaviour. It is important to note that nurses are perhaps only able to care for others if they are also able to care for themselves.

An important strength of the humanistic perspective for nursing is that it has a number of values which are congruent with those of professional nursing. High regard is given to human beings as individuals who need to be viewed holistically in order to be understood. The approach is very accepting of, and indeed celebrates, individual differences and rejects all notions of prejudice. Emphasis upon autonomy lends support to the facilitation of independence and taking responsibility for one's own health care to the extent to which this is feasible. This poses a challenge to nurses, other health care professionals and patients as it requires the shifting of the traditional power base in care from therapist to patient.

There are, however, challenges that can be levelled at the humanistic perspective's idiographic underpinnings similar to those directed at the psychodynamic perspective. Humanism, being idiographic, is based on case studies of people who tend to be sufficiently articulate to report their feelings in in-depth interviews. As such, a selective research sample may be of the élite and not generalisable to a wider, more diverse population. While this is not an issue if the purpose of knowing a person is to respond to them as a unique person, a positivist critique of the humanistic perspective is that it is untestable and therefore impossible to prove or falsify.

ACKNOWLEDGING PEOPLE AS INDIVIDUALS

A review of human development perspectives suggests that, although there are a number of ways in which human beings are similar, there are even more ways in which individuals are very different. Assumptions made about people which are not based on a thorough assessment are likely to be inaccurate, and yet it is claimed by Boney & Baker (1997) that nurses frequently base clinical decisions on inadequate information, tending to be influenced by stereotyping, cultural bias and a desire to make rapid decisions. Greater understanding of the diversity and individuality of people by nurses could improve communication between themselves and their patients. Two areas to assist nurses to be more effective in acknowledging people as individuals are those of recognising the diversity of lay health beliefs and understanding the influence of the self-concept on health behaviour.

DIVERSITY OF HEALTH BELIEFS

It is well established that health and ill health are often interpreted differently by health care professionals and patients. Dines (1994) has reviewed research which suggests that there are frequently marked disparities between the way in which non-health care professionals (lay people) and health care professionals interpret health and ill health. It is argued that lay and professional

health differences must be identified and acknowledged between a nurse and those for whom she is caring, particularly in the context of the enhancement of health promotion. In her research, Stainton Rogers (1991) has identified eight alternative accounts of health in Britain. These are summarised in Table 7.4.

A nurse who is able to ascertain her own accounts of health and those of others will be much better placed to effectively communicate using a shared schema.

THE SELF-CONCEPT

The self is an abstract concept which, at the same time as being at the very centre of each person's existence as an individual, is difficult to define and operationalise. Burnard (1992) divides self-awareness into the inner aspects of self (how a person feels inside) and the outer aspects of self (what others see) (Table 7.5). It is by means of the outer aspects of self that individuals communicate their inner self, but the relationship between the two dimensions is not transparent. Sometimes a person will feel it necessary to transmit an outer message which is different to their inner feelings, for example a parent who puts on a 'brave face' when helping a child to prepare for surgery. An important skill in nursing is to attend to the whole person, not just the most obvious messages being given out at a particular time.

The Johari window (Luft 1970) is a useful way to represent the relationship between the inner and outer aspects of the self (Box 7.3). The boundaries between the four windows are sometimes moveable and it may be that health care professionals see a different aspect of a person to that seen by others. For example, health visitors advising parents on weaning may sometimes have to sensitively inform them about their poor food hygiene standards and the risks of gastroenteritis (thereby moving from the parents' blind selves to their public selves). A mother who is stressed about coping with a new baby may reveal to a health visitor that she has feelings of anger towards her baby (thereby moving from her private self to her public self).

Table 7.4   Alternative accounts of health (from Stainton Rogers 1991)

Health belief	Examples in practice
The body as a machine Confidence in, but also perhaps dependence on, the skills of health care professionals to repair bodily damage	Replacement surgery, e.g. heart valve replacement, hip replacement
The body under siege Awareness of harmful effects in the environment and the need to protect the body	Infectious diseases, stress, radiation hazards
Inequality of access Confidence in the power of health care, but critical of the unequal distribution of resources which results in health differences	Health and social factors; concerns about rationing and the inequalities of the 'inverse care law'; a political view of health
Cultural critique of medicine A challenge to the assumption that health care professionals are the experts; concerns about over-medicalisation	Iatrogenic illness, e.g. steroid induced diabetes mellitus; cultural intolerance of differences labelled as mental illness
Health promotion Social and personal responsibility for health	Government policy to promote health, e.g. anti-smoking legislation; personal responsibility for health, e.g. choosing to attend a stopping smoking programme
Robust individualism Personal rights to select a particular lifestyle	Rejection of the 'nanny state', health is regarded as the responsibility of the individual; freedom to choose a particular lifestyle is more important than restrictive health-related legislation
God's power Health is regarded as a spiritual gift and linked to the power of personal faith; health care professionals seen as the agents through which God works	Emphasis upon the power of external forces and prayer upon health outcome; external health locus of control
Willpower Control of health is in the hands of the individual to follow appropriate advice	Internal health locus of control; health is regarded as the responsibility of the individual to act responsibly

Table 7.5   The self-concept (from Burnard (1992))

Inner aspects of self	Outer aspects of self
Thinking	Eye contact
Feeling	Facial expression
Sensing	Gesticulation
Intuition	Touch
Bodily sensation	Proximity to others
	Movement
	Dress
	Language
	Paralinguistics

A reflective practitioner may enhance her own self-awareness about an aspect of practice (thereby moving from her unknown self to her private or public self).

Self-concept and self-esteem

Self-esteem is a feeling of self-worth and is considered to be a function of satisfaction with one's personal performance in relation to an issue which is valued. Hence a high self-esteem reflects a close fit between an individual's self-concept of his worth and his personal aspirations. Self-esteem may be compromised if a person sets himself unrealistic targets and this has the potential to influence behaviour. Egan (1994) suggests that people will tend to take action in relation to an issue if two conditions are satisfied:

1. they believe that particular behaviours are likely to lead to certain desirable consequences (outcome expectations)

Box 7.3 **The Johari window** (from Luft 1970)

Public self: known to self and known to others (what is known about self which is presented to others so that they know it as well)	*Blind self:* unknown to self but known to others (aspects about the self of which the individual is unaware, but which others see)
Private self: known to self but unknown by others (what is known about self, but which is not revealed to others)	*Unknown self:* unknown to self and others (what is unknown to self and unknown by others)

2. they are reasonably confident of their ability to engage in such behaviour (self-efficacy expectations).

This is of relevance to nurses in that health advice will be more likely to result in appropriate action if these two conditions are incorporated into the plan of care. For example, when advising a pregnant woman to stop smoking cigarettes the woman needs to be helped to understand that stopping smoking will be better for the development of her baby (outcome expectation), and a strategy to assist her to stop smoking in which she has confidence must also be made available (self-efficacy expectation). Each of these factors in isolation is likely to be less effective than both of them presented together as an integrated package of care, because self-esteem is maintained through the facilitation of a sense of control over health related behaviour options.

HEALTH LOCUS OF CONTROL

A person's notion of self-efficacy has implications for health advice strategies linked to beliefs about locus of control and health (Norman & Bennett 1996). Dimensions of health locus of control are reported as internal, external (others) and external (luck). Internal locus of control is linked to a sense of personal empowerment which is likely to lead to proactivity in self-care, for example self-managing a dietary and exercise regimen to control obesity. External (others) locus of control is associated with attributing responsibility for

one's health care to others, which frequently results in passive reliance upon health care professionals with little sense of personal autonomy, for example expecting a dietary and exercise regimen to control obesity to be supplied by people perceived to be experts, with little sense of responsibility to work in partnership and relate advice to personal lifestyle. External (luck) locus of control relates to the adoption of a passive and fatalistic perspective which attributes health status to be beyond the control of self or others, for example believing that obesity is determined by luck and is not amenable to change by an appropriate balance of healthy eating and exercise.

The difficulty of making use of lay health beliefs in relation to locus of control is discussed by Furnham & McDermott (1994), whose research demonstrates that lay interpretations about whether to be self-reliant or to seek external help are often contrary to accepted professional opinion about treatment. They conclude that although caution should be exercised regarding the use of lay notions of locus of control, it is appropriate to access this component of self-concept as these notions are likely to assist communication when giving health advice. Nurses who are aware of a patient's orientation towards health locus of control as part of their assessment are well placed to make use of this understanding in the planning and implementation of health advice strategies. A skill required in this context is to judge whether to work within the patient's health locus of control schema or whether to challenge it with an alternative perspective.

MAKING ASSESSMENTS

Having appreciated the extent to which people are different, and recognising that understanding a person as an individual is central to effective health care, it is not difficult to accept that assessment is fundamental to nursing. Without accurate and comprehensive assessment the other elements of the nursing process (planning, implementation and evaluation) will be informed by flawed information. Even before assessments are made, however, it is necessary to direct conscious attention to what is going on around the patient at any particular point in time and to direct attention to that which is deemed important.

Although empirical measures are a feature of nursing assessment (e.g. blood pressure measurement, neurological observations and urine testing), much useful assessment data are at an interpretive level of analysis (e.g. judgements about stress, pain and motivation) and frequently require evaluative or impressionistic assessment. These latter types of data collection are highly skilled and dependent upon an understanding of attentional and perceptual processes.

ATTENTION

Attention is a cognitive process and so can be explained by the representation of concept and data driven processing in Box 7.2. All around every person is a flood of information arriving at the sensory organs which would be overwhelming if it were all responded to at the same time. It is the function of attention to select that which is considered to be most important at a particular time. Hence human attention is an active process which is concerned with the collection of data but in a selective way. This selective nature of human attention is illustrated on a paediatric ward when a sleeping parent will not respond to general ward noise, but will awaken to sounds made by his own child. Although attention is often automatic, it can be experienced as selective conscious awareness by undertaking Activity 7.3.

It should be recognised that human attention is not passive like a video recording. Human beings

Activity 7.3 Selective attention

Get together with a friend and experience a short interaction in a busy place such as the waiting area of a general practice. Have conversation for a few minutes about a topic in which you are both interested. Next split up for a few minutes and sit on your own paying attention to what is going on around you. I expect that you will notice a great deal of detail that you were unaware of when deep in conversation with your friend, because you have taken the trouble to actively attend to the stimuli around you. Now imagine yourself to be a patient waiting to hear the results of some recent tests. What are the strengths and limitations of the environment as a place for waiting to learn important information that could affect the rest of your life? Discuss your thoughts with your friend.

attend to their environment in different ways because the focus of attention is influenced by external factors such as colours, novelty and humour (as used by the advertising industry). It can therefore be helpful to make health education messages as attention-grabbing as possible. Internal factors may be physical, for example sensory function, and nurses can enhance these by ensuring spectacles are worn and hearing aids are working where appropriate. Other internal factors are related to mental processes, for example level of motivation to be receptive to information. Encouraging patients to be interested in their health so that they are receptive to information may assist them to improve their health status. Finally, the importance of expertise in attention must be recognised. It is often noticed how more experienced nurses are able to notice details about a patient that have been initially overlooked by those who are less experienced. For example, because mouth care has been effective and the patient is not complaining of thirst, an inexperienced nurse may not attend to the potential for clinical dehydration. However, once a collection of facts is pointed out – such as the presence of a tissued intravenous infusion, low-volume dark urine, nil by mouth sign, skin inelasticity and slight confusion – the clinical picture becomes more obvious.

Hence attention is not just dependent on what is seen, heard, smelt, touched and tasted; it is also underpinned by what is known, thought, considered to be of interest and which reflects personal expertise. Much of the time attentional processes go on automatically and unconsciously and only come to consciousness when an unfamiliar situation is encountered. Nurses who generally feel comfortable in their familiar surroundings when on duty need to remind themselves of their first few days in a new practice setting and how different they then felt. It is important to keep in mind that patients are frequently undergoing an experience which is unfamiliar for them. If a patient is coming to terms with a new experience which is demanding much of their attentional capacity, it is not surprising if they have little spare to respond to information from nurses. It is essential to be prepared to repeat important information on subsequent occasions.

PERCEPTION

Perception is the process by which people organise and give meaning to that which is attended. This is an active process and influenced by expectations, so that sometimes there is a perception of what is *expected* to be there, not of what is really there. For example, with the drugs prednisolone and prednisone or dipyridamole and disopyramide it can be seen how an error might occur if a nurse was relying on unconscious attention to check a prescription rather than actively scrutinising the prescription chart. A nurse working in an orthopaedic setting may perceive the initials PID to refer to a prolapsed intervertebral disc, while a nurse more used to working in women's health may interpret the same shorthand as pelvic inflammatory disease. The key to accurate assessment is to perceive that which is there, rather than to seek confirmation of that which is expected to be seen.

Expectations are a function of experience and may overlap with those of others or, on the other hand, be highly individual. It is important for nurses to accept that their personal way, or indeed a generalised nursing way, of perceiving something may be entirely different to the way in which individual patients or colleagues perceive the same topic. For example cancer may be

perceived by some as being treatable in many instances with the reasonable expectation of a curative outcome, but others may interpret a cancer diagnosis as a death sentence. It is important to attempt to understand differing perceptions before entering into a discussion as different schemas may inhibit communication if they are not clarified. It is not essential to agree about an issue, but it is very helpful to understand another person's expectations so that differences are acknowledged.

PERSON PERCEPTION

A number of research studies have consistently demonstrated that nurses and other health care professionals sometimes make judgements about patients which are inappropriate (see, e.g., Rosenhan 1973, Simpson 1976, Jeffrey 1979, Kelly & May 1982, Ganong et al 1987, Walsh 1995). These studies are concerned with first impressions that can be made of people and how conclusions are sometimes rapidly drawn about an individual's personality on the basis of inaccurately perceived qualities or traits.

The notion of the 'halo and horns' effect is central to person perception. With the halo effect an expectation of positive attributes within a person, or what they represent, leads to that person being perceived favourably, which in turn further supports the continuance of the self-fulfilling prophecy. The horns effect is the same process except with unfavourable expectations. For example a nurse who expects all people who have a mental illness to be aggressive may inaccurately interpret assertive behaviour as being aggressive and consequently respond with counter-aggression, which may provoke greater assertion on the part of the patient, which in turn perpetuates the escalation of the horns effect. Given the potential of the halo and horns effect to distort the accuracy of person perception, it is important for nurses to avoid using powerful labels such as 'aggressive', 'unintelligent', 'difficult', etc. Rather than categorising individuals with a label such as 'poorly motivated', assessments and reports will be much more accurate if there is a description of observable behaviour, for example 'is reluctant to get out of bed', 'reacts to ideas, but does not offer suggestions', or 'expresses pessimistic expectations of recovery'. Accurate observation and reporting of behaviour will avoid the need to label a person. Others involved in the assessment will be able to compare and contrast their observations using the same criteria and this promotes more reliable assessment.

Although studies of person perception have yielded a great deal of information on how people use impressions to perceive others, they do not address the question of how people perceive the causes of others' behaviour. The issue of better understanding the reasons behind behaviour is important to nurses because much of disease causation and recovery is dependent upon adopting particular patterns of behaviour. Explanations of reasons behind behaviour are provided by attribution theory.

Attribution theory

Attribution theory is discussed in detail by Gross (1996). The attribution theory of correspondent inferences developed by Jones & Davis (1965) is based upon the assertion that people tend to infer an external disposition in another person which explains their actions. For example, it might be believed that a young child is angry because he is going through a fractious phase, there tending to be an undervaluing of situational factors such as being hungry. In contrast, a hungry person is likely to attribute his own short temper to the situational factor of low blood sugar rather than consider himself to have the disposition of an angry person. This fundamental attribution error highlights how causal attributions of the reasons behind behaviour of self and others is biased and unreliable in a characteristic way which tends to support a preferred self-image which is usually to regard the self-concept in a positive light. Hence, according to attribution theory, we tend to, automatically and unconsciously:

- attribute our successes to dispositional factors (e.g. the ward is running well because I am a good leader)

- attribute our failures to situational factors (e.g. the ward is chaotic because we have too many patients and we are short-staffed)
- attribute others' successes to situational factors (e.g. my colleague's shift ran well because it was quiet and she had plenty of staff on duty)
- attribute others' failures to dispositional factors (e.g. my colleague's shift was chaotic because she is a poor leader).

According to the covariance model of attribution developed by Kelley (1967), we calculate the permutations of three factors and decide upon the most likely attribution from the relationships between these variables:

Distinctiveness

- If the person behaves in a particular way in similar situations, then the behaviour is more likely to have a dispositional cause (e.g. if a particular staff nurse always seems to be angry, then she is probably a bad tempered person irrespective of where she is).
- If the person behaves in a particular way only in a specific situation, then the behaviour is more likely to have a situational cause (e.g. if a particular staff nurse only seems to be angry when on duty, then anger is probably provoked by the situation of being on duty).

Consistency

- If the person does not behave consistently in a particular way in a specific situation, then the behaviour is more likely to have a situational cause (e.g. if a staff nurse only seems to be angry when she is in charge, and not when someone else is in charge, then anger is probably provoked by the situation of being in charge when on duty).

Consensus

- If there is consensus about the behaviour of others in the same situation, then the behaviour is likely to have a situational cause (e.g. if everyone is angry when they take charge on a particular ward, then anger is probably provoked by the situation of being in charge on that particular ward).

• If there is not consensus about the behaviour of others in the same situation, then the behaviour is likely to have a dispositional cause (e.g. if no other person is angry when taking charge on a particular ward, then anger in one individual is probably because that person is prone to bad temper in any situation).

Gross (1996) comments upon the nomothetic nature of attribution theory and argues that the largely laboratory-based studies lack external validity. Are human beings as rational as they are portrayed to be in attribution theory? It can be argued that any number of factors may influence behaviour, and that the very essence of being human is the potential to be idiosyncratic and illogical. Despite these limitations, it is important to recognise the common sense plausibility of attribution theory. Nurses who understand attribution theory are usefully reminded to question the attribution bias by giving consideration to the range of personal and dispositional factors operating in a given situation. Greater attention to more eclectic assessment will yield more informed conclusions.

USING MEMORY EFFECTIVELY

The efficient use of memory is essential to nursing practice in order to cope with the processing of the copious amounts of information encountered both by nurses in the course of their work and by patients in the course of their treatment (Wilkinson 1997c). Much of the information which is supplied to individuals is not remembered, the implications of this being impaired communication and ineffective patient participation in care. Memory is often conceptualised as having three interlinked stages, registration, storage and retrieval, an understanding of which is useful for nurses in order to enhance both their own memory function and that of those in their care.

Memory registration

It has already been established how human attention is an actively selective process. That which is perceived is determined by the clarity of the stimulus, the functioning of the sensory organs and the importance of the message to the individual (see Box 7.2). In order to remember anything, the information needs to be received and understood meaningfully, and the use of skilful communication strategies is fundamental to enhancing the accessibility of information to human attention.

Using the storage files of schemas, memories are organised in ways which reflect the uniqueness of an individual, common experiences and cultural norms. Schemas, as already established, can be thought of as files of knowledge and understanding. The development of a complex schema system with cross-referencing links to other related schemas enables new information to be filed in relation to what is already known and understood. Schema development through accommodation and assimilation is a much more mentally efficient system than constantly opening a new file for every new piece of data encountered.

It is because of the central role of schemas in memory processes that information which is meaningful to an individual is more effectively stored than that which is less relevant (Activity 7.4).

Rote learning, or the use of some form of mnemonic, may enable a person to register information in their memory which is not personally meaningful. However, long-term storage and subsequent retrieval of material considered to be unimportant is very difficult for most people. If the information becomes more meaningful, most people become more efficient at storage and retrieval as they are more motivated to devise a more effective storage system. The more active and deeper the mental effort employed in the registration of information, the more effective the encoding into memory becomes. Rote learning and the use of mnemonics have their uses, but most meaningful memory storage is dependent upon understanding rather than simply trying to store something for no particular reason. For example people who are not interested

Activity 7.4 Memory

Take steps to remember the following 12-digit number: 181510661966.

You are much more likely to store the information in a way that will enable you to access it if you split it up into chunks which relate to existing schemas, i.e.

1815 – Battle of Waterloo
1066 – Battle of Hastings
1966 – England wins the World Cup (the only time to date!)

Compare how much more difficult it is to store the following 12-digit number: 161985160616.

I expect that this number (the same digits but in random order) appears more difficult to memorise, the reason being that you are less likely to have a term of reference to store this seemingly meaningless list of digits.

in learning about safe sex and contraception may subsequently put more effort into registering information about these topics if they anticipate becoming sexually active and need to make informed choices about their sexual behaviour.

There are two key implications for nurses in relation to enhanced memory registration. First, it is essential to understand one's own schema system, and to try to store new information and experiences in the context of this by means of accommodation and assimilation. Second, when assisting others to store something to be remembered it should not be assumed that they share the same schema system. It is important to take time to assess how someone stores related data and to make use of this to present new material in a way which is congruent with their schema or to assist them to develop a new schema. For example a person who has become pregnant when this is neither planned nor desirable for them may have a poorly developed schema of methods of contraception. A nurse advising this person would need to ascertain whether help was required with selecting contraception and/or with negotiating the use of preferred methods of contraception with the person's partner.

Memory storage

The capacity of memory storage is enormous, and in day-to-day interactions people use a considerable number of stored memories which are brought into conscious attention as and when they are needed. To be able to function in a way that enables selective attention to the issue in hand, rapid access is needed to the vast supply of information and experiences which can be recalled as necessary from the preconscious (you are probably not thinking about the last time you contributed to developing a patient's care plan, for example, but you can access your stored memory of this event now that it has been mentioned). As previously outlined, the psychodynamic perspective emphasises the importance of the unconscious repository of memories which are hinted at in the form of dreams and may become manifest through psychoanalysis.

As people develop knowledge, experience and understanding of health related issues, they are likely to develop associated schemas structured around their experiences. These schemas will be most meaningful if they are related to existing understanding and memory frameworks and the challenge to nurses is to assist those in their care to make these links. Hence, when advising a person about safe sex it is necessary to be explicit about measures to prevent cross-infection as well as undesired pregnancy because the schema of the recipient of the information may not necessarily include both components.

Memory retrieval

Memory retrieval – the process by which memories are accessed from storage – is a complex process and frequently subject to omissions and distortion. In a classic experiment Sir Frederick Bartlett (1932, cited by Eysenck & Keane 1996) demonstrated that memory retrieval is not the same as extracting a document from a file or replaying a tape, arguing that human memory retrieval is highly subjective, being influenced by numerous factors such as mood, value systems, personality and personal interest. When individuals remember a particular event or experience they frequently construe a representation of what they would like to believe occurred or what they feel is most likely to have occurred. This phenomenon – termed 'memory construction' – accounts for the fact that memory is often unreliable.

Memory construction has two important implications for nurses. First, given that there is a human tendency to remember that which is desired or expected, it is important to give particular stress to that which is undesired and unexpected when imparting information which needs to be remembered. A person who considers himself immune to sexually transmitted disease because he is heterosexual may not remember safe sex advice because, inappropriately, he believes he was told that safety precautions do not apply to him. Second, when conducting an assessment, the potential for suggestion should be recognised. A nurse in a sexually transmitted disease clinic who assumes that patients will have urinary frequency may inadvertently cue their patients into reporting this symptom because they are expected to have it, rather than because of actual experience.

Recall which is unaided by any memory hints is much more difficult than recognition which is triggered by memory aids and contextual cues. When discharging a patient from hospital into the community it is important to consider that the contextual cues that have been used in hospital will not be available at home and therefore a patient may need to develop new memory retrieval strategies. The best forms of cue are those which are part of established behaviour patterns. If you wished to advise a woman to take an oral contraceptive regularly, it might also be helpful to recommend that the tablets are kept next to her toothbrush. This is because, if cleaning teeth is an already established routine, then the sight of the contraceptive pill packet will cue taking the contraceptive at the appropriate time.

PROBLEM SOLVING

Clinical practice is a series of problem-solving challenges which need to be tackled by active information processing strategies rather than being responded to passively. This is relevant for patients as well as for nurses because of the emphasis placed upon the empowerment of patients to be actively engaged in their own health care. Nurses need to make use of problem-solving strategies in their clinical work, and to facilitate patient engagement in solving the problems they may face in taking responsibility for their own health and its management.

PROBLEM SOLVING AND EVIDENCE-BASED DECISION MAKING

Problems faced in clinical practice are on a continuum of well defined to ill defined, but mainly focused towards the latter. Well-defined problems are those with clearly established start and end points and explicit procedures for effecting a solution. An example of a well-defined problem is a cardiopulmonary arrest (Box 7.4).

Reducing resuscitation to the level of a well-defined problem is useful to clarify the appropriate application of solutions. Resuscitation algorithms have developed from research, clinical experience and professional consensus and as such have the status of being evidence- rather than opinion-based. It is the former which is

---

Box 7.4   An example of a well-defined problem: cardiopulmonary arrest

Start point
- sudden collapsed state
- not rousable to shaking and calling
- absence of breathing
- absence of major arterial pulse

Solution rules
- initiation of basic life support and/or advanced life support in the form of recommended procedures termed algorithms, or
- a predetermined decision to not intervene with life support

End point
- resuscitation and restoration of cardiopulmonary functioning with or without physiological support, or
- a decision to withdraw life support measures and death, or
- patient is allowed to die without the initiation of life support measures

required as the basis of clinical decision making in modern health care (Gray 1997). However, although cardiopulmonary arrest can be managed in the way described, in practice the process is also complicated by the associated decisions made about the ethics surrounding decisions about resuscitation. Hence, even though some problems encountered in health care may appear well-defined, closer scrutiny reveals that in practice clinical problem solving demands the tackling of ill-defined and complex problems.

Clinical governance is a statutory framework to strengthen evidence-based decision making within health care (DoH 1997) and great emphasis is being placed upon the development of guidelines for practice from the National Institute for Clinical Effectiveness (NICE) and in the form of the national service frameworks. However, Hands (1999) comments that many clinicians place value on the need to be responsive to the uniqueness of how individuals respond to health care and disease management. It is therefore necessary to consider the use of problem-solving strategies which draw upon professional expertise in combination with evidence-based protocols.

EXPERTISE AND PROBLEM SOLVING

Expertise is domain specific and is on a continuum, which means, for example, that a person may simultaneously have expertise in dealing with challenging behaviour, be developing some expertise in writing reports and be a complete novice at first aid. These activities may all be important to the work of a nurse who works with a specific individual with a learning disability and, therefore, if this were the case, it would be necessary for the nurse to increase expertise in the last two skills in order to become expert at caring for that person. According to Crow and colleagues (1995), domain specific expertise consists of knowledge which is developed through learning from experience. The complex nature of knowledge is analysed by Quinn (1995), who subdivides it into three elements: cognitive, affective and psychomotor (Box 7.5).

Self-evaluation of level of expertise can be undertaken by tackling Activity 7.5, which is a self-assessment of expertise at giving an intramuscular injection.

Box 7.5 Different forms of knowledge

Cognitive knowledge (head)
- knowing facts
- thinking by processing information
- developing schemas

Affective knowledge (heart)
- attitudes as the consequence of value and belief systems
- feelings and intuition
- tacit knowledge, i.e. knowing something but being unable to explain it to someone else

Psychomotor knowledge (hands)
- skilled behaviour (often practised without conscious attention)
- an ability to adapt a skill to novel circumstances

 Activity 7.5 Self-assessment of intramuscular (i.m.) injection knowledge

Please answer the following questions:
Cognitive knowledge (head)
- Are you able to interpret and record on a prescription chart?
- Are you able to calculate drug dose administration using the appropriate formula?
- Are you aware of legal and safety measures to be taken regarding drug administration?
- Do you understand about the i.m. route of drug administration including relevant anatomy and physiology?
- Are you familiar with a drug which may be prescribed via the i.m. route including clinical effects and any side-effects?
- Do you feel able to monitor patients appropriately after they have received a given i.m. drug?

Affective knowledge (heart)
- How do you feel about giving drugs via the i.m. route?
- How would you assess how another person feels about receiving a drug via the i.m. route?

Psychomotor knowledge (hands)
- Are you able to draw up, administer and dispose of the i.m. injection equipment with safety and dexterity?

Discuss your responses with someone who can be expected to have i.m. injection expertise, such as a qualified nurse. How do your responses compare and contrast? Are you an expert or are there deficits in your knowledge?

As well as being dependent upon breadth of knowledge, expertise is associated with having depth of understanding. In her research into nursing expertise, Benner (1984) argues that expert practitioners are able to learn from their considerable experience and develop as a consequence. The characteristics of expert problem solving are summarised in Box 7.6.

Developing problem-solving expertise

The key to developing expertise in any domain is to gain experience and to learn from it. Experience alone will not lead to expertise – this can be confirmed by witnessing someone who has done the same thing for a long time but continues to perform poorly. It is important, therefore, to adopt strategies to enable effective learning from experience. Two significant ways to do this are through personal introspection and by working with established experts.

Personal introspection has become popular in nursing in the guise of reflective practice. However, as already shown in this chapter, there are limitations to the process because of difficulties in accessing the unconscious and because of the potential for distortions through memory construction. Frequently there is poor self-awareness of the determinants of behaviour and hence, in order to provide an explanation for action, there is a tendency to make up plausible but erroneous explanations post hoc. Reflection based upon introspection is best facilitated through structured means (Burns & Bulman 2000) within a framework of clinical supervision (Morton-Cooper & Palmer 2000).

In addition to reflection, Eraut (1994) suggests that there is a need for professionals to value and develop the more intuitive parts of decision making through learning from colleagues. For example a student nurse who accompanies a community psychiatric nurse (CPN) may not notice any clinical difference in two separate visits to the same client. This is a wasted learning opportunity unless an attempt is made to understand what has informed, for example, the CPN's decision to seek a second opinion in a particular instance. In order to develop her problem-solving skills, the student nurse needs to adopt a questioning stance. When working with a health care professional who has greater expertise in a particular domain, steps should be taken to enquire about the breadth and depth of her knowledge and understanding. The suggestions in Activity 7.6 are designed to be helpful to structure learning from experienced practitioners.

Activity 7.6 Learning from an expert

When you are in practice, be alert for an example of an effective clinical intervention which was beneficial, but you were unable to say why. If it is appropriate to take some time out, ask the person who instigated the practice (the expert) if she minds being interviewed about her problem-solving processes to assist your learning:

- Ask the expert to tell you about the cognitive, affective and psychomotor knowledge she brought to bear on the problem (see Box 7.5 and Activity 7.5).
- Use the list in Box 7.6 ('Characteristics of expert problem solving') to discuss with the expert whether she can recognise her use of any of these processes.
- Ask the expert about any factors which underpinned her decision-making processes.

In working through these points, be aware that much expertise is tacit and hence will require much mental effort to access into conscious attention. Reassure your expert that much expertise is difficult to express, but it is worth persevering as careful questioning can make us aware of what we know but cannot easily say.

Box 7.6 Characteristics of expert problem solving

Experts:
- use rich domain-specific knowledge which is sufficiently broad to include all relevant types of knowledge, i.e. cognitive, affective and psychomotor
- integrate their knowledge so that there is unified, rather than fragmented understanding
- draw upon experiences and use analogies with previous experiences
- identify underlying principles and filter out irrelevant or peripheral distractions
- use intuitive as well as analytic thinking
- attempt to access and express tacit knowledge through reflection

STRESS

Stress is a complex and abstract phenomenon which is explained and experienced by different people in many different ways (Ogden 1996). It is for these reasons that any attempt to develop a universal definition is of limited use. In order to understand stress it is necessary to give consideration to the different ways in which it may be interpreted, as this is the key to gaining an insight on how it is experienced, stress responses and coping strategies (Edelmann 1996). Classically, stress is delineated and represented by three different approaches: an environmental approach, a physiological approach and an interactional approach (Kent & Dalgleish 1996). Each of these approaches will be considered in turn.

An environmental approach to stress

In the environmental approach, stress is defined as something external to the individual in the environment which impinges upon the person. Examples are factors which can be perceived by the senses, such as unpleasant sights, sounds, smells, temperatures and tastes. Examples of stressful environments include: living in poor housing, working in a 'sweat shop' factory, being unable to sleep on a noisy ward or perhaps even the smells of a hospital. For nurses in particular, environmental stressors might be: caring for critically ill patients, competing demands upon time, visiting patients at home in areas with a high incidence of crime or being sent to work in a practice setting with a reputation for being particularly challenging.

A strength of the environmental explanation of stress is that it can usefully direct attention to stress-provoking factors. Stressful environmental stimuli which are generally accepted as undesirable, such as excessive noise, bright light, workloads and knowledge base, are measurable, and steps should be taken to address potential causes of patient or staff stress. However, it must be recognised that different people perceive their environment in different ways. For example, in a coronary care unit one patient and his visitors may regard the presence of high tech equipment as reassuring, while in another it may induce a stressful response. The way in which potentially stressful environments are interpreted is more important than the nature of the environmental stimuli themselves.

Coping within the environmental approach to stress can be direct in terms of taking steps to tackle the environmental stressors. Hence ward environments and care routines can be organised so that patients are disturbed as little as possible at night. In the community, legislation attempts to improve housing and working environments. Indirect measures include time out arrangements so that nurses are on a rotation to enable a break from particularly physically and/or emotionally demanding areas of practice. Respite care is designed to give a break and change of scene to carers and chronically ill or disabled people who are usually cared for at home by a family member.

Despite its practical applications, an interpretation of stress as being attributable to the environment alone is reductionist and static. A serious limitation is its failure to acknowledge individual differences in the perception of what might be stressful. The assumption of linear and progressive causality of stress is additionally flawed because there is poor acknowledgement of the variation of human capacity to adapt and cope. A coping measure that works for one individual may not have a similar effect in another.

A physiological approach to stress

The physiological approach defines stress as the individual's responses to perceived threat in an effort to maintain homeostasis. This is mediated principally through the actions of the autonomic nervous system to release the catecholamines adrenaline and noradrenaline from the adrenal medulla, and the endocrine system to release glucocorticoids from the adrenal cortex.

If homeostasis is not achieved there may be local pathological consequences termed the local adaptation syndrome (LAS). Examples of LAS responses to stress are headaches, cold sores, rashes, respiratory wheezing or intestinal upsets. Ironically, many people report experiencing such symptoms at the end of a stressful period, such as at finishing work to start a holiday. This is explained by homeostasis becoming unbalanced because the physiological defences are relaxed due to the physical end of the stress seeming to be coming to an end at a time when the psychological effects are still present.

Uncontrolled LAS or overwhelming stress may trigger a more pathologically disseminated response termed the general adaptation syndrome (GAS) which comprises three phases. In the alarm phase there is an initial rapid physiological response due to catecholamine release which is sustained through endocrine activity. This may lead to a resistance phase where homeostasis has been restored, but with reduced physiological reserve capacity to respond to sustained or additional demands. As a consequence, the person is more vulnerable to the third phase which is exhaustion as a result of prolonged exposure to stressors. Exhaustion is associated with deterioration in physiological functioning which can have serious health consequences.

As with other representations of stress, direct coping strategies are those which tackle any known causes of stress head on. Indirect coping includes relaxation techniques such as meditation and biofeedback designed to control the physiological effects of the stress response. Many nurses have become interested in therapies such as aromatherapy massage to assist patients to gain some mastery over stress-related symptoms such as idiopathic hypertension.

Strengths of this understanding of stress are that there is the establishment of a relationship between stress and disease, although the nature of this is unclear. Whatever the relationship, it is important for nurses to be able to recognise the effects of LAS and GAS so that early intervention can be initiated. Like the environmental approach, the physiological approach can be criticised for being an overly deterministic explanation of stress which fails fully to allow for individual interpretation and response to circumstances which might yield stress.

An interactional approach to stress

According to this approach, stress is defined as the result of an interaction between the individual and understanding of their situation. The key to the model is a person's unique and idiosyncratic interpretation of threat and perception of what can be done in response in the form of coping strategies. The model has three phases.

Primary appraisal involves the initial assessment of challenge or demand. In this phase people may ask questions such as: 'What is happening?' and 'How will this affect me?'. In other words, it is suggested that each individual makes an assessment and evaluates whether he feels threatened or not. Secondary appraisal is an estimation of personal resources to counter, or coping resources to deal with, any perceived threat. In this phase the person may ask questions such as: 'What can I do?', 'What help do I need?'. Coping in response to appraisal may be to address a problem directly, or to seek emotional release of tension. Finally, the reappraisal phase is an evaluation of the subsequent outcome in the light of the primary and secondary phases. Here the questions asked may be: 'How am I coping?', 'Is the situation better or worse now?'.

Coping, according to the transactional approach, is centred around how stress is perceived and notions of self-efficacy to exert control. Direct coping may involve the use of assertion skills or having a sense of personal autonomy to effect change. Indirect coping strategies are through denial and other forms of mental defence. A third mode of coping, palliation, is the adoption of behaviours which do not tackle the stressor but which provide temporary escape or diversion. Examples of palliative coping are reliance upon alcohol, drug misuse and time out.

The strengths of this model lie in its highly individualistic and dynamic representation which allows for differences and change both within and between people. It offers an explanation for stress in the absence of an apparent stressor, such as in the case of covert phobias or anxiety states. The model serves well to remind nurses that the way they interpret a given situation may differ from that of those they care for, or their colleagues. Practice can be guided by the model if the questions associated with each phase are used as a basis for assessment. A limitation in the application of the interactional approach to stress is that it requires a degree of articulacy to be able to voice the thought processes linked to each phase – not all individuals will be able to express this.

A composite explanation of stress

It has been suggested elsewhere (Wilkinson 2000) that all representations of stress have relevance to nursing. Assessment of the environment will indicate avoidable stress-inducing factors. Assessment of the patient will indicate physiological responses which will potentially confound other physical pathology. At the heart of stress, however, are the interpretations and responses made by each individual linked to their perceptions of their situation. In this context communication skills are as important as environmental audit or physical examination.

CONCLUSION

In this chapter a range of psychological theories have been highlighted and their relevance to nursing has been demonstrated. In the recently published commission for nursing and midwifery education it is argued that: 'Nursing and midwifery are no longer routinised, task-orientated roles; they are patient and client-centred, based on holistic, partnership approaches to care' (UKCC 1999, para 2.28). It has been the intention of this chapter to illustrate the important role that a knowledge of psychology has in this process.

REFERENCES

Barber P 1993 Developing the 'person' of the professional carer. In: Hinchliffe S, Norman S, Schober J (eds) Nursing practice and health care, 2nd edn. Edward Arnold, London, ch 14, pp 344–373

Barber P 1997 Caring: the nature of a therapeutic relationship. In: Perry A (ed) Nursing: a knowledge base for practice, 2nd edn. Edward Arnold, London, ch 6, pp 171–211

Benner P 1984 From novice to expert: excellence and power in nursing practice. Addison Wesley, Menlo Park

Boney J, Baker J 1997 Strategies for teaching decision making. Nurse Education Today 17: 16–21

Burnard P 1992 Know yourself! Self awareness activities for nurses. Scutari, London

Burns S, Bulman C (eds) 2000 Reflective practice in nursing, 2nd edn. Blackwell Science, Oxford

Conner M, Norman P (eds) 1996 Predicting health behaviour. Open University Press, Buckingham

Crow R, Chase J, Lamond D 1995 The cognitive component of nursing assessment: an analysis. Journal of Advanced Nursing 22: 206–212

Department of Health 1997 The new NHS, modern, dependable. Stationery Office, London

Department of Health 1998 Saving lives: our healthier nation. Stationery Office, London

Dines A 1994 A review of health beliefs research: insights for nursing practice in health promotion. Journal of Clinical Nursing 3: 329–338

Edelmann R 1996 Stress. In: Aitken V, Jellicoe H (eds) Behavioural sciences for health professionals. W B Saunders, London, ch 2, pp 22–33

Egan G 1994 The skilled helper, 5th edn. Brookes/Cole, Pacific Grove

Ellis R 1996 The psychological self. In: Kenworthy N, Snowley G, Gilling C (eds) Common foundation studies in nursing, 2nd edn. Churchill Livingstone, Edinburgh, ch 2, pp 43–61

Eraut M 1994 Developing professional knowledge and expertise. Falmer Press, London

Eysenck M, Keane M 1996 Cognitive psychology, 2nd edn. Lawrence Erlbaum, London

Falconer D 1999 The emotional labour of nursing. Assignment 5(1): 11–15

Fatchett A 1998 Nursing in the new NHS: modern dependable? Baillière Tindall, London

Ferlie E 1999 Clinical effectiveness and evidence based medicine: some implementation issues. In: Lugon M, Secker-Walker J (eds) Clinical governance: making it happen. Royal Society of Medicine Press, London, ch 5, pp 49–60

Furnham A, McDermott M 1994 Lay beliefs about efficacy of self-reliance, seeking help and external control as strategies for overcoming obesity, drug addiction, marital problems, stuttering and insomnia. Psychology and Health 9: 397–406

Gabe J, Kellaher D, Williams G (eds) 1994 Challenging medicine. Routledge, London

Ganong L, Bzdek V, Manderino M 1987 Stereotyping by nurses and nursing students: a critical review of research. Research in Nursing and Health 10: 49–70

Gray J 1997 Evidence based health care. Churchill Livingstone, Edinburgh

Gross R 1996 Psychology: the science of mind and behaviour, 3rd edn. Hodder and Stoughton, London

Hands D 1999 Integrated care. In: Lugon M, Secker-Walker J (eds) Clinical governance: making it happen. Royal Society of Medicine Press, London, ch 4, pp 33–48

Jeffrey R 1979 Normal rubbish: deviant patients in casualty departments. In: Black N, Boswell D, Gray A, Murphy S, Popay J (eds) 1984 Health and disease: a reader. Open University Press, Milton Keynes, ch 5.3, 249–254

Jones E E, Davis K E 1965 From acts to dispositions: the attribution process in social perceptions. In: Berkowiz L (ed) Advances in experimental social psychology, vol 2. Academic Press, New York

Kelley H H 1967 Attribution theory in social psychology. In: Levine D (ed) Nebraska symposium on motivation. University of Nebraska Press, Lincoln, NB

Kelly G 1979 A psychology of man himself. In: Potter D, Anderson J, Clarke J, Coombs P, Hall S, Holloway C, Walton T (eds) 1981 Society and the social sciences. Routledge, London, p 360

Kelly M, May D 1982 Good and bad patients: a review of the literature and a theoretical critique. Journal of Advanced Nursing 7: 147–156

Kent G, Dalgleish M 1996 Psychology and medical care, 3rd edn. W B Saunders, London

Leddy S, Pepper J 1993 Conceptual bases of professional nursing, 3rd edn. Lippincott, Philadelphia

Luft J 1970 Group processes: an introduction to group dynamics. Mayfield, Palo Alto

Martin L 1997 Talking point. Nursing Standard 11: 19

Menzies I 1961 The functioning of social systems as a defence against anxiety. Tavistock, London

Morton-Cooper A, Palmer A 2000 Mentorship, preceptorship and clinical supervision, 2nd edn. Blackwell Science, Oxford

National Health Service Executive 1998 Making a difference: a strategy for nursing midwifery and health visiting. NHSE, Leeds

Niven N 2000 Health psychology for health care professionals, 3rd edn. Churchill Livingstone, Edinburgh

Norman P, Bennett P 1996 Health locus of control. In: Conner M, Norman P (eds) Predicting health behaviour. Open University Press, Buckingham, ch 3, pp 62–94

Ogden J 1996 Health psychology: a textbook. Open University Press, Buckingham

Payne S, Walker J 1996 Psychology for nurses and the caring professions. Open University Press, Buckingham

Pervin L 1978 Am I me or am I the situation? Personal dispositions, situationism and interactionism in personality. In: Barnes P, Oates J, Chapman J, Lee V, Czerniewska P (eds) 1984 Personality development and learning: a reader. Hodder and Stoughton, Sevenoaks, ch 3.1, pp 169–187

Quinn F 1995 The principles and practice of nurse education, 3rd edn. Stanley Thornes, Cheltenham

Rogers C 1974 On becoming a person, 4th edn. Constable, London

Rosenhan D 1973 On being sane in insane places. Science 179: 250–258

Simpson M 1976 Brought in dead. Omega: Journal of Death and Dying 7: 243–248

Stainton Rogers W 1991 Explaining health and disease: an exploration of diversity. Harvester Wheatsheaf, London

Stevens R 1983 Freud and psychoanalysis. Open University Press, Milton Keynes

United Kingdom Council for Nursing Midwifery and Health Visiting 1996 Guidelines for professional practice. UKCC, London

United Kingdom Council for Nursing Midwifery and Health Visiting 1999 Fitness for practice: the UKCC commission for nursing and midwifery education. UKCC, London

Walsh M 1995 Why patients get the blame for being ill. Nursing Standard 9(37): 38–40

Wilkinson J 1997a Developing a concept analysis of autonomy in nursing practice. British Journal of Nursing 6(12): 703–707

Wilkinson J 1997b Understanding motivation to enhance compliance. British Journal of Nursing 6(15): 879–884

Wilkinson J 1997c Understanding memory to enhance nursing practice. British Journal of Nursing 6(15): 741–744

Wilkinson J 1999 Understanding patients' health beliefs. Professional Nurse 14: 320–322

Wilkinson J 2000 Interpersonal issues in high dependency care. In: Sheppard M, Wright M (eds) Principles and practice of high dependency nursing. Baillière Tindall, London, ch 3, 35–51

FURTHER READING

Gross R 1996 Psychology: the science of mind and behaviour, 3rd edn. Hodder and Stoughton, London
An excellent general text in terms of clarity of expression and comprehensiveness of the material included, but specific links to health care applications are limited.

Niven N 2000 Health psychology for health care professionals, 3rd edn. Churchill Livingstone, Edinburgh

Payne S, Walker J 1996 Psychology for nurses and the caring professions. Open University Press, Buckingham
The above two specialist psychology texts are written for a health professional readership and merit looking at if you wish to follow up in more detail the topics raised in this chapter.

8

The sociological basis of nursing

Kevin Gormley

CHAPTER CONTENTS

Introduction 226

Sociological theory 226
Structuralism and interpretative
  approaches 227

Health as a social construct 229
Biomedical concept 229
Socially constructed concept 230

Health beliefs 231

Socialisation 232
Anticipatory socialisation 233
Professional socialisation 233

Social roles and role sets 234
Stereotyping and role conflict 235
The sick role 236

Culture 237
Cultural heritage 237
Universal culture 238

Social policy 238
What is social policy? 239
Social and health problems 239
Welfare 239
Universality and selectivity 240

Community care 240
Assessment of need and care
  management 241
Services in the community 242
Hospitals 242
Day centres 242
Residential and nursing homes 242
Home care services 243

Primary health care: a new direction 244
New Labour and inter-agency
  cooperation 245
Royal Commission on old age 246
Primary health care groups and health
  education 247

Conclusion 248

References 249

Further reading 250

If nurses are to be able effectively to meet the needs of their patients, it is essential that the sociological and social policy influences that determine personal and culturally related responses to ill health are fully understood. It is from this premise that the purpose and objectives for this chapter emerge; they are to:

- highlight the nature of sociology and social policy, and their value to nursing practice
- introduce some of the key concepts that underlie sociological and social policy theories
- explore health as a sociological and social policy construct
- consider the current direction of government policy for the care of frail older people and those who are physically dependent.

INTRODUCTION

In the past, the preparation and education of health care professionals tended to concentrate on disease and the biological reasons for its presence. Nursing, as a supportive profession within this model, was essentially task orientated, and any theory used to underpin practice was usually biologically based. However, more recently nursing education has begun to address the social aspects of disease as well as the social influences that both maintain and enhance individual well-being. The concept of holism (that man is a bio-psycho-social-economic and spiritual entity in which each component is interdependent) is a key determinant in the development of nursing curricula. Consequently, nursing students are able to consider the existence of patients' problems, and ways of resolving them, from a much broader perspective.

Although sociology remains a marginal subject in nurse education compared to, for instance, the biomedical sciences, its value and importance is fairly well acknowledged. There is even a suggestion that sociology can act as a humanising

factor in education programmes for nurses, not just in terms of the acquisition of knowledge but also in the development of new ways of interpreting the world – and the people who occupy it (Cooke 1993). This chapter should provide a fundamental appreciation of basic sociological and social policy concepts. However, to increase an appreciation of the subject to a satisfactory level, full use should be made of the references provided and the further reading suggested throughout and in the Further reading list at the end of the chapter. Organising discussion groups with fellow students and lecturers in order to tease out these issues even further will be a useful activity.

SOCIOLOGICAL THEORY

Sociology is concerned with the interactions that occur as people engage with one another and with the many dynamics that operate as part of social living, such as relationship building, communication, cooperation and conflict. Sociology can provide us with an appreciation of the roles that social structures such as religion, families and health and social care services play within society. Through scientific investigation it is possible to begin to appreciate how these structures have emerged as integrated components of society, decide whether they are useful, and possibly consider alternative or critical views of their value or importance in terms of day-to-day living.

Most sociological analysis operates at a number of different levels. These include:

1. The micro-level: ideas are put forward as to how individuals may feel about, and react to, different circumstances that constitute their world. This may be the existence of stigma, labelling or inequality in treatment from the law or health care.

2. The institutional level: ideas provide an insight into the workings and operationalising of a range of essential services and structures that interact and dovetail together to create the modern society we often take for granted. For example, it is possible to consider the linkage between economic growth and development

with the mechanisms through which government and business choose to redistribute wealth creation to ensure a healthy living standard for all.

3. The macro-level: at this level ideas emerge that cross international boundaries and can be said to reflect a given society or group of societies at a point in time. Probably the works of early theorists such as Auguste Comte (1798–1857), Karl Marx (1818–1883) and Émile Durkheim (1858–1917) would essentially be in this domain, since they attempted to come to terms with and analyse the social, industrial and economic upheavals of their time.

Structuralism and interpretative approaches

Having identified the levels within which sociological analysis usually operates, an examination of a number of theoretical perspectives that operate within society at one or more of these levels can be undertaken. For the purpose of simplicity and ease of understanding, it is useful to summarise sociological theory into two broad sociological domains, structuralism and the interpretative approach.

The first theoretical domain addressed in this chapter is structuralism. Within this school of thought, theorists examine large groups of people, communities or nations to find out how they function. Within the structuralist domain two distinct groups have emerged. One view held by theorists is that society is a functional entity and is like a giant jigsaw in which everybody, knowingly or unknowingly, plays their part. Over a period, the jigsaw will adjust to changing circumstances. Some roles may become obsolete, while others may require simple adjustments to meet new situations. Classically, Talcott Parson's (1951) work on the sick role and the functional part that dependent people play in society would reflect this view of structuralism. The alternative view of structuralism is that it interprets functionalist ideas as merely a means of social control and a way of maintaining existing social systems. Following the French revolution, and using this period of major political upheaval as a theoretical source, Karl Marx put forward a view that

conflict was a necessary dynamic in any social system in order to provoke change and correct injustice. Marx argued that without conflict or revolution, social inequalities and unfair social systems remain unchecked.

The second broad theoretical domain that would seem to be the opposite of a structuralist view is interpretative sociology. Interpretative theory operates principally at the micro-level and is mainly concerned with the social interactions and dynamics that operate between and within individuals as they continue to experience and feel the effects of an unfolding social world around them. Eminent theorists within this domain, such as George Herbert Mead (1934), play down the value of the group or society and, instead, focus on the lived experience of the individual.

In Activity 8.1 the reader is presented with two sets of apparently opposite statements. They illustrate two comparative and contrasting approaches to the study of man and society: structuralism and interpretative approaches. Structuralism views man as an entity that is, in many social circumstances, controlled by the economic infrastructure of society. The rules, roles, customs and laws that relate to the structures, systems and institutional frameworks serve to constrain, enable or regulate the existence of man. Although man has a choice of action, a relatively passive role is adopted with the individual being a receiver of, and responder to, society. The interpretative approach, in contrast, would consider man as an agent who actively changes and manipulates society in face-to-face interactions within all forms of social organisations. Its emphasis lies in the belief that man is the creator of society and the social world.

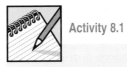 **Activity 8.1**

Answer the following questions:

1. Does society make man, or man make society?
2. Is sociology about man in society, or society in man?
3. Why do you think you replied in the way in which you did?

The structuralist approach takes a macro-sociological view, as its focal point is society as a set of interrelated, interdependent parts or systems. These include the political, economic, educational and medical systems. Within the medical system, the actors (nurses and patients) are depersonalised into passive role-receivers. Using this example of a structuralist organisation, it is possible to understand how social relationships and actions are either adapted or coerced by the system into a harmonious and cooperative structure. Conversely, the interpretative approach tends to be micro-sociological, where the sociological self is symbolic in a world where meanings are constructed and shared rather than externally imposed. The individual negotiates and constructs future roles with others in society. He interprets the culture in which he lives in a unique and distinctive manner, and is active in the construction of meaningful relationships during the process of giving and receiving care.

There is within the sociology departments of many universities a constant debate about the relative merits of the structuralist and interpretative approaches to the understanding of phenomena. Rather than become entangled in this debate in terms of deciding which domain is 'right' or 'wrong' or of most value to health care, nursing seems to have engaged both theories and to consider both to be equally valuable and useful in terms of their scientific contribution to the improvement of nursing practice. Bennett (1992), for example, proposes that it is particularly relevant to nursing to have some awareness of the two approaches. If prospective nurses are familiar with the approaches, it will assist them in understanding their future roles within the health care system and help them more fully to appreciate the social and cultural origins of their patients.

Although the two approaches (structuralist and interpretative) would appear to be poles apart, they are in fact closely connected and complementary, as they both represent different ways of observing the same social world, albeit through the use of different conceptual frameworks. The difference permits the use of a variety of investigative approaches and the adoption of different methods of data collection and data analysis,

which in turn provides for richer explanations about the social world within which we live. An interactionist approach is probably more relevant and immediate to the work of health care professionals as it concentrates on the micro-sociological processes such as the dynamics and relationships within families, whereas the structuralist approach would be to look at family in the context of family patterns that result from, for example, unemployment (Case example 8.1 and Activity 8.2). As the effectiveness of nursing depends very much upon the formulation and management of interpersonal relationships, knowledge of how the patient feels about being a patient appears more appropriate than, for example, knowing what percentage of single parents suffer physical ill health.

Case example 8.1 Social change

It was the first time that Helen, a third-year student nurse, had been given management responsibility for a group of patients in one of the bays in the ward, under the supervision of an experienced qualified nurse who was her mentor during that clinical placement. The reason for assigning the responsibility to Helen was to give her an opportunity to experience the complexities involved in the provision of holistic and individualised care for a group of patients.

One of Helen's patients was Trevor, a 36-year-old married man who had three young children. He was a happy, contented man, despite the fact that he had been made redundant from his job nearly 2 years ago and had not been in paid employment since. His wife, Vicky, was a very attractive woman who had returned to full-time employment a year ago in a large national company where she had worked before and where she was now a well-respected management consultant.

Trevor had been admitted to hospital following an accident in which he had sustained burns to the right side of his body, particularly his arm and leg, and to his left hand. The latter were comparatively minor, but the former required extensive skin grafts. However, he had fully recovered from his operation and was due to be discharged home in the next couple of days, although he would need care as an outpatient for a considerable time.

Helen had been organising appointments for Trevor that morning. She had remembered to make appointments for him to attend his local health centre for twice weekly dressings, to see the dietician who would explain and advise him on the special dietary needs that had resulted directly from the extensive tissue damage caused by the burns, and to attend the consultant's outpatient clinic in 4 weeks' time.

Although Helen was finding the management responsibilities quite challenging, she had certainly not found it difficult to sort out times for Trevor's appointments as he was not working and could, therefore, attend at any time. Quite pleased with her achievements, Helen proudly went to a review meeting with Joan, her mentor, and felt that she would surely get a 'well-done' pat on her back rather than the usual 'Did you consider...?'. This time she had thought of everything. She had not needed prompting but had used her initiative instead and organised all the necessary follow-up care. Or so she thought!

Flustered and red-faced Helen emerged from the seminar room where she had met her mentor. How could she have been so stupid? Now she would have to sort out all those appointments again, as well as organising home-help services. It had never occurred to her that the nature of the roles of the individuals within Trevor's family had reversed. He was a 'househusband'; he was quite content to look after the children and do all the housework while his wife went out to work. They had long since mutually agreed that, because of the better career prospects and job opportunities, Vicky would return to full-time employment, whereas he would take on the responsibility of running the home. It made no difference to him what 'certificated' sickness he had. He still had the children to look after, to take to and fetch from school, and so on, and would not, therefore, be able to attend his appointments at just 'any time'.

Helen had come to realise that change in society is a major component in any change in nursing. For health care workers to be able to provide holistic and individualised care, they must be fully conversant with the elements of current and foreseeable social change.

Activity 8.2

Using Case example 8.1:

Discuss with your colleagues what could be learned in terms of social change.

How should nursing adapt to this change?

The area of health promotion and health education can be used as another example. Health promotion is clearly a function of nurses in terms of educating large groups of people at community level about the importance of, for example, safe sex as a means of reducing the spread of HIV. Conversely, nurses also use health education programmes to address the same social issue. The

difference here is that programmes are specifically designed for particular individuals and, following careful planning, they are offered in a meaningful way that best suits their discrete social circumstances (Gormley 1999).

HEALTH AS A SOCIAL CONSTRUCT

When continuing to question and understand the complexities associated with sociological phenomena, it becomes apparent that there are close links to theories that directly relate to health care. The provision of good quality nursing care can be more effectively realised if health care practitioners can base their practice on empirical data relating to, for example, changing patterns of disease, dependency and death, and to people's perception of and responses to illness. The images of health through the ages have varied. In the past, a state of health was linked to the practice of medicine, scientific or technological developments or beliefs systems. This idea can be represented in a continuum, the extreme ends of which are biomedical concepts and health as socially constructed states (Fig. 8.1). However, it is also clear that one did not evolve from the other, but rather they both developed in tandem and still continue to coexist as such today.

Biomedical concept

The biomedical concept emerged as a mechanistic perspective, based on the belief that to be healthy was to be free from recognisable disease. The role of the physician was to treat disease and to restore health by correcting any imperfections caused by the accidents of birth and life (Dubos 1960). It is this concept that informed the ideology of traditional medical education. The study of the structure and process of disease became a predominant feature in the education of physicians. This trend persists today, but social sciences are gaining a stronger hold. However, it appears that the development of medical services based on biomedical concepts of surgery, immunological responses to transplants, chemotherapy and the molecular

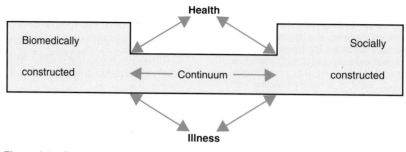

Figure 8.1   Conceptions of health.

basis of inheritance are given priority, not only in the provision of sciences, but also in medical and nurse education (Townsend & Davidson 1982).

Socially constructed concept

Similarly, nursing and nurse education had a biomedical emphasis until the 1970s. Then, with the emergence of a professional reform movement, 'the new nursing', the focus of nursing moved away from a medical, disease-orientated approach to become more person-centred and individualised. Where the caring role of the nurse had previously centred around the biological functions of the patient, it now began to extend to the psychosocial aspects of the individual and the recognition of the patient as an active participant in, rather than a passive recipient of, care (Corbett 1995). Thus, with the changing emphasis of care, the study of the sociological self has become a predominant feature in the education not only of nurses, but also of other health care professionals, including doctors.

Health as a socially constructed state had its origins in Ancient Greece. The teachings of the goddess Hygeia advocated that rational social organisation and rational behaviour by an individual were the most important commodities in the promotion and maintenance of health. The World Health Organization (WHO) gave credence to this approach at its foundation at the end of the Second World War. WHO, the current authoritative agency on health, included the social perspective as an important component of health. This brought about an increased awareness of the need

to include social and socio-economic factors not only within education related to health, but also within the design and provision of health services.

In societies where health and illness present as social categories, health is seen in the context of the distribution of illness, epidemiological patterns and class structures of that society. The existence of bacteria, viruses and 'injury' to mind and body are acknowledged. However, the real meaning that is afforded to them, while making sense of them, is social.

Helman (1992) describes how, for example, the presentation of illness and the way in which an individual responds to it is largely determined by sociocultural factors. These factors influence the perception of which symptoms and signs are abnormal in a given culture, and shape the physical and emotional changes that occur into a pattern with which the individual sufferer, and people around him, identify. The gap between subjective feelings of altered health status and their social acknowledgement is connected by what Helman calls 'its own language of distress', which also describes the term 'folk illnesses'. These can be 'learned' in the sense that a child growing in a particular culture learns how to respond to, and express, a range of physical or emotional symptoms, or social stresses, in a culturally patterned way (Helman 1992). Cultural and social forces such as television, newspapers and magazines and the dominant ideology of the society further shape these. It is through this language that a consensus of what constitutes the presence of illness and wellness among the members of a particular culture occurs. An awareness

Case example 8.2 Healthy eating

In response to the Health of the Nation strategy (DoH 1992), a fundholding GP practice in a city in northern England provides opportunities at the health centre for mothers to learn about diet and nutrition. A special meeting is organised once a month at the end of one of the bi-weekly baby clinics. Mothers are invited to bring with them any members of their family who might be interested. The health visitors who usually run the clinics choose a topic that they consider to be particularly pertinent or that has been requested by mothers. Sometimes they deliver the talk themselves; sometimes they invite an expert on the topic to talk about it. Whatever the case, the health visitors take it in turn to prepare an information sheet on the subject of the talk and make it available for the mothers who were unable to attend.

In a recent practice management meeting, it had been noted that quite a number of babies and children, particularly West Indian babies and children, appeared to be overweight. Because of this, and in order to emphasise the importance of healthy eating, it was decided to invite a dietician from the local hospital to talk about the prevention of obesity.

The event was extremely well attended, perhaps because a few mothers were concerned about their children being teased and bullied at school and being called names such as 'Michelin tyre man'. The talk, and especially the discussion that followed, proved to be very enlightening. The dietician, Angela, was very charismatic and appeared to have a great deal of insight to the variations that existed in the beliefs and practices about food in different cultural groups. The audience immediately warmed to her, as she did not just tell them not to eat this or that, but seemed to be able to understand the issues that were of concern to individuals, particularly those belonging to ethnic minorities.

Angela explained how food is much more than a source of nutrition: it is a social convention. Although all human societies process their food supply in some way, a great many cultural variations exist in terms of what substances are regarded as food and, indeed, how food may be grown, gathered, presented and consumed. Substances that may be acceptable as food in one society or culture may be rigidly forbidden in another. She gave an example of the unacceptability of dogs, cats and mice being used as food in the UK, despite the fact that they may well be edible, and how religious groups have strict taboos about not only the ingestion, but also the handling of certain foods.

In a similar vein, Angela demonstrated through the use of slides how there are variations in what is considered to be healthy and beautiful in different cultures, as had been found by anthropologists studying physique and body images within different societies. She gave examples of: how wealthy men in some West African cultures send their daughters to 'fattening houses' where they are fed with fatty foods and denied exercise to make them plump and pale, to indicate both wealth and fertility; and of how some West Indian mothers, because malnutrition has been so common in the communities from which they have come, appear to desire to see their offspring as big fat babies, because they believe that a plump, cherub-like baby immediately gives the impression of an affluent family. Angela also explained how scientists had found a great deal of evidence to suggest there to be an extremely strong desire to maintain cultural continuity through the adherence to traditional beliefs and practices relating to food, particularly among immigrant ethnic minority groups. She hastened to add, however, that such things as unemployment, low income, social isolation, long working hours, lack of leisure time and cultural change itself, issues often beyond the control of individuals, also influence health and nutrition.

It was only after this that Angela told her extremely captive audience about the importance of healthy eating and what makes up a healthy diet. The talk had been a great success and, as it transpired later, produced a number of positive outcomes, including a reduction in the number of potential 'Michelin tyre men'.

Activity 8.3

Place yourself in the position of a Polish student, a qualified nurse in Poland, who has come for an orientation programme in your college before being allowed to register as a qualified nurse in the UK.

Describe what would you need to do, as her mentor, to ensure that she is competent to deliver culturally sensitive care in this country.

of this by health care professionals is paramount in enabling them to provide culturally sensitive care, as can be seen in Case example 8.2 (see also Activity 8.3).

HEALTH BELIEFS

Clearly, perceptions of health and illness vary in different cultural and social groups. Health behaviour, like all other behaviour, is determined by the values and beliefs that the members of a society hold. Indeed, Townsend & Davidson (1982) propose that the pursuit of health is

Box 8.1   **The key components of a health belief model** (adapted from Abraham & Shanley 1992)

- How susceptible we are to the illness in question
- The seriousness/severity of the illness
- The potential costs
- The effectiveness of this action in relation to possible alternatives

Activity 8.4

Discuss with colleagues your views on alternative therapies.

Is it possible to accommodate different demands for treatment via the NHS?

increasingly acknowledged as a social and not merely a technical enterprise. However, despite health promotion and the wide availability of preventative health programmes (such as well woman and well man clinics), health behaviour varies greatly, even within a single society whose members acknowledge the same cultural heritage. To make sense of this, Abraham & Shanley (1992) propose the use of a health belief model which lists the four key components of a person's belief about his own health (see Box 8.1).

The significance of this model is that it provides a useful tool in assessing and making sense of the patient's health beliefs. Having done this, the nurse could then identify, together with the patient, a plan of action to promote health behaviour, not only in the individual patient, but also in the individual's society. The latter, in a small way, addresses some of the inequalities in health as identified by Townsend & Davidson (1982).

As economic and transport systems bring different cultures and communities closer, the goals of health care need to be even more culturally sensitive. Health care professionals need to be fully aware of the health beliefs, traditions and practices of the different cultural and ethnic groups coexisting in the particular society in which they practise (for example the religious practices of Orthodox Jews, Catholics or Muslims). Lynman (1992) proposes that seeking knowledge of the patient's perspective on health is imperative to be able to provide culturally sensitive care. This is because the patient normally uses his lay 'carers' – family, friends, spouse or partner – for initial advice, and thus important decisions which may have great relevance for subsequent

health care may be made outside of the formal health care system.

There are cultural variations in terms of the relevance and value of 'scientific' health care. Alternative medicine or therapy seems to be gaining in popularity among the general population. Old methods of healing considered obsolete decades ago appear to be in demand again. This does raise issues about the nature of health care. It could be that people who believe in naturopathic health care are absenting themselves from conventional care and not accessing alternative care because of the cost (Activity 8.4).

SOCIALISATION

Socialisation is a process that preserves the cultural heritage of society and provides a bridge between generations throughout an individual's life cycle. It is most intense in infancy ('primary socialisation'), the most formative years of an individual's life. Each child is unique, an individual who acquires different values, attitudes and beliefs and develops a personality of his own. Societies differ widely in their socialisation practices. However, provided that the process proceeds reasonably well, the individual will eventually be able to fulfil his social role functions, making adjustments as he moves along in a changing society. During primary socialisation the most important agents of socialisation are contained within the immediate family unit, i.e. the carers of the child with whom the child can form a lasting bond. The importance of maintaining the bond cannot be overemphasised. For example, when a child is hospitalised, parents are encouraged to involve themselves in providing care.

The child gradually learns the behavioural characteristics of his parents or carers and, to a lesser extent, those in his immediate community. The influence of people other than the family is more important today than previously because of the altered working patterns of women. The peer group at a day-care centre may assert an influence during what sociologists call the 'secondary socialisation' phase. Other agents of secondary socialisation include schools. Here, alongside the formal curriculum, a hidden curriculum exists whereby children learn to accept and respond to the teaching staff and their authority. According to Giddens (1993), schools can be extremely influential agents of socialisation, especially for underprivileged children, in that they allow them to escape from the restricting aspects of the social backgrounds from which they come. The influence of the media, particularly the television, as an agent of socialisation is very important. A lot of delinquent behaviour among adolescents is often a result of uncontrolled exposure to violence on television. Conversely, Giddens (1993) proposes that access to the media has many beneficial effects, as it conveys information to which people would not otherwise have access.

Both primary and secondary socialisation are influenced by a variety of social factors, including social class, agents of socialisation, economic relationships to the community, critical points in the life of an individual, residence patterns and household structures. It is becoming increasingly difficult to determine when primary socialisation ends and secondary socialisation begins because of the changes in family structures, particularly in the employment patterns of parents. Gomm (1982), however, proposes that primary socialisation is about learning the basics, and secondary socialisation is about applying the basics to specific roles, without there being any age divide.

Anticipatory socialisation

Although the major analysis of socialisation has focused on child development, other milestones in an individual's life can be identified as specific socialisation periods. One such period is the anticipated entry into a professional life, which

Activity 8.5

How did you prepare yourself for entry into the nursing profession?
How, if at all, did your values and beliefs about society change?

sometimes calls for a shift in the individual's beliefs and values (e.g. to fulfil entry criteria).

Sometimes, anticipatory socialisation can be problematic and create role strain, as, for example, if an individual has formed an erroneous impression about an occupation and reality does not match his expectations. No scientific evidence for this exists yet, but it is suggested that beliefs, attitudes, values and motives of adults are evolving continuously, although gradually, throughout their working lives (Gahagan 1980) (Activity 8.5).

Professional socialisation

Professional socialisation is a continued form of anticipatory or preparatory socialisation. It is about learning shared meanings of the professional culture. Students acquire the intricacies of the role of the nurse and knowledge of the rights, responsibilities, obligations and values of the profession. Abraham & Shanley (1992) identify that there may be feelings of bewilderment during initial encounters – with a hospital or other institution, for example – until such time as language becomes shared between professionals. Little by little, new ways of talking become new ways of thinking. Socialisation is gradual and students often find a difficulty in adapting to and understanding what is expected of them. They may well experience this socialisation phase as they learn to adjust to the different role requirements of the professional culture of nursing and conform to its expectations.

It is appropriate here to recognise that a structuralist approach to professional socialisation differs from that of the interpretative approach. The structuralist approach views it as the making of the professional and the acquiring of the professional culture through the process of socialisation, which reconciles the opposition between the functioning of the social system and the actions of individual members of society. The core values are internalised through this process so that there is a correspondence between the norms and values of the system and the subjective meanings of the actors within (Bond & Bond 1994). In accordance with the interpretative view, an individual does not become a professional during the process of preparatory education programme but while actually occupying the role and status of a qualified professional and negotiating with individuals and situations that he meets. It is only then that the organisation of the environment begins to influence professional behaviour.

SOCIAL ROLES AND ROLE SETS

The concept of social role refers to a role that is enacted within a group and incorporates appropriate behaviours – role-appropriate behaviour. This behaviour includes the accepted rules and expectations assigned to that role, which denote the functions that an individual undertakes while within a particular role. There are kinship roles (mother/son), gender roles (male/female), age roles (child/adult) and occupational roles (doctor/nurse). Each role is derived from social structures. Although individuals assume the roles, they do not exist in isolation but are complementary to the social structure. They are intertwined within social systems; for example, parents and children are in a family, students and teachers are in an education system, and nurses and patients are in a health care system.

As can be seen from Activity 8.6, an individual may have several concurrent roles in his social life, within each of which he behaves in a certain way. If an individual has learned – generally through the process of socialisation – the role-appropriate behaviour, the uncertainty and trauma of social life are minimised. A social role informs the individual of the appropriate dress, duties, talk, obligations, privileges and rights (Smith 1981). To take a contrary example, it is unlikely that a ward

Activity 8.6

Read the account below:

Gary was delighted! After weeks of trying, he had finally managed to get tickets to a rare concert of his favourite pop group. His wife and children found the determination with which he had set about ringing ticket agents and even approaching the 'black market' amusing.

However, Gary's friend and long-standing golf partner, with whom he played in a weekly match, was annoyed. 'Your fanaticism will do you no good if you want to renew your position as a club secretary for next season. Besides, your doctor won't be pleased either. He told you to stop rushing about, because of your blood pressure.'

Gary had been sure that he would succeed in the end; he had even cancelled the day out in his business diary so that his secretary could not book any appointments that would prevent him from attending the concert. Gary's mother had been equally convinced of her son's eventual success: 'I knew he would do it; he'll turn heaven and earth to get something that he wants. I am just surprised that he hasn't convinced his next door neighbour to go with him! He'll have to leave home early, though, to travel from Brighton to Glasgow and back in one day.'

Now, make a list of the different roles that you can identify Gary to have.

manager would go on duty dressed in a jogging suit, address the staff in a manner similar to a sergeant major in the army addressing new recruits during drill practice, be disrespectful towards doctors or patients, or accept personal gratuities from patients or their relatives.

Gahagan (1980) supports this by claiming that there are certain expectations affiliated to social roles in relation to the degree of general consensus of expectation, the penetration of the role into all the behaviour of an individual, the legal sanctions associated with the roles and, in the case of professional roles, the code of conduct. For example, there is a consensus that the role of a student is to learn. In an education system where the central tenet was adult education there would be occasions where the student would be expected to teach. This might, to a person with a traditional view of education, present a difficulty and result in only marginal consensus about the nature of a teacher–student relationship.

Some roles can 'infiltrate' an individual's total behaviour. A religious leader, for example, is required to be an ardent believer, benevolent and moral in both public and private life. In contrast, no such demands are made of a plumber. As long as he carries out the job safely and to an agreed specification, he can do so dressed in shorts or singing the latest pop song. The role of a plumber makes no demands on the person outside the job.

Role expectations may also involve legal sanctions. If a parent fails to provide satisfactory care for a child, it can result in a period of imprisonment. If, however, the parent fails to provide recreational facilities for the child, this would not result in any form of punishment. Similarly, a code of conduct, which is one of the hallmarks of a profession, will provide guidelines of behaviour within a professional role. Any deviation from the guidelines, as in the case of nurses, may result in the removal of the offending individual's name from the professional register, with the consequence that the individual ceases to practise in that role.

STEREOTYPING AND ROLE CONFLICT

New entrants to nursing may come into the profession with a distinct view of the role of a nurse based on a stereotypical view. Stereotyping, however, may extend beyond the role itself. The personality characteristics of the role occupants can be portrayed in either a positive or a negative way. The latter carries with it an inherent problem, not necessarily for those entering a particular profession, but for those outside it. To illustrate this, the person with a view of a nurse as a sex-symbol – as frequently depicted in caricatures and comic films – or someone who enters nursing with a romantic notion of continually 'soothing the fevered brow' of patients will undoubtedly encounter problems.

A role function and the role occupant may also present as a mismatch. Generally, an individual is appointed to a role because he appears to have the aptitudes and personality to enact the role. If, however, it transpires that the individual and his role partners (fellow workers) do not perceive the role function in the same way, or the individual simply does not have the ability to carry out the function, role strain will result. For example, a student nurse who has chosen a particular branch of nursing may find out during the 'sampling' of the branch in the common foundation programme that the choice of branch is not appropriate. Unless the mismatch is rectified, the outcomes will be unfavourable, not only for the student, but also for potential employers and patients.

In exploring the concept of role strain, it is evident that role strain relates to internal antagonism between an individual and a particular role. Any one individual, however, generally has multiple roles. There are times when it may be difficult to enact competing roles comfortably. For example, it may be problematic for a nurse to combine her usual work role with that of being a patient. A person in a powerful position in local government and used to being totally 'self-directing' may find it hard to accept and enact a dependent role. The role conflict that results may be so strong that it may even make the individual discharge himself from hospital against medical advice.

Some role functions often have conflicting demands. It is possible to appreciate the dilemma faced by an army chaplain during a time of war. On the one hand, he may preach the ideals of peace and tolerance, while on the other he is also involved in a war situation where loss of life is expected. The roles that individuals may have in both their private and public lives have a powerful influence on social life. However, a role is frequently more stable than is the role occupant (Groenman et al 1992). It provides guidelines for appropriate behaviour in different circumstances. Individuals tend to have a strong sense of conformity. Sometimes they even conform against their better judgement. It may be much easier for students to approach their duties during clinical placement in a task-orientated way – if that is common practice in the area – rather than attempt patient-centred holistic care which they know to be more beneficial to the patient. It can be very stressful for a new role occupant to differ greatly from customary behaviour, because social pressures exerted by those who control entry into a particular role are very strong (see Case example 8.3).

THE SICK ROLE

Given that the effectiveness of a social system depends on the effectiveness of the role functions it contains, a text for students engaged in health-related studies must explore the concepts of 'wellness' and 'sickness'. Being well implies that an individual is able to function appropriately in the context of his bio-psycho-social self and in the roles that he occupies. There are times, however, when an individual may need to withdraw from the obligations and activities that these roles imply. He may be either temporarily or permanently unable to enact his 'normal' roles and assumes, as Parsons (1951) proposes, a sick role in a health system.

Society does not allow for the adoption of a sick role without regulation. It is the physician who is involved with the authority to admit and discharge individuals in their passage through the sick role (Mann 1983). In doing so, the physician keeps a social and emotional distance and deals with each sick role occupant on equal terms. In return, the sick individual is exempt from his normal role obligations and is not held responsible for his condition. This is conditional. The individual is expected not to use sickness for gainful purposes, either in terms of using the system fraudulently or of prolonging the period of sickness. He must also seek and act on the advice of qualified professionals. The above forms the basis of what could be termed a contract between the physician or nurse and the patient in the sick role. There may be a lack of role compliance on behalf of the patient, particularly if the advice given by the professional does not coincide with the patient's wishes and expectations.

Parsons (1951), acknowledging that becoming ill is a natural event, categorises sick role behaviour as deviant. Deviance in a sociological sense should not necessarily contain negative aspects. The enactment of the sick role, providing it adheres to the contract previously mentioned, will improve the functioning of social systems. This is because the health system is designed, ideally, for the purposes of optimising the health status of the nation as a whole. The latter begs the question that the reader may wish to explore: how forceful is medicine as an agent of social control?

Whatever the response to the questions in Activity 8.7, each member of society has a unique view relating to the concepts of health and sickness. This view will be an integral part of the cultural beliefs and values of the individual in the context of the society in which he lives. George's experience in the sick role (Case example 8.3) was unhappy. He had obviously achieved a great deal by rolling a cigarette, despite the fact that he could use only one hand. However, the structural constraints imposed on him almost negated not only his positive experience, but also the experience of

Case example 8.3
(reproduced from Bennett 1992)

George, a 72-year-old man recovering from a stroke, had just spent an hour making three of his own cigarettes with one hand. The nursing staff were thrilled to see his achievement, while gently and appropriately admonishing him for smoking. George wheeled himself to the day room and was about to light his cigarette when a physiotherapist arrived to take him for his treatment. George refused to move and a row ensued. He was taken for treatment and was later returned in an angry and unrepentant mood by an equally angry physiotherapist. The nurse and the physiotherapist presented a united professional approach to the patient but argued in the ward office about the relative merits of forcing a patient to undergo treatment.

Activity 8.7

Many conditions (e.g. sexually transmitted diseases, smoking related diseases) are morally 'loaded'. How do you think this moral perspective may affect:

- the sick role?
- the interaction between the doctor and the potential sick role occupant?
- the relationship between the nurse and the potential sick role occupant?

Attempt to substantiate your conclusions with evidence from the media (television, radio and newspapers).

the individuals enacting the professional roles. The adoption of a more interpretative approach, whereby George, the nurse and the physiotherapist would take a negotiating approach to designing the treatment schedule for George, would have made it a much happier and a more satisfactory situation for everybody within the context of their respective roles.

CULTURE

In addition to the physical and psychological component of the self, each individual has a degree of social integrity through which the cultural heritage of his society is safeguarded. Cultural determinants are a major factor in shaping the way that individuals behave as members of a particular society. However, it is also essential to appreciate that there may be considerable variations not only within different societies, but also within the varied cultures that exist in any one society. In order to provide an appropriate and a quality caring service, health care professionals must be able to differentiate between cultural variations of behaviour of individuals. For example, interaction patterns often vary greatly between cultures. In a number of Asian societies, maintaining a large interpersonal space, averting the eyes and keeping the head low during periods of interaction demonstrates respect for others. Europeans or Americans would suggest that this behaviour would imply that the person is being distant, submissive or evasive. Even from this rather simple example, it is clear that health care professionals who are not consciously aware of cultural differences between individuals could come to an incorrect conclusion when assessing the health status of a patient.

Giddens (1993) proposes that a highly illuminating perspective can be achieved through the study of sociology for its 'scope is extremely wide, ranging from the analysis of passing encounters between individuals in the street up to the investigation of global processes'. Increasingly, cultural changes and their importance to individuals within given societies are becoming very far-reaching. Issues such as language, diet,

lifestyle and attitude to health care provision are now in many cases culturally driven. It would seem that social phenomena that could previously be understood by nurses through common sense would now require a more rational and scientific investigation if nurses are to fully understand what is occurring and, ultimately, its effect on patient care. Case example 8.1 illustrated how, for example, a change in the economic status and the nature of the relationships between individuals within a family may directly influence the provision of care. If a nurse is unaware of such change, the care may be inappropriate or obsolete, particularly if the nurse is committed to the idea of holistic and individualised care as a way of nursing.

There are two distinctive definitions of the word 'culture'. Most people use the word in the context of art, literature or music. An appreciation of art and other cultural pursuits used to be the preserve of the sophisticated – normally the 'élite' and middle-class intellectuals. Media coverage, however, has changed all that: all members of society now have access to this kind of 'culture'. Sociologists, while recognising the above, have extended the use of the term 'culture' to embrace the values members of a given group hold, the norms they follow and the material goods they create (Giddens 1993). Indeed, Martin & Belcher (1986) consider culture to be a philosophy of life and death in society. It contains the human heritage of a society in the form of rules, values and beliefs of that society. These are passed from one generation to the next during the process of socialisation. Individuals learn to act in accordance with role-appropriate behaviour in human practices such as child rearing, marriage, dress, work and religion. They learn values of what is right and wrong in their culture and beliefs about the world and the nature of society.

CULTURAL HERITAGE

Cultural heritage is not about the physical environment: it is about the way in which the environment is used (for example, issues such as preventing global warming or protecting whales).

Nor is cultural heritage about such things as genetically determined characteristics such as skin colour: it is about the way in which the members of a group sharing, among other things, the same skin colour behave. Culture is pervasive at all levels of human functioning in society. Because of its profound effects, there is a tendency to assume that the culture an individual 'owns' is the best one. This is not so. For example, monogamy is the natural form of marriage in Western industrial societies, and polygamy is considered deviant and against the law. Yet in a number of tribal societies of Africa the only accepted form of marriage is polygamy. The polygamous society would struggle to exist within a monogamous structure. Gender-related issues (e.g. women politicians and priests) are mostly culturally determined. Other matters associated with gender such as equal opportunities in pay also often provoke heated debate. Such issues as paternity leave have a direct relevance to marriage and family patterns in society, and will in the future become part of the cultural heritage.

There is universal recognition of the fact that food and water are essential to sustain life. However, there are great cultural diversities in terms of 'what' and 'how'. Food that is acceptable, and even a delicacy, in one culture may be considered inedible by another. Feelings of hunger generally produce images of food and these images, frequently 'informed' by religious beliefs and practices, have variations from one culture to another as well as from one individual to another. Some people prefer thick beefsteaks cooked to a crisp, while others savour raw fish.

Variations exist not only between different cultures, but also within the subcultures of a dominant culture. In modern Britain, many subcultures – Italian, Pakistani and Chinese among others – live side by side. The cultural diversity predominant in industrialised societies presents its own challenges. When children from a minority culture encounter norms, beliefs and values beyond their own culture they may well encounter difficulties with school or with accepting the practices relating to courtship and marriage. Their own cultures often make demands on them in terms of

their dress and their gender roles that may result in what their parents would identify as culturally deviant behaviour.

UNIVERSAL CULTURE

Thus far, this chapter has concentrated on cultural diversity. However, there are universal cultures that apply to all societies. All people use language to communicate; it is only the specific languages that differ. Each culture has some form of family and marriage system, religious ritual and medicine based either on scientific methods or on the supernatural. There is universal recognition of the importance of hospitality, be it expressed by offering food and drink to guests or – as in some Inuit groups – by lending the wife for the night to keep a visitor warm. Whatever the diversities or universals, the individual's total view of the world is culturally determined, whether the earth is considered to be round or flat, at the centre of the universe or not, whether the cosmos is believed to be inhabited by one deity or many, by ghosts, demons or ancestral spirits, it is all determined by culture (Winefield & Peay 1980).

SOCIAL POLICY

The second half of this chapter examines the role of social policy and its effect on the provision of health care. Modern curricula that are used as a basis for teaching and preparing health care professionals focus on introducing to the student a sense of self-enquiry and flexibility, alongside a sound understanding of the practice of health care from a basis of research and societal appreciation. It is within this framework that the importance of social policy as a curricular subject is best understood. Social policy is a broad subject. It is vital that the content of a social policy unit in pre-registration curricula is placed within pre-existing maps of knowledge. In health care, the most appropriate focus is the patient and the divergent needs and backgrounds from which they come (Gormley 1999) (Activity 8.8).

Activity 8.8

Discuss with your teacher and fellow students the value of studying social policy when preparing to become a health care professional.

WHAT IS SOCIAL POLICY?

Social policy studies are focused on the study of social welfare and health and social services. Social policy determines how the nation's resources are organised for the perceived benefit of society. Ideas of what benefits society most are dependent on who is in charge of policy and what they perceive as beneficial. The main areas of social policy studies are:

- policy and administrative practices in health, social security, education, employment services, community care and housing management
- the circumstances in which people's welfare is likely to be impaired, including disability, unemployment, mental illness, learning disability and old age
- social problems such as crime
- issues relating to social disadvantage, including race, gender and poverty
- the range of collective social responses to these circumstances (Spicker 1995, p. 4).

The core elements of policy are its origins, goals, the process of implementation and the results or net effects. Social policy does not study a subject, but how it is provided and achieved; for example, it is not concerned with physical health but with policies that promote health and the provision of health care services.

The study of social policy as an academic discipline has its roots in the early years of the 20th century, a time when fundamental moral and social questions were debated with a sense of vigour and purpose. Titmuss (1963) described how the focus of enquiry moved from 'Who are the poor and neglected in society?' to 'Why are they poor and what are the resultant effects of poverty in terms

of health and well-being?'. As an area of academic study, social policy is underpinned by many other subjects from which it creates its discrete body of knowledge, including sociology, politics and philosophy. Through these subjects, social policy theorists question the nature and philosophy of government interventions that protect and provide a reasonable lifestyle for all citizens.

SOCIAL AND HEALTH PROBLEMS

Social policy is sometimes depicted as a response to social problems. Social problems present issues to which some response is required. However, it is not always the case that everyone will agree on what constitutes a problem. The definition of a problem varies and the nature of that problem needs to be understood in order to respond to it. The broad health and social care needs of the most dependent members of society, and the ways in which government responds to meet them, are important areas of examination.

Social problems may affect not just individuals but society as a whole, though the problems tend to arise from individual human needs. Some are obvious, such as the need for food and clothing, whereas some are conceptual, for example the need for status in society. These common human needs are largely met by personal and family action. Individuals work for a living, find accommodation, establish friendships and obtain care, security and a sense of purpose within family and social groups. When these needs are unmet, this gives rise to problems. The basic need to subsist leads to the social problem of poverty, if family and individuals are unable to meet the need themselves. Likewise, the common need for shelter is the basis of housing problems (Brown & Payne 1994).

WELFARE

Social policy is also concerned with welfare. Welfare can mean well-being, and social policy can be represented as being concerned with well-being in general and with people who lack well-being – people with particular kinds of problems or needs and the services which provide for them. The boundaries are indistinct because people's needs have to be understood in terms of facilities that are available to them and others; good housing and adequate income or good health affect the view of what people need or what is a problem. What is judged as being poor housing in one society will not necessarily be the same in other societies.

UNIVERSALITY AND SELECTIVITY

Policy can largely be divided into two types, a universal policy or a selective policy. A universal social policy is one that aims to provide services to everyone, or at least everyone within a broadly defined category, such as the old, the mentally ill, children or those individuals with a learning disability. A selective policy is one that focuses resources just on the people in need. The arguments for and against universality and selectivity concern the focus of policy. Universality is seen as a way of making resources available to everyone irrespective of need (e.g. child benefit). The main problem with this approach is that resources are wasted on those who are not in need. The argument for selective policies is that if benefits were targeted, less money would be spent, and with greater effect. One problem with targeting individuals is that, first, they need to be identified and second, of course, how they can be identified. If the process is self-selection, then the people in that situation have to know that they are eligible for help and how to go about applying for benefits. Along with this there is a problem of defining limits: falling below a certain level makes a person eligible for certain benefits; being just above the limit means one is ineligible. This can result in a worse position for those

people just above the limit than for those just below it (Spicker 1995) (Activity 8.9).

COMMUNITY CARE

The term 'community' is a vague term, and often means different things to different people. A community is regarded as an area within which people live, i.e. the local neighbourhood. This definition of community can be more applicable to some areas than others, depending on the degree of social interactions within the neighbourhood. Another way of looking at community is to define it in terms of interactions between people, even though there may not be a common geographical boundary. This would cover such communities as those defined by religious convictions. Other communities can have what may seem on the surface to be little linkage, such as the business community, which refers to a large number of diverse organisations over a vast geographical spread (Spicker 1995).

The Conservative government's 1990 National Health Service and Community Care Act provided the strategic framework for the introduction of community care in the UK. It encouraged statutory agencies to form positive partnerships with consumers of services, informal carers and the voluntary and independent sectors in order to afford a positive choice in the provision of services. This Act was the result of three White Papers that were particularly influential: *Working for Patients* (DoH 1989a) and *Caring for People* (DoH 1989b). These White Papers provided clear guidelines for the introduction of community care policies. The net effect of the White Papers was the emergence of a new philosophy of care that was based on the idea that the responsibility for care should be shared with consumers and that, wherever possible, care should be provided as close to the person's home as possible. The introduction of community care has had a dramatic effect on the nature of care and on the provision of services for most client groups who require medium- to long-term assistance, including young people, older people and

Activity 8.9

Discuss with your friends whether social policies tend to discriminate against specific groups in society, for example, young people or ethnic minorities.

those with a learning disability or mental health problems.

Assessment of need and care management

Assessment and care management are the core changes associated with the implementation of community care in the UK. A comprehensive assessment enables an accurate and objective identification of the needs of dependent individuals. Having clearly identified the existence of needs, a care manager is able to provide a comprehensive range of services, a care package, and where possible restore the independence and autonomy of the person. Since the introduction of community care in 1990, all patients who are not self-funding must receive a full assessment from a care manager or care coordination team. Assessment is the cornerstone to identifying individuals whose needs require further assessment or intervention, or identifying more complex needs that remain unmet. The White Paper *Working for Patients* (DoH 1989a) advised that a needs assessment should determine the development of a programme for overcoming individual deficits and must focus on what the individual is able to do independently. An assessment of need is not an exercise in determining the suitability of a user for a particular service. Instead it is a process involving active consideration of the wishes of the individual and the primary carer and of the carer's ability to provide care and then to respond in a creative and innovative way to ensure that these needs are addressed (DoH 1989a).

Having put in place a comprehensive system of assessing the needs of dependent and frail older people, local authorities also provided a strategy for the provision of care. The Griffiths Report (Griffiths 1988) suggested that social services tended to slot people into a limited number of inflexible and traditional services that often failed to satisfy their needs. The report went on to provide guidelines for implementing, among other changes, the idea of care management. It proposed that a care management system should respond flexibly and sensitively to the needs of clients and their informal carers and allow for a range of options to permit choice when selecting services. Intervention is only necessary to foster independence and to prevent deterioration (paragraphs 3.1–3.26). A reiteration of this definition appeared in the government's acceptance of care management as the way forward for community care policy in the White Paper *Caring for People* (DoH 1989b).

Care management emerged in North America as a mechanism for assisting people to obtain the best and most appropriate care from an extensive range of health and social care agencies (Beardshaw & Towell 1990). In the US model the care manager is not a professional but rather an independent broker or advocate acting on behalf of the client between health and social care agencies or informal carers of dependent relatives. The policy guidance for the implementation of care management (DoH 1991, p. 23) suggested that care management should meet three objectives:

1. to ensure the effective utilisation of available resources
2. to focus on restoring individual independence with the ability to live in the community
3. to promote choice and empowerment in individual decision making.

Care management within the UK community care programme operates at the interface between the user and the service provider. It involves the construction and implementation of a package of services that will meet the identified needs of the patient following a rigorous user and informal carer assessment (Audit Commission 1992). The White Paper *Caring for People* (DoH 1989b) states that care managers are facilitators of care. They ensure the provision of care rather than providing the service. Unlike the position in the USA, the care manager is usually a health or social care professional assigned to this role. Care management is expected to adopt a *needs led* strategy as a replacement for a *service led* organisation. A service that is needs led should be able to respond more flexibly and creatively in assisting people (Audit Commission 1992) (Activity 8.10).

Activity 8.10

Consider the benefits for frail older people and people with disabilities in conducting an assessment and arranging a care package for them.

Services in the community

The NHS and Community Care Act (1990) established a new framework for the provision of health and social services in the UK. The Act, along with the preceding White Papers (DoH 1989a, 1989b) and the Griffiths Report (Griffiths 1988), facilitated a change in the mix of service provision between the voluntary, private and statutory sectors. These changes aimed to enhance the cost-efficiency of services and increase the choice of care available to the public (Nolan & Caldock 1996). It is clear that care should not be measured in terms of eliminating disease, but by the effect it has on the individual's ability to fulfil certain roles and activities of daily living (Reed & Watson 1994).

Hospitals

Throughout the last two decades there has been a steady decline in the number of hospital beds designated for the provision of long-term care for frail or disabled people (DoH 1994a). According to national statistics, within the UK between 1985 and 1994 there was a net loss of approximately 20 000 long-term hospital beds, which is approximately a 35% reduction (DoH 1994b). A similar net loss has occurred in the number of psychogeriatric hospital beds; these fell by about 5000 between 1991 and 1994 (DoH 1994b). The introduction of community care has therefore facilitated the development of new and supportive services and at the same time allowed Trusts to reduce the amount of long-term hospital care for sick and disabled people. Nevertheless, hospitals do retain a vital role in the care of dependent individuals, but the focus of care is directed towards rehabilitation and to provide support for community-based services through the provision of respite and palliative services.

Day centres

In the context of older people and individuals with differing disabilities, day care services offer a wide range of services. Day centres are able to assist in alleviating many of the physical, psychological and emotional problems that can make it difficult for individuals to continue to live at home. They also assist in improving the quality of life among frail and disabled individuals as well as providing support for carers. Day centres have close links with health and social care professionals who are able to access them more easily and provide support for residents during their stay (Booth & Waters 1995).

Day centres also promote the idea of interagency cooperation between the many different providers of services (statutory, private and voluntary health and social care service, social security, housing authorities, recreational services and other voluntary organisations). Patterns of care can thus be better coordinated and gaps or overlaps can be eliminated (Brearley & Mendelstam 1992). Aside from the opportunity of company and regular meals, people who attend a day centre can engage in a range of social activities including bingo and craft exercise. They can also avail themselves of support provided by visiting or on-site services such as hairdressing, chiropody and occupational therapy.

Residential and nursing homes

Residential and nursing homes in the private sector for older people and many other forms of disability have, since the early 1990s, assumed the role once held by local authority homes and long-stay hospital wards. Compared to 1973 the amount of money allocated as income support for residents in private nursing homes rose from £10 million to £2374 million in 1993 and the number of claimants increased from 12 000 to 268 000. This amounted to a per capita support of £8800 in 1992–3. Residential and nursing homes have become particularly influential in meeting the needs of frail older people. The number of older people entering private residential and nursing homes each year was about 60 000 in 1983 compared to 92 000 in 1994 (Laing & Buisson 1994). Laing & Buisson (1994) estimated that about 8500 of these older people were self-funding and the average length of stay for each resident was thought to be about 2–3 years.

Darton and colleagues (1991) carried out an independent study of older people who were resident in private residential and nursing homes. This study confirmed that there were similarities in the levels of disability between residents in nursing homes and in residential care. Darton's study conceded that, for the most part, the levels of dependence among residents living in nursing homes was higher than their counterparts in residential accommodation. Dependency levels were measured in terms of individual ability to carry out self-care tasks, the existence of physical disability or disease, and the presence of incontinence, antisocial behaviour and mental confusion. In Darton's study, among the nursing home residents, 14% could walk a distance of up to 200 metres compared to 36% of those in residential homes; 22% of nursing home residents were more or less totally immobile compared to only 4% in residential homes; and 38% of residents in nursing homes were experiencing problems with elimination compared to only 16% of those people living in residential homes. The study demonstrated that nursing homes tended to provide care for a larger proportion of frail older people with severe disabilities, although significant minorities of residents in both forms of service were in equal need of care and support. In their discussion about the survey, Darton and colleagues (1991) focused on the existence of this minority to form an argument that questioned the need for different forms of care. They also took the view that continuity in care is as important in planning services as the need for appropriate placement.

People who require care in a residential home are supported in an environment wherein they can live as independently as possible, with respect, dignity and security. However, this does not guarantee the older person long-term security of residence because there is a proviso that if the older person becomes too dependent then they must transfer to a nursing home. It is possible to avoid compulsory relocation if the local community nursing service contractually agrees to provide the required nursing support. However, since the implementation of the community care and statutory assessments, the likelihood of this happening has decreased. On the one hand, the statutory assessment provided before admission ensures that the older person qualifies for a specific service. If the older person selects an alternative service, this can compromise any agreed assistance with funding. On the other hand, George & Snell (1993) found that the number of older people moved to a nursing home because of deterioration in their condition remained quite small.

George & Snell (1993) also argue that there have been moves towards providing more homes that are multipurpose. In the longer term, this should contribute to the elimination of this problem. The increase in the number of nursing and residential homes that occurred throughout the 1980s began as an alternative to traditional long-stay hospital care and to statutory managed old people's homes. However, since the introduction of community care it is becoming more evident that their role requires further integration with existing community-based services. In doing so, the care that is provided within these facilities will take on a more active function and the stereotype that has grown around them as miniature forms of institutional care will, in the longer term, gradually disappear.

Home care services

Home support services for frail older people and people with other forms of disability have developed considerably from the traditional services that were once limited to a home help, a district nurse, a general practitioner and a social worker. Throughout the last two decades, the government has pursued a programme of policies to enable increasing numbers of dependent people with higher levels of disability to continue living at home. To achieve this the government has engaged from the statutory, private and voluntary sectors an extensive range of professional and non-professional personnel to provide services for disabled and frail older people.

The White Paper *Caring for People* (DoH 1989b, paragraph 11), placed as a priority: 'the promotion and development of domiciliary, day and respite services to enable sick and dependent people to continue living in their own homes wherever possible and sensible'. The document further suggested that pre-existing services had worked against such objectives, and it went on to state that, 'in future, the Government will encourage the targeting of home-based services on those people whose need for them is the greatest'.

Home care teams provide support, advice and information, including housing, benefits and home help services. Additionally, in some areas, as part of a home care package, home care teams provide meals on wheels, warden schemes, luncheon clubs and sometimes social centres (Waters 1996). The Office of Population, Census and Surveys reported in 1995 that home care assistants represented the largest domiciliary service, nationally, for older people. The report showed that they provided assistance with basic activities of living for approximately 3% of all older people aged between 65 and 75 years who were living at home and 18% of all of those aged over 75 years (OPCS 1995).

Voluntary services make a vital contribution to the needs of frail and dependent people living at home. For example, organisations such as the Fold Housing Association and Age Concern contribute through the provision of sheltered accommodation, supervision and alarm services. These organisations have also extended their range of services to include day care services, home care services and practical support in repairing, renovating or adapting older people's homes. Trusts give financial assistance and advice to some voluntary organisations and assist in the purchase of buildings, vehicles for transporting clients and professional support where necessary. Local groups and church groups also provide assistance to reduce the social isolation of dependent individuals as well offering support for carers.

Activity 8.11

Discuss with your colleagues what more could be done in terms of service provision for disabled and frail older people to help them become fully integrated members of society.

For many relatively independent people this sort of service provides a chance to be of use or to talk about loss and this may be more important than other physical or financial needs (Activity 8.11).

PRIMARY HEALTH CARE: A NEW DIRECTION

The WHO's official launch of primary health care as an internationally recognised and accepted mechanism for providing health and social services took place at the Alma Ata conference in 1978. During the first few years that followed the Alma Ata conference, the UK government moved very slowly towards its implementation. There was a view that the introduction of primary health care required only rudimentary adjustments to the existing health and social services. However, throughout the 1990s there has been a growing realisation that the introduction of primary health care would lead to root and branch changes to all health and social care services. Inter-agency and professional collaboration will provide an important underpinning for health and social services as they develop a commitment to the maintenance of public health and the prevention of disease, alongside their traditional association with the treatment of disease.

The first phase of the government programme for refocusing the National Health Service towards primary health care began in the mid-1990s. The Department of Health created a revised role for health authorities and published guidance to the essential elements of their new function (NHSME 1994). Health authorities were instructed to

Activity 8.12

Visit your library and borrow the government White Papers (DoH 1996a, 1996b,) outlining the plans for implementing a health service structured around primary care. Make short notes about the main recommendations and then organise a debate with your colleagues to discuss the merits or otherwise, of this policy.

continue to assess health care needs, implement local strategies, develop partnerships with local agencies and monitor the quality and effectiveness of service delivery. The guidelines also required health authorities to agree priorities with general practitioners and with local people and agencies in order to meet the needs of a community through a GP-led purchasing of services.

The government also launched a series of White Papers. Together these documents formed a framework for the government's intentions with regard to the creation of a National Health Service that is structured around the concept of primary health care (DoH 1996a, 1996b). The White Papers proposed that managerially the NHS should encourage teamwork, flexibility and inter-professional partnerships to maximise knowledge and expertise. The government argued that improved teamwork would enable the most appropriate professionals to take the lead in organising care for specific groups, such as frail older people. In doing so, services would become more sensitive and better able to meet the actual needs of clients (Activity 8.12). In the foreword for one of the White Papers (DoH 1996a), the Health Minister, Mr Dorell, stated that 'among the key demands made by professional staff during the consultation period was a call for partnership and community development to create a seamless service'.

NEW LABOUR AND INTER-AGENCY COOPERATION

When the Conservative government introduced community care, significant funding was set aside as a community care grant to aid its implementation. An additional £140 million was also allotted to local districts for the same purpose. Despite this extra funding, resources remained limited and insufficient and there is increasing evidence that community care is proving difficult to implement. A survey undertaken by the *Observer* newspaper in March 1997 revealed that local authorities are finding it harder to meet their commitments to older people who are in need of any form of social support. The survey reported that services in East Sussex have not increased commensurately with the increase in need. This means that the offer of home care support (or a place in a private nursing home) has become dependent on an existing recipient no longer requiring that service.

Other regions in the *Observer* survey reported substantive reductions in day centre services, home care support, transport arrangements and closures of statutory residential accommodation. To offset the effects of these financial restraints several councils are opting for two measures. They are increasing the eligibility criteria through which people qualify for assistance and are introducing charges (day centre meals, emergency on-call systems or transportation). A report by the Audit Commission (1997a) supported the findings of the *Observer* survey. The Audit Commission's report identified significant depreciation in social support services for frail older people. It also stated that the number of people over the age of 75 years who received assistance had fallen by 1% from the previous year.

On election in May 1997, the new Labour government committed itself to further develop primary health care. According to the government's first White Paper, *The New NHS* (DoH 1997), primary health care is the preferred mechanism for the organisation of services. The government asserted that it offered the best way of meeting the long-term care needs of dependent members of society, especially frail older people. The White Paper (DoH 1997) described the government's future intentions for the NHS. First, integrated care should replace the internal market. Second, equity should be encouraged in the provision and accessibility of care as a means of improving the quality of the care. Third, the development of primary care groups would harness the expertise of skilled practitioners, such as community nurses and general practitioners, together to meet health and social care need. Fourth, the government would remain committed to the promotion of research or evidence-based care. Concurrent to these proposals the government also launched a major investigation, via a Royal Commission, into the needs of frail older people.

ROYAL COMMISSION ON OLD AGE

Secretary of State for Health Frank Dobson established the Commission in 1997 and appointed Sir Stewart Sutherland as chairperson. The Commission's terms of reference were to examine the short- and long-term options for a sustainable system of funding and the provision of care for older people, both in their own home and in other settings. The Royal Commission's report, entitled *With Respect to Old Age*, was published on 8 March 1999 (Royal Commission on Long Term Care 1999). In the report the Commission arrived at a number of overall conclusions and recommendations, some of which are particularly influential concerning the broader policy of meeting the needs of dependent individuals (Box 8.2 lists a selection).

From the beginning of the Commission's work, the membership identified a lack of available information with regard to the total expenditure on care for older people by all of the various agencies. The Commission recommended an improvement in the availability of reliable, consistent and universally acceptable data in order to inform debate and identify problems in providing services. One such problem was the apparent overlap between health and social care services for frail older people.

The Commission argued that an overlap in the division of services has caused a degree of confusion among health and social care staff with regard to their areas of responsibility. To ameliorate this, it proposed the introduction of an intermediary service called personal care. Personal care is described as care that directly involves touching an older person's body, but is distinct

---

Box 8.2 **Some of the recommendations of the Royal Commission on Long Term Care** (1999)

- For the UK, there is no 'demographic time-bomb' as far as long-term care is concerned and, as a result, the costs of care will be affordable.
- Private insurance will not deliver what is required at an acceptable cost, nor does the industry want to provide that degree of coverage.
- The costs of care for those individuals who need it should be divided between living costs, housing costs and personal care.
- Personal care should be available after an assessment and should be paid for from general taxation.
- The government should establish a National Care Commission to monitor longitudinal trends, represent the interests of consumers, encourage innovation and set benchmarks, now and for the future.
- Further research on the cost-effectiveness of rehabilitation should be a priority.
- There should be an increase in the amount of care given to older people in their own homes. The role of housing will become increasingly important in the provision of long-term care.

---

both from treatment and other forms of indirect care such as home helps or the provision of meals (Royal Commission on Long Term Care 1999, paragraph 6.43). The Commission suggested that personal care should be available when the fundamental needs of a frail older person (e.g. bathing, mobilising or dressing) also involve further issues such as intimacy, personal dignity, prescribed care or confidentiality.

This clearly identified area of care has nurtured considerable debate between health and social services. Although this service is very much part of the world of nursing, in reality it is often delivered by people who are not nurses. The Commission proposed that the provision of personal care should be free at the point of use and decisions about how, when and by whom it should be provided would be discussed during the course of the older person's assessment of need. The report of the Royal Commission proposed that the introduction of personal care would require periodic review and, if necessary, its boundaries should be adjusted. First, this would eliminate the difficulties in separating an older person's need for health care from social care, and second, it would support the further development of a seamless service and encourage interdisciplinary collaboration.

The Commission accepted the need for an increase in joint working arrangements between health and social care staff. It did not agree with a suggestion that these two forms of service should become a singular and integrated structure. It examined and supported the integrated arrangements that currently exist in Northern Ireland but believed that formal integration across the remainder of the UK is unnecessary. The Commission took the view that the guidelines for further collaboration between services, contained within *Partnership in Action* (DoH 1998), and the development of primary care Trusts provide sufficient scope to enable flexible and cooperative working practices.

The Royal Commission recognised that, for the near future, there will remain a need for some forms of institutional care. It commended the high standard and quality of care that is provided by nursing and residential homes and other supported dwellings, but proposed that they pursue a greater community focus. The Commission believed this would help to reduce many of the negative attitudes currently associated with institutional living (paragraphs 17–35). In retaining this form of service, the Commission accepted that a minority of frail older people would continue to require protection from the extreme effects of isolation and loneliness. However, it went on to make clear its overall view of services for frail older people, stating that, 'with appropriate safeguards, care in the home is feasible and should be available for as long as possible, for most frail older people' (paragraph 6).

The primary function of the Royal Commission's report was to inform government of a possible direction for policy that could lead to a modernisation of the current system of funding the care of frail older people. In meeting this aim, the Commission's recommendations also represent a new relationship between government and society. The Commission believed that the recommendations were a means of ensuring that the services for older people would become

 Activity 8.13

List five reasons why the government set up the Royal Commission on Long Term Care.

Find out what the terms of reference were for the Commission team.

Write a brief resume of the major administrative changes and services that will be in place for disabled and frail older people by the year 2003.

more effective and would promote social cohesion and inclusiveness among all generations (p. 19). To this end, it recommended the setting up of a National Care Commission to represent consumer interests in monitoring the implementation of the Commission's proposals. The Health Committee supported this idea and suggested that a Care Commission should also assume responsibility for promoting further policies that would ensure a qualitative improvement in the lives of frail older people.

The government's response to the proposals contained in the Commission's report was published in July 2000. Most of the recommendations were accepted, and a planned 2-year programme of implementation was set to commence in the autumn (DoH 2000) (Activity 8.13).

PRIMARY HEALTH CARE GROUPS AND HEALTH EDUCATION

The introduction of primary care groups provides a further opportunity to address the health and social care needs of frail older people living in the community. Primary health care groups (PHGs) will contribute to extending the availability of supportive services for the very frail and thus further reduce the need for institutional care for some of these people. The report of the Royal Commission proposed that primary care groups should become the contact point for frail older people. It also recommended that PHGs should assume the responsibility for the process of assessment and assume responsibility for the commissioning of care (Royal Commission on

Long Term Care 1999). Whether this is achievable, especially in terms of ensuring objectivity in the provision of services, remains to be seen.

The issues of health promotion and the prevention of disease for older people and other dependent people has been addressed in the past by government, but the two issues have been less evident as a combined strategy. Age Concern (1992) argued that the White Paper failed to address the health promotion needs of older people satisfactorily. Age Concern believed that older people should have been identified as an important group and that they should have been allocated appropriate resources to respond to a range of specific issues (cancer screening, incontinence, the prevention of osteoporosis and strokes, and dementia).

The Audit Commission anticipated that the demand for health education among frail older people and other dependent groups would increase as the policy of primary health care develops (Audit Commission 1997b).

This view is supported by the government in the proposals contained in *Partnership in Action* (DoH 1998). The government contends that health care should re-focus towards the prevention of ill health among frail older people and improve the rate of detection and treatment of presenting conditions. These publications also address other issues such as:

- providing quality care and services for frail older people through the development of preventative measures (e.g. health education programmes)
- the need for partnership between agencies, local communities and individuals.

The government believes that the establishment of 'healthy neighbourhoods' is an appropriate way of creating such services for frail older people. According to the consultative report *Better Government for Older People* (DSS 1998), the concept of a 'healthier neighbourhood' proposes the development of integrated strategies for the provision of services for frail older people. The planning of integrated strategies should involve older people, personal social services and health

services (DoH 1997, 1998; Royal Commission on Long Term Care 1999).

CONCLUSION

The study of policy examines both formal decisions and actions. A decision by itself is not an action; the result of that decision is the action. What happens in practice may be different from what was intended by decision makers, indeed the implementation of a policy may have the reverse effect of what was intended, so the implementation of a policy can be as important as how that policy was decided on in the first place. Policy implementation may involve a number of decisions as opposed to one main decision, or it may be the selection of one possibility from a number of others. A policy may be chosen not for its effectiveness at alleviating a problem, but often for its cost-effectiveness. Policy tends to be defined in terms of a number of decisions which, taken together, comprise an understanding of what the policy is. Along with this, policies can, for various reasons, change over time. Yesterday's policy goals may not be the same as today's; policy can change as perceived attitudes change, or due to those previous goals having been met. After a mass vaccination programme has been carried out, for example, and the number of cases of the disease has reduced to a tiny amount, then there is no need to continue the policy on such a massive scale.

Along with policy implementation there is policy stagnation. This is where political activity is concerned with maintaining the status quo and resisting attempts to upset the apple cart by re-allocating existing resources to what may be seen as an unpopular policy. The promotion of good health and the prevention of disease require the creation of a social and economic environment within which people can live healthier lives. In order for this to come about they must be able to exert the necessary pressure on local and central government to ensure the provision of health education, proper nutrition, safe water, basic sanitation and adequate housing in addition to the preventative, curative and rehabilitative services that the health service already provides (Gormley 1999).

REFERENCES

Abraham C, Shanley E 1992 Social psychology for nurses: understanding interaction in health care. Edward Arnold, London

Age Concern 1992 Other people's money. Age Concern, London

Audit Commission 1992 Community care: managing the cascade of change. HMSO, London

Audit Commission 1997a Local authority indicators. HMSO, London

Audit Commission 1997b The coming of age: improving care services for older people. HMSO, London

Beardshaw V, Towell D 1990 Assessment and case management: implementation of caring for people. Kings' Fund, London

Bennet K R 1992 The sociological self. In: Kenworthy N, Snowley G, Gilling C (eds) Common foundation studies in nursing. Churchill Livingstone, Edinburgh, pp 59–74

Booth J, Waters K R 1995 The multifaceted role of the nurse in the day hospital, Journal of Advanced Nursing 22: 700–706

Bond J, Bond S 1994 Sociology and health care, an introduction for nurses and other health care professionals, 2nd edn. Churchill Livingstone, Edinburgh

Brearley P, Mandelstam M 1992 A review of literature 1986–91 on day care services to elderly people: a report prepared by the Disabled Living Foundation for the Social Services Inspectorate. HMSO, London

Brown M, Payne S 1994 Introduction to social administration in Britain. Routledge, London

Cooke H 1993 Why teach sociology? Nurse Education Today 13: 210–216

Corbett T M 1995 The nurse as a professional carer. In: Ellis R B, Gates R J, Kenworthy N (eds) Interpersonal communication in nursing. Churchill Livingstone, Edinburgh

Darton R, Sutcliffe E, Wright K 1991 Private and voluntary residential and nursing homes: a report of a survey by the Personal Social Services Research Unit and the Centre for Health Economics. Personal Social Services Research Unit, University of Kent at Canterbury

Department of Health 1989a Working for patients. Comnd 55. HMSO, London

Department of Health 1989b Caring for people: community care in the next decade and beyond (comnd 849). HMSO, London

Department of Health 1991 The health of the nation. Cmnd 1523. HMSO, London

Department of Health 1994a Bed availability for England: financial year 1993–94. HMSO, London

Department of Health 1994b The F factor: reasons why some older people choose residential care. HMSO, London

Department of Health 1996a Primary care: delivering the future. Cmnd 3512. HMSO, London

Department of Health 1996b The NHS: a service with ambitions. HMSO, London

Department of Health 1997 The new NHS. White Paper. Comnd 3807. HMSO, London

Department of Health 1998 Partnership in action: new opportunities for joint working between health and social services. HMSO, London

Department of Health 2000 The NHS plan: the government's response to the Royal Commission on Long Term Care. HMSO, London

Department of Social Security 1998 Better government for older people: a consultative report. HMSO, London

Dubos R 1960 Mirage and health. Allen and Unwin, London

Gahagan J 1980 The foundations of social behaviour. In: Radford J, Govier E (eds) A textbook of psychology. Sheldon Press, London, pp 577–601

George S L, Snell P H 1993 Is there consensus on the placement of older adults? Public Health 107: 97–100

Giddens A 1993 Sociology, 2nd edn. Polity Press, Cambridge

Gormley K (ed) 1999 Social policy and health care. Churchill Livingstone, Edinburgh

Gomm R 1982 Health as a social product. In: Gomm R, McNeill P (eds) Handbook for sociology teachers. Heinemann Educational, London, pp 86–92

Griffiths R 1988 Community care: an agenda for action. HMSO, London

Groenman N H, Slevin O D'A, Buckenham M A 1992 Social and behavioural sciences for nurses. Campion Press, Edinburgh

Helman C G 1992 Culture, health and illness, 2nd edn. Butterworth-Heinemann, Oxford

Laing W, Buisson J 1994 Care of elderly people. Laing and Buisson, London

Lynman M J 1992 Towards a goal of providing culturally sensitive care: principles upon which to build nursing curricula. Journal of Advanced Nursing 17: 149–157

Mann M 1983 The Macmillan student encyclopaedia of sociology. Macmillan, London

Martin B, Belcher J 1986 Influence of cultural background on nurses' attitudes and care of the oncology patient. Cancer Nursing 9(5): 230–237

Mead G H 1934 Mind, self and society. University of Chicago Press, Chicago

NHS Management Executive 1994 Developing NHS purchasing and GP fundholding: towards a primary care-led NHS. HMSO, Leeds

Nolan M, Caldock K 1996 Assessment: identifying the barriers to good practice. Health and Social Care in the Community 4(2): 77–85

Office of Population Censuses and Surveys 1995 Population trends. HMSO, London

Parsons T 1951 The social system. Routledge and Kegan Paul, London

Reed J, Watson D 1994 The impact of the nursing model on nursing practice and assessment. International Journal of Nursing Studies 31: 57–66

Royal Commission on Long Term Care 1999 With respect to old age: long-term care, rights and responsibilities. HMSO, London

Smith J P 1981 Sociology and nursing, 2nd edn. Churchill Livingstone, Edinburgh

Spicker P 1995 Social policy themes and approaches. Prentice Hall/Harvester Wheatsheaf, Hemel Hempstead

Titmuss R 1963 Essays on the welfare state. Allen and Unwin, London

Townsend P, Davidson N 1982 Inequalities in health: the Black report. Penguin, Harmondsworth

Waters J 1996 How care in the community has affected older people. Nursing Times 92: 29–31

Winefield H R, Peay M Y 1980 Behavioural science in medicine. Allen and Unwin, London

FURTHER READING

Elston M A 1997 The sociology of medicine, science and technology. Blackwell, Oxford
This text discusses in detail the impact of technological development on health and social care provision.

Fraser D 1984 The evolution of the British welfare state, 2nd edn. Macmillan, London
This text provides a useful analysis of the emergence of health and social care services in the aftermath of the Second World War.

Giddens A 1993 Sociology, 2nd edn. Polity Press, Cambridge
This text provides a critical view of some of the important sociological concepts and their value to an ever-changing society.

Lynan J 1992 Towards the goal of providing culturally sensitive care: principles upon which to build nursing curricula. Journal of Advanced Nursing 17: 149–157

Porter S 1998 Social theory and nursing practice. Macmillan, London
This text provides a useful critique of the position and function of nursing in society and as part of the health and social services team.

3 Fundamental nursing principles and skills

SECTION CONTENTS

9. The nurse as communicator   253

10. The nurse as health promoter   279

11. Accountability in practice   309

12. Evidence-based practice   331

13. Nursing theory and nursing care   365

14. Safe nursing practice   391

15. Caring for the person with pain   457

16. Palliative care and care of the dying   483

9 The nurse as communicator

Andy Betts

CHAPTER CONTENTS

The importance of communication in nursing 254
    The nurse–patient relationship 255
    The inevitability of communication 255
    Relating 255

The complexity of communication and potential for misunderstanding 256
    The nurse's relationships 257
    Personal flexibility 257

What is communication? 257
  Channels of communication 258
  Modes of communication 259
    Different modes for different uses 259
    Channels of non-verbal communication 259

Self and communication 261
    The conscious and the unconscious mind 261
    Self-awareness 262
    Increasing self-awareness 262
    Learning about self, relationships and communication through reflection 263

Matching communication to different contexts 263
    Taking action 264
    Advising 265
      Principles of giving advice 266
    Challenging 266
      Principles of challenging 266
    Teaching 267
      The educational role of the nurse with patients and carers 268

      The educational role of the nurse with colleagues 268
    Clinical supervision 268
Informing 269
    Principles of giving information 269
    Use of accessible language 270
    Giving and receiving feedback 270
Counselling skills 271
    Defining counselling 271
    Counselling within the context of nursing 271
    Requirements for effective counselling 271
    From dependence to independence 272
    Focusing on the personal world of the patient 272
    Commitment 273
    Listening and responding skills 273
Supporting 275

Conclusion 276

References 276

Further reading 277

The United Kingdom Central Council for Nursing Midwifery and Health Visiting (UKCC) states that, to be 'fit for practice', a registered nurse must be competent to 'engage in, develop and disengage from therapeutic relationships through the use of appropriate communication and interpersonal skills' (UKCC 1999). At the end of this chapter the reader will be able to:

- discuss the importance of communication in nursing
- integrate the behavioural and relational aspects of communication in a nursing context
- identify evidence-based enquiry relating to problems in nursing communication
- discriminate between the different verbal and non-verbal channels of communication
- reflect on her own use of communication skills using critical incidents and a communication diary (Activity 9.1)
- relate communication theories to nursing in her selected branch
- summarise the different types of therapeutic communication
- relate the significance of self-awareness and reflection to communication.

THE IMPORTANCE OF COMMUNICATION IN NURSING

Nursing, by definition, takes place in the presence of others and can be viewed as essentially an interpersonal process (Peplau 1988). If one accepts this perspective, then nurses' competencies and sensitivity as communicators will largely determine the effectiveness of nursing care, wherever it takes place. This is recognised by the UKCC in its recently published core competencies for entry to the Nursing Register (UKCC 1999).

This chapter addresses these communication skills and is grounded in the belief that we can

 Activity 9.1 Communication diary

It is highly recommended that readers start and maintain a communication diary to enable reflection on critical and personally significant interactions, both as a participant and as an observer. This will prove useful in some of the other activities included in this chapter.

all become more effective communicators than we are today. The pursuit of effectiveness in communication is a frustrating process; frustrating because it is lifelong and everyday experiences remind us of just how complex and elusive effective communication actually is; frustrating because to become more effective requires that we first realise our inadequacies. There is a risk in only perceiving communication as a repertoire of skills, so that the activity is reduced to an over-mechanistic process (Hartrick 1997). The contents and activities of this chapter are designed to achieve a balance between the behavioural and relational aspects of nursing communication. The relational element is an acknowledgement of the phenomenological or subjective nature of human encounters. In other words, the nurse and the patient are unique individuals, with their own constructed views of the world, who bring their perceptions, values, interpretations and experiences to any interactions.

A view is sometimes expressed that communication skills are more significant in mental health nursing than other specialities. This would seem to undervalue the significance of communication with other client groups and implies that relating to patients is not central to nursing. It is certainly the case that mental health nurses engage in complex relationships in their working lives, but communication is equally as important for all of the other care groups. Nurses working in an intensive care unit (Activity 9.2) or in an operating theatre still require sophisticated communication skills, as do nurses trying to relate to an individual with severe learning disability or to families in a children's ward. Each context has its own challenges but a consistent feature is the need for effective communication. It follows from

Activity 9.2

Consider a nurse caring for an unconscious patient in an intensive care unit. Why is it important that this nurse is an effective communicator? Think of aspects of the nurse's role that require effective communication skills.

these general remarks that nurses are expected to take seriously the communication aspects of their work and to develop key professional communication skills alongside more obvious practical or technical competence.

Contextual and demographic changes impact on the nurse as communicator. The significantly rising ageing population presents a challenge for nurses. Older people often feel isolated in society and, if they are to be included and heard in a comprehensive health system, a shared responsibility lies with nurses and other health care professionals. Shorter stays in hospitals and an emphasis on a community-based service also change the context of nursing communication. Hospital staff often express the view that they have insufficient time to get to know the patients and community staff sometimes feel they have insufficient time to meet the demands of increasing caseloads. Communication between hospital and community, and between different community agencies, largely dictates whether community care works or does not work. The other demographic change concerns the increasing multicultural diversity of society in the UK. This, too, presents challenges to nurses in respect of communication.

The nurse–patient relationship

It has become commonplace to say that nursing has shifted its emphasis from the treatment of illness in a patient to the treatment of the patient as a person who happens to be ill. The implication of this shift is that both nurse and patient are now seen as people who bring their full humanity to their relationship, the quality of which contributes significantly to the therapeutic

effectiveness of any treatment the patient receives. This can be both reassuring and daunting for a nurse: reassuring, because *all* personal resources, and not only the competence achieved as a direct result of training, are relevant to the professional role; daunting, because there is no opting out of recognising the relevance of the nurse's whole personality and behaviour to the treatment of a patient.

The inevitability of communication

Human beings have a basic drive to relate to one another which is expressed through communication. When two or more people are together they cannot help but communicate (Watzlawick et al 1968). It is difficult to imagine strangers on a train sitting together for any length of time without some form of communication taking place between them, even if no one speaks. Smiling is a communication, as is not smiling. One cannot *not* communicate as there is no opposite of 'behaviour'. All behaviour has message value even when this is not consciously intended, and once a message has been sent it cannot be retracted.

Relating

Babies cannot survive without someone relating to them. Their bodies are made out of the bodies of their closest relatives. Their capacity to be fully human in an emotional sense is realised through relationships with others. As children mature, this external relating gradually becomes internalised, so that the quality of their earliest relationships with others profoundly affects the way in which they relate to themselves. In turn, this inner world of relating is projected onto the outside world, affecting the way they relate to other people. It is helpful for a nurse to be aware of this basic pattern of relating and of how the present is built on the past.

The human need to relate remains fundamental and universal. It does not go away with time or maturity. Its very intensity and permanence give rise to the multifarious ways in which it is expressed – in love, in sex, in marriage, in friendship, in work, in social activities, in sport, in religion – and is the glue that holds families, communities, organisations and nations together. It can also be suppressed or hated. Nevertheless, the 'me–you' issues of life never go away; they determine our happiness and sense of fulfilment.

THE COMPLEXITY OF COMMUNICATION AND POTENTIAL FOR MISUNDERSTANDING

Shortcomings of both intimate and work relationships are often similar, centering around poor communication: not being listened to, not knowing what is going on, not being valued for one's individual self, not being taken into account. Statements such as 'We live in the same house but we just don't communicate' or 'No one tells me anything around here' suggest the feelings of anger, frustration and even helplessness that are aroused by poor communication. They also show that sending a message is not, in itself, communication. The message has to be received and understood by the receiver for communication to take place. Perhaps it is not surprising that users of the NHS have consistently highlighted dissatisfaction with communication. Indeed, it seems there is a significant correlation between the general satisfaction of patients and their specific satisfaction with nursing communication (Ricketts 1996)

Many studies have identified communication problems in the delivery of health care (some of the most influential are listed in Box 9.1). Nurse education has responded to these findings to some extent but there is no room for complacency (Activity 9.3). The reasons for the problems are complex and often specific to the area being researched but include: lack of skills and training; lack of resources and time; emotional vulnerability; the location of power; and even some deliberately perpetuated bad practices between agencies. This has to be seen within the complicated and elaborate network of relationships with patients, colleagues, informal carers and multidisciplinary agencies (Fig. 9.1).

Box 9.1 A summary of influential research into communication and health care

1972 Stockwell found that nurses viewed some patients as 'unpopular' and spent less time with them.

1975 Hayward established a relationship between the amount of information patients have and the amount of pain they experience.

1979 and 1985 Faulkner reported on levels of patient dissatisfaction with communication generally.

1980 Menzies-Lyth noted that nurses sometimes maintain emotional distance from patients and close down interactions with them as a defence against their own anxiety and stress.

1980 Gerrard and colleagues established that patients were more critical of the interpersonal dimension between patients and staff than any other facet of experience in hospital.

1981 and 1984 Macleod-Clark noted poor information giving, insufficient listening time, an overemphasis on factual information and the use of inaccessible language. These were seen as symptomatic of tactics that discouraged communication.

1988 Ley reported a dissatisfaction rate with communication in an average of 37% of patients.

1990 Bradley & Edinberg observed that many nurses preferred to maintain communication in a one way direction. They thought that this was done partly to retain control over communication and to save time to do other tasks.

1991 Burnard & Morrison found that many nurses self-rated their facilitative communication skills as less well developed than their authoritative skills.

1991 Davis & Fallowfield reported common specific failings in the communication skills of health care workers, such as a failure to elicit available information, worries, expectations; acceptance of imprecise information; failure to encourage questions; neglect of covert/overt cues provided by patients; avoidance of personal information; failure to elicit information about feelings, perceptions of illness; a directive style; failure to provide enough information; lack of empathy.

1991 Graham described a breakdown in mutual respect among some health and social care disciplines resulting in intentional failure to communicate on occasions.

1992 Wilkinson recognised that nursing environments were often not conducive to open communication even if the nurses were highly skilled in it.

1995 Brereton suggested that the increased emphasis on communication in nursing curricula had less influence on developing practitioners than did the socialisation process in clinical areas.

1995 Hewison highlighted the power dimension inherent in the nurse-patient relationship that constituted a barrier to open and meaningful communication and that nurses exert power through the use of language, persuasion and terms of endearment.

Activity 9.3

Consider the research listed in Box 9.1 that has high-lighted different failings in communication in the NHS. Based on your own experiences, is this a realistic or over-pessimistic picture today?

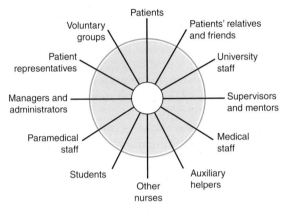

Figure 9.1 A web of relationships.

The nurse's relationships

Figure 9.1 gives a general picture of the variety of relationships that a nurse is likely to have. The nurse's relationships with such a wide range of people give rise to a need for the sensitive use of a variety of communication styles, depending on the context and position of the other person or persons involved. Young children have normally not acquired the capacity to make the subtle judgements needed to adopt appropriate ways of communicating in different circumstances. Such naivety is charming in children but less so in adult professionals.

Consider the dimensions of communication identified in Figure 9.2. Any communication is likely to be biased towards one end of each dimension, depending on the context and the people involved. For example, a doctor who says, 'And this patient's blood pressure?' is likely to expect an answer of objective information rather than an expression of personal feelings about the patient's treatment.

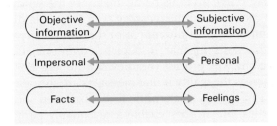

Figure 9.2 Dimensions of communication.

Personal flexibility

Some people are flexible in their use of different communication styles and manage to respond to different contexts in an appropriate way. Others find it difficult to adjust so that, for example, they always talk impersonally and factually even when an expression of feelings and subjective views is of pressing importance. Another person might be emotional and subjective when a cool look at the facts is what is really needed. The multifaceted role of the nurse within a complex social context necessitates nurses' flexibility in matching the appropriate communication to the individual(s) and the set of circumstances.

The way in which we communicate can be seen as dependent on our whole personality. Certainly, what is communicated between two people is a product of the interaction of the three basic components: sender, receiver and message (see Fig. 9.3). A patient who is asked the question 'How are you?' by two different nurses might pick up quite different meanings. From one, it might be an empty phrase, said perhaps while the nurse was attending to something else. From the other, it might be a genuine empathic enquiry into the patient's thoughts and feelings at the time. Which message is received will depend on the patient processing all of the information available. The judgement about the meaning of that information will depend on the patient's own expectations and personality.

WHAT IS COMMUNICATION?

As stated above, communication has three funda-mental components, all of which are necessary for it to live up to its name: these are the sender, the receiver and the message (Fig. 9.3). This diagram does not fully represent the complexity of interactions in that it depicts communication as a one way process (Bradley & Edinberg 1990), whereas the reality is that messages are simultaneously going back and forth between both parties, but it does enable a reasonably simple analysis. The message is encoded into a symbolic representation of the thoughts and feelings of the sender and then, in turn, decoded and interpreted by the receiver. Communication is judged as successful when the received message is close enough to that of the sender. The potential for things going wrong at any of these stages is considerable. The coding of the message is achieved through a number of channels.

CHANNELS OF COMMUNICATION

Because of the power of human language, it is easy to equate the message with words and overlook other ways in which we communicate, for example with our bodies, with posture, with gestures, and with tone of voice and intonation. Non-verbal communication consists of all forms of human communication apart from the purely verbal message (Wainwright 1985). While verbal communication is perceived mainly through the ears, non-verbal communication is perceived mainly through the eyes, although it is occasionally supplemented by other senses.

Humans are the only species to have developed elaborate systematic language and we tend to concentrate on verbal messages. Other species use sound, colour, smell, ritualistic movements, chemical markers and other means to transfer information from one member to another. Scientists are constantly discovering how complex and subtle are communication systems, even in the lowliest of species, and how necessary these systems are for survival. Non-verbal communication is often of a more primitive and unconscious kind than is verbal communication, and powerfully modifies the meaning of words.

In face-to-face communication, verbal and non-verbal channels are open and carrying information. When they give a consistent message (congruence), the receiver is likely to receive the message at face value as being sincere. When there are inconsistencies, non-verbal communication is normally taken to be more reliable than the words spoken (Case example 9.1). This is summed up in the cliché 'Actions speak louder than words'. We commonly hear people say: 'It's not so much *what* he said, it's *how* he said it', or 'Even though she's tough with you, you know she really cares'.

The subtlety of human communication arises from the interplay of these various channels. The capacity to be ironic or sarcastic, or to mean the opposite of what is said, depends on the exploitation of this rich resource in human communication.

Case example 9.1 Incongruence in communication

As David prepared to leave the acute psychiatric ward where he had spent the past 3 weeks, everything that he said to the nurse suggested that he was confident about managing his own life after his discharge home. Despite David's words, the nurse sensed that, far from being confident, David was actually apprehensive about leaving the ward. At first, the nurse was unsure of the basis for this interpretation but when asked to justify the assessment by a colleague, realised what had been observed. David had avoided eye contact by looking down at the floor, he was hesitant in packing his belongings and, as he turned to leave, his shoulders dropped slightly and he adopted a heavy posture as he walked away. It was the non-verbal communication that reflected his true feelings, and David was given the opportunity to talk about his fears and address the issues involved before being discharged.

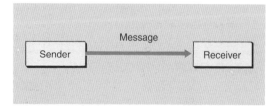

Figure 9.3 The three components of communication.

MODES OF COMMUNICATION

Not all communication is face-to-face with all channels open. Consider the variety of communication modes that a nurse might use in the course of a day's work:

- rules and procedures
- memos
- reports
- letters
- information technology (email, discussion forums, internet sites)
- telephone calls
- face-to-face contact.

Written rules of procedure or safety regulations may be referred to as impersonal and faceless, because they are sent from 'the authorities' to a generalised person of no particular identity. A memo can have personal or impersonal qualities, depending on whether it is sent from one person to another or is of a general nature. A report is a more formalised method of information-sharing and may be written to selected individuals or for general access. A letter is more commonly a communication between two individuals, the writer having in mind a particular person when it is written, though it can, of course, also be generalised and public.

Information technology is increasingly being used as a method of communication in all walks of life. It may take the form of direct messages, such as electronic mailing systems, or data files that are accessible to others. There are an increasing number of nurse discussion forums which offer topical debate and information on contemporary issues. A telephone call allows for the immediate interaction that is missing from the written word, so that the message is not only in *what* is being said but also in *how* it is said. If a telephone message is written down, it is reduced to the verbal channel only, thus losing the meaning carried by the other channels. Only in face-to-face contact are all channels open. That is why, when important matters are being discussed, there is no substitute for face-to-face meetings. Lovers have always known this!

Different modes for different uses

Everyday experience shows that we gradually learn the subtleties of each mode of communication and use them to suit our purposes. Making a complaint about an aspect of one's health care, for example, is most easily done for some people by writing a letter, so that the complainer is in sole charge of the language used. Another person might prefer the fuller contact of a telephone call but avoid face-to-face encounter. All of this points to the complexity of human communication.

Channels of non-verbal communication

Use of touch

Touch has been said to:

- connect people
- provide affirmation
- be reassuring
- decrease loneliness
- share warmth
- provide stimulation
- improve self-esteem.

On the other hand, not all touch is interpreted positively, even when so intended by the nurse (Davidhizar 1997). Because of these potential positive or negative effects, nurses need both to understand touch and to value the ability to use it therapeutically. Touch, in a nursing context, may be either instrumental (which includes all functional touch necessary to carry out physical procedures such as wound dressing or taking a pulse) or expressive (used to convey feelings). Nurses are unusual in that they are 'licensed touchers' of relative strangers. This legitimised transgression of the normal social code requires that nurses are sensitive to the reaction of patients.

Cultural uses of touch vary from country to country. Murray & Huelskoetter (1991) note that cultures such as Italian, Spanish, Jewish, Latin American, Arabian and some South American countries typically have relationships that are more tactile. Watson (1980) identifies England, Canada and Germany as countries where touch is more taboo. These cultural differences in social codes heighten further the need for sensitivity when judging if touch is appropriate. Whitcher & Fisher (1979) found that the use of therapeutic (expressive) touch by nurses preoperatively produced a positive response to surgery among female patients, but not males. There is some evidence that males may perceive touch differently to females in relation to aspects of status or dominance (Henley 1977) (Activity 9.4).

Proxemics

Proxemics refers to the spatial position of people in relation to others, such as respective height, distance and interpersonal space. Hall (1966) originally identified four different interactive zones for face-to-face contact and considered anything less than 4 feet as intrusive of interpersonal space in most relationships other than intimate ones. The four zones are used differently according to the topic of conversation and the relationships of the participants. Patients in hospital settings may not perceive that they have any real personal space. French (1983) suggests an area 2 feet around a patient's bed and locker could be viewed as personal space. One's spatial orientation and respective height to the other person are also significant and should be considered when engaging with others.

Posture

Posture conveys information about attitudes, emotions and status. For example Waxer (1997)

Activity 9.4

Reflect on any recent experiences that involved you touching patients.
Determine if your touch was instrumental or expressive.
How sensitive were you to how the patient interpreted your touch?
Consider the respective age, gender, ethnic background and social class of the patients and yourself.
How appropriate was your touch?

suggests that depressed and anxious patients can be identified purely by non-verbal communication. A person who is depressed is more likely to be looking down and avoiding eye contact, with a down-turned mouth and an absence of hand movements. An anxious person may use more self-stroking with twitching and tremor in hands, less eye contact and fewer smiles. Of course the nurse's posture carries just as many social messages. The ideal attending posture to convey that one is listening has been variously described in the literature (Egan 1998).

Kinesics

This includes all body movements and mannerisms. Gestures are commonly used to send various intentional messages, particularly for emphasis or to represent shapes, size or movement, or may be less consciously self-directed and sometimes distracting to others. Head and shoulder movements are used to convey interest, level of agreement, defiance, submission or ignorance.

Facial expression

Facial expressions provide a running commentary on emotional states according to Argyle (1988), and Ekman & Friesen (1987) identified six standard emotions that are universally recognisable across all cultures by consistent movement of combinations of facial muscles, namely happiness, surprise, anger, fear, disgust and sadness.

Gaze

Eye contact is a universal requirement for engagement and interaction. In Western society listeners look at speakers about twice as much as speakers look at listeners (Argyle 1988), although there are cultural variations to this. When people are dominant or aggressive they tend to look more when they are speaking. The absence of eye contact may indicate embarrassment, disinterest or deception.

Appearance

Our self-presentation makes statements about our social status, occupation, sexuality and personality.

Activity 9.5

Think about your chosen branch of nursing and the different contexts in which it takes place.

How does the wearing of a uniform affect relationships with others?

What are the advantages and disadvantages of wearing uniforms in these different settings?

Activity 9.6 Observation of channels of communication

1. Next time you are in a public area, take time to observe the non-verbal messages that are being used. Identify the channels and functions of the messages that are exchanged.
2. If you have access to recording equipment, arrange to both audiotape and videotape a short conversation with a fellow student. Replay the interaction in the following order:
   – audiotape (alternatively you could listen to the videotape, facing away from the TV)
   – videotape with the sound turned right down
   – videotape with the sound.

Make notes as you replay each stage. In particular, contrast the different stages, noting limitations of the first two playbacks. Identify how meaning is changed by additional data.

Some aspects of appearance can be easily manipulated, for example our dress and hairstyle, but other features are beyond our control, such as height. Both types of presentation communicate messages about who we are. Nurses have often discussed the merits and disadvantages of wearing a uniform. Uniforms and other forms of regalia make nurses easily identifiable to others and provide additional information about seniority and qualifications. In some contexts uniforms may be seen to present a barrier to establishing therapeutic relationships by reinforcing the power of the professional in the relationship (Activity 9.5).

Paralanguage

Paralinguistics includes those phenomena that appear alongside language, such as accent, tone, volume, pitch, emphasis and speed. It is these refinements of the lexical content that provide meaning to spoken communication. It is possible to use the same actual words but with contrasting paralanguage and convey an entirely different meaning.

Physical environment

The nature and organisation of the physical environment in which any communication takes place will have significant impact on the interaction. One clear example is the difference between visiting patients in their homes and nursing them in a hospital ward. The experience for both parties is significantly altered. This example sheds some light on issues of power and control. The nurse has less control over the environment in the patient's home setting and is a guest. Hospital buildings are unusual settings for most patients and provide consistent reminders that the health care professionals are in control of the environment to a large extent. Wilkinson (1992) recognised that nursing environments were often not conducive to open communication, even if the nurses were highly skilled in it. Making the most strategic use of facilities available according to the nature and purpose of the exchange is an important aspect of nursing communication.

All of the above are extremely important and may constitute up to 90% of communication taking place. They do of course occur in combinations with each other, not separately as above (Activity 9.6). The various functions of non-verbal communication are summarised in Box 9.2.

SELF AND COMMUNICATION

The conscious and unconscious mind

Another distinction is between the conscious and unconscious aspects of the psyche. Put simply, the conscious mind is aware that it knows; the

Box 9.2 The functions of non-verbal communication

- To replace speech. A meaningful glance, a caring touch, a deliberate silence. Also specific symbolic codes such as Makaton.
- To complement the verbal message. The main function and used to add meaning to speech. If we say we are happy we are expected to look happy. We use gestures to provide clarification and emphasis.
- To regulate and control the flow of communication. We generally take turns in conversation by prompts indicating 'I am finishing – you can take over'. Some may use non-verbal communication to dominate.
- To provide feedback. We monitor others' non-verbal communication to interpret their reactions, e.g. are they listening, worried? Have they understood? There is evidence that patients place great emphasis on non-verbal communication because of the technical nature of some verbal messages given by health carers (Friedman 1982).
- To help define relationships between people. An example is the wearing of uniforms in hospital settings to indicate role, function and status.
- To convey emotional states. Emotions and attitudes are recognised primarily on the basis of non-verbal communication.
- To engage and sustain rituals. Argyle (1988) identified an additional function, namely ritualistic. Certain meaningful behaviours are expected at ceremonies such as weddings and graduations.

unconscious is not aware that it knows. Sigmund Freud was the first to study the unconscious mind seriously and has greatly enriched our understanding of human nature, although many of his views are still controversial. The common experience of not knowing why we do things, or of saying things contrary to our conscious wishes, suggests the working of the unconscious mind as, of course, do dreams.

Self-awareness

One reason why communication may be ineffective is lack of awareness of aspects of ourselves which significantly affect our interactions with others. Facets of ourselves which are beyond our consciousness are also beyond our control and may adversely impact on the best of intentions. Aspects of ourselves which inevitably affect communication consist of attitudes, values, beliefs,

feelings and behaviours. Increasing self-awareness in these domains is likely to result in more productive interactions and a more intentional use of self. This increased self-understanding serves to convert potential pitfalls into potential assets.

These ideas require commitment to continual self-exploration, growth and development. Greater self-awareness nearly always results in an individual being clearer about what feelings and thoughts originate from his internal world, in contrast to what has originated from other people. Such clarity makes personal responsibility more realistic.

The realisation that the image that one has of self may contrast greatly with how one is perceived by others is significant learning and lies at the heart of development as a communicator. Each individual constructs a subjective view of the world which is different to how others perceive it. This subjectivity, plus the fact that our behaviour is partly unconsciously motivated, means that nurses, who are directly involved in interpersonal relationships, need to maximise their self-awareness and conscious use of self. Stein-Parbury (1993) states:

Nurses need to develop acute self-awareness whenever they engage in interactions and relationships with patients, because the primary tool they are using in these circumstances is themselves. Without self-awareness nurses run the risk of imposing their values and views onto patients.... Through self-awareness nurses remain in touch with what they are doing and how this is affecting patients for whom they care. (p. 60)

Increasing self-awareness

Rogers (1967) emphasised the view that the degree to which we understand ourselves is the degree to which we are able to understand and help others. The first point to make is that this is a pursuit of the unachievable. The idea that we achieve complete self-awareness on a certain day sounds ridiculous. The concept of self-awareness is best thought of as a continuum. The lifelong task is to inch our way along that continuum in the realisation and acceptance that we will never reach the end. This progress is achieved through introspective processes such as reflection, self-exploration and self-assessment and by interactive activities such as self-disclosure, discussion and feedback.

Burnard (1985) defines self-awareness as a process:

> self awareness refers to the gradual and continuous process of noticing and exploring aspects of self, whether behavioural, psychological or physical, with the intention of developing personal and interpersonal understanding ... to have a deeper understanding of ourselves is to have a sharper and clearer picture of what is happening to us. In a sense it is a process of discrimination. (pp. 15–16)

Case example 9.2 illustrates this process in action.

Learning about self, relationships and communication through reflection

Since Schon (1983) coined the term 'reflective practitioner' it has appeared frequently within nursing literature. The suggestion is that nurses incorporate 'reflection' into their practice, but confusion exists regarding the meaning of the word. Boud and colleagues (1985) state succinctly that 'reflection' in this context refers to 'turning experience into learning'. This is a purposeful and conscious activity requiring structured time and effort rather than an automatic process. Different methods can be used to achieve this such as introspection, writing,

Case example 9.2 Increasing self awareness (from Betts 1995)

Julie, a student on the learning disabilities branch, watches the replay of a video recording of herself interacting with a fellow student. She is both fascinated and disconcerted by what she observes. Seeing herself from the outside presents a contrasting image to her 'internal' view of herself.

She notices repeated mannerisms which previously she had no idea she used. She is able to check out later with her peers how they had experienced these behaviours and is not too surprised to discover that others had perceived them as a distraction. As a result of this experience Julie is aware of aspects of herself which were previously beyond her consciousness. This learning experience has increased her options and further refined her capacity to communicate effectively with others.

discussion or clinical supervision. One common misconception of reflection is that it consists purely of historical analysis (Fig. 9.4). Kemmis (1985) stresses that reflection is not an end in itself but that it leads to informed, committed action. Development as a reflective communicator eventually leads to the ability to process what is happening during an interaction rather than only after it has finished. Accurate processing of communication as it occurs increases options and results in a more intentional use of self. Schon (1983) referred to processing experiences as they happen as 'reflection in action' and retrospective reflection after the event as 'reflection on action' (see Fig. 9.4).

For some people, reflective writing is productive as a medium for the recording and analysis of interactions. The use of learning journals or communication diaries to record, analyse and evaluate specific experiences may suit some people. Walker (1985) suggests that writing provides an objectivity and clarity to experiences by removing elements of subjective feeling that can obscure issues. These written records also provide data for further review in tutorials, supervision sessions or with peers (Activities 9.1, above, and 9.7). Some examples of reflective questions are given in Box 9.3.

MATCHING COMMUNICATION TO DIFFERENT CONTEXTS

On a conscious level, communication is concerned with making choices. Effective communicators have a high success rate of making appropriate choices in the situations that are

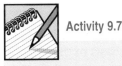

Activity 9.7

During your next placement keep a communication diary. Record any significant interactions in which you are involved, or that you observe. You may find it helpful to use the questions in Box 9.3 to reflect on the personally significant interactions in which you were involved.

Figure 9.4 Three dimensions of reflection (adapted from Betts 1995).

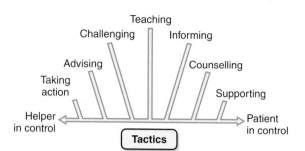

Figure 9.5 Strategies for helping. Adapted from the NICEC (National Institute for Careers Educational and Counselling) model.

Box 9.3 Examples of reflective questions (adapted from Betts 1995)

What was the context of the interaction?
What was the purpose of the interaction?
What actually happened?
What were my behaviours, thoughts, feelings at the time?
What were the other(s)' behaviours?
What do I imagine were the other(s)' thoughts and feelings at the time?
What were my thoughts and feelings afterwards?
What do I imagine were the other(s)' thoughts and feelings afterwards?
How successful was the interaction?
What skills did I use well/not so well?
Given the opportunity, how would I do it differently?

Case example 9.3 Adaptability as a prerequisite for effective communication

Simon is an experienced nurse on a children's ward. He is the supervisor of a common foundation programme student who is on placement. The student is required to write up observations of nurse–patient interactions to meet the learning outcomes of one of the modules.

What impresses the student about Simon is his versatility as a communicator. At one point he demonstrates a close rapport with a 6-year-old girl, and at another he listens attentively to the concerns of a worried mother. The student notices that Simon matches his intervention to the individual in a seemingly effortless manner. He recognises when it is appropriate to advise or give information to patients and relatives, and also when it is more appropriate to encourage self-disclosure or emotional expression through the effective use of counselling skills.

The student reflects on the crucial importance of developing the ability to be adaptable and intentional in nursing interactions and hopes to achieve Simon's level of competence, judgement and confidence.

---

encountered because they are clear about the aims or purpose of each interaction (Heron 1990). This decision process requires sensitivity and empathic understanding to read the situation accurately and respond appropriately. The nurse's choice of intervention is determined by the needs and resources of the other person at the time.

Nurses are likely to choose to use any one of the range of helping strategies illustrated in Figure 9.5 (TACTICS) according to context. From one extreme tactic of 'taking action' to the other extreme of 'supporting', the basis of the helping relationship changes by degrees from 'helper in control' to 'patient in control'. The issue of where the balance of control lies between helper and patient distinguishes one strategy from another and gives each its own special characteristics. None of these tactics or strategies is intrinsically

superior to others. The art of effective communication in nursing concerns diversity and choosing the appropriate strategy according to the needs of the patients or carers at the time (Case example 9.3).

TAKING ACTION

The taking action tactic implies that the nurse is working on behalf of the individual. This type of strategy is indicated when a patient is incapacitated through some aspect of ill health or loss of function. This type of communication is by nature directive. The rationale for such helping is founded in a judgement that patients are unable, temporarily or permanently, to perform an action or represent themselves. Consequently nurses need to either take this responsibility themselves or refer on to another who is more able to do so (Case example 9.4).

The decision to take action for others (to take control) is a significant judgement that should be based on careful consideration of all the factors. As a general principle, it is preferable to negotiate and empower patients in their own decision making, but situations arise where a more paternalistic approach is required in the interests of the patient.

Case example 9.4 Two situations requiring nurses to take action for others

Dean, a 21-year-old man, is in an intensive care unit (ICU). He has been unconscious for 2 days since his car accident. The chances of Dean surviving his injuries are slim. All of his physical care is undertaken by the ICU staff and the technical equipment that supports his functions. He is entirely reliant on the actions of others for his survival. The ICU staff are by necessity in total control. Even though he is unconscious, each of the nurses who attend to his physical needs converse with Dean as they go about their work, either giving information to explain their actions or just chatting to pass the time of day.

Maria has schizophrenia. She was admitted last night under an emergency section of the Mental Health Act, after being found wandering the streets, shouting at passers by and trying to get into people's houses. She is fearful that she is being followed by two women who are out to do her harm. Her psychotic state of mind makes it difficult for her to make rational decisions or to look after herself. The nursing staff consider her to be a danger to herself and to others on the ward. A nurse takes on the task of staying with Maria wherever she goes. This causes even more suspicion on Maria's part but the decision is made that she needs this constant observation to protect her from harming herself or others. There is no negotiation about this care plan because it is judged that Maria is not in a position to understand the reality of her situation. The nurses are taking action on her behalf until she is able once again to make decisions for herself. Despite Maria's acute illness, the nurse tries to begin to communicate with her in an attempt to establish some kind of relationship with her.

An alternative form of taking action for others involves an advocacy role for nurses. Gates (1994) defines advocacy as: 'the process of befriending, and where necessary representing a patient … in all matters where the nurse's help is needed, in order to protect the rights or promote the interests of that person' (p. 2). Nurses sometimes find themselves in a position to represent the patient's interests, for example in a multidisciplinary team meeting. Alternatively, for some issues it may be more appropriate to refer the patient to an 'outside' advocacy agency.

ADVISING

The most crucial aspect of giving advice is first of all to assess if advice is appropriate. Inappropriate advice-giving may have more negative consequences than doing nothing. Advice comes from the adviser's frame of reference and usually consists of what the adviser would do in the given situation. Stein-Parbury (1993) notes that offering advice and suggesting solutions is a common response to others who present problems. She warns that this response may be habitual rather than based on considered choice and that nurses may need to unlearn this customary response and refrain from their usual way of responding.

Inappropriate advice can undermine the self-determining competence of others and may also encourage dependence rather than autonomy. The other potential problem is that the advice may not work out well in practice, resulting in a loss of confidence in the nurse. As a general rule, advice is inappropriate in the case of personal issues but sometimes more appropriate in specialist issues. The medical model relies on the expertise of the doctor and sometimes views the patient as a passive recipient of advice who is expected to comply with the solution that is offered. This is changing, largely as a result of lobbying from patient and carer representative groups to move towards partnership and greater empowerment of patients in their treatment.

Having warned against excessive use of advice, there is clearly a need for such interventions within a nursing context. Consider the scenarios in Activity 9.8 and decide in each case if advice is appropriate or not.

Principles of giving advice
(Activity 9.9)

When advice is indicated there are a number of factors to consider. First, it is important to assess the person's level of knowledge and understanding of their situation along with their emotional and physical states. These will influence the starting point, the language used and the timing and amount of advice given. It is possible

Activity 9.8 To advise or not to advise?

Respond to each of the following scenarios, indicating if advice is appropriate or not – think carefully about why you arrive at the decision you make:

- A 21-year-old male university student, has an extreme episode of anxiety that is mainly related to his impending final examinations. He asks the community psychiatric nurse if he should give up his degree studies.
- A woman, caring for her partner who is recovering from a stroke, contacts the community nurse because she is struggling to help her partner transfer from the bed to a chair.
- A 10-year-old boy wants to know when he can start playing football again following an appendicectomy.
- A female resident with a learning disability lives in a group home and asks one of the care staff for advice about a sexual relationship she is considering starting with another resident.

Activity 9.9 Reflection on advice

Think of an occasion when you were given advice. Recall the context and nature of the experience. Reflect on the following questions:

- Was the advice appropriate at the time?
- How well was it given?
- How would *you* have delivered such advice if roles were reversed?
- Finally, in the light of your reflections, list what you think are the principles of giving advice effectively.

to prescribe advice at different levels. Heron (1990) identifies 19 different types of prescription, ranging from directive approaches through to more subtle influencing. This is a question of matching the level of influence to individuals and their circumstances and resources. Finally, it is important to evaluate the response to the advice, by judging the other's level of understanding and degree of acceptance or rejection of the suggestions.

CHALLENGING

Egan (1998) discriminates between the word 'challenge' and the term 'confrontation'. Many construe confronting and being confronted as unpleasant experiences, ones to be avoided. Egan (1990) defines challenge as 'an invitation to examine internal or external behaviour that seems to be self-defeating, harmful to others, or both and to change the behaviour if it is found to be so' (p. 184). Successful challenges increase awareness and promote insight by enabling others to come face to face with aspects of themselves or their behaviour. Heron (1990) emphasises that, in a helping context, challenge is a non-aggressive and non-combative intervention, unlike the meaning of the term in some other situations. Sensitive challenging is an advanced communication skill but necessary within the repertoire of strategies available to nurses. Case example 9.5 illustrates scenarios where challenging is appropriate.

Principles of challenging

There is a difference between a constructive and a destructive challenge. Constructive challenges throw a searchlight on alternatives and leave the other person with something on which to build or change. Destructive challenging is delivered unskilfully and leaves the other person feeling bad or put down, with nothing to build on. The goal is to raise the consciousness of unused strengths and potential.

Another principle of the effective challenge is specificity or being unambiguous about the focus

Case example 9.5 Challenging situations

During a particularly hectic shift on a children's ward, a nurse observes one of her colleagues expressing her frustration in an angry exchange with a 14-year-old male patient. The nurse thinks that her colleague's response is excessive and takes the opportunity at a quieter moment in the coffee room to challenge her about what happened. The firm but sensitive intervention highlights the unacceptable nature of the exchange without alienating the colleague.

Sarah, a 28-year-old woman, has been an in-patient on the mental health unit for 3 weeks. Her depression has started to lift and she is now more able to engage in therapeutic dialogue with one of the nurses. She talks about her life, in particular the things that have gone wrong. The nurse listens carefully and notices that there is a theme running through all of Sarah's life situations. She describes events as if she has no power or control over how things turn out. It is as if life is all down to fate rather than to choice. The relationships that have gone wrong and the missed opportunities she has experienced are the fault of others. She sees herself as a victim of circumstances with no resources to influence the outcomes of these situations. The nurse uses a skilful combination of empathy and challenge to bring into relief this pattern of victim that runs through Sarah's life situations. Together they explore ways in which Sarah could take more responsibility and control over life events.

of the challenge. To be clear about the message one wants to give rather than generalising.

Empathic understanding is a crucial element of challenging. This involves listening carefully to the other's perspective and acknowledging their position while encouraging an alternative. Challenging without empathy is brutal and destructive because it invalidates the subjective reality of the other person. Assertiveness is a feature of effective challenging. The message should have sufficient strength without being apologetic or over zealous. Aggression is destructive and passivity is ineffective. Non-verbal communication should be congruent with the spoken message, as suggested earlier in this chapter.

The context of the challenge is important, both in terms of timing and setting. The first scenario in Case example 9.5 demonstrates this well. The nurse did not challenge her colleague at the time

of the incident but selected a strategic moment and setting with the desired result. Finally, Egan (1998) suggests that effective challengers are open to challenge themselves by not immediately rejecting or disputing any challenge, but instead, clarifying and considering the alternative perspective before deciding how to respond.

TEACHING

There is an increasing recognition of the educative role of nurses. This role comprises the promotion of health and independence of patients, and the facilitation of learning of colleagues in a variety of contexts. The impetus for a change in emphasis away from patient compliance to co-operation between patients and health care workers (Council of Europe 1980) is partly dependent on nurses being skilled educators. Other initiatives such as the general raising of the academic profile of nursing, the introduction of clinical supervision and an emphasis on evidence-based practice require that nurses share knowledge and promote reflection throughout their careers.

Figure 9.5 locates teaching at the midpoint of the continuum of control. This position is indicative of the diversity of possible teaching approaches ranging from strategies that are authoritative in nature, where the teacher is in control, through to methods that are facilitative and leave more control with the learner. The authoritative approach assumes the teacher is expert and is concerned with imparting knowledge to a learner who is seen as a passive recipient of information. At the other end of the spectrum is the facilitative approach which is characterised by active participation on the part of the learner who engages in discovery and retains more control over the way that the interaction proceeds. The communication skills required of the educator are substantially different in each case. The former relies mainly on information giving and the latter on the softer or facilitative skills of the educator (Case example 9.6). Neither approach is superior to the other, but both are valid structures according to the aims, context and preferred learning styles of the participants.

Case example 9.6 Two contrasting styles of learning

In the school of nursing a session has been arranged in the large lecture theatre entitled 'An introduction to the nervous system'. Roughly 100 common foundation programme students will be attending. The nurse teacher only has a 60-minute time slot to address a list of learning outcomes relating to the topic. The large number of students, the limited time available and the nature of the content prompt the teacher to plan a 45-minute lecture using diagrams displayed from a data projector, leaving 15 minutes for any questions and clarification. A handout including recommended further reading is prepared for the session. The method of delivery will be didactic and consist primarily of factual information giving.

In the small classroom next door a learning disability teacher has a 90-minute session with a group of six students who are attending for a reflection day relating to their current placement. The learning outcomes are less precise and relate to the process as much as the outcomes of the session. The planned method is radically different to the lecture next door. The teacher is quite unobtrusive in the group conversation as different students are given the opportunity to recount their experiences on placement. The communication skills used are facilitative, mainly comprising listening, prompting and clarifying. A complex scenario is also used to stimulate a problem-based learning discussion. The session runs similarly to a group clinical supervision meeting.

The educational role of the nurse with patients and carers

As previously suggested, this function is an important element of nursing in all four branches. The work may involve teaching skills of self-care or preparing relatives to carry out tasks involved in caring for a patient. Orem (1985) believes that patients have a responsibility to maintain their own health by extending their self-care functions as necessary. She suggests that if an individual is unable to do this, the next logical care giver is an immediate family member or close friend. It is estimated that there are 6 million non-professional carers in the UK (NHS 2000). For many of these carers, nurses are the front line in terms of finding out information and gaining new skills in caring for their relatives.

There is a danger in teaching skills in isolation of the theory that informs the practice. For example, teaching a carer the practical skills of an aseptic technique with no attention to the principles of asepsis will not help the carer if, for some reason, he has to adapt the procedure due to a shortage of resources. This requires that nurses have some understanding of educational psychology and the principles and practice of teaching and learning.

The educational role of the nurse with colleagues

In addition to teaching patients and relatives, nurses have a responsibility to educate other health care workers. These may be students, health care assistants, other nurses or associated disciplines involved in health care delivery. A potentially confusing collection of terms are used to describe the various educative activities in this area, such as mentorship, preceptorship and clinical supervision. The topical emphasis on lifelong learning is a pertinent one within a career characterised by the rapid accumulation of new knowledge and continuous exposure to different experiences. With regard to learning, nurses cannot afford to stand still, irrespective of seniority or experience, a fact recognised by the UKCC in promoting the introduction of clinical supervision for all nurses on the Register.

Clinical supervision

Clinical supervision has been variously defined but there is a general agreement that it is a learning dialogue, for example the King's Fund states that it is: 'A formal arrangement that allows nurses, midwives and health visitors to discuss their work with another experienced professional ... [clinical supervision] involves reflecting on practice in order to learn from experience and improve competence' (Kohner 1994).

Proctor (1987) identifies three main strands to effective clinical supervision, namely formative, normative and restorative (Fig. 9.6). It is the formative element that explicitly acknowledges the learning function within clinical supervision, although, as previously stated, learning is integral

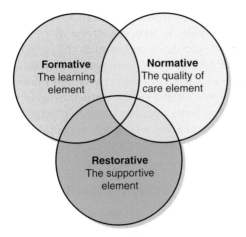

Figure 9.6 The three elements of clinical supervision (Proctor 1987).

to the whole activity. Clinical supervision is essentially a mechanism for reflection and can occur in pairs or groups. The educative skills required of the clinical supervisor are predominantly facilitative and are aimed at enabling the supervisee to explore, clarify and increase options. As clinical supervision becomes more established within the culture of nursing, the communication skills required of clinical supervisors can be seen as an important element in the nurse's role.

INFORMING

Many studies over the past 20 years have highlighted shortcomings of information giving in health care settings (see Box 9.1). Perhaps in such a large and complex system it is inevitable that the exchange of information is not always as good as it could be. The potential for information to get lost or become corrupted as it journeys between agencies, departments and individuals is considerable. We live in the information age, new technologies, better education, lobbying groups and increased expectations have resulted in greater and more immediate access to all kinds of information. The health arena is no exception and patients, carers and professionals rightly expect to receive relevant, accurate and understandable information. Information empowers patients and elevates them to partnerships in care, rather than passive recipients of treatment.

It is easy to confuse information with advice. On one level the distinction is clear in that information is neutral and non-prescriptive whereas advice involves suggesting or presenting solutions. On a second level things are more complex. The informer may believe that the message is given in a non-prescriptive way but may underestimate the social influence that is inherent in the way that it is given, or the very fact that it is provided by a person who is seen as an expert.

Principles of giving information

A starting point is to determine the other's readiness to receive information. Benner (1984, p. 79) considers that 'capturing the patient's readiness to learn' is an advanced judgement that is characteristic of expert nursing practice. This involves picking up and determining cues from patients to judge if, when and how much information should be given. This will vary with individual patients, some of whom will be eager to gather every scrap of information about their condition while others would prefer not to know very much at all. These same cues give indications of the timing of the information giving.

Having ascertained that information sharing is the appropriate intervention, it is important to clarify what the patient already knows and to assess the accuracy of this knowledge. This demonstrates that information sharing begins with open questioning rather than the imparting of facts and allows the informer to pitch the information at the right level and to keep it relevant. At this stage it may become clear that the type of information required means that a third party is in a better position to provide it.

When it comes to the actual information giving, there is some evidence that people recall opening statements (primacy effect) and attach high significance to these messages. This is particularly likely if the opening statement is emotionally significant to the patient, such as a confirmation of a diagnosis. An example of this is the confirmation of a positive HIV test result.

Staff working in this speciality have learned that the capacity to absorb information directly following the receipt of this news is poor. The need for follow-up interviews and back-up written information is clear in these circumstances. This relates to another working principle, to limit the amount of information to the capacity of the patient to absorb it. Too much detail can result in confusion and misunderstanding.

Use of accessible language

Health care jargon and technical language often exclude patients and carers from meaningful communication. Nurses are socialised to use a language that identifies them with other nurses. Gumperz (1968) states that they belong to a 'speech community' within which there is a sharing of verbal signs and professional jargon. Jargon, by definition, is an unfamiliar, restricted code to those who are external to the parameters of the specialism. It is basically used as a form of shorthand between professionals but sometimes used as an inappropriate style of speech with patients and carers (Kagan et al 1986). Case example 9.7 is illustrative of such an exchange. Usually this is not an intentional attempt to exclude, but a careless choice of words that may have the same effect. Taking time to clarify others' understanding of the information given and prompting for any questions usually resolves the issues.

Other examples of inappropriate language include times when assumptions are made by

Case example 9.7 Inappropriate use of language

Information given by a psychiatrist to a patient's partner:

'Your partner's symptoms are characteristic of a bipolar affective disorder. This condition is typified by fluctuating episodes of hypomania and periods of depression. Your partner's pre-morbid personality is cyclothymic, which is not uncommon in these cases. Symptoms are usually fairly well controlled by lithium carbonate, although neuroleptics or antidepressants may be required at certain times. Any questions?'

health care professionals that all people have literacy skills or that patients and carers from different ethnic backgrounds have sufficient English to understand what they are being told. Access to interpreters and to written information in different languages is more accessible than it was some years ago, but remains patchy in some geographical areas where different ethnic groups are not as well represented.

Giving and receiving feedback

Providing feedback to others is a refined communication skill that can fit into either the information or challenging tactic. Learning to provide constructive feedback adds value to many types of interactions, for example appraisal interviews, learning structures, clinical supervision, evaluations, meetings, patient and carer interactions in different settings. The principles identified in Box 9.4 apply in the giving and receiving of constructive extrinsic feedback.

Box 9.4 Principles of giving and receiving feedback (from Betts 1995)

Principles of giving feedback
- Be specific. A clear statement of what precisely was observed is more helpful than a wide generalisation.
- Achieve a balance. Highlight the strengths but also include aspects which require attention. Praise alone may make the person feel good but is not as helpful as balanced feedback.
- Offer possible alternatives. Comment tentatively on how things could have been done differently. Avoid dogmatic advice giving.
- Refer to behaviour rather than personal characteristics. Behaviour can be changed; personal characteristics cannot.
- If a contract exists, stay within its boundaries, i.e. if specific feedback is requested then this should be the focus of your comments.
- Think what your feedback says about you.

Principles of receiving feedback
- Have an open mind. Avoid becoming defensive, rejecting or argumentative.
- Ask for clarification.
- Listen, consider and decide what you will do in the light of the feedback.

COUNSELLING SKILLS

Defining counselling

Counselling is a professional activity in its own right, and it may be more appropriate in the nursing context to think of nurses using counselling *skills* rather than being counsellors to their patients. Each person brings his internal world and outward behaviour into a common space in which the counselling work is carried out. This can happen only if the space is protected from intrusion or distraction and the two people are engaging with each other in a voluntary way. In the past, for nurses, the word 'counselling' has been incorrectly linked to disciplinary procedures, and it is important to extract it from such a context and place it within the general framework of supportive one-to-one contact between people.

The basic aim of counselling is to help individuals help themselves. The British Association for Counselling (1992) makes the following comments on the nature of counselling:

The overall aim of counselling is to provide an opportunity for the client to work towards living in a more satisfying and resourceful way. . . . Counselling may be concerned with developmental issues, addressing and resolving specific problems, making decisions, coping with crisis, developing personal insight and knowledge, working through feelings of inner conflict or improving relationships with others. The counsellor's role is to facilitate the client's work in ways which respect the client's values, personal resources and capacity for self-determination.

The goal of counselling is to enable people to be in closer touch with their own resources so that they can move towards greater freedom, autonomy and independence. It assumes that any conflict or anxiety arising within the personal world of the individual can only be dealt with using the resources within that person. An individual may ask for help or advice from another person but until such assistance is actually accepted, it cannot be used for self-help.

Counselling within the context of nursing

Most nurses are not counsellors but are professional helpers whose work includes, to a greater or lesser extent, providing psychological support and assistance in problem solving to people who are experiencing a diversity of personally significant life events (Betts 1995). The British Association of Counselling (1990) states clearly that unless both the user and recipient explicitly contract to enter into a counselling relationship, then the helper is using counselling skills rather than counselling. A detailed examination of the use of counselling skills in nursing is beyond the scope of this chapter (for a more comprehensive account, see Betts 1995).

A frequent comment from health carers is that they do not have the time to engage in this type of helping. In these days of economic restraint and limited resources the counselling relationship may be viewed as costly in terms of human resources. An alternative perspective is that time spent using counselling skills may actually be less demanding of resources in the long term. If the interaction results in a more accurate understanding of the client's world, self-empowerment and independence, then this may be time profitably spent.

Requirements for effective counselling

Carl Rogers (1967) has suggested that for counselling to be effective, three core conditions are necessary:

1. empathic understanding
2. congruence or genuineness
3. unconditional positive regard.

These values are the foundation for a trusting relationship. Without trust in the capacity of clients to help themselves, the counsellor is joining forces with those who would keep the client exactly where he is. Respect for the client is linked to trust. It suggests that the individual's rights, beliefs and resources are respected for what they are, without judgement.

Empathic understanding

Empathy is often seen as the most critical ingredient of the helping relationship. Carkhuff (1970) argues that without empathy there is no basis for helping. Kalisch (1971, p. 203) defines empathy as: 'the ability to sense the client's world as if it were your own, but without losing the as if quality'. This short definition contains some complex ideas. Empathic understanding is often described as 'standing in somebody else's shoes', but this is not the full story. Imagine how you may feel at the end of a day if you stand in the shoes of each person you meet in your helping role – experiencing their thoughts and feelings. Empathy involves retaining your own separateness while trying to understand the world from the other person's perspective. In order to do this, it is necessary to understand the client's world as if you were inside it, attempting to see it with the client's eyes, but at the same time keeping in touch with your own world. In this way the helper remains in a position to help – to get close enough to the client's experience to make a difference while retaining a sense of objectivity in order to hold on to the process and not become overwhelmed.

Genuineness

This is sometimes referred to as congruence or authenticity. All three of these terms refer to the helper being consistently real in the helping relationship. Corey (1986) suggests that congruent helpers are without a false front and that their inner experience matches their outer expression of that experience and vice versa. In other words, what clients see is who the helper really is. Relating deeply to others is a part of the effective helper's lifestyle rather than a role that is switched on and off. Inauthentic helping may appear as 'plastic counselling', or cloned behaviour learned from a counselling trainer or textbook where helpers mechanistically use behaviours and responses that disguise their own integrity, personality and communication style. It is the very qualities that make the helper unique as an individual which serve the relationship. The nurse who switches into 'helping mode' upon the sight of an individual in distress may be perceived by the client as patronising and untrustworthy.

Unconditional positive regard

Unconditional positive regard refers to the idea that there should be no conditions laid down by the counsellor for his acceptance and care for the client. So often we are brought up to believe that we will be accepted if we are good, successful and pleasant, and rejected if we are bad, unsuccessful and unpleasant. The 'unconditional' nature of Rogers's approach means that we are accepted whatever we are, and in our entirety. 'Positive regard' is an attitude of optimistic expectation, stemming from the unconditional acceptance of the person. The three words together, if translated into practice, create a quality and atmosphere in the 'counselling space' that facilitates growth in clients, allowing them to get in touch with the more positive aspects of themselves over time, so that they become more able to help themselves. If we have been lucky, we have experienced the positive effect of someone else who is benign, who believes in us, who accepts us and who is on our side. Such experience releases the potential in us, which otherwise may have remained dormant and unrealised.

From dependence to independence

The paradox that is central to counselling stems from the basic human need to relate, the theme throughout this chapter. It is out of relating to another person that the individual is able to develop a surer sense of 'I, myself' – a common outcome of successful counselling. The individual can have no clear sense of identity without relating to others, just as he can have no real independence without having had, at some time, the experience of dependence.

Focusing on the personal world of the patient

The focus is on the person and the personal world, especially feelings. Nurses need to listen, think, imagine and feel in the counselling space between themselves and the patient, so that they get as good an idea as possible of what it is like to be that person, as he is, in the present. This empathy has a 'with you' quality about it, which goes beyond intellectual understanding and sympathy, concentrating as it does on 'being there' with and for the patient rather than 'doing something' for him. It enables the nurse to 'hold' a patient's fears and anxieties, without being tempted to try to give answers or solutions. The following exchange illustrates the quality of interaction referred to here:

Patient: Why did this happen to me?
Nurse: (Silence, then:) It's difficult to understand.
Patient: But why *me*?
Nurse: (Silence, then:) I can see how angry you feel.
Patient: That's not much use, is it?
Nurse: (Quietly accepting the expressed feelings.)

This kind of exchange allows for an acceptance of the patient's feelings (unhappiness and anger in this case) rather than brushing them aside, retaliating or referring to people who are worse off.

Commitment

All this requires a commitment to patients – to their well-being and best interests. A word such as 'commitment' can sound heavy and serious, but it describes quality rather than quantity. Such real human contact can happen over a few seconds of time or over a much longer period. In this type of intervention the nurse is available and open, rather than distant or insincere. It immediately becomes clear that such a commitment involves the resources of the inner private world of the nurse as well as skills and knowledge. It necessarily involves a willingness to be affected emotionally by the patient and to be somewhat vulnerable (which is often confused with being weak), but it also involves a certain toughness and resilience. It hardly helps the client if the counsellor is overwhelmed by the feelings that are expressed and becomes *too* involved, losing the objectivity that is also needed. There is an optimum 'therapeutic distance' between nurse and patient that allows the best possible helping to take place.

Listening and responding skills

These skills are transferable to all types of helping but are included in this section because of

their paramount importance in counselling interventions. What are now examined are the *skills* of communication, i.e. what nurses might actually do and how they might behave with other people, in practical rather than theoretical terms. It has been noted that a nurse might be called on to make contact with several categories of people during the course of a day: doctors, patients, fellow nurses, relatives. The focus in what follows is the particular relationship and communication between a nurse and patient. It is assumed that the nurse regards relating to the patient as part of the patient's total care.

The context in which an interaction takes place affects its content and quality. This seems obvious when gross differences are considered, such as the difference between talking to someone in a bar as opposed to in his own home, but more subtle differences may be overlooked, for example the contrast between a ward in a hospital and a day room: a move from one to the other may be beneficial. Community nurses may complain that the television set is left on during home visits, but they also find it difficult to suggest that it be turned off.

Certain features of the setting may militate against effective communication. The principles that are urged here are for nurses to be sensitive to the ways in which the setting affects any interaction, and for them to endeavour to make the most strategic use out of what are often far from ideal settings.

Listening and attending

To listen to someone with attention and commitment is a caring response that is all too rare. It is the basis of all effective communication on a one-to-one basis and requires hard work on the part of the listener. This work involves much more than accurate recording of what is said. It involves making accurate perceptions through several senses, looking for patterns and checking creative ideas against new information. It also requires flexibility and a willingness to give up preconceptions about the person in the face of the evidence. To some extent, listening and attending are insufficient in themselves. A further component involves the transmission of the message that one is listening and attending to the other person. This is achieved through a combination of verbal and non-verbal channels.

Silence

The possibility of silence is often referred to with anxiety by those wishing to help others. Paradoxically, the capacity to be comfortable with silence is often a good indicator of listening skill. It normally means that listeners are able to contain their own anxiety (if any) and to concentrate on the other person. The rush to 'help' another person with words or gestures is often misplaced and can have its roots in our attempt to deal with our own feelings of awkwardness. An acceptance of silence, on the other hand, can be an eloquent recognition of the patient's need for someone to *be* there rather than for something to be *done*.

Encouraging

Some people who are able to talk freely about their ideas and feelings need only the slightest encouragement to explore these further. This encouragement may be given by minimal prompts such as 'Mm' or 'Aha', a nod or smile, depending on the listener's own conversational style. Other people will falter without such feedback, needing reassurance before they continue talking. Some seem to need no encouragement at all, but a compulsive way of talking may indicate that real relating is difficult for the patient and may cover painful feelings.

Responding

The two empathic responding skills of paraphrasing and reflection of feelings are paramount to effective listening.

Paraphrasing. Paraphrasing consists of a repetition of the core message communicated by the other person translated into the listener's own words. This involves attention to the emphases and meaning of content of what has been said and allows for some personal interpretation and imaginative input on the part of the listener. It can often be helpful to use an image that catches the emotional force of the message: 'It's as

though you feel trapped, with no way out.' The patient may accept the image and elaborate further or may wish to modify it in some way to make it more suitable.

Reflecting. To reflect back to patients their own expressed emotional reactions is a potent form of empathic responding. It gives clear feedback that what has been said and felt has been received and understood. It lets the patient know that any implied message that has not been directly expressed has also been understood. The patient's question 'How long will I be in here, nurse?' may have several layers of meaning behind it. The nurse's answer, if the several layers have been successfully decoded, will reflect back something of the underlying feelings as well as giving a direct answer to the question. This response might be: 'It's normally about 3 days ... You seem a bit concerned about it.'

Summarising. Summarising what has been said after a suitable interval serves a similar purpose, i.e. consolidating information and verifying whether or not the sense the listener has made of it coincides with the intended message: 'Let me see if I've got this right. What you seem to be saying is ...'. To some degree a summary is an extended form of paraphrasing but requires a broader perspective. The key to effective summaries is a filtering process that highlights the significant experiences, reactions and themes expressed in the patient's dialogue. For patients to hear what they have just been saying in summary form from somebody else often feels reassuring but may also offer fresh insights as different experiences are connected in a thematic way, a process that Egan (1998) terms 'connecting islands'.

Asking open questions. Asking open rather than closed questions – as in 'Can you say a little more about how you felt when ... ', rather than 'Did you feel angry when ... ' – can help patients to explore their experiences. The first form of question makes a demand on patients to examine experience and to express it in their own language. The second invites a yes/no response, which is less exploratory and potentially less useful to the patient. Often students on counselling skills courses will start by assuming that asking a lot of questions of the individual will somehow help understanding. Such questioning may be a way of coping with the uncomfortable feeling of being unskilled by *doing* lots of things verbally. The idea that a timely open question indicates more skill in communication than does asking a large number

Case example 9.8 A dialogue illustrating listening and responding skills

The GP has referred Mr White to the practice nurse. Mr White has been under pressure at work over the past 18 months, resulting in a series of minor ailments and conflict within his relationships with his family. The GP thought that the nurse might be able to help with stress management strategies. The following dialogue is an extract from the interaction:

Practice nurse: How has this increased pressure affected you? (*Open question*)

Mr White: The worst part is that I feel tired all the time. When I get home in the evenings, I don't feel like communicating with my family. All I want to do is go to sleep. I used to be so full of life, but now I'm not much company.

Practice nurse: It's as if your batteries are run down and you have nothing left at the end of the day. (*Paraphrase – repeating back the core message in her own words*)

Mr White: Yes, but I feel so bad about it. I don't like what I'm doing, but I can't seem to stop it. It's not my family's fault, and I feel guilty about the way I treat them.

Practice nurse: So it's like you feel powerless but you still blame yourself for what is happening. (*Reflection of feelings*)

Mr White: I suppose it's like I'm putting my job before them. I'm sure my children see it that way … it's like a battle between work, and what's expected of me there, and my family …

Practice nurse: Mm, mm. (*Minimal encouragement*)

Mr White: It's such a difficult balance. If I slack off at work, I run the risk of losing my job, and that would be of no use to my family. If I don't, my family and my health suffer …

Practice nurse: (*Remains silent for some time – she can sense that the silence is far from empty*)

Mr White: It's like a no-win situation … I can't think how things could be improved.

Practice nurse: So far you have talked about the difficulty of balancing work and home life, of how exhausting your lifestyle is at the moment, and of how little control you seem to have over changing things. You seem to feel stuck and pessimistic about finding any solution. Is that how you see things? (*Summarising the main points that have been brought up and checking her understanding is accurate*)

of closed questions is difficult for the relative novice to accept. Of course, closed questions do have their place, such as requests for factual information during an admission interview.

Case example 9.8 illustrates some of the listening and responding skills in action.

SUPPORTING

Heron (1990) asserts that a supportive intervention is an exchange that affirms the worth and value of other people. He regards it as an attitude of mind that underlies all the different communication strategies previously mentioned. In many ways this relates to the values or qualities previously discussed such as unconditional positive regard, empathic understanding and warmth or respect. Rogers (1974) saw this type of helping as 'a way of being present with another person' and sometimes this is simply what is needed. Nurses are often required to be pragmatic and this can lead to an over-reliance on being active in doing things for patients. A pure supportive interaction is as much about *not* doing the things that are habitually accessible, but merely being present with another in a qualitative way as they experience their particular situation (see Case example 9.9). In some ways this tactic is simple, but the difficulty is learning as a professional helper that sometimes the most helpful intervention is to do nothing more than communicate one's presence to the patient or carer. In this spirit, the supporting tactic is placed

Case example 9.9 Being present as a form of supportive communication

Kelly is a 35-year-old woman with a learning disability. The extent of her learning disability is quite severe, although she can communicate verbally in a limited capacity. Kelly lives in a small community home and has recently been told by a relative that her mother has died following a long illness. Since receiving this news, she has spent most of the time alone and very quiet. Her isolation is plain for all to see. One of the female carers has a particularly close relationship with Kelly. She instinctively knows that Kelly's needs can be best met by just sitting with her, holding her hand and letting her know that she is with her as she goes through the pain of her recent loss.

at the extreme end of the continuum illustrating that the patient is in control.

CONCLUSION

With the increasing recognition of the patient as a person who happens to be ill, the therapeutic interaction is now being viewed as a combination of key communication skills and a human, personal relationship between two or more people, the quality of which significantly affects any treatment or caring interventions. These behavioural and relational aspects of communication, when combined, enable a therapeutic relationship to be established.

The communication process has three components – the sender, the receiver and the message – and for communication to take place, the message must be not only received but also understood. The style of the interaction will be influenced by personality, but nurses must be encouraged to be flexible to the needs and communication style of patients, colleagues and family, in order to strengthen their relationships with them.

The key factor in effective communication is making the right choice of intervention based on an empathic assessment of the individual, the situation and resources. It is possible to classify the available strategies using the acronym TACTICS, standing for: taking action, advising, challenging, teaching, informing, counselling and supporting. Having made the correct choice, nurses need to utilise developed micro-skills to ensure the communication is effective.

The nurse who is developing the quality of interaction within the work setting is one who has realised both the importance of communication skills and their place in professional effectiveness.

REFERENCES

Argyle M 1988 Bodily communication, 2nd edn. Methuen, London
Benner P 1984 From novice to expert: excellence and power in clinical nursing practice. Addison-Wesley, Menlo Park, CA

Betts A 1995 The counselling relationship. In: Ellis R, Gates R, Kenworthy N (eds) Interpersonal communication in nursing: theory and practice. Churchill Livingstone, Edinburgh
Boore J 1978 Prescription for recovery. Royal College of Nursing, London
Boud D, Keough R, Walker D 1985 Reflection: turning experience into learning. Kogan Page, London
Bradley J, Edinberg M 1990 Communication in the nursing context. Appleton-Century Crofts, Connecticut
Brereton M 1995 Communication in nursing: the theory–practice relationship. Journal of Advanced Nursing 21: 314–324
British Association of Counselling 1992 Code of ethics and practice for counsellors. British Association of Counselling, Rugby
Burnard P 1985 Learning human skills: a guide for nurses. Heinemann, London
Burnard P, Morrison P 1991 Nurses' interpersonal skills. Nurse Education Today 11: 24–29
Carkhuff R R 1970 Helping and human relations. Holt, Rinehart and Winston, New York
Corey G 1986 Theory and practice of counselling and psychotherapy. Brooks Cole, Pacific Grove, CA
Council of Europe 1980 European Public Health Committee. The patient as an active participant in his own treatment: final report. Council of Europe, Strasbourg
Davidhizar R, Newman J 1997 When touch is not the best approach. Journal of Clinical Nursing 6(3): 203–206
Davis H, Fallowfield L (eds) 1991 Counselling and communication in health care. Wiley, Chichester
Dickson D, Hargie O, Morrow N 1989 Communication skills training for health professionals: an instructor's handbook. Chapman and Hall, London
Egan G 1990 The skilled helper, 4th edn. Brooks Cole, Pacific Grove, CA
Egan G 1998 The skilled helper, 6th edn. Brooks Cole, Pacific Grove, CA
Ekman P, Friesen W 1982 Measuring facial movements with the facial action coding system. In: Ekman P (ed) Emotion in the human face. Cambridge University Press, Cambridge
Ellis R, Gates R, Kenworthy N 1995 Interpersonal communication in nursing. Churchill Livingstone, Edinburgh
Faulkner A 1985 The organisational context of interpersonal skills in nursing. In: Kagan C (ed) Interpersonal skills in nursing. Croom Helm, London
French P 1983 Social skills for nursing practice. Croom Helm, London
Friedman H 1982 Non-verbal communication in medical interaction. In: Friedman H, Di Matteo M (eds) Interpersonal issues in health care. Academic Press, New York
Gates B 1994 Advocacy: a nurse's guide. Scutari Press, Harrow
Gerard G, Boniface W, Love B 1980 Interpersonal skills for health professionals. Reston Pub. Co., Reston
Graham R J 1991 Understanding the beliefs of poor communication. Interface 11: 80–82
Gumperz J 1968 The speech community. International encyclopaedia of the social sciences, 2nd edn. Macmillan, London
Hall E 1966 The silent language. Columbia University Press, New York

Hartrick G 1997 Relational capacity: the foundation for interpersonal practice. Journal of Advanced Nursing 26(3): 523–528

Hayward J 1975 Information: a prescription against pain. Study of Nursing Care Project Reports. Series 2, No. 5. Royal College of Nursing, London

Henley N 1977 Body, politics, power, sex and nonviable communication. Prentice Hall, Englewood Cliffs, NJ

Heron J 1990 Helping the client. Sage, London

Hewison A 1995 Nurses' power in interactions with patients. Journal of Advanced Nursing 21: 75–82

Kagan C, Evans J, Kay B 1986 A manual of interpersonal skills for nurses: an experiential approach. Harper and Row, London

Kalisch B J 1971 An experiment in the development of empathy in nursing students. Nursing Research 20(3): 201–211

Kemmis S 1985 Action research and the politics of reflection. In: Boud D, Keough R, Walker D (eds) Reflection: turning experience into learning. Kogan Page, London

Kohner N 1994 Clinical supervision in practice. King's Fund, London

Ley P 1988 Communication with patients: improving communication, satisfaction and compliance. Croom Helm, London

MacLeod-Clark J 1981 Nurse–patient communication. Nursing Times 77: 12–18

Macleod-Clark J 1984 Verbal communication in nursing. In: Faulkner A (ed) Recent Advances in Nursing 7. Communication. Churchill Livingstone, Edinburgh

Menzies-Lyth E P 1980 The functioning of social systems as a defence against anxiety. Tavistock, London

Murray R, Huelskoetter M 1991 Psychiatric/mental health nursing. Appleton and Lange, Los Altos, CA

National Health Service 2000 Help available to carers from the health service. <http://www.nhs50.nhs.uk/healthy-atoz-i4011c230.htm> (accessed 16.7.00)

Orem D E 1985 Nursing: concepts of practice, 3rd edn. McGraw Hill, New York

Peplau H 1988 Interpersonal relations in nursing. MacMillan Education, Basingstoke

Proctor B 1987 Supervision: a co-operative exercise in accountability. In: Marken M, Payne M (eds) Enabling and ensuring. National Youth Bureau for Education in Youth and Community Work, Leicester

Ricketts T 1996 General satisfaction and satisfaction with nursing communication on an adult psychiatric ward. Journal of Advanced Nursing 24: 479–487

Rogers C 1974 On becoming a person, 4th edn. Constable, London

Rozelle R, Druckman D, Baxter J 1986 Non-verbal communication. In: Hargie O (ed) A handbook of communication skills. Croom Helm, London

Schon D A 1983 The reflective practitioner: how professionals think in action. Temple Smith, London

Stein-Parbury J 1993 Developing interpersonal skills in nursing. Churchill Livingstone, Edinburgh

Stockwell F 1972 The unpopular patient. Study of Nursing Care Project Reports. Series 1, no. 2. Royal College of Nursing, London

United Kingdom Central Council for Nursing Midwifery and Health Visiting 1999 Fitness for practice. UKCC, London

Wainwright G 1985 Body language. Hodder and Stoughton, London

Walker D 1985 Writing and reflection. In: Boud D, Keough R, Walker D (eds) Reflection: turning experience into learning. Kogan Page, London

Watson O 1980 Proxemic behaviour: a cross cultural study. Monitor, The Hague, Netherlands

Waxer P 1997 Non-verbal cues for depression. Journal of Abnormal Psychology 83: 319–322

Whitcher S, Fisher J 1979 Multi-dimensional reactions to therapeutic touch in a hospital setting. Journal of Personal and Social Psychology 37: 87–96

Wilkinson S 1992 Confusions and challenges. Nursing Times 88(35): 24–28

FURTHER READING

Bond M, Holland S 1998 Skills of clinical supervision for nurses. Open University Press, Buckingham
A practical book on clinical supervision for nurses. Includes aspects of communication and provides a general overview of clinical supervision within a nursing context.

Egan G 1998 The skilled helper, 6th edn. Brooks Cole, Pacific Grove, CA
The skilled helper is one of the most widely used models of counselling in the world. This book examines the skills and stages of counselling and offers pragmatic guidance for nurses in the use of counselling skills.

Ellis R, Gates R, Kenworthy N (eds) 1995 Interpersonal communication in nursing. Churchill Livingstone, Edinburgh
This text integrates theoretical concepts of communication into the analysis of everyday nursing situations. It provides an excellent grounding in the important aspects of communication and expands on some of the ideas in this chapter.

Heron J 1990 Helping the client. Sage, London

Nicklin P, Kenworthy N 1995 Teaching and assessing in nursing practice: an experiential approach, 2nd edn. Scutari, London
A general introduction to teaching and assessment in nursing practice.

Rogers C 1974 On becoming a person, 4th edn. Constable, London
Sets out Carl Rogers' thinking in relation to the therapeutic relationship. Rogers' ideas have been massively influential within all helping contexts, including nursing. Encourages the reader to reflect on the values of a helping relationship.

Stein-Parbury J 1993 Developing interpersonal skills in nursing. Churchill Livingstone, Edinburgh
Uses exercises and examples from nursing to encourage reflection on the nurse as a communicator. Examines skills and principles involved in establishing and maintaining effective relationships in nursing practice.

Stewart I, Joines V 1987 TA today. Lifespace, Nottingham
A very readable introduction to transactional analysis. The fundamental ideas of TA are presented in straightforward language and illustrated by examples. Includes reflective exercises.

10

The nurse as health promoter

Diana Forster

CHAPTER CONTENTS

Introduction 280

The Ottawa Charter 280

New strategies 281
The health promoting hospital 282
Disabled people 282
Health choices 283

An integrated approach 284
Defining health 284
Holistic health 285
Health as a quality of life 285
Environmental health 286
Unhealthy neighbourhoods:
 inequalities in health 286
The Acheson Report 287
Saving Lives: Our Healthier Nation 287
Healthy schools 288
The healthy workplace 288
Health improvement programmes 289

Psychology and health promotion 290
The health belief model 290
The theory of reasoned action 291

Health promotion and health education 291
Communication 291
Learning and teaching 292
Types of learning 292
Holistic health education 294
Reflection 295
Getting the message across 295
Planning: setting aims and objectives 296
Implementing learning and teaching 296
Strategies for achieving aims and
 objectives 297

Learning in groups 297
Assessing learning outcomes 297

Health education models 298
The preventive model 298
Staying healthy: primary prevention 298
Secondary health education 301
Tertiary health education 303
The radical option: healthy public policy 304
The empowerment model 305

Health for everyone 306

References 306

Further reading 308

Health promotion is the process of helping people to increase control over and improve their health. It is an essential component of nursing today. Goals for nursing and health promotion are clearly linked as the context of health care widens. After reading this chapter, nurses should be able to:

- **understand the wide array of factors that impact upon health**
- **enable patients and clients to improve their health status**
- **enable the wider community to choose to enhance its health and health care**
- **apply current government health policies to promoting health.**

INTRODUCTION

'The aim is to achieve adequate health for all, rather than simply to achieve still better health for those whose health is already adequate' (WHO 1999a).

THE OTTAWA CHARTER

According to the Ottawa Charter for Health Promotion (WHO 1986), health promotion is the process of helping people to increase control over and improve their health. This charter was the result of the First International Conference on Health Promotion, held in Ottawa, and arising out of the theme of 'Health for all by the year 2000' (WHO 1978). Based on principles of equity and social justice in striving for health for all, the charter focused on the creation of environments which are supportive to health and on developing personal skills within communities so that people may take increased responsibility for their own health. It identified health as a resource for everyday life, not just an end in itself. The strategies for action were meant to make health choices easier for individuals, organisations and

groups. These strategies have withstood the test of time, spearheading new health promotion initiatives and principles as indicated in Box 10.1.

One of the main objectives laid down by the European Community on future action in the field of public health is to promote a healthy lifestyle and healthy physical and social environments (WHO 1999a). This chapter aims to explore issues of health improvement, promotion and health education in relation to the practice of nursing and health care. Many things affect our health – where we live, where we work, what we have to eat, the air we breathe, the germs we are in contact with and our genetic inheritance. For instance, the links between nutrition and health are well documented. People with poor nutrition have greater health risks throughout life, with increased incidence of coronary heart disease,

---

Box 10.1 Principles of health promotion
(Tones & Tilford 1994, Tones 1998)

If we are to improve health, we must consider all influences on human behaviour and daily living:

- Health should be viewed holistically. It is a positive state and an essential commodity which people need in order to achieve a socially and economically productive life.
- Health will not be achieved, nor illness prevented and controlled, unless existing health inequalities between and within nations and social groups have been eradicated.
- A healthy nation is not only one which has an equitable distribution of resources, but also one which has active empowered communities which are vigorously involved in creating the conditions necessary for a healthy population.
- Health is too important to be left to medical practitioners alone; there should be a reorientation of health services, recognising that a wide range of public and private services and institutions influence health. Medical services do not always meet the needs of the public and they may treat people as passive recipients of care. The focus of health promotion should be on cooperation rather than on compliance and should aim to enable and not coerce people.
- People's health is not just an individual responsibility – physical, social, cultural and economic aspects of our environment also govern our health. Cajoling people into taking responsibility for their health while ignoring the social and environmental circumstances which may make them ill is 'victim blaming' and unethical. The process of 'building healthy public policy' is at the very heart of health promotion.

diabetes, some cancers and higher rates of still-birth and infant mortality. Good housing is of paramount importance for health (Box 10.2), and transport policies can be health promoting – or not – for the communities they serve. Public expectations of health care are rising, and challenging new policy agendas place health promotion in even greater prominence.

Life expectancy is increasing rapidly. Since 1970 the life expectancy of 60-year-olds has risen from 78 to 84 years in men and from 82 to 88 years in women of 60 (Office for National Statistics 2000). Britain is now a multicultural, multiethnic society with many people speaking different languages, having various different beliefs and practices, eating a wide variety of foods and viewing life from within different cultural frameworks.

Today's nursing students will be working in a variety of settings and dealing with all factors affecting health. They need preparation for work with individuals, families, groups and whole populations.

NEW STRATEGIES

Goals for nursing and goals for health promotion are now clearly linked as the context of health care is becoming wider. The focus is upon health and well-being alongside clinical care. Nurses need to develop new strategies to respond to changes in society and in patterns of health and disease. Trends in disease patterns show a rise in chronic non-communicable diseases, in obesity and its consequences, in mental illness and in some new infectious diseases as well as familiar long-standing ones such as HIV/AIDS (Box 10.3) and tuberculosis. Health promotion therefore is an increasingly important part of all branches of nursing. It broadens the way in which health services are viewed, going beyond medical services to consider the wider influences that can affect health positively or negatively. In the past nurses have traditionally focused on individual patients, without recognition of the social context of behaviour and of their own responsibility for facilitating change at the social, economic and political level. Health promotion advice on important lifestyle issues such as nutrition, exercise, consumption of alcohol and stopping smoking is most effective if

---

Box 10.2 Housing and coronary heart disease (Hicks & Crowther 2000)

Why is housing relevant to health?
Cardiovascular changes increase the risk of myocardial infarction and stroke when room temperature falls below 12°C.

What is the evidence?
Excess mortality in winter: about 40 000 more people die in Britain in winter than in summer; most are older people.

Excess deaths are mostly due to respiratory and cardiovascular diseases, not hypothermia; risk to health increases as temperature falls.

What action/intervention is needed?
Standards should be set so that an acceptable indoor temperature, say 20°C, can be achieved at no more than 10% of the household income.

Any excess needed should be paid for in social benefits.

Who will benefit?
The poorest in society: the unemployed, the chronically sick, older people.

'Fuel poverty' describes those with least to spend on heating but living in houses that are hard to heat.

Many low-cost houses are prone to cold and damp.

What are the key targets?
Indoor temperature of local authority housing stock to be kept at a minimum of 20°C.

Box 10.3 AIDS/HIV in children (BMA 1999)

AIDS and HIV is seen as an emerging infectious disease of increasing concern to children's health in the UK. By the end of April 1998, 334 cases of AIDS in children under 14 had been reported. Of these 50% had died; 84% were infected by transmission from mother to infant, 10% by blood factor treatment (e.g. haemophilia), 5% by blood or tissue transfer and 1% were of undetermined origin. A total of 817 children were reported infected with HIV by the end of April 1998, of whom 61% had acquired the infection through mother to infant transmission. Of the 1234 children known to have been born to HIV infected mothers, 40% are known to be infected, 36% uninfected and 24% undetermined. There is now clear evidence that transmission of HIV from an infected mother to her child can be greatly reduced by avoiding breastfeeding and giving antiretroviral treatment in pregnancy and the perinatal period.

Box 10.4 **Nurses' contribution to the fight against coronary heart disease** (DoH 1999b)

Evidence suggests that nurses, midwives and health visitors can make a significant contribution in the fight against coronary heart disease through:

- nurse-led blood pressure clinics to identify and help manage hypo/hypertension and medication compliance
- smoking cessation clinics using national smoking cessation guidelines
- 'healthy lifestyle' clinics in collaboration with other health professionals to address factors such as diet, nutrition and exercise
- cholesterol clinics to assist in risk identification and management
- care for patients with congestive cardiac failure under home-based initiatives
- nurse-led chest pain clinics or risk factor screening and reduction clinics
- the coordination and delivery of cardiac rehabilitation programmes in conjunction with other health care professionals.

Box 10.5 **The health promoting hospital** (Tones 1998)

Main principles:

- There should be a focus on health rather than on disease.
- The environment should be conducive to health promotion: there should not only be complementary health policies regarding issues such as nutrition and smoking, but the hospital should also set a good example to other workplaces by having a model occupational health service catering for the needs of all its staff.
- Extending (quite considerably) the notion of a patient's charter, patients and their relatives should be the beneficiaries of good communication and sound health education.
- There should be a concerted effort to actively empower patients and staff.
- The hospital should have an epidemiological database. It should be outward looking, seek support from voluntary bodies and establish a 'healthy alliance' with the community which it serves.

it is persistent, consistent and continuous, and if it is offered to families and communities at all levels. Within this population context, individual advice can be given, when the opportunity arises, to those who attend hospitals and other health services for whatever reason. It has been shown that interventions such as brief advice and counselling about exercise in the prevention of heart disease are very cost-effective and clinically effective (WHO 2000). Broader strategies are outlined in Box 10.4.

THE HEALTH PROMOTING HOSPITAL

The notion of the health promoting hospital has been developed as part of the 'settings' approach to health promotion (Ashton & Seymour 1993). Its principles are summarised in Box 10.5.

Safeguarding health can improve the quality of life, benefiting the individual and society as a whole. The health strategy for England *Saving Lives: Our Healthier Nation* (DoH 1999a), discussed below, recognises the potential of all nurses, midwives and health visitors to play a major part in promoting health and preventing illness. They

have contact with people at critical points in their lives, for instance during pregnancy or acute illness, when people may be particularly receptive to advice and support about healthy lifestyle choices. With the onset of chronic illness there are important opportunities to help people manage and take control of their condition, minimising their dependence and maximising their mental and physical well-being. Nurses are exceptionally well placed to identify patterns and causes of ill health and to join with others to tackle them. Through their work with people who are vulnerable, those who are socially excluded and those at greatest risk of ill health, nurses can help tackle health inequalities, targeting those in greatest need (Box 10.6 describes one example).

Disabled people

Disabled people should have every opportunity to lead socially and economically fulfilling and mentally creative lives. The health of people with disabilities can be improved if social and health policies create equal opportunities for them, so that they can be fully integrated into the normal social and economic life of their community.

They should be able to enjoy family life, education, employment, housing, access to public facilities and freedom of movement. They need to be enabled to create homes, rear children and engage in intimate and caring relationships with others. For this to happen, more needs to be done nationally and locally to ensure that all people receive the appropriate level and type of support they prefer.

Health promotion for psychiatric clients also reflects a changing emphasis. Evidence suggests that there is a high level of unrecognised medical problems among psychiatric clients and patients. Cigarette smoking, poor physical fitness and poor nutritional status are more likely to be found in this group than in the general population. Environmental factors such as reduced social networks and support, limited housing options and poverty may all contribute to their poorer physical health status. In addition, the stigma of being mentally ill, lack of knowledge of services and lack of opportunities to learn how to manage their own health care are factors contributing to the great need for community- and hospital-based health promotion activities to be made available. In the past, health education programmes for people with chronic mental illness have concentrated on symptom control and issues related to medication. However, more recently there has been a focus on health, wellness and quality of life experiences. There has also been a shift from hospital-based to community-based programmes.

Box 10.7 **How to help people stop smoking** (RCN 1999)

About half of those who give up smoking do so as a result of a health problem or crisis, so a medical setting is an ideal place to offer help. Many nurses who smoke feel that they would be hypocritical to raise the issue. Equally, non-smoking nurses fear that they may be the wrong people to promote stopping smoking as they cannot fully empathise with the subject. For these reasons smoking is not often discussed by hospital or community nurses, and patients who want to give up may not be offered the support they need. Even if you smoke yourself, your advice is valuable. You may not be able to quit the habit yourself, but your patient may be. Follow the national guidelines and use the four As – ask, advise, arrange and assist (see p. 300).

 Activity 10.1 Making healthy choices

What choices do you make that are comforting but are not necessarily healthy?
Think through why you make these choices, and perhaps discuss your reasons with colleagues.

Health choices

It is vital to consider that:

- making choices about being healthy or not is more complex than it seems
- many factors are outside an individual's control
- healthy choices are easier for some people to make than others
- the health choices that people make are affected by their cultural background and by the social and physical environment in which they live
- nurses and other health promoters need to acknowledge their own difficulties in making healthy choices (see Box 10.7 for an example) (Activity 10.1).

In order to develop a leading role in health promotion the nursing profession should free itself from subordination and increase its autonomy and self-determination. There may then be more evidence of nurses lobbying, networking and working collaboratively with others in order to influence policies and environments in the interest of health (Tones 1998). Inequalities and difficulties with making healthy choices, as we have seen, underpin many aspects of health. 'Nurses witness daily the effects of poverty and the wider environment on the health of individuals and families' and 'nurses have much to contribute to the public health movement' (RCN 1994).

AN INTEGRATED APPROACH

An integrated approach to health promotion is involved in:

- increasing access to health
- the development of an environment, in its broadest social and physical sense, that is conducive to health
- strengthening social networks and support
- promoting positive health behaviour and coping strategies
- increasing knowledge and making information widely available (as shown in the example in Box 10.8).

Health promotion is characterised as:

- involving the population (or specific subgroups) as a whole
- using many different but complementary methods and approaches
- being aimed at public participation, addressing problems that people themselves define as important
- being an activity in the health and social fields
- being often rooted in popular struggles and movements for social change
- valuing lay knowledge and not relying on expert-designed interventions in problem solving and decision making (in self-help groups, for example) (Activity 10.2)
- working best when in harmony with a healthy public policy.

Nurses and other health educators need to be able to work with clients in various settings, communicating to people the process of making health-related decisions relevant to themselves,

> **Box 10.8 Outreach** (Arora et al 2000)
>
> Outreach may be a useful way of ensuring some access to health promotion. In Peterborough, for example, an annual 'mela' or fair is held. This includes many opportunities for health promotion in a family-oriented way.

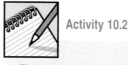

Activity 10.2

Find out the range of self-help groups that are available in the area where you live or work. Identify places where such information is available, e.g. public libraries, health centres, health promotion offices, etc., or the internet. Can you suggest other self-help groups that might be beneficial in your area?

rather than telling them what those decisions ought to be.

DEFINING HEALTH

How can health be defined? It is commonly thought of as a state of feeling well and not being ill, but health and sickness are not entirely separate concepts – they overlap. There are degrees of wellness and illness.

A positive view may be used to define health as a state of physical, mental and social well-being – not simply the absence of injury or disease – that varies over time along a continuum. A high level of wellness is at one end of this continuum, with disease or illness and its characteristic signs, symptoms or disabilities at the other. Our position along the continuum varies, but there is no clear demarcation between health and ill health. Blood pressure, for instance, may be described as low, normal or high, but the degrees merge into each other and the appropriate point at which treatment is necessary may be difficult to determine. Similarly, senile dementia is widely regarded as a distinct entity, and much research effort goes into the search for its causes. However, studies of cognitive function in elderly people show that 'normality' merges imperceptibly into 'dementia', progressively affecting a minority of this age group. The identification of early dementia is a notoriously difficult clinical area, and diagnostic criteria differ widely.

A large proportion of people rate their health as 'good' or 'fairly good' in spite of suffering from some form of chronic disease or disability. People with impairments move along the health continuum, sometimes feeling at their peak of health and on other occasions feeling less so. One study in which older women were interviewed found that health problems were often played down. The women would typically say, 'Oh I'm fine in myself, it's just this … stiff knee/high blood pressure/trouble with my waterworks … ' (Bernard & Meade 1993). Health was therefore being assessed not just in terms of the presence or absence of disease, or in terms of function; the women felt well in spite of their illness or disability. We therefore need to understand what people themselves mean when they discuss 'health'. It is also possible for people who are terminally ill to experience a sense of well-being; their bodies may be diseased, but they are at peace with themselves and are well adjusted to the ending of their lives. Nurses working in hospices or caring for terminally ill people at home may be familiar with such examples; it is not a contradiction to refer to a healthy attitude towards illness or death. Professionals need not impose their own values on those whose health they are trying to promote. It is vital to consider people's own ideas of health, their perceptions of need and the cultural influences upon them. Healthy choices depend upon people's value systems and there are links between a person's lifestyle health aspects and the social and environmental context of their lives.

Holistic health

Attempting to understand the web of influences upon someone's health and well-being involves taking a 'holistic' approach (from the Greek *holos*, meaning 'whole'). The holistic health approach incorporates a belief in people's responsibility for their own lives, a willingness to cooperate with others, and an emphasis on developing meaningful relationships and a positive outlook on life.

Nurses applying the holistic approach to health care place emphasis on the whole person, taking

---

> **Box 10.9 Participation in health promotion**
> (McNeish 1999)
>
> The holistic definition of health as a 'state of complete physical, mental and social well-being', as set out in the constitution of the World Health Organization (1946), supports the view that participation is an important element of good health because:
>
> - participation contributes to self-esteem which in turn affects physical and mental health
> - it helps people to feel more in control of their lives and their health
> - it increases access to information and skills
> - it increases the responsiveness of service providers
> - it contributes to a more accurate assessment of need
> - it engenders a sense of ownership
> - in young people it capitalises on the importance of peer influence.

into account each one's physical, emotional, intellectual, spiritual and sociocultural background (Box 10.9). The nurse's focus is on prevention and well-being, and on helping individuals to take responsibility for their own health. For example, although some people with particularly challenging behaviour still require residential care, most people with learning disabilities now live in the community. Learning disability nursing is probably the best example of holistic care (Jones 1999).

Health as a quality of life

Health promotion and education are concerned with health as a quality of life, and viewed in this way five main components can be identified:

1. *Social health*: the ability to interact well with people and the environment; having satisfying interpersonal relationships.

2. *Mental health*: the ability to learn; a person's intellectual capabilities.

3. *Emotional health*: the ability to control emotions so that someone feels comfortable expressing them when appropriate and expresses them appropriately; the ability not to express emotion when it is inappropriate to do so.

4. *Spiritual health*: a belief in some unifying force; for some that will be nature, for some it will be scientific laws, and for others it will be a god-like force.

5. *Physical health*: the ability to perform daily tasks without undue fatigue; biological integrity of the individual (Greenberg 1992).

These five aspects of health need to be balanced and integrated with each other for a high level of 'wellness' to be present. In the past, many health education programmes have provided information for people in the hope that they will change their behaviour in the light of knowledge about risks to their health. Now, with an increased holistic and whole-person approach, more health education addresses the importance of self-esteem, personal skills and social support in developing healthy lifestyles.

Environmental health

Environmental health covers those aspects of human health and disease that are determined by factors in the environment. These include both the direct pathological effects of chemicals, radiation and some biological agents, and the effects (often indirect) on health and well-being of the broad physical, psychological, social and aesthetic environment. This includes housing, urban development, land use and transport (WHO 1999a).

When hampered by factors such as poor health, low income, inadequate housing and lowered self-esteem, people may not believe themselves able to take control or have any power to alter the conditions affecting their health and well-being. It is difficult for people to take responsibility for their health where healthy foods are too expensive, where housing is inadequate and telephones vandalised, where working conditions are unhealthy or unemployment is common. An elderly, frail person who is physically disabled and lives far from shops or a young, unsupported mother with little money and poor housing may require extra resources but not know how to gain access to them, or may not find them appropriate.

Unhealthy neighbourhoods: inequalities in health

Trends in both child and adult health in the UK show that although health status has improved

---

> Box 10.10   **Inequalities and child health**
>
> Maternal and fetal health are adversely affected by poverty, poor housing, unemployment and smoking. Homeless mothers and their children face particular difficulties regarding health from birth and in later life. Mothers living in bed and breakfast accommodation in Hackney were the subjects of a study that showed 25% of their newborns had a birth weight below 2500 g compared with 10% among babies of local area residents and 7.2% in England (Parsons 1991). Poor housing can also affect maternal health by contributing to depression, higher rates of respiratory infection, poor nutrition (many homeless women staying in bed and breakfast accommodation do not have access to a kitchen), and an increased risk of smoking, alcoholism or drug abuse (BMA 1999).

---

over past decades, those in non-manual occupations and their families have benefited most from these improvements. Mortality rates for most major causes of death are higher amongst the poorest in society, including infants and children (Box 10.10).

Poverty – whether defined by income, socioeconomic status, living conditions, age, ethnic group, gender or educational level – is the largest single determinant of ill health. Living in poverty is correlated with higher rates of substance abuse (tobacco, alcohol and illegal drugs), depression, suicide, antisocial behaviour and violence and a wide range of physical complaints. Perhaps the easiest way of seeing intuitively what the socioeconomic differences in death rates mean is to:

Imagine two people, each with a similar sized circle of friends and relations – let us say 50 personal contacts – but living in separate rich and poor areas. For every death that occurs among the circle of friends of the person in the rich area, the person in the poor area will know of two, three or even four times as many deaths among his or her circle of friends. (Wilkinson 1996, p. 57)

Health care and related services have not always been made accessible to those most needing them, including refugees and displaced people. Taken as a whole, ethnic minority groups are more likely than the rest of the population to live in poor areas, be unemployed, have low incomes, live in poor housing, have poor health and be victims of crime. However, it is important not to stereotype those from ethnic groups as passive victims: many do not fit these categories and are among the wealthiest groups in society.

It was over 20 years ago that Sir Douglas Black (1980) set up his committee that demonstrated unequivocally the link between poverty and ill-health. Those in social class V experience worse health than those in higher social classes in non-manual occupations. Many recent studies demonstrate that poverty is increasing and the inequalities gap is widening (Office for National Statistics 2000). The more affluent members of society continue to live longer and enjoy better health and quality of life than do those who are less advantaged, as the following quotation illustrates:

> To feel depressed, cheated, bitter, desperate, vulnerable, frightened, angry, worried about debts or job and housing insecurity; to feel devalued, useless, helpless, uncared for, hopeless, isolated, anxious and a failure: these feelings can dominate people's whole experience of life, colouring their experience of everything else. It is the chronic stress arising from feelings like these which does the damage.
> (Wilkinson 1996, p. 215)

Paradoxically, health promotion initiatives that fail to pay attention to low income and material disadvantage may increase health inequalities by improving the health of high-income groups, who are more likely to attend screening sessions or read health promotional literature, while failing to reach low-income groups and help them to improve their health.

The Acheson Report

In 1997 the Secretary of State for Health invited Sir Donald Acheson to review and summarise inequalities in health in England. The resulting report (Acheson 1998) shows that poor neighbourhoods are characterised by poor health. The report vividly illustrates the ways in which every aspect of health – mortality, years of life lost and morbidity – is measurably worse for people living in deprived circumstances.

Three key areas for action were identified:

1. There should be evaluation of all policies likely to have an impact on health inequalities.

2. High priority should be given to the health of families with children.
3. Further steps should be made to improve the living standards of poor households and reduce income inequalities.

The report stated that all policies likely to have a direct or indirect effect on health should be evaluated in terms of their impact on health inequalities. All policies should also be formulated so that less well off people are favoured as much as possible. The recommendations cover income, education and employment, food, environment, gender, ethnicity and older people. The report also recommended some direct measures, including the abolition of tobacco advertising and promotion, the availability of nicotine replacement therapy on prescription and the reduction of sodium in processed foodstuffs.

One of the great strengths of the Acheson Report (Acheson 1998) is its in-depth analysis of the range of inequalities which have an impact upon health, including age, gender, race and culture, housing and poverty. It sets out an ambitious agenda for action to improve health. In relation to the neighbourhood, the report considers the role of housing and the environment in shaping health, and highlights the importance of social networks. It also places schools firmly in the context of the broader community, and points out the contribution that health promoting schools can make by tackling issues such as poor nutrition, stress and truancy.

SAVING LIVES: OUR HEALTHIER NATION

The 1999 English White Paper on public health, *Saving Lives: Our Healthier Nation* (DoH 1999a), is a major innovation in policy. It presents an action plan for tackling poor health and improving the health of everyone in England – especially the worst off in society.

Four priority areas for action, each with specified targets, are identified:

1. *Cancer* – to reduce death rates in people aged under 75 by a fifth, saving 100 000 lives

2. *Coronary heart disease and strokes* – to reduce death rates in people aged under 75 by at least two-fifths, saving 200 000 lives

3. *Accidents* – to reduce death rates by at least a fifth and to reduce the rate of serious injury from accidents by at least a tenth, saving 12 000 lives

4. *Mental health* – to reduce death rates from suicide and undetermined injury by at least a fifth, saving 4000 lives.

In setting these targets, the government requires intermediate national milestones to be met by 2005. Local targets are required to be set to achieve national priorities and specific local issues, including health inequalities. Practical proposals include a £100 million anti-smoking programme and broader cross-government plans to reduce unemployment, tackle pollution problems and improve housing, benefits and wages through legislation to promote a minimum wage policy. In addition, a range of new developments are proposed, for example health skills for parents will be initially linked to 'Sure Start' programmes to ensure that children get the best possible start in life. Other wider action areas identified that need to be addressed are summarised in Box 10.11.

The identification of settings as a focus for improving health has long been advocated by the World Health Organization. Most recently, target 13 of *Health 21* (WHO 1999a), 21 targets for the 21st century, states: 'By the year 2015, people in the region should have greater opportunities to live in healthy physical and social environments at home, at school, at the workplace and in the local community' (WHO 1999a).

These three particular settings, home, school and workplace – also identified in *Saving Lives: Our Healthier Nation* (DoH 1999a) – are seen as providing a focus for interdepartmental government action and local partnerships.

Healthy schools

Healthy schools are intended to improve the health of children, not only through health education but also by equipping them with the life skills and knowledge to take care of their health throughout their lives (Case example 10.1 and p. 301).

The healthy workplace

The healthy workplace setting has two aims:

1. to improve the overall health of the workforce
2. to ensure that people are protected from workplace hazards.

Case example 10.1 A health promoting school (Moore 1998)

Lansdowne school in Staffordshire is an example of the government's initiative to develop a national healthy schools scheme. It has already demonstrated how targeting health can improve educational attainment through its health promoting culture. Results have improved and the school has won praise in its evaluation. The school has added an official target on promoting health to its statutory literacy and numeracy targets. Healthy messages are incorporated into every part of the curriculum aiming to emphasise self-esteem and awareness of the mind as well as the body. During 'circle time' the children and their teacher discuss their feelings about issues that arise at school or at home. Respect for one another is encouraged as solutions are considered.

At appropriate stages in their school life children learn about healthy eating, exercise, safety, dental hygiene and other traditional health education topics which are still regarded as important. However, the school's approach has evolved into an all-embracing drive to improve the physical and emotional health of its pupils, involving parents, staff and the local community. Specific events are planned throughout the year encouraging pupils to develop confidence, knowledge and awareness of current health issues.

Box 10.11

Wider action areas identified in *Saving Lives: Our Healthier Nation* (DoH 1999a) include:

1. Sexual health, for which a national strategy is being developed to encourage more comprehensive sex and relationship education, more coherent disease prevention and more effective service interventions.
2. A move away from dealing with the consequences of drug misuse towards prevention and treatment through
   - helping young people to resist drug misuse
   - protecting communities from drug-related antisocial and criminal behaviour
   - enabling people with drug-related problems to overcome them and live healthy, crime-free lives
   - reducing the availability of illegal drugs.
3. To reduce heavy drinking that is harmful to the individual, families and society.

It is therefore:

- a place where health risks are recognised and controlled if they cannot be removed
- a place where work design is compatible with people's health needs and limitations
- an environment that supports the promotion of healthy lifestyles
- a place where employees and employers recognise their responsibility for their own health and that of their colleagues (Gowman 1999).

Health improvement programmes

All health authorities are required to produce health improvement programmes (HImPs) for their populations (Box 10.12). They are local strategies for improving health and health care, drawn up by health authorities in consultation

---

Box 10.12 Health improvement programmes
(NHS Executive 1998)

A 'health improvement programme' is a local strategic plan designed to improve health and health services through working in partnerships or networks.

Good public health is rooted in a supportive environment developed within the framework of a sustainable physical environment. A supportive (and thus healthy) social environment requires:

- opportunities for people to make a rewarding, useful and rewarded contribution to society
- easy and equitable access to services, including childcare, education and training
- available, affordable housing
- an equitable distribution of wealth across the society
- a range of local cultural and community activities that people are connected to and engaged in
- local participation in decision making, such that individuals feel that they have a say in, and an appropriate degree of control over, their lives
- facilities for encouraging active lifestyles, so that activity, and with it the benefits of exercise, becomes a normal part of daily life
- access to affordable, healthy foods
- a social environment where people can live without fear of violence, either in their personal or public lives
- social networks to help prevent exclusion or marginalisation.

Community development is public participation in public health.

---

with health professionals, local authorities, local businesses, patient groups and representatives of the wider community. HImPs should provide the framework in which all NHS bodies operate.

Acheson (1998) recommended that HImPs should be used for reducing inequities in access to effective health care. They are 3-year programmes and will be evaluated particularly with regard to their impact on the population's health. Local HImPs should address any significant health and health care issues in which improvement is possible, including, for example, developing a programme to tackle drug misuse, a problem that is not only widespread but the number one public health problem in many Western countries. Coronary heart disease, teenage pregnancy, child health improvement, promoting the health of the expanding population of older people and mental health issues are also subjects for HImPs.

Partnership is an essential ingredient for HImPs, the main challenge being to move away from current fragmented approaches to health improvement towards an integrated approach.

Health promotion = health education × healthy public policy (Tones 1998)

Tones is saying that health education operates in a kind of partnership with policy development, having a twofold role:

1. It seeks to influence individual lifestyle, but not in order to coerce, cajole or persuade. Its main purpose is to facilitate choice by providing people with the support and competencies they need to make health choices. This empowering function also helps people to use health services according to their needs and to interact assertively with practitioners.

2. This challenging function is concerned with influencing policy by raising people's awareness and concern about matters which affect their own health and that of their community. Health education seeks to address the problems of inequalities in health and to create concern for others' rights to be healthy. It aims to give people a fairer

share of power. This equates with the radical approach to be considered in more detail later (see p. 304).

PSYCHOLOGY AND HEALTH PROMOTION

People's own behaviour can have an important effect on their health. A healthy lifestyle can help to prevent the risk of illness, for example not smoking, exercising, practising safe sex and eating a healthy diet. How can people be encouraged to take care of their health through appropriate preventive action and compliance with health care advice? A number of psychological theories have found widespread acceptance in certain types of health promotion, including the health belief model and the theory of reasoned action.

The health belief model

Research suggests that four elements influence the likelihood of someone engaging in a healthy habit or changing a detrimental one (Bandura 1977, Becker 1984). Individuals must believe that:

- the disease or disorder is serious (e.g. 'How likely am I to suffer from breathing difficulties or contract lung cancer if I smoke?')
- they are susceptible to the disorder
- the response will be effective in reducing the dangers and protect them from the threat (i.e. they believe in the efficacy of the response – such as giving up smoking)
- they will be able to carry out the recommended preventive health action (i.e. they believe that they could respond successfully by stopping smoking).

Changing behaviour

Modifying health behaviours and beliefs is, however, not a simple matter; for example, the immediate costs of changing diet to avoid heart disease may not seem worth the effort. It may involve

changing from preferred methods of cooking, eating less-favoured foods and perhaps increased shopping expenses.

Besides health teaching for individuals and groups, behavioural changes in relation to diet may be motivated by:

- advertising health aspects of foods
- labelling foods, as, for example, having a high or low fat content
- health warnings to raise awareness.

People often need to pass through stages of changing attitudes and assimilating information before they make actual changes in their behaviour. Those wishing to avoid the risk of HIV infection, for example, may need help in developing social skills enabling them to adopt safer sexual practices, such as effective condom use.

The motivation to change practices depends partly upon the social and cultural groups to which people belong, and how far HIV and AIDS, for example, are seen as threats to health. Successful helping requires that habitual practices are viewed from the client's own perspective. Actions that involve the risk of HIV infection, with its potential life-threatening, long-term consequences, may be regarded by outsiders as irrational and irresponsible, but to some clients unsafe sex may seem to offer security, love and the satisfaction of desire. The possible threats to health in an already uncertain and unpromising future then seem less important (Anderson & Wilkie 1992).

An understanding of health beliefs suggests that encouraging responsible attitudes towards sexuality involves empowering young people to resist social pressures – including sexual advances and advertising – and to act upon informed choices. Education in parenting skills and empowerment education in schools may be the best long-term solution. People are more likely to undertake a health-related behaviour when they believe that:

- their health is important
- they are susceptible to a health threat which could be serious for them
- the proposed action will be successful and does not involve too many costs

- other people approve of the action and this is important
- they can effectively carry out the action.

The theory of reasoned action

Another model that has been found to be relevant to health promotion is the theory of reasoned action (Ajzen & Fishbein 1980). This separates beliefs from attitudes, for example, in relation to making decisions about health, and emphasises the influence of significant others on a person's intention to act. The theory is based on the assumption that most health-related behaviour is under voluntary control. Behaviour is considered to be governed by two broad influences:

1. people's attitudes towards a certain behaviour (each attitude consists of a belief, e.g. that smoking can cause cancer, and a value attached to that belief, i.e. how important this is to the person concerned)
2. people's ideas of what significant others will think of their behaviour.

These two influences combine to form an intention to act. People do not always behave in accordance with their expressed attitudes because of the influences upon them. Bennett & Hodgson (1992) provide the example of an ex-smoker who may have a number of negative attitudes towards smoking. However, when out for a drink with friends who smoke, he may himself smoke, because smoking is an acceptable norm for the group and drinking alcohol may also interfere with the previous intention of not smoking.

Similarly, a person may jump out of an aeroplane attached to a flimsy length of silk or nylon, despite having a negative attitude towards jumping – including fear at the point of leaving the aircraft – because he does not want to lose face with friends by going against the norms of the group.

The ability successfully to change habitual practices is influenced by the social and cultural groups to which people belong, and the extent to which HIV and AIDS, for instance, are viewed as threats to health. Active participation and approaches that seek to raise self-esteem as well as provide factual information have been found to be the most effective ways of imparting health knowledge and promoting healthy lifestyles.

Nurses should ensure that each patient is treated as an individual by focusing on the person's health beliefs and needs and working towards an achievable set of goals.

HEALTH PROMOTION AND HEALTH EDUCATION

Health education remains a vital tool concerned with the sharing and learning of knowledge, values and attitudes – with clients in partnership with their health educators. It is one component of the broader, umbrella concept of health promotion.

A definition of health education, in the context of empowering and supporting individual choice, is offered by Tones & Tilford (1994):

Health education is any intentional activity which is designed to achieve health or illness related learning, i.e. some relatively permanent change in an individual's capability or disposition. Effective health education may, thus, produce changes in knowledge and understanding or ways of thinking; it may influence or clarify values; it may bring about some shift in belief or attitude; it may facilitate the acquisition of skills; it may even effect changes in behaviour or lifestyle.

Communication

Nurses need to be skilled facilitators; health education is a communication activity. It is not enough simply to relay information: the beliefs, attitudes and behaviour of individuals and communities must be considered if health education is to be effective. In working with an interpreter, for example, it is important to:

- check that the interpreter and patient speak the same language
- allow time for discussion with the interpreter before and after the interview
- ask the interpreter how to pronounce the client's name correctly
- allow time for the interpreter to introduce and explain his own and your role to the client

- encourage the interpreter to intervene when necessary
- use plain English, avoiding jargon
- actively listen to the client and the interpreter
- allow enough time for the interview
- check that the client has understood everything and whether he wants to ask anything else (Kai 1999).

LEARNING AND TEACHING

Types of learning

Learning is a process resulting in some modification, relatively permanent, of the learner's way of:

- thinking
- feeling
- doing.

Learning theorists identify three types of learning:

1. cognitive
2. affective
3. psychomotor.

Cognitive learning

This is concerned with thinking, knowing and working with information that has been acquired. It includes the processes of critical, reflective and creative thinking, decision making and problem solving.

An outpatient's health education programme described by Byrne et al (1994) was developed for people with chronic mental illness. Its focus was to increase cognitive knowledge about how to:

- maintain health and fitness
- use and apply information about safety
- prevent common health problems
- gain access to health services that were needed.

In any learning activity the nature of the material to be learned should be considered as well as the abilities and characteristics of the learners themselves. This is illustrated in Case example 10.2.

Case example 10.2 Evaluation of the London Dance Safety Campaign (Branigan & Wellings 1998)

Approaches using the 'Just say no to drugs' type of message have been criticised because they ignore the pleasure principle in drug use. A campaign was developed by 26 London drug action teams using the principle of 'informed choice', in which the target audience is given access to accurate facts about drugs and can choose whether or not to use them. Drugs have been associated with music and youth culture for many decades, but in the 1990s the appearance of ecstasy and the increased scale of illicit drug use in London dance venues prompted this particular campaign. A multi-levelled approach was adopted, and included:

- A poster campaign using the London public transport system. Posters featured cannabis, cocaine, ecstasy, LSD, poppers and speed.
- A booklet campaign throughout London clubs. This provided in-depth information about dance drugs and health and safety measures and was known as the 'Vital Information Pack' or VIP booklet.
- Training of club professionals. One-day training programmes were organised for club managers, door staff, outreach workers and paramedics.
- A campaign phone line. Operators provided information about the campaign and dance events, and provided VIP booklets on request.

Results showed that the majority of respondents in the study recognised that the main message of the campaign was harm minimisation through providing information. One male club member is quoted as responding: 'I think it's the kind of thing which everyone who ever has anything to do with drugs, or is thinking about doing drugs, or knows people who do drugs should have and read, 'cause if you know about drugs then you can actually make a decision based on proper evidence and understanding of drugs.'

Other methods appropriate for developing cognitive information include lectures and lecturettes, reading assignments with study guides, audiovisual aids, interactive computer-supported learning, quizzes and self-paced programmed learning.

Affective learning

This is the aspect of learning that includes values, attitudes, beliefs and emotions. Adults bring to their learning a store of established attitudes, thought patterns and fixed ways of doing things. Although this may help them to adapt to new situations, it may also make it difficult for them to readjust attitudes. Attitude change depends upon knowledge and information being viewed as important and relevant to the person concerned. Health educators need to recognise that they cannot 'instil' confidence or 'motivate' people. However, they may help others to develop their own confidence and plan to change aspects of their behaviour in a health promoting way.

Graham (1993) reported that mothers in her study found smoking a difficult habit to break, although they realised that their own health and that of their children might be harmed by it. Bringing up children in disadvantaged circumstances, such as inadequate housing and being in debt, meant that smokers clung to the support their habit provided for them, and they graphically described smoking as a help in coping 'when life's a drag'. The emotional state of learners will influence how they learn – and may either help or hinder successful outcomes. Taking learners' emotional needs into consideration involves helping them to acknowledge and explore their own feelings. A relationship based on respect, empathy and genuineness helps to develop an atmosphere of mutual trust and equality between teacher or facilitator and learner, making health choices more accessible.

Methods of teaching which may be successful in the affective domain include role play and group discussion and interaction, so that attitudes and beliefs can be explored in relation to other people, and feelings may be shared in a supportive environment.

Psychomotor skill learning

This is the acquisition of a motor skill that may be learned and developed through practice once the necessary tasks and movements have been taught. Appropriate methods of teaching in this domain include demonstration, coaching and individual supervised practice. Examples include managing a stoma appliance; storing and administering insulin; breast self-examination; the safe use of condoms; and techniques of applying a dressing. People with learning difficulties find it difficult to learn a variety of skills including skills such as reading and writing, handling money, cooking and using public transport. This group also presents a particular challenge to health educators in needing to learn, for example, when and how to talk to strangers and how to express their feelings in words or ask for what they want.

Demonstration

People learn best from a combination of seeing, hearing and doing. When teaching someone to perform a skill, the activity should be broken down into basic steps or movements, and as each step is carried out the demonstrator should clearly explain the actions. The stages should be as follows:

1. Explain the activity involved and its purpose or outcomes.
2. Arouse and maintain the learner's interest.
3. Reveal the main steps of the activity and identify likely problem areas.
4. Inspire confidence in learners so that they themselves will be willing to try.
5. Enable learners to undertake individual practice afterwards and receive feedback about their performance.

It is essential to check that learners understand each stage of the activity and how it fits into the whole demonstration. A discussion aimed at encouraging people to try for themselves leads into individual practice, support and supervision. A psychologically safe environment needs to be provided so that learners feel comfortable and are not embarrassed by failed attempts at performing new skills. The amount of practice varies according to the complexity of the task, and the capabilities, physical limitations and past experiences of the learner. Most children are eager to practice, but adults may easily lose interest and motivation if not immediately successful. Developing self-care by self-catheterisation or learning to give oneself an injection will probably take many practice periods. Rewards, praise and successes work as reinforcers, leading to further success and skill development (Activity 10.3).

Activity 10.3

Plan a learning programme for a friend, client or patient designed to teach a particular skill.

HOLISTIC HEALTH EDUCATION

A holistic approach to health education encompasses all three types of learning discussed – cognitive, affective and psychomotor. Emotional, social and spiritual aspects of health are as important as physical ones. People learn best when:

- they feel secure and can try out things in safety
- their needs are being met in ways that they can see are relevant and appropriate
- they know what they have to do; especially when they have been involved in setting their own goals
- they are actively involved and engaged
- they know how well they are doing
- they see and experience that they are welcomed and respected as individuals in their own right (Daines et al 1992).

Using the educational approach, nurses provide knowledge and information from which people can make informed choices about their health. Individuals have a right to choose, to be given information, to understand the risk factors associated with their lifestyle and to decide whether or not to change any aspect of it. Tackling one aspect of behaviour at a time is usually more successful than trying to remove several risk factors at once. In encouraging patients to stop smoking, for example, they may be invited to state or write down their personal goals as a powerful step towards ownership. A person is more likely to act on something personally said aloud or written down. It is important to develop a partnership with learners so that they remain in control of the choices made and feel supported.

'Whether working in a hospital or the community, nurses care for everyone – from schoolchildren to older people. This means they are in a

---

Box 10.13   Teenage pregnancy (Social Exclusion Unit 1999)

In England there are nearly 90 000 conceptions a year to teenagers; about 7700 of these are to girls under 16 years of age and 2200 to girls aged 14 or under. About 56 000 result in live births. However, more than two-thirds of under 16s do not have sex, and most girls reach their 20s without getting pregnant. The Social Exclusion Unit's report on teenage pregnancy (Social Exclusion Unit 1999) states that teenage pregnancy rates in the UK are the highest in Western Europe. A 10-year action plan was launched in 1999 to:

- halve the rate of conceptions among under-18s by 2010
- encourage more teenage parents into education, training or employment to reduce their risk of long-term social exclusion

Risk factors for teenage pregnancy include:

- *Poverty:* a girl whose family is in social class V (unskilled manual) is 10 times more likely to become a teenage mother than a girl whose family is in social class I (professional).
- *Looked after by local authorities:* young women who had been in care were more likely than those brought up with both their natural parents to become teenage mothers.
- *Education:* low educational achievement, truancy and exclusion from school are linked with being a teenage mother. In a survey of 150 teenage mothers more than 40% left school with no qualifications compared to the national average in England in 1997–8 of 6.6%
- *Employment and training:* teenage parenthood for women aged 16 and 17 years is linked with not being in employment, education or work.
- *Daughters of teenage parents* were more likely to be teenage mothers and at increased risk of living in poverty, poor housing and having a poor diet.

Studies show that 75% of these pregnancies are unplanned and tend to be at risk of:

- *Lower birth weight babies:* their babies are 25% more likely than average to weigh less than 2500 g.
- *Higher infant mortality rates:* babies of teenage mothers are more likely to die in the first year of life than babies of older mothers (the death rate is 60% higher).
- *Children of teenage mothers* are twice as likely to be admitted to hospital as the result of an accident, especially poisoning or burns.

---

prime position to encourage smokers to think about giving up and provide them with the information they need to kick the habit. As a nurse, your intervention to help a patient quit smoking may be the most important single influence you can have on their health' (RCN 1999).

Holistic health and wellness programmes may include exercise, meditation and stress-reduction techniques. A day hospital activity programme for people with chronic mental illness described by Perry & Kirmer (1990) emphasised 'holistic wellness', and sought to develop clients' self-assessment skills, identify personal goals and increase their knowledge of self-care and self-evaluation. Topics included nutrition, sexuality, fitness, managing harmful habits and stress management. The goal was that through taking greater responsibility for their own health needs, clients would manage more successfully outside the hospital. A 10-year campaign to reduce teenage pregnancy is described in Box 10.13.

Reflection

Reflecting on what we do involves consciously noticing thoughts, feelings and changing attitudes as new skills are carried out. Experience alone is not enough to ensure that learning has taken place; new experience needs to be made sense of by reflecting and thinking about past experience (Boud et al 1993) (Activity 10.4).

Getting the message across

General principles for teaching and learning in health education involve identifying:

- the aims of the intervention (the WHY)
- the audience (the WHO)
- the content (the WHAT)
- the learning method (the HOW)
- the learning environment (the WHERE).

The educational cycle

The steps of the educational process are similar to those of the nursing process:

- assess
- plan
- implement
- evaluate.

Both are circular in form with ongoing assessment and evaluation constantly redirecting the planning and teaching.

Activity 10.4 Active reflection

Individual exercise:

1. *Preparing.* Think about an activity in which you will be taking part and try to anticipate what you might learn from participating.
2. *Experiencing.* Engage in the activity, noticing your behaviour, thoughts and feelings, other people and the environment surrounding you – this is reflection in action.
3. *Reflecting.* Return in your thoughts to the experience, noticing feelings in particular, and re-evaluate the experience, planning how to apply your new perspectives in future.

Reflection may be carried out individually or it may be part of a group process, when sense is made of experiences through group discussion.

Box 10.14 Nutritional needs of people with learning disability (Barker 1996)

- Overcoming underweight
- Correction and prevention of specific nutritional problems
- Specific medical condition requiring special dietary treatment, for example diabetes, hyperlipidaemia
- Special diets for the inborn errors of metabolism, for example phenylketonuria, galactosaemia
- Help in overcoming feeding problems
- Specialist advice for treatment of Prader–Willi syndrome.

Assessing needs

The decision to carry out some form of health education rests on the identification of a to do so. For example, a healthy diet is essential for the good health and well-being of everyone, and those with learning disabilities should not be excluded from its benefits. Certain people in this population group will have specific nutritional needs (Box 10.14).

In assessing what learners need to know, it is important to find out what they already know and what relevant skills they may already possess. It is then time to move on to the planning stage.

PLANNING: SETTING AIMS AND OBJECTIVES

Effective planning and preparation begins with establishing overall aims. These are general statements that indicate the purpose of the individual session, course or programme. If possible, clients, patients or groups should be involved in this goal setting. An elderly patient recovering from a cerebral vascular accident for instance may not be able to take part initially in setting goals, but as the condition improves then involvement can increase. Examples of aims are:

- to improve understanding, general skills or physical coordination
- to modify attitudes, beliefs or standards
- to impart information, knowledge or ideas
- to stimulate action
- to encourage changes in behaviour.

Educational objectives may be defined as 'things that the learner will be able to do at the end of the session or course'. 'An objective is a description of a performance you want learners to exhibit before you consider them competent' (Mager 1990). These may be written down and agreed by learners and teachers. Objectives should be realistic, achievable and able to be measured and evaluated. They are linked to learning outcomes, as shown in Case example 10.3 (see also Activity 10.5).

IMPLEMENTING LEARNING AND TEACHING

It is always worth taking the time and effort to talk to patients about stopping smoking because every year over 120 000 people die prematurely because of the habit. These unnecessary deaths could be prevented – stopping smoking prolongs life regardless of the age at which a person quits. Remember that brief interventions have an impact, each time you raise the subject, give information and offer a follow up you are helping your patients who smoke to consider stopping. (RCN 1999)

This quote illustrates the importance of opportunistic health education – being ready to raise health education issues during health care activities. A formal plan is not appropriate at such a time, but having considered the possibilities and

Case example 10.3 Helping children to learn about their diabetes (Greenhalgh 2000)

Greenhalgh (2000) set up an educational programme to help young children with diabetes and their families learn about their condition and how to manage it daily, so that the risk of future problems was reduced. Six sessions were developed with the aim of introducing the children to the principles of diabetes management and self-care techniques. Each session had specific learning outcomes. At the end of each session the children should:

1. Understand why they need insulin injections; know the signs and symptoms of high blood sugar.
2. Identify the sites where insulin can be injected; know why it is important to rotate injection sites; demonstrate the correct technique for injecting insulin.
3. Know why they need to have their blood sugar levels monitored; know why it is important to prick a different finger each time; know which blood sugars are too low, just right, a bit too high and too high by a number or a colour.
4. Know the names of different food groups; be able to identify at least one food from each group.
5. Know the signs and symptoms of a hypo; know how to prevent a hypo; know what they need to do to treat a hypo.
6. Have had a good time.

Activity 10.5

Choose a topic related to your own expertise or health interest. Develop a set of learning outcomes for a person or group who would benefit from a health education programme teaching aspects relevant to them.

having acquired background knowledge, nurses can encourage this aspect of health promotion (Box 10.15).

Whether you are teaching a group, family, patient or client in a one-to-one setting, it is helpful to have your material organised into a logical framework (Ewles & Simnett 1999). A straightforward, logical approach for a talk or lecture may be based on:

- an opening
- a set of key points
- a summary.

Box 10.15   **Assisting someone to stop smoking**
(RCN 1999)

If the smoker would like to stop, help should be offered. A few key points can be covered in 5–10 minutes (RCN 1999):

- Set a date to stop; stop completely on that day.
- Review past experience: what helped, what hindered?
- Plan ahead: identify likely problems, make a plan to deal with them.
- Tell family and friends and enlist their support.
- Plan what you are going to do about alcohol.
- Try nicotine replacement therapy using whichever product suits best.

Careful preparation is necessary so that clarity and interest are maintained in both the material and the presentation. An outline plan may be transferred to paper or cards and the talk given from these. Participative activities should be built into the presentation using well-prepared learning resources and visual aids. A visit beforehand to the venue for a talk ensures that seating, lighting, electrical power points and heating arrangements can be checked.

STRATEGIES FOR ACHIEVING AIMS AND OBJECTIVES

When deciding how to facilitate learning, the health educator should choose appropriate methods and materials. A session plan is the teacher's practical working document and contains a selection from the following:

- date and time of session
- venue and room
- type of group and what they already know
- number in group; seating plan
- topic
- aims and objectives
- learning resources (e.g. nursing equipment, models and simulation devices, flip charts, transparencies for overhead projector, books and handouts, videos/films, computer assisted educational materials)
- arrangement of the environment (heating, lighting)

- session timing, content and methods
- evaluation.

Introducing a talk. The opening should gain and hold attention from the beginning, perhaps using a relevant anecdote, a thought-provoking question, a request for listeners' own experiences or using a picture, photograph or other visual image. Let the audience know whether you will take questions of clarification during your talk or at the end.

Key points. These should be arranged in logical order, beginning with a brief outline of what is to follow. Main points may be emphasised by repeating them in a different way or going over them again. Discussion can be used to encourage people to participate, and then the session concluded by summarising the points and perhaps challenging learners to continue developing their knowledge.

Learning in groups

Being part of a group satisfies people's need for feeling safe and favourably regarded, and for giving and receiving attention. The term 'group' may be defined in a variety of ways relating to its function, to the kinds of people who belong to it, to their reasons for joining it and whether membership is voluntary or not. Each member in such a collection of people influences and is influenced by every other member to some extent. Attitudes may be reconsidered and modified and new skills can be developed and practised. More varied and more stimulating ideas can be produced in a group than by individuals working alone. Teaching plans should provide opportunities for group members to learn and develop through their interaction with each other. Larger groups may be divided into smaller units of six to eight people to allow for interaction between all members. In a diabetic clinic, for example, families or small groups could learn about food exchanges and dietary management. A school-based sex education project is outlined in Case example 10.4.

Assessing learning outcomes

Evaluation of health education activities helps to determine how well the objectives have been achieved – has effective learning taken place?

Case example 10.4 A PAUSE project
(Social Exclusion Unit 1999)

The A PAUSE ('added power and understanding in sex education', University of Exeter) project was established in 1990. It is a new approach towards effective, school-based sex education that involves close collaboration between teachers, health professionals and young people trained as peer educators. A PAUSE seeks to reduce the increasing medical and social problems associated with some teenage sexual behaviour. It is funded by the North and East Devon Health Authority and is planned to be delivered to all secondary schools in the area. The project has also been adopted in North Essex, Teesside and Sandwell.

Aims. The long-term goal is to promote positive aspects of emotional and physical relationships, and specifically to:

- increase tolerance, respect and mutual understanding
- enhance knowledge and counteract popular teenage myths
- improve effective contraceptive use by teenagers already sexually active
- provide effective skills to those wanting to resist pressure to become sexually active.

Delivery. Parts of the programme are delivered throughout students' secondary school years, some by specially trained and supported teachers and some led jointly by teachers and school nurses.

Peer education: peer educators aged 16–19 are recruited and trained to present four peer-led sessions in year 9.

Approach. A PAUSE uses a variety of classroom techniques that include role play and small group discussions and presentations.

Audit. The A PAUSE programme is continually evaluated using data from a student questionnaire administered in year 11.

Outcomes. Results evaluating the overall effects of the school programme, compared to local and distant control schools, showed that 16-year-olds:

- increased their knowledge about sex, contraception and sexually transmitted infections
- were less likely to believe that sex is important in relationships
- were less likely to be sexually active
- were more tolerant of the behaviour of others
- were nearly twice as likely to say that sex education was 'OK'.

Evaluation, as the final step in the teaching and learning process, also restarts the programme, providing direction for changes and modification in the assessing–planning–implementing–evaluation cycle. However, evaluation is part of the ongoing learning and teaching process, not just the final point, and it should involve learners and facilitators or teachers alike. The terms 'process' or 'formative' are applied to evaluation used as a continuous check or process of feedback during the learning activities. Am I talking too fast? Am I making my points clear? Is the environment comfortable or are there too many distractions?

HEALTH EDUCATION MODELS

Tones & Tilford (1994) describe three approaches to health education:

1. the preventive model
2. the radical model
3. the empowerment model.

THE PREVENTIVE MODEL

The preventive model may be considered under the headings of primary, secondary and tertiary health education.

Staying healthy: primary prevention

Primary health education encourages people to behave in ways that will help them to reduce the risk of disease or injury and adopt a healthy lifestyle, for example promoting dental health (Box 10.16). Parents who take their children to be immunised against such infectious diseases as diphtheria, polio, whooping cough, measles, mumps and rubella are seeking to prevent them contracting these potentially harmful illnesses. Nurses and other health educators could teach parents that immunisation is designed to prevent the onset of certain diseases, and encourage them to undertake the appropriate immunisation schedules.

Infection control

Good and effective control practices are fundamental in protecting patients, health care professionals and the public from infection. Understanding the principles of infection control

Box 10.16   Primary prevention: dental health

The Hall Report, *Health for All Children* (Hall 1996), recommends that the issues listed below should be covered. Suggestions about when to give this advice (Fuller 1998) follow each point:

- Avoid the use of sugared dummies and juices in a dinky feeder or night comforter.

Give this advice any time after birth, but before the practice begins and the habit becomes established.

- Wean babies onto a diet that, as far as possible, is free from non-milk extrinsic sugars.

Give this advice before weaning begins.

- Discourage the use of a bottle after 12 months.

It may be helpful to encourage the use of a cup as soon as a child can hold it.

- Restrict the intake of any sugary food to mealtimes.

Give this advice with other weaning advice.

- Read labels carefully and beware of 'hidden sugars' in food and drink, even in commercially prepared baby foods.

Give this advice as soon as possible after birth, to discourage the giving of sweetened drinks, and reinforce when weaning begins.

- Restrict the intake of acidic drinks, such as fruit juices, to mealtimes and dilute any fruit juices with water.

Give this advice with other advice on starting weaning.

- Brush babies' teeth, once they appear, using a small toothbrush with a smear of toothpaste.

Give this advice when the baby is 6–8 months old.

- Commence early and regular dental visits.

Six months of age is the ideal time to seek advice from a dentist on whether or not a child needs fluoride supplements.

- Advise the use of sugar-free children's medicines.

Give this advice as soon as possible after birth.

is the key to their successful application. Health education and health promotion help prevent the spread of infection by encouraging safer behaviour, for example, safer food preparation, safer sex and reducing needle sharing by drug users.

Primary health education also involves genetic counselling and antenatal care. Counselling may be offered, for example, to couples whose future baby might be at risk of developing a genetic disorder such as sickle cell anaemia or Down's syndrome.

Children's accidental deaths

An important cause of childhood mortality is accidental death. It was therefore included as a *Health of the Nation* target for England (DoH 1992). The target to achieve a reduction in accidental deaths among children under 15 by at least 33% between 1990 and 2005 has already been met. However, although death rates from injury and poisoning have fallen, there is an increasing difference between social classes. The introduction of child resistant containers for medicine has been associated with a steep drop in childhood poisonings, and there are many other small- and large-scale possibilities in which preventive efforts reflecting environmental rather than behavioural changes alone could be effective. However, the decline in rates between the 1981 and 1991 censuses shows a much smaller decline for those children in social classes IV and V (21% and 2% respectively) than those in social classes I and II (32% and 37% respectively). Motor vehicle accidents accounted for half of all childhood injury deaths and showed a similar social class gradient to that for all accidental deaths in childhood. Children from social class V are more than four times as likely to die as pedestrians than children in social class I. One of the steepest social class gradients occurs in deaths from fire and flames, mostly residential fires. Between 1981 and 1991 death rates actually increased in children from social classes IV and V while decreasing for those in social classes I and II (Drever & Whitehead 1997).

Although accidents are a major cause of childhood death, they are fortunately relatively rare. However, accidents which result in injury are more common and are also class related. Injuries to children in social classes IV and V are also likely to be more severe. Factors that partly account for this include:

- overcrowding leading to higher risks of falls or burns and scalds
- relative deprivation leading to older and less safe cooking equipment, fires, wiring, furniture and safety equipment
- unprotected roads, particularly fast arterial roads

Activity 10.6

Discuss the suggestion that attempts to educate parents about the risk of accidents and to encourage them to take more responsibility for supervision leads to victim blaming, and to feelings of guilt and defensive anger. How would you plan a health education activity relating to accidents in an appropriate, non-blaming way?

- inadequate play facilities
- difficulties in supervising children in high-rise blocks (Porter et al 1999).

Primary health education can help to reduce the number of such accidents in many different ways (Activity 10.6). Accident prevention includes campaigning for safer roads and vehicles, as well as teaching people about safe practices. Nurses can encourage others to use child safety seats, never to drink and drive and not to leave children unattended at home. Why should nurses not also become involved in changing laws where they think this is necessary, for instance by making their views about penalties for driving offences, or about potentially dangerous situations for pedestrians, widely known?

Accident and emergency departments

Growing numbers of accident and emergency (A&E) departments have computerised systems for booking in patients. Monthly accident statistic reports, detailing the occurrence and severity of injuries, could be used to identify areas with a high percentage of accidents, perhaps by using postcodes. Nurses could then develop health promotion strategies with outside agencies such as city council road safety units, road traffic police, city council home safety units, trading standards offices and other statutory and voluntary organisations (Broomfield 1999).

Examples of educative efforts directed towards primary prevention also include:

- weight control to prevent the onset of diabetes

- nutrition education to help maintain normal systolic and diastolic blood pressures
- education concerning the danger of over-exposure to sunlight as a risk factor for skin cancer
- 'stop smoking' programmes to help to prevent cancer of the lung and cardiovascular disorders.

One of the target areas for *Saving Lives: Our Healthier Nation* (DoH 1999a) is to reduce the death rate from coronary heart disease and stroke. The UK has one of the highest premature death rates from circulatory disease (including heart disease and stroke) in Europe, after the Irish Republic and Finland (Office for National Statistics 2000). For those under 65, the rate for men in the UK is two and a half times greater than that in France, the country with the lowest death rates, while for women the rate is over four times higher. A number of risk factors have been identified which are known to increase a person's risk of circulatory disease, including the lack of regular exercise, high blood pressure, obesity and smoking.

Because smoking often starts in adolescence, health promoters have tried to tackle the problem by studying ways to keep teenagers from smoking. The most successful programmes seem to be those which provide anti-smoking information in formats that appeal to adolescents, portray a positive image of the non-smoker as independent and self-reliant, and use peer-group techniques (popular peers serve as non-smoking role models) and skills development to help teenagers to resist peer pressure. The essential features of individual smoking cessation advice are: ask, advise, assist, arrange (the four As).

- Ask about smoking at every opportunity
- Advise all smokers to stop
- Assist the smoker to stop
- Arrange follow-up to monitor progress.

Smokers who need additional help should be referred to a specialist support service (RCN 1999).

Primary health education also has a major part to play in the area of mental health. Counselling individuals and families can help them to recognise or avoid problems such as anorexia nervosa in adolescents, to deal constructively with many situations that may cause stress and, more generally, to cope with life's crises as they arise. Health education and support may be available in local self-help groups or voluntary groups, advice centres or social or health services for people at risk of becoming depressed or suicidal, including those who are:

- unemployed (particularly young men)
- bereaved
- physically disabled
- elderly
- socially isolated
- suffering from chronic, painful or life-threatening conditions.

School health

Much health education that takes place in schools is primary in nature, that is, designed to promote a healthy lifestyle and to prevent, for example, the misuse of drugs, alcohol and tobacco (particularly during pregnancy). Stress, life events and family life are also topics for discussion. Programmes and activities can be developed to teach children and young people how to take responsibility for their own health and lifestyle, not only to prevent illness, but also to enhance the quality of life itself. The characteristics of a healthy school are outlined in Box 10.17. However, it is easy for those teaching health education merely to pass on knowledge and skills to their pupils, without evaluating the changes in pupils' outlook and behaviour. 'How can I motivate these young people to want to know what a healthy diet might be; and how do I encourage them to avoid such conditions as anorexia nervosa, bulimia and obesity?': these are questions that teachers, nurses and other health educators need to ask themselves when planning programme activities. Suggestions for developing a policy for school snacks are given in Box 10.18.

Secondary health education

Secondary health education is concerned with halting or reversing the development of an existing disease, minimising its severity and reversing its

---

Box 10.17 **What is a healthy school?**
(Moore 1998)

A healthy school:

- is a learning community, where education is the core business
- is committed to ongoing school improvement, improving teaching and improving learning
- is explicit about values, which are supported by all school staff, pupils, parents, governors and local communities
- provides clear leadership and direction
- is committed to meeting the personal, social and health education (PSHE) needs of pupils and staff in a systematic manner
- gives pupils a voice which influences policy and practice
- develops effective partnerships with parents, community groups and others
- gives consistent responses to pupil needs
- provides a supportive, challenging learning environment
- celebrates diversity and achievement
- is keen to learn what works well and engages in self-monitoring evaluation.

Box 10.18 **Developing a policy on snacks**
(Fuller 1998)

Producing a policy on snacks can involve teachers, governors, catering staff, school nurses and parents. A written policy confirms the school's commitment to developing a healthy school environment, and it may be written into the school's prospectus. Such policies may recommend what is stocked in tuck shops, what snacks are available for younger children and what drinks children are allowed to bring to school.

Some schools make a profit from selling healthy, sugar-free snacks in their tuck shops – for example easy-to-store items such as low fat crisps and fruit. Children can also benefit by learning valuable business skills through running tuck shops. They may also enjoy special projects involving preparing and selling a wider variety of healthy snacks.

---

progress. It aims to encourage people to seek early diagnosis and treatment and to comply with medical treatments and recommendations.

Health screening

People may be encouraged to undergo health screening procedures so that a condition or disease can be identified at an early stage, often before any signs or symptoms have been noticed. The appropriate treatment or management of the condition can then begin.

HIV testing

The NHS Executive (1999) recommends that all pregnant women should be offered and recommended an HIV test along with other antenatal screening tests as an integral part of their care. By December 2002 the uptake of antenatal HIV testing should be 90%, with 80% of HIV infected pregnant women being identified and offered advice and treatment during antenatal care.

For screening to be effective for the condition or disease (Naidoo & Wills 1994):

- it should have a long pre-clinical phase so that a screening test will not miss its signs
- earlier treatment should improve the outcomes
- the test should be sensitive (i.e. it should detect all those with the disease)
- the test should be specific (i.e. it should detect only those with the disease)
- the test should be acceptable, easy to perform and safe
- the test should be cost-effective (i.e. the number of tests performed should yield a number of positive cases).

Screening programmes for hypertension, diabetes, glaucoma and sexually transmitted diseases are examples of other vital aspects of secondary health education in which nurses can become involved. The community setting is the venue for essential preventive programmes, such as vision and hearing testing, screening for scoliosis and the assessment of children for disabilities or developmental delays (Box 10.19).

Nurses are also taking the lead in tackling growing problems such as hospital acquired infection. By taking the initiative and drawing on expert knowledge, they can make a real difference to the way in which services are coordinated to improve outcomes (Case example 10.5).

Box 10.19 **Developmental screening** (Hall 1996)

The performance of one or more developmental examinations on apparently normal children at specified key ages in infancy and early childhood. The aim is to examine *all* apparently normal children in order to identify those who may have some undetected abnormality.

Developmental examination
A clinical procedure which evaluates the level of development reached by a child at a particular age and detects any deviations from the normal. It may include an interview with parents, structured observations, physical and neurological examination and the administration of specific tasks. A comparison is made between the abilities of the child being examined and those of other children of the same age. Various developmental tests, charts and scales contain the data needed to make such comparisons.

 Case example 10.5 Infection control (Department of Health 1999b)

In a district general hospital in Wiltshire the infection control nurse has established an infection control link nurse network, recruiting 65 link nurses from acute hospitals and the community. Infection control knowledge, compliance with policies by health care workers and within the wider environment has been assessed through a quality and audit framework. It has clearly demonstrated quality improvements including lower rates of hospital acquired infection.

Cancer

There is an increase in testicular cancer in young men, and breast cancer accounts for 30% of all female cancers and will affect 1 in 12 English women at some time in their lives. Individuals can detect cancer of the breast or testicles in its early stages by self-examination, which can be taught by nurses either to groups or on an individual basis. People can also be taught to recognise early melanoma and to attend for treatment at a stage when prospects for cure are good – as is the case with several other types of malignancy. People can be encouraged to attend well man and well woman clinics, where health education and health promotion activities, including breast and cervical screening, are carried out.

Tertiary health education

The function of this aspect of health promotion is to prevent deterioration, relapse and complications where disease or a condition already exists, thus promoting rehabilitation of the patient, so that the best possible level of health might be achieved. Case example 10.6 shows how a successful support group was set up for pregnant teenagers. Nurses taking part in tertiary health education may also be involved in helping patients to adjust to terminal conditions, and in providing counselling for patients and their relatives and carers. In the treatment of incurable forms of cancer, the health education goal may be to help the patient remain as comfortable as possible.

HIV/AIDS

There is clear evidence that transmission of HIV from an infected mother to her baby can be

Case example 10.6 Teenage pregnancy support group, St George's Hospital, Tooting (Social Exclusion Unit 1999)

A teenage support group was set up by a midwife who noticed that pregnant teenagers often felt anxious attending clinics when older mothers were present. Many young mothers were therefore possibly missing important antenatal care. The teenage support group continues to offer support, education and continuity of care to pregnant girls under 18.

Range of services. Clients are referred from GPs, are looked after by one consultant and see the same midwife throughout their pregnancy where possible, to allow continuity of care. Group or individual advice and education is provided on contraception, parenthood, health and diet and other relevant topics, helping to promote a positive approach to pregnancy and allow informed decisions and choices to be made. Families are encouraged to give support to the expectant mothers and fathers.

Education. Involvement with school or college education is encouraged until as near the birth as possible.

Outcomes. Although formal evaluation is difficult, project workers consider that the number of those presenting late in pregnancy for care and monitoring has been reduced. The clinic has become an integral part of the maternity services and the improved obstetric care reduces health dangers to the young mothers and their babies.

greatly reduced by interventions such as antiretroviral treatment in pregnancy and the perinatal period and the avoidance of breastfeeding. The development of new effective combination therapies for treatment of HIV in adults means that there are increasing benefits for the woman herself in knowing she is infected. In the public perception, AIDS is the territory of the young, its cause rooted in youthful behaviour, and its tragedy being the cutting short of young lives. However, in the UK, some 11% of people with AIDS are aged 50 and over (Kaufmann 1993). Those diagnosed as HIV-positive may have parents and grandparents who are, in their turn, deeply affected by the virus, and who need the kind of support usually only offered to younger people who need information, care and counselling.

Patients with chronic conditions such as diabetes need to adjust their dietary intake to ensure maximum health, and health education for them would include the stimulation of positive attitudes towards altering their diet. Nurses can help those whose illness is disabling to adopt a lifestyle that minimises limitations, for example, through the introduction of mechanical and electronic aids. Simple adaptations, such as using easy-to-hold cutlery or modifying the living environment with ramps or rails, may be needed in addition to nursing and dietary advice. In the case of patients who have overcome an illness, nurses may need to provide support in the adjustment to a former state of health and in the abandonment of the 'sick role'.

Tertiary health education in mental health may involve helping individuals and their families to deal with the stress and management of established mental illness or handicap. Helping families to cope with current crises and to manage problems associated with learning disabilities or long-standing illness can make a significant contribution to the rehabilitation of the whole family unit. The aim is to help patients and families to reach and maintain an optimum level of functioning. Support and education for the family is especially important in cases of handicapping conditions and long-term psychotic illnesses such as schizophrenia (Case example 10.7).

Case example 10.7 Caring for Tony
(Finlayson & Forster 2000)

This case example describes the care of Tony, a man with severe and enduring mental health problems. It illustrates the use of a psychosocial model of care and multidisciplinary teamwork to promote rehabilitation. Tony is a 39-year-old patient in a mental health high dependency unit (HDU), a locked unit which caters for complex health problems and needs. In Tony's case these include challenging behaviour such as aggression and a past history of fire-setting. He appears to have developed schizophrenia at an early age; there is a possibility of a genetic component to his illness as other family members have also experienced mental health problems. He suffered respiratory problems as a baby and developmental delay was noted in childhood. At 14 years of age Tony took time off school to help care for his dying father. This was a major life event as Tony lost the role model he idolised and the person who had provided much of his social interaction. Adolescence was stressful as he was bullied at school and did not do as well as his older siblings. He is thought to have suffered from low self-esteem and lack of confidence in managing everyday tasks. He became increasingly disruptive and aggressive, often towards his mother, and was admitted to a psychiatric hospital. He was convicted of threatening his mother and a policeman with his father's shotgun, and detained in a regional secure unit. After an unsuccessful attempt at returning to the community in a hostel, continuing assaults on others and twice setting fire to bedding, Tony was transferred to a special hospital for care in conditions of high security.

Various psychotic symptoms were identified, including delusions that UFOs had landed, that he had a religious mission and that he was a fictional television character. He experienced disturbing auditory hallucinations in which he heard voices from television shows of his youth. Tony's behaviour did not respond well to treatment for some years, until he was given the novel antipsychotic drug clozapine and improved enough to be transferred to the HDU. While Tony was calmer and no longer assaulted others, his conversation revolved around the same delusional ideas and his motivation, personal hygiene and social skills remained poor.

Interventions to improve the quality of Tony's life and health

Multidisciplinary case management was introduced into the HDU and gradual progress was made in areas identified as priorities. He was safely maintained on clozapine. No further assaults and fire-setting occurred, suggesting they were indeed a response to psychotic symptoms. Tony was escorted by staff to activities first within the hospital, then outside it. He was gradually introduced to situations new to him such as supermarkets and public transport. In time, he was allowed unescorted visits to the town, and would sometimes go out with his mother. He was accepted for a place in a high dependency nursing home. Tony's mother, as the most important person in his life, has been involved, supported and kept informed. In the unit's relatives' support group she played a key role in supporting other relatives. Having felt marginalised by services in the past, she came to develop confidence in her relationships with Tony and with the team.

Training initiatives had taken place to introduce all the unit's staff to psychosocial approaches to complement the model of care. They were encouraged to modify the unit's atmosphere by employing a low level of expressed emotion in their day-to-day interactions with service users, avoiding criticism and intrusiveness. Remaining tolerant and sensitive to the effects of illness and stress on behaviour enabled the planning of consistent, systematic interventions to bring about improvements. As all team members had contact with Tony, suitable responses to undesirable behaviour were discussed and agreed to be used by all. Inappropriate speech was sensitively pointed out, and suitable alternatives were suggested, modelled and practised. Appropriate speech and actions were positively reinforced with praise and increased periods of leave off the unit. Tony's self-esteem gradually increased and as his confidence grew new goals were agreed with him.

Tony's freedom of choice and movement have increased, and he is less frustrated as he can express and discuss his needs. His behaviour and conversation have become more socially acceptable, although his hygiene remains poor. His future care will need careful planning to maintain support for him and his mother, monitoring his risk management as re-introduction to community living is pursued.

THE RADICAL OPTION: HEALTHY PUBLIC POLICY

Tones (1998) discusses criticisms of the preventive approach to health education. It may disregard the social context and environment in which a person's health occurs and assume that people have free choice regarding health behaviour. To advocate individual lifestyle change is to blame the victims of the social and environmental factors which create the unhealthy circumstances in the first place. The radical option is fully compatible with the Ottawa Charter (p. 280). This brought the matter of health policy to centre stage, and argued that there would be global improvement in health only when governments made serious efforts to deal with the environmental and social circumstances which promoted ill-health and nurtured disease. Building healthy public policy requires political will to bring about the necessary legislation and create healthy environments. The preventive model also assumes that people will act rationally when given information and advice by nurses and other health educators. In contrast, the radical approach seeks the roots of health problems and finds them in social, economic and political factors. The radical approach rejects the so-called victim blaming stance of the preventive model and attempts to 'refocus upstream'. This term refers to a parable that describes a doctor busily dragging drowning people from a flooding river who remarks, 'You know, I am so busy jumping in, pulling them to shore, applying artificial respiration, that I have no time to see who the hell is upstream pushing them all in'. The radical model seeks to focus not on the individual and his behaviour but on those social, economic and political factors that promote unhealthy practices and produce unhealthy food and hazardous products.

A large amount of information that was collected and analysed in a national survey (Blaxter 1990) arrives at an inescapable conclusion: circumstances have greater weight than does behaviour in determining health status. This is not to suggest that a person's health would not be improved if he stopped smoking for instance, but that, in some circumstances, the improvement might only be a modest one. The avoidance of unhealthy behaviour, such as smoking and eating a poor diet, offers much more protection to health in parts of the country where the environment is already more conducive to good health, for example, in non-industrial suburban or rural areas. Moreover, adopting a healthy lifestyle is much more difficult for those living in poverty.

The radical model applied to the prevention of coronary heart disease would focus not upon the individual, but upon the various social, economic and political factors that promote unhealthy products and practices. Public awareness of the ways in which commercial interests can be at odds with health interests, such as dangers from factory emissions of smoke, might be heightened. A local campaign consistent with the radical approach might unite a parent–teacher association and a school's governing body to influence the school canteen to provide healthy food, in line with the 'health promoting school' initiatives discussed earlier.

THE EMPOWERMENT MODEL

This third health education approach reflects the idea that the individual's ability to choose for himself and determine his own lifestyle is an important aspect of both psychological and physical well-being. The aim is to encourage personal growth by developing self-esteem and self-assertiveness. Health educators support change through the individual's own choices, rather than by coercion. True empowerment not only requires a basis of knowledge to support informed choices, but also demands the clarification of values and the chance to practise decision-making skills. People also need to be able to influence their own environment and to seek to change it, perhaps by working together in groups to influence policies at a local or national level.

People who view themselves as having little control over their circumstances have higher rates of mortality and illness. Research also shows that health promotion approaches that involve people in defining their own needs and engage them in a participatory way are more effective than those which apply a 'top-down' approach (Gillies 1997). Many self-help groups and patients' organisations have been set up, for instance associations of patients with chronic renal failure, Crohn's disease, haemophilia, thalassaemia, diabetes and asthma, and associations of relatives of patients suffering from mental disorders. They play an important role in health promotion by sharing information and acting as advocates of improvements in the services provided. They also contribute to monitoring the quality of services and to improving the management of the condition concerned or its prevention. One explicit aim of health care systems in the future should be to provide citizens and patients with information, in order to empower them and improve their health (WHO 1999b).

In order to reach this level of empowerment, people will need support and guidance in acquiring the necessary skills (see, for example, Case example 10.8). The ability to motivate patients to

Case example 10.8 Health promotion among ethnic minorities: colorectal cancer

Carcinoma of the large bowel is a common malignancy that occurs mainly in older people. There are 31 000 new cases each year in the UK, with an annual death rate of about 18 000. It is more prevalent in highly developed countries such as the UK, the USA, Australasia and Western Europe than in central Africa and Asia. However, when black Africans adopt a Western diet their incidence of colorectal tumours increases.

Swan (1999) discusses the implications of a rising incidence of bowel disease in the relatively high Asian population in Walsall. She points out that nurses need to understand Asian culture and health beliefs so that health education is culturally sensitive and will encourage people to present with symptoms early. Many people perceive a social stigma attached to bowel disease, especially in Asian cultures where it has up to now been rare. Patients may delay seeking treatment, relying on home remedies and herbal medicine, resulting in advanced disease when treatment is finally sought. Positive steps taken in Walsall to overcome the unmet needs of some sections of the population include the establishment of local networks which aim to:

- provide information and support
- increase health resources
- implement more appropriate policies and actions
- improve uptake of health services to meet local needs, for example, by offering easier access or translation services
- generate more information about the health of the local population
- identify areas of inequality.

The hospital trust has also sought to achieve fair ethnic minority representation in the workforce and developed other successful initiatives that include:

- investigating courses for local people who want to work in health care but feel they lack literacy skills
- auditing recruitment and selection procedures annually
- providing education and training
- organising a cultural awareness group that uses the skills and knowledge of ethnic minority staff to improve services
- sending health professionals to local meetings of ethnic minority groups to explain and answer questions through translators about medical conditions and hospital services.

These measures aim to increase knowledge about services such as breast screening and why they are offered and to promote awareness of bowel conditions through education and the provision of information. Thus Asian and other ethnic minority groups may be empowered to take control and seek advice regarding appropriate, relevant services (Swan 1999).

change their substance abuse behaviour, for example, is one of the most challenging skills that nurses need to develop. Through working with individuals, families and community organisations, nurses can help to influence change and promote health. On a one-to-one basis, nurses can motivate the patient by gradually building a therapeutic relationship in which they help the patient to set goals and to assume responsibility for his own recovery.

HEALTH FOR EVERYONE

Health promotion is concerned with the full range of modifiable determinants of health – not only individual behaviours and lifestyles, but also factors such as income and social status, education, employment and working conditions, access to health services and the physical environment. These, in combination, affect the lives and health of all of us. One of the greatest challenges facing nurses today is how to promote the health of people who live in conditions of social, economic and environmental deprivation. The health divide between rich and poor, the employed and the unemployed, is getting wider. The key to effective health promotion lies in looking beyond individual behaviours to the personal circumstances in which people find themselves. The essence of health promotion is choice. People should be free to participate in promoting and improving their own health, while acknowledging social responsibilities towards others and the wider community.

REFERENCES

Acheson D 1998 Independent inquiry into inequalities in health. Stationery Office, London
Ajzen I, Fishbein M 1980 Understanding attitudes and predicting social behaviour. Prentice-Hall, New Jersey
Anderson C, Wilkie P (eds) 1992 Reflective helping in HIV and AIDS. Open University Press, Milton Keynes
Arora S, Coker N, Gillam S, Ismail H 2000 Improving the health of black and minority ethnic groups: a guide for primary care organizations. King's Fund, London
Ashton J, Seymour H 1993 The setting for a new public health. In: Beattie A, Gott M, Jones L, Sidell M (eds) Health and wellbeing: a reader. Macmillan/Open University, Milton Keynes

Bandura A 1977 Self-efficacy: toward a unifying theory of behavioural change. Psychological Review 64(2): 191–215

Barker H M 1996 Nutrition and dietetics for health care, 9th edn. Churchill Livingstone, New York

Becker M H 1984 The health belief model and personal health behaviour. Slack, New Jersey

Bennett P, Hodgson R 1992 Psychology and health promotion. In: Bunton R, Macdonald G (eds) Health promotion: disciplines and diversity. Routledge, London, pp 23–41

Bernard M, Meade K 1993 Women come of age. Edward Arnold, London

Black D 1980 Inequalities in health: report of a research working group. HMSO, London

Blaxter M 1990 Lifestyle, health and health promotion: proceedings of a symposium on health and lifestyle. Health Promotion Research Trust, Cambridge

Boud D, Cohen R, Walker D 1993 Using experience for learning. Open University Press, Milton Keynes

Branigan P, Wellings K 1998 Dance drug education in clubs: evaluation of the London Dance Safety Campaign. Health Education Journal 57(3): 232–240

British Medical Association 1999 Growing up in Britain: ensuring a healthy future for our children. BMJ Books, London

Broomfield R 1999 Health promotion in A&E. Nursing Times Clinical Monographs No 8. NT Books, London

Byrne C, Isaacs S, Voorberg N 1994 Assessment of the physical health needs of people with chronic mental illness: one focus for health promotion. Canada's Mental Health 39: 7–12

Daines J, Daines C, Graham B 1992 Adult learning, adult teaching. University of Nottingham, Nottingham

Department of Health 1992 The health of the nation: a strategy for health in England. Cmnd 1986. HMSO, London

Department of Health 1999a Saving lives: our healthier nation. Stationery Office, London

Department of Health 1999b Making a difference: strengthening the nursing, midwifery and health visiting contribution to health and healthcare. Department of Health, London

Drever F, Whitehead M 1997 Health inequalities. Stationery Office, London

Ewles L, Simnett I 1999 Promoting health: a practical guide, 4th edn. Baillière Tindall, Edinburgh

Finlayson S, Forster J 2000 Addressing institutionalisation. In: Mercer D, Mason T, McKeown M, McCann G (eds) Forensic mental health care: a case study approach. Churchill Livingstone, Edinburgh

Fuller S S 1998 Oral health promotion: a practical guide for health visitors and school nurses. Health Education Authority, London

Gillies P 1997 Partnerships for health and the potential for social capital. Paper presented at World Health Organization health promotion conference, Jakarta. WHO, Geneva

Gowman N 1999 Healthy neighbourhoods. King's Fund, London

Graham H 1993 When life's a drag: women, smoking and disadvantage. Department of Health/HMSO, London

Greenberg J S 1992 Health education: learner-centered instructional strategies, 2nd edn. Brown, Iowa

Greenhalgh S 2000 Helping children to learn about their diabetes. Professional Nurse 15(12): 755–757

Hall D 1996 Health for all children, 3rd edn. Oxford University Press, Oxford

Hicks N R, Crowther R 2000 Coronary heart disease: a practical tool and structured approach to developing and implementing a HImP. In: Rawaf S, Orton P Health improvement programmes. Royal Society of Medicine, London

Jones S 1999 Learning disability nursing: holistic care at its best. Nursing Standard 13: 52, 61

Kai J 1999 Valuing diversity: a resource for effective health care of ethnically diverse communities. Royal College of General Practitioners, London

Kaufmann T 1993 A crisis of silence: HIV, AIDS and older people. Age Concern, London

Mager R F 1990 Preparing instructional objectives, 2nd edn. Kogan Page, London

McNeish D 1999 From rhetoric to reality: participatory approaches to health promotion with young people. Health Education Authority, London

Moore W 1998 Making the healthy option the easy option. Healthlines 58: 12–14

Naidoo J, Wills J 1994 Health promotion: foundations for practice. Baillière Tindall, London

NHS Executive 1998 In the public interest: developing a strategy for public participation in the NHS. NHS Executive/Institute of Health Service Management/NHS Confederation, Leeds

NHS Executive 1999 Reducing mother to baby transmission of HIV. Health Service Circular 183. NHS Executive/Institute of Health Service Management/NHS Confederation, Leeds

Office for National Statistics 2000 Social trends 30. Stationery Office, London

Parsons L 1991 Homeless families in Hackney. Public Health 105: 287–296

Perry K, Kirmer D 1990 Wellness education for clients receiving psychiatric care in a partial hospital program. Holistic Nurse Practitioner 4: 72–78

Porter M, Alder B, Abraham C 1999 Psychology and sociology applied to medicine. Churchill Livingstone, Edinburgh

Royal College of Nursing 1994 Public health: nursing rises to the challenge. RCN, London

Royal College of Nursing 1999 Clearing the air: a nurses' guide to smoking and tobacco control. RCN, London

Social Exclusion Unit 1999 Teenage pregnancy. Stationery Office, London

Swan E 1999 Equal care for all. Nursing Standard 13(27): 42–44

Tones K 1998 Health education and the promotion of health: seeking wisely to empower. In: Kendall S (ed) Health and empowerment: research and practice. Arnold, London, ch 3, p 57

Tones K, Tilford S 1994 Health education: effectiveness, efficiency and equity, 2nd edn. Chapman and Hall, London

Wilkinson R G 1996 Unhealthy societies: the afflictions of inequality. Routledge, London

World Health Organization 1946 Preamble of the constitution of the World Health Organization. WHO, Geneva

World Health Organization 1978 The Alma Ata Declaration. WHO Chronicle 32: 28–29

World Health Organization 1986 Ottawa Charter for Health Promotion. WHO, Geneva

World Health Organization 1999a Health 21: the health for all policy framework for the WHO European region. WHO, Copenhagen

World Health Organization 1999b World health report 1999: making a difference. WHO, Geneva

World Health Organization 2000 World health report 2000: health systems: improving performance. WHO, Geneva

FURTHER READING

Ewles L, Simnett I 1999 Promoting health: a practical guide, 4th edn. Baillière Tindall, Edinburgh
This popular text provides a readable, comprehensive introduction to both the theory and practice of health promotion. It features an active learning approach incorporating case studies, practical exercises, quizzes and questionnaires. Many useful suggestions for further reading and resources are given, and practice points are summarised at the end of each chapter.

Kendall S (ed) Health and empowerment: research and practice. Arnold, London
This text focusses on research and issues relating to empowerment in nursing and health care, providing valuable insights into the background and current aspects of this topical concept.

Naidoo J, Wills J 2000 Health promotion, 2nd edn. Baillière Tindall, London
These experienced health promotion authors provide students with a comprehensive, critical framework for their study of theoretical and practical aspects of promoting health. Many in depth discussions of reflection, planning, evaluation and similar crucial aspects relating to a wide variety of practice are included. It is a reader-centred text and an invaluable resource.

World Health Organization 1999 Health 21: the health for all policy framework for the WHO European region. WHO, Copenhagen
The WHO European programme features the need to understand the wider social influences on health and this text brings the latest targets for public health and health promotion up to date in a highly readable format.

11

Accountability in practice

Cynthia Gilling

CHAPTER CONTENTS

Nursing as a profession 310

Changes in the concepts of professionalism 310
Reflective practice 311
The decision process and patient empowerment 312
Supporting practice and standards of care 312
Collective responsibility and specialisation 312

Accountability and the nurse 312

The Code of Professional Conduct 313
Purpose 313
Students and the Code 313
Applying the Code 313
Clause 1: Promoting well-being 315
Clause 2: Responsibility 315
Clause 3: Professional Development 316
Clause 4: The limits of competence 316
Clause 5: Patients' and clients' rights 317
Clause 6: Collaboration with other health carers 317
Clause 7: Respect for cultural differences 317
Clause 8: Conscientious objection 318
Clause 9: The proper use of privilege 318
Clause 10: Maintaining confidentiality 319
Clauses 11 and 12: The environment of care 320
Clause 13: Protecting colleagues 321
Clause 14: Teaching colleagues 321
Clause 15: Dealing with gifts 322
Clause 16: Qualifications and advertising 322

The role of the statutory bodies 322
The UKCC 322
Improving standards of training 323
Meeting EC guidelines 325
Admission conditions 325
Further training 326
Standards of professional conduct 326
Minority groups within the profession 326
The National Boards 326
The UKCC and the National Boards 327

Professional organisations and trade unions 327
The Royal College of Nursing 327
Developments since 1916 327
Benefits of membership 327
Other activities 328
Unison 328
Joining an organisation 328

The international setting 328
The European Community 328
The International Council of Nurses 328

Conclusion 329

References 329

Further reading 330

This chapter describes different aspects of the professional role of the nurse and discusses issues relating to accountability in the nursing profession and the role of the bodies concerned with its regulation. At the end of the chapter, the student should be able to:

- discuss the status of nursing as a profession
- interpret and apply the sixteen clauses of the Code of Professional Conduct
- describe the role of the statutory bodies governing nursing, and the professional organisations and trade unions, both domestic and international, that represent nurses.

NURSING AS A PROFESSION

On entering nursing as a student it is soon obvious that you are not only following an academic and practical course but also learning how to be part of the nursing profession. But what does this mean? The word 'profession' and its adjective, 'professional', are used in a number of different ways today. 'Professional' is often used as the opposite of amateur, as, for example, professional footballers or professional actors who are paid to play or perform rather than doing it unpaid. We also talk about 'professional behaviour', usually perceived as acceptable to society, but particularly involving ethical and/or moral behaviour. If we use the term 'professional judgement', we expect the person to be knowledgeable about a certain subject and to be able to give expert advice.

Society has, through the centuries, tried to develop definitions of particular professions. The earliest of these covered law, medicine and the church, primarily because people practising these professions first underwent a lengthy period of theoretical study and members followed a certain code of behaviour. In the 17th and 18th centuries education was only for those who could afford it, and this enabled these new 'professionals' to guard their knowledge and thus gain great respect, power and influence over the majority of people. The concept of a profession or professional has, however, changed with the growth of education and development of society.

Pyne (1998) quotes Benson's (1992) five key elements of a profession:

1. Register of members, standards of conduct and compliance
2. Control of admission
3. Preparation and dissemination of advice and guidance
4. Maintain fitness for purpose
5. Having the authority for removal from the Register.

The United Kingdom Central Council for Nursing, Midwifery and Health Visiting (UKCC) was set up as the regulating council for nurses as a result of the Nurses, Midwives, and Health Visitors Act passed in 1979. The Council maintains a Register of members and defines professional standards. It controls admission to the Register of all those licensed to practise by defining the educational programme of theory and practice students must achieve prior to registration. It maintains fitness for purpose through issuing guidance on the education required to maintain professional knowledge and practice through regular updating. This is also a requirement for renewal of the licence to practise (see also p. 316 and Ch. 1).

The UKCC also meets the third element, to disseminate advice and guidance, through its quarterly journal *Register* and through various booklets on specific nursing and midwifery issues.

Finally the UKCC has a Professional Conduct Committee composed of council and lay members. If misconduct is proved, the committee has various options regarding disciplinary action, depending on the severity of the offence and the effect on patient care (see also p. 326).

CHANGES IN THE CONCEPT OF PROFESSIONALISM

In looking at the history of nursing (Ch. 1) we have seen how nursing developed in the shadow

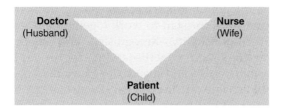

Figure 11.1   The nurse within a patriarchal triad (Gamarnikov 1978).

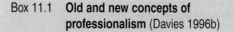

Box 11.1   **Old and new concepts of professionalism** (Davies 1996b)

Old professionalism
Mastery of knowledge
Unilateral decision process
Patient as dependent
Colleagues as deferential
Autonomy and self-management
Individual accountability
Detachment
Interchangeability of practitioners

New professionalism
Reflective practice
Interdependent decision process
Colleagues involved
Support practice
Collective responsibility
Engagement
Specificity of practitioners' strengths

of medical practice and the masculine dominance of society. This was particularly strong in the patriarchal system of the Victorian era. Prevailing attitudes encouraged the devaluation of women and as the medical profession became more powerful it became one of the major producers and enforcers of gender roles in our society. Nurses in the early part of the last century were predominantly women and were seen as handmaidens or subordinates to the doctor. The patriarchal element was acted out in the ward situation and its legacy is still with us today (Gamarnikov 1978). The strictly defined roles identified in Figure 11.1 endorsed the hierarchical structure in both medicine and nursing, producing communication problems and role conflict within the nurse–patient–doctor triad. While such roles can still be recognised, particularly in the hospital setting, this is changing.

It is these changes in today's society and in health care that have made writers look at new concepts of professionalism for nurses (Davies 1996a, Abbott & Meerabeau 1998). Economic stringencies, reorganisations in the NHS and increased knowledge and demands by patients and clients have undermined some of the doctor's power and influence.

Davies (1996b) argues that the old ideas of a professional, developed in the early 1900s, were in fact created and dominated by the male-orientated society of that period. In this century, new concepts of professionalism may be the way forward for nursing (Box 11.1). If we explore some of these new ideas of professionalism, it is obvious that such changes are already taking place within the nursing profession.

Reflective practice

Whereas previously the person with specialist knowledge – usually the doctor – had the higher status, more recently, nursing has begun to explore the concept of reflective practice. Reflective practice is essentially learning from practice. As a student you will gradually see how the knowledge you have gained in the classrooms can be put into practice once you start nursing. As you gain experience your skills in aspects of nursing will develop. Such skills will be enhanced if you think back on how or why you took a particular action and how you might improve the care you gave. Schon (1983) explains how professionals think in action; this is termed reflection IN practice, whereas evaluating care afterwards would be reflection ON practice. In this way nurses can use knowledge and research as well as formal and intuitive experience to improve skills and standards of care. Eraut (1994) explains how educationally, professional knowledge and competence can be developed. This includes using a problem-solving approach when reflecting on practice, in other words identifying a problem and using theory to inform and enhance practice rather than just gaining further knowledge from study. See Chapter 14 for details about reflective practice.

The decision process and patient empowerment

The decision processes within the care setting have also changed from that described earlier when the doctor dominated. Patients, patient support groups and other health care workers are part of the decision-making process. Doctors now have to be open with patients and discuss all options of treatments and recognise the rights of patients to make an informed choice or even to decline treatment altogether. Recent government policies and guidelines set out patients' rights to standards of care. The nurses' Code of Conduct (Clauses 1 and 5) encourages nurses to be the patient's advocate in upholding such rights.

Supporting practice and standards of care

Professionals have always claimed that autonomy and self-management is an essential part of practice. Self-regulation and peer review are seen as the only appropriate means of monitoring because no one else is versed in the specialist knowledge and practice. For many years this has worked well, and it still continues to work well. However, recent tragedies within the NHS have demonstrated that the method is not foolproof. The General Medical Council is now looking at how its self-regulating mechanism is failing to pick up incompetence or poor standards of doctors at an early stage. Nursing can have similar problems (Clothier Report 1994), but a move to preceptorship for newly qualified nurses, mentoring and clinical supervision should help nurses to recognise their responsibilities in upholding and developing better standards of care. Recent developments within medicine on identifying evidence-based practice has demonstrated the need for a joint approach by the professions within the NHS in setting and maintaining standards (Taylor 1996).

Collective responsibility and specialisation

With the development of more specialisms within medicine – and consequently within nursing – and the reduction in junior doctors' hours, there is a greater need for staff to work together and take joint responsibility. Recognising and sharing knowledge and expertise with, for example, physiotherapists and speech/language therapists should enable care to be better planned and coordinated. This is particularly pertinent in the area of learning disabilities where nurses work very closely with personnel from social services.

Nurses have always been more involved with patients than other members of the caring professions, simply because they are with patients 24 hours of the day. Instead of nurses being given tasks to do to all patients (e.g. a bedpan round), they are now responsible for the total care of a certain number of patients, and this has altered the relationship between nurse and patient. This is particularly so in treating the mentally ill where the nurse develops a therapeutic relationship with the patient.

In looking at Davies's old and new concepts of professionalism (see Box 11.1) and the old criteria, it is obvious that old and new coexist. However, new developments and roles within nursing, for example the clinical nurse specialist, emphasise some of these new concepts and point the way to the development of nursing as a profession in the future. In this instance the specialist nurse (sometimes called a nurse practitioner or surgeon's assistant) has taken a course of further study in a particular speciality in order to expand the boundaries of their practice (ENB 1997). In all cases the emphasis is on holistic nursing care.

ACCOUNTABILITY AND THE NURSE

As we have seen in this chapter, for many years nursing was set in a hierarchical structure, and accountability was with either the doctor or the matron. Personal accountability within nursing is growing, particularly as nurses take on new roles and often find themselves working on their own without supervision. This is particularly so in the community. However, there can be no accountability without responsibility. Similarly patients have rights but also have responsibilities with regard to how they utilise the services provided.

In the last decade there has been an enormous increase in litigation against hospital and community personnel. It is therefore essential for all nurses to be aware that accountability means taking responsibility for your own actions and decisions. No one else can answer for you and it is no defence to say that you were acting on someone else's orders. You must be able to justify the decisions and judgements you make. Harris & Redshaw (1998) raise concerns regarding the increase of specialist nurses, the ambiguity of role and lack of guidelines or protocols that make the nurse's accountability role difficult. The UKCC Code of Conduct for nurses, midwives and health visitors (UKCC 1992a) acts as a guide in helping the profession take on its role of accountability. A useful publication is *Guidelines for Professional Practice* (UKCC 1996).

THE CODE OF PROFESSIONAL CONDUCT

The first code of ethics for nurses was produced by the International Council of Nurses (ICN) in Brazil in 1953 and was subsequently revised in 1965 and again in 1973. This code was similar to the one now used in the UK, the *Code of Professional Conduct* (UKCC 1992a), formulated by the UKCC in 1983 and revised in 1992.

PURPOSE

The UKCC Code of Professional Conduct aims to define and improve professional standards and grows out of a clear background of law, in particular Sections 2(1) and 2(5) of the Nurses, Midwives and Health Visitors Act 1979. The Code makes ethically-based statements regarding the value of life, justice, honesty and individual freedom (see Ch. 3). It therefore assists in safeguarding the public and provides guidance regarding appropriate conduct to the profession. This is summarised in the statement introducing the Code: 'Each registered nurse, midwife and health visitor shall act, at all times, in such a manner as to:

- Safeguard and promote the interests of individual patients and clients
- Serve the interests of society
- Justify public trust and confidence
- Uphold and enhance the good standing and reputation of the professions'.

The UKCC (1996) guidelines for professional practice have been produced to help practitioners with the many challenges they face in day-to-day practice.

STUDENTS AND THE CODE

Before we turn to its individual clauses, we must consider how the Code of Professional Conduct affects the student nurse. The overall responsibility for a student's actions lies with the qualified member of staff supervising the practice. In reality, however, the supervisor is not able to watch the student every minute of the day. As the student gains more knowledge and experience, she may be able to undertake some aspects of care without being closely supervised. A student is accountable under the common law of negligence. Any action considered as negligent would, of course, take into account the standard of care expected of the student at her stage of training.

The student should, therefore, guard against undertaking care for which adequate instruction has not been received or in which her role is unclear or inappropriate. The UKCC has produced a very useful guide for students which covers many key issues (UKCC 1998a). The Code of Professional Conduct is also a guide to students in developing their professional role.

Registration as a nurse, midwife or health visitor by the UKCC gives the holder the legal right to practise in that speciality. This too, through the UKCC, helps to safeguard the public and the profession.

APPLYING THE CODE

The following sections will take each of the 16 clauses of the UKCC Code of Professional

Conduct in turn, considering their interpretation and application. Heywood Jones (1999) debates the clauses of the code and provides a number of case studies involving issues of professional conduct and accountability which make salutary reading for any member of the profession.

The present code (Box 11.2) is being revised by the UKCC. It is unlikely to change much in content but hopefully will be less 'wordy'. Vousden's (1999) suggested wording will therefore be used to identify each clause (for patients read, also, clients).

Box 11.2 UKCC Code of Professional Conduct (reproduced with kind permission from UKCC 1992a)

Each registered nurse, midwife and health visitor shall act, at all times, in such a manner as to:

- safeguard and promote the interests of individual patients and clients;
- serve the interests of society;
- justify public trust and confidence; and
- uphold and enhance the good standing and reputation of the professions.

As a registered nurse, midwife or health visitor, you are personally accountable for your practice and, in the exercise of your professional accountability, must:

1 act always in such a manner as to promote and safeguard the interest and well-being of patients and clients;
2 ensure that no action or omission on your part, or within your sphere of responsibility, is detrimental to the interests, condition or safety of patients and clients;
3 maintain and improve your professional knowledge and competence;
4 acknowledge any limitations in your knowledge and competence and decline any duties or responsibilities unless able to perform them in a safe and skilled manner;
5 work in an open and co-operative manner with patients, clients and their families, foster their independence and recognise and respect their involvement in the planning and delivery of care;
6 work in a collaborative and co-operative manner with health care professionals and others involved in providing care, and recognise and respect their particular contributions within the care team;
7 recognise and respect the uniqueness and dignity of each patient and client, and respond to their need for care, irrespective of their ethnic origin, religious beliefs, personal attributes, the nature of their health problems or any other factor;
8 report to an appropriate person or authority, at the earliest possible time, any conscientious objection which may be relevant to your professional practice;
9 avoid any abuse of your privileged relationship with patients and clients and of the privileged access allowed to their person, property, residence or workplace;

10 protect all confidential information concerning patients and clients obtained in the course of professional practice and make disclosures only with consent, where required by the order of a court or where you can justify disclosure in the wider public interest;
11 report to an appropriate person or authority, having regard to the physical, psychological and social effects on patients and clients, any circumstances in the environment of care which could jeopardise standards of practice;
12 report to an appropriate person or authority any circumstances in which safe and appropriate care for patients and clients cannot be provided;
13 report to an appropriate person or authority where it appears that the health or safety of colleagues is at risk, as such circumstances may compromise standards of practice and care;
14 assist professional colleagues, in the context of your own knowledge, experience and sphere of responsibility, to develop their professional competence, and assist others in the care team, including informal carers, to contribute safely and to a degree appropriate to their roles;
15 refuse any gift, favour or hospitality from patients or clients currently in your care which might be interpreted as seeking to exert influence to obtain preferential consideration; and
16 ensure that your registration status is not used in the promotion of commercial products or services, declare any financial or other interests in relevant organisations providing such goods or services and ensure that your professional judgement is not influenced by any commercial considerations.

Notice to all Registered Nurses, Midwives and Health Visitors

This Code of Professional Conduct for the Nurse, Midwife and Health Visitor is issued to all registered nurses, midwives and health visitors by the United Kingdom Central Council for Nursing, Midwifery and Health Visiting. The Council is the regulatory body responsible for the standards of these professions and it requires members of the professions to practise and conduct themselves within the standards and framework provided by the Code.

Clause 1

Promote and safeguard the well-being of patients.
Chapter 13 illustrates aspects of the relationship between the patient and the nurse, and the need to respect patients as individuals. The chapter develops this theme through the concept of individual care and illustrates the reciprocal nature of the nurse–patient relationship, i.e. the nurse takes on certain responsibilities in the delivery of care in return for the trust and confidence that the patient freely gives.

The move away from routine care to a more individualised approach heightens the awareness of this special relationship and may present the nurse with new difficulties in upholding this part of the Code. For instance, how can a nurse have an equally trusting and warm relationship with every patient, when nurses, like anyone else, relate better to some people than to others? Nurses often 'categorise' patients to the detriment of their well-being. For instance, they may refer to patients as 'difficult' or 'awkward', and this will influence their attitudes and relationships and the care they give (see Chs 7 and 9). Nurses should be able to make better judgements regarding patients through exploring their own values, beliefs and attitudes and by having discussions with peers, seniors and patients on this subject.

The nurse's relationship with patients has also changed from the maternal role discussed earlier to that of patient's advocate. Patients often now know more about the diagnosis through the media and in many instances can make an informed choice regarding treatment. While the nurse's role is often to explain treatments or the consequences of taking one option rather than another, her role is also to uphold patients' interests and not coerce them into a particular course of action. This is particularly relevant with the elderly, the mentally ill or those with learning disabilities who do not always understand options and implications. In this instance the nurse would act as the patient's advocate in helping him to voice his needs.

Clause 1 of the UKCC Code calls upon the nurse to 'promote' the well-being of the patient as well as to 'safeguard' it. The nurse's role in promoting

healthy lifestyles is described in Chapter 10, and this applies to any nursing speciality, both within hospitals and in the community.

Clause 2

Ensure that no action for which you are responsible will harm or potentially harm patients.
Responsibility can be viewed as falling into the following categories:

- Legal: relating to the law
- Ethical: relating to an informed sense of right or wrong
- Moral: relating to society in general
- Professional: relating to standards in our work
- Contractual: relating to agreements
- Personal: relating to how we feel and think about the welfare of others.

For the nurse, all these aspects have to be considered, as her prime responsibility is to deliver the highest standard of care to her patients. Crow (1983) suggests that the nurse's responsibility includes four main aspects:

1. Responsibility for all nursing care. This includes delegation to others and confirmation that care is carried out satisfactorily.
2. Responsibility to ensure through research and evaluation that the care given is effective and safe.
3. Responsibility to deliver care in a caring manner, i.e. with compassion, competence, confidence, conscience and commitment (Roach 1982).
4. Responsibility to deliver care within the framework of agreed moral principles, for instance those reflected in the Code itself.

The nurse may on occasion be asked to give an account of her actions – for instance if legal action is taken as a result of an action or omission that was detrimental to a patient. In such circumstances, the nurse's knowledge and experience would be called into question and any written evidence examined. This emphasises the importance of recording correct and relevant details of all nursing care given to patients. UKCC guidelines (1998b) suggest that good record keeping helps to protect the welfare of patients and clients by promoting:

- high standards of clinical care
- continuity of care
- better communication and dissemination of information between members of the inter-professional health care team
- an accurate account of treatment and care planning and delivery
- the ability to detect problems, such as changes in the patient's or client's condition at an early stage.

Another area under this clause is patient safety. To use equipment in an unsafe manner may be harmful to the patient and result in an accident. For example, lifting equipment to help patients in and out of bed or bath must always be used according to the manufacturer's instructions. Such things as failure to observe the principles of cross-infection such as hand washing between tasks may also bring harm to the patient by introducing infection. The alarming increase of patients picking up infections in hospital points to a decline in standards of care and the cleanliness of wards and departments. (See Ch. 11 in relation to safe practice.)

Clause 3

Maintain and improve your professional knowledge and competence.
The UKCC has introduced compulsory updating for all qualified staff (UKCC 2001). There are already numerous and flexible ways of maintaining competence within one's own specialism. Study days, courses and clinical experience will, through the Credit Accumulation and Transfer Scheme (CATS), go towards a diploma or degree. Post-registration programmes are provided by hospitals and by health departments in higher education. They offer study days and courses ranging from orientation of new staff, clinical updating, and courses (e.g. renal nursing and community psychiatric nursing) to special skills based courses (e.g. 'Introduction to counselling

skills' and 'Preparation for management'). The assessment of the knowledge gained through clinical practice and experience can also be used as evidence of maintaining knowledge and competence.

Such programmes are designed to meet the needs of the service as well as those of the professional. Some courses may be run on a multi-disciplinary basis to enhance understanding and teamwork among health care workers.

Clause 4

Carry out only those duties that you can perform in a skilled way.
Both students and qualified nurses need to be aware of their limitations in carrying out procedures or giving information. Either of these actions, performed badly, could put a patient in jeopardy. Most methods of competence assessment include a self-assessment component, which helps the learner to explore her limitations. Part of knowing one's limitations is having self-awareness, and teaching and developing this has been a key element in many nursing courses.

Another difficult area, often called the 'extended role', refers to the nurse undertaking procedures usually (in the UK) carried out by a doctor, for example giving intravenous drugs or performing a simple suture. Patients could use the dangers associated with such procedures, for example damage to the vein or poor scar formation through faulty suturing technique, as examples of negligence. The UKCC's document *The Scope of Professional Practice* (UKCC 1992b) is a position statement on the issue of extended role. It stresses that accountability rests firmly with the registered nurse. The document sets out six principles:
The registered nurse, midwife or health visitor:

1. must be satisfied that each aspect of practice is directed to meeting the needs and serving the interests of the patient
2. must endeavour always to achieve, maintain and develop knowledge, skill and competence to respond to those needs and interests
3. must honestly acknowledge any limits of personal knowledge and skill and take steps

to remedy any relevant deficits in order effectively and appropriately to meet the needs of patients and clients

4. must ensure that any enlargement or adjustment of the scope of professional practice must be achieved without compromising or fragmenting existing aspects of professional practice and care and that the requirements of the Council's Code of Professional Conduct are satisfied throughout the whole area of practice

5. must recognise and honour the direct or indirect personal accountability borne for all aspects of professional practice and

6. must, in serving the interests of patients and clients and the wider interests of society, avoid any inappropriate delegation to others which compromises those interests.

This area of practice has recently undergone further debate with the reduction in junior doctors' hours and thus an increase in some areas of responsibility for the nurse (Greenhalgh Report 1994, discussed elsewhere in this chapter under accountability).

Clause 5

Encourage patients to be independent and involve their loved ones in their care.
This clause emphasises the importance of involving patients in their own care and this has already been discussed under the new concept of professionalism. The recent NHS Plan (2000) sets out a new relationship with patients and promises better information for patients and carers. The use of integrated care plans should lead to greater patient/client involvement and continuity of care. This is important in the care of children. New designs of children's wards and accident and emergency departments cater for mothers to stay with their children so that they can be involved in caring for them. In caring for the elderly, the involvement, where possible, of the next of kin in decisions on treatment, rehabilitation and supportive care when discharged helps elderly people to still feel in control of their lives.

Clause 6

Work collaboratively with all those providing care.
Many people with specialist knowledge and skills contribute to the care of the patient. The doctor, nurse, physiotherapist, occupational therapist, speech/language therapist and others form what is often referred to as a 'health care team'. This collaboration works well when each team member respects the others' knowledge and skills and considers the patient's welfare to be the prime objective. In the areas of learning disabilities and mental health, nurses work closely with social workers and colleagues in the community and would be unable to achieve their patients' objectives without their assistance.

'Collaboration' does not always have to mean 'acquiescence', and the nurse should feel able to contribute on an equal basis with other colleagues. Nurses who have extended their knowledge and expertise in a particular area will feel more confident in challenging and contributing to the decision-making process (Activity 11.1). Small units, such as intensive care, palliative care or in elderly care, work well through team collaboration. Perhaps teamwork is also easier in such units because objectives are clearer and more easily defined.

Clause 7

Give equal care to all patients.
It is quite easy to forget this aspect of the Code even though we live in a multiracial, multicultural society. For many years there was a distinct lack of input into the nursing and medical curricula on these very issues (Mares et al 1985). This deficiency is lessening, partly due to the great

Activity 11.1

The doctor states that a certain patient should be discharged (his bed is required for another patient). The occupational therapist feels that the patient is not ready to cope on his own. How would you, as the nurse, contribute to a solution?

increase in the non-European, non-Christian population living in the UK and working in the health care setting. An increased awareness of the nature of different customs and beliefs through the media and the introduction of equal opportunities legislation has assisted in raising awareness on these important issues. There are many textbooks and pamphlets now available to help staff and patients understand different religions and gain insight into different customs and rituals. Having more knowledge assists the nurse not only to respect the patient's beliefs but also to recognise the associated rituals and customs. Particularly distressing to some bereaved families is the failure to observe certain customs and beliefs surrounding death. Many hospitals give guidance on this, and it is usually possible to seek advice from the hospital chaplain or an official of the particular religious group concerned (Activity 11.2) (see also Ch. 5).

Clause 8

Make known any conscientious objection.
The law prevents a practitioner from registering conscientious objection to participation in any care and/or treatment *except* with respect to the termination of pregnancy under the terms of Section 4 of the Abortion Act 1967 and the Human Fertilisation and Embryology Act 1990. It is therefore advisable for students or trained staff to check with nurse managers of operating theatres and gynaecology day wards on the extent to which nursing staff are involved in abortion procedures. They can then decide whether to

Activity 11.2

Sister asks you to prepare Mr Shah, who is a practising Muslim, for surgery. Mr Shah insists that he must get out of bed to pray to Mecca several times a day and that he will not undress for a female nurse. Mr Shah is second on the operating list and you need to give him his premedication in half an hour. How would you uphold Mr Shah's wishes and have him prepared for his operation in time?

exercise this right or to seek employment elsewhere within the hospital or unit.

There may also be other times when a nurse may question her participation in certain forms of treatment, for example electroconvulsive therapy (ECT) or resuscitation of the elderly. If this is the case, the nurse should consider carefully why she objects to such forms of treatment and discuss this with senior staff in good time, so that, if appropriate, arrangements can be made for others to care for the patient during the treatment.

Refusal to give treatment on professional rather than conscientious grounds calls for a different approach. An example might be when a nurse feels that a drug should not be given, although it is due, because the patient's condition has changed. If the nurse then decides not to administer the drug, she must record carefully the reasons for this decision, discuss the issue with the prescribing doctor and request a visit to the patient. Following this discussion, if the nurse still feels that the doctor was wrong, she should confirm again to the doctor, in writing, why she decided not to give the drug.

It is not acceptable under the Code of Conduct to refuse to care for patients with acquired immune deficiency syndrome (AIDS) or who are HIV-positive. There is no difference between caring for these patients and caring for patients suffering from an infectious disease (e.g. open tuberculosis, gastroenteritis or methicillin-resistant staphylococcus infection) as long as the principles underlying infection control are observed. The UKCC (1989) states: 'To seek to be so selective is to demonstrate unacceptable conduct. The UKCC expects the practitioner to adopt a non-judgemental approach in the exercise of their caring role.' In January 1991, a registered nurse was removed from the register for refusing to care for a patient with AIDS (Activity 11.3).

Clause 9

Do not abuse your privileged access to patients, their person, property, residence or workplace.
The relationship built up between nurse and patient is very different from normal relationships: as Burnard & Chapman (1999) state, it is in

Activity 11.3

You are asked to look after a patient while he is having ECT. You have been observing and talking to Mr Brown for the last 4 weeks, since his last treatment, and feel that there is an improvement in his depressive state, and you are personally against the use of such treatment. How would you solve this problem to the benefit of Mr Brown?

fact unique. It is different from normal social relationships because the nurse cannot choose the patient, nor the patient the nurse. The patient may be different from the nurse in age, culture and religion, and may have little in common with her socially. Yet the nurse is expected quickly to gain a rapport with the patient and put him at ease. Not only does the nurse have to forge this relationship, but at the same time she must also perform intimate care that in normal social/ ethical circumstances would not be acceptable. In the case of the mentally ill, the nurse listens to detailed accounts of very personal feelings and actions. Such situations put the nurse in a privileged position because the patient is demonstrating his trust in the nurse at a time when he is at his most vulnerable. It is therefore the nurse's duty to treat the patient's disclosures with the utmost confidentiality. This includes not discussing one patient with another and not discussing nursing details in public places, such as restaurants or when travelling in public transport, where one might be overheard.

A nurse may have access to the patient's property in hospital or in the home. If patients' property is left in the hospital for safe-keeping, local procedures must be adhered to in detailing every item, be it jewellery, money or clothing. The same applies to any items used in personal care kept on or in the patient's locker, or in their home.

Just as they cannot choose their patients, nurses cannot choose which homes they visit. Consequently, they may come across, in their work, standards and ways of life that are very different from their own and which go against

their own values and beliefs. Unless the situation is such as to endanger the health of the individual, such issues should not be discussed either with the patient or with anyone else.

The occupational health nurse who cares for patients within their work setting has a particular role to play and one in which the importance of confidentiality must be emphasised. This is particularly so in relation to management. The question may arise of whether certain information regarding an employee's health status should be divulged, particularly if it has a bearing on work performance. This is for the occupational health nurse to judge; such decisions are usually discussed with the employee before the minimum details are relayed to the manager in confidence.

Clause 10

Respect patient confidentiality, except where disclosure is required by a court order, or justified in the public interest.

The respect by nurses of confidential information has always been stressed but has been emphasised with the Data Protection Act 1984 and computer filing systems. Confidentiality, as already discussed in Clause 9, implies a trusting relationship and the patient has a right to believe that the private and personal information he gives will only be used for the purposes for which it is given and will not be released to others without his permission. It is obviously important that patients understand that some information needs to be available to others involved in the delivery of care, and who those people are (UKCC 1996). Problems arise from the number of people who may have legitimate access to notes, i.e. not just doctors and nurses but also paramedical staff and, of course, students. Students are sometimes required to use patient information for assignments; in such cases care must be taken to obtain permission, protect the identity of the patient and ensure that notes are not left lying around in public places where access cannot be monitored. This also applies to those engaged in research and audit (see Chs 3 and 12).

It is often a difficult decision as to when to withhold or disclose information. It is preferable to discuss the matter fully with other professional colleagues and, if appropriate, consult the UKCC or your professional organisation. You always need to obtain the explicit consent of a patient before disclosure of specific information. The death of a patient does not give you the right to disclose information or to break confidentiality. Disclosure of information should only occur:

- with the consent of the patient
- without the consent of the patient when the disclosure is required by law or by order of court
- without the consent of the patient when the disclosure is considered to be necessary in the public interest (UKCC 1998a).

'In the public interest' covers matters such as serious crime, child abuse, drug trafficking and other activities that place others at serious risk. If you have made a decision either to withhold or release information, then you should record the reasons for your action in the appropriate file or record (Activity 11.4) (see also Ch. 4).

With the Access Modification (Health) Order 1987 and the Access to Health Records Act 1990, patients can ask to see their records. Whether they are written down or on a computer, where anyone is involved with access to records, statements regarding confidentiality are included in the contract of employment. It is important that all records, written or computerised, must clearly indicate the identity of the person who made the record and that systems are protected from inappropriate access. The UKCC issues further guidance on both these points in the booklets *Confidentiality and Use of Computers* (1992c) and *Standards for Records and Record Keeping* (1993a).

Activity 11.4

What other matters should the nurse disclose that would be 'in the public interest'?

Clauses 11 and 12

Report to an appropriate person, any circumstances which could jeopardise standards of practice or in which safe care cannot be provided.

These clauses have implications of a political and ethical nature and point to the fact that it is really not possible to separate the private and personal from the public and political (Clay 1987). The clauses raise the question of acting upon conscience – something that is often more easily said than done. The Public Interest Disclosure Act (1998) requires organisations such as NHS Trusts to have a 'speaking out' or 'whistleblowing' policy which details the procedure for raising concerns at work. These concerns may be about patient care and services, professional practice, dishonesty, financial malpractice, patient or staff safety and many other issues. Raising concerns about the conduct of another employee is particularly difficult but the new Act, which was brought into force in 1999, is intended to make it a little easier. This type of policy is expected to assist professionals to comply with aspects of their professional codes of conduct such as Clauses 11–13 in the UKCC Code.

The most vulnerable groups of patients include the mentally ill, older people and people with learning disabilities. Such patients cannot readily articulate physical and mental abuse, lack of privacy or a want of social stimulation (Activity 11.5). Individualised care, the change in the role of those working with the mentally ill from custodian to a more therapeutic function and specific courses in caring for older people have done much to improve standards. Standards of care and principles of nursing practice are now based on research rather than on conventional practice. Research can help to guide

Activity 11.5

What action would you take if you were contributing to the care of patients who were mentally ill and resident in the community but were not being accepted by the local population?

our judgements when standards are reduced. However, without documented evidence a complaint may be ignored or dismissed. This emphasises once again the need for accurate and relevant records.

The environment of care embraces not only safe nursing practice and the physical surroundings, but also the atmosphere of the ward or department (Activity 11.6). This will have an effect on the patient's physical and mental state and on his capacity to get better.

Adequacy of resources is certainly a political issue in these days of financial restraint. Too often, new surgical techniques or complex medical investigations are introduced without any consideration of the extra workload they create for the staff involved. Current staffing levels are frequently deemed adequate to accommodate these developments when, in reality, extra staff are required. Before putting a case forward for additional staff, it is the duty of the nurse to know what resources are available and to question whether or not these are being used effectively and efficiently. Nursing costs are among the highest expenditure in the NHS and, when resources are strained, are the first to be questioned and therefore frequently have to be justified. Recent developments in the area of quality of care will also be a useful tool in measuring standards of nursing care. (See Ch. 2 for information about how the NHS encourages setting and maintaining standards within a national framework).

Clause 13

Report to an appropriate person any circumstances in which the health or safety of colleagues is at risk.

Activity 11.6

During a practice placement, make a note of changes that could be made to enhance the environment. These may vary from devising a more comfortable seating arrangement in a GP's waiting room to creating a more homely atmosphere in the day-room of an elderly care ward.

Clause 13 ties in with Clause 6 in its emphasis on respecting and working in a collaborative and cooperative way with other health care workers. The purpose of the NHS is to care for others, but it sometimes fails to acknowledge the stress it creates for its employees. This may be due partly to it being such a large organisation (the largest employer in Europe) and partly to the traditional view of medical and nursing staff as being different from other people in their ability to cope with anything and everything that comes along.

There is now more recognition of nurses as individuals and of the fact that they have different capacities to cope with different workloads and pressures. Many hospitals have created support groups in areas of clinical care such as intensive care and accident and emergency. These are usually multidisciplinary and help in exploring issues and coping with problems as a team. What is stressful to one person may not be to another, and joint problem solving will go a long way towards reducing the pressures of colleagues.

Managers need to recognise that they are breaking this clause of the Code of Conduct when they leave second-level nurses and students to cope with heavy workloads without sufficient supervision. This could result in mistakes being made and standards being reduced. If adequate cover cannot be provided, admissions should be reduced, and if staffing problems cannot be surmounted, the ward should be closed.

Clause 14

Help colleagues develop their professional competence and assist others, including informal carers, to contribute safely to patient care.

Traditionally, after the initial introduction into nursing, students take on the teaching role of introducing nursing skills to the next new intake of students. This continues and increases with the individual's level of knowledge, experience and authority. Hence the sister/charge nurse role has always contained a teaching element. With the development of a more individual approach to learning, students are involved in identifying their own learning needs against specific objectives. It is usually the senior staff who have made the greatest contribution in developing the clinical competence of students and the newly qualified nurse. Using their experience and knowledge, senior staff can contribute to the development of nursing practice through the setting of policies and standards and through the implementation of research. However, in order to achieve this, they must keep up to date themselves with developments in the profession and within their sphere of practice.

This clause is emphasised through the concept of 'preceptorship' for the newly qualified nurse, and of clinical supervision and its contribution to developing nursing practice (Faugier & Butterworth 1994) (see also Ch. 1).

Clause 15

Do not accept any gift, favour or hospitality that will influence your nursing care.

Many patients naturally wish to express their gratitude for the care and attention they have received and offer gifts or money to staff. As this clause implies, accepting favours or hospitality could be interpreted by the patient as a promise of preferential consideration. Most hospitals and community units have local policies regarding gifts, particularly if they involve money. In most cases, gifts go into a general fund to help with extras for patients that cannot be provided through the usual channels.

Care should be taken when accepting gifts from pharmaceutical companies that they are not a means of seeking preference in the purchase of their products against those of another (Activity 11.7).

Clause 16

Do not promote commercial products or services from which you stand to benefit and ensure that your professional judgement is not influenced by commercial considerations.

It is inadvisable to use a professional qualification in a commercial context as it may cast doubt upon the independence of professional judgement, on which patients rely. Advertising is in fact a form of propaganda and seeks to influence people to buy certain products. Firms seek to use nurses in

Activity 11.7

What would you say to a patient who offered you money or an expensive present?

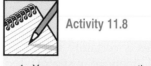

Activity 11.8

1. You are a nurse currently working as a sales representative for a pharmaceutical firm. Would it be permissible to use your nursing qualifications on your business card?
2. You assist with making a video on patient care and your name appears on the credits. Can it be followed by your registration status?

their advertisement of products because nurses are seen by the public to have a high level of knowledge and reliable judgement. For a nurse to recommend just one product, over many others, is not advisable. Nurses used in advertisements for medical products are usually models.

The UKCC guidance on this clause is included in *Guidelines for Professional Practice* (UKCC 1996). For example, a qualified nurse who owns a nursing home may use her qualification in advertising the home (Activity 11.8).

THE ROLE OF THE STATUTORY BODIES

THE UKCC

The Nurses, Midwives and Health Visitors Act 1979 provided for the establishment of the UKCC, which replaced six previous statutory bodies representing the nursing, midwifery and health visiting professions in England, Scotland, Wales and Northern Ireland. By the terms of the Act, the UKCC also took on responsibility for the organisations concerned with post-registration clinical practice, such as short courses in intensive care and renal nursing.

The main functions of the UKCC (set out in Section 2 of the Act) are as follows:

(1) The principal functions of the central Council shall be to establish and improve standards of training and professional conduct for nurses, midwives and health visitors.

(2) The Council shall ensure that the standards of training they establish are such as to meet any Community obligation of the United Kingdom.

(3) The Council shall by means of rules determine the conditions of a person being admitted to training, and the kind and standard of training to be undertaken, with a view to registration.

(4) The rules may also make provision with respect to the kind and standard of further training available to persons who are already registered.

(5) The powers of the Council shall include that of providing, in such manner as it thinks fit, advice for nurses, midwives and health visitors on standards of professional conduct.

(6) In the discharge of its functions the Council shall have proper regard for the interests of all groups within the professions, including those with minority representation.

Each of these functions will now be considered in turn.

Improving standards of training

The UKCC initiated the proposals set out in *Project 2000: A New Preparation for Practice* (UKCC 1986). This document followed a number of working papers relating to the reform of nursing education and training. Areas of discussion included the number of nursing levels needed, manpower and costing. The UKCC proposals also used previous reports on nursing education, for example the Briggs Report (DHSS and Scottish Home and Health Department 1972). The case for change, as urged by the Project 2000

document, was based at that time on three general concerns:

1. changing patterns of health care
2. potential difficulties in recruitment/manpower
3. the need to update education and training.

Changing patterns of health care. That health care patterns are changing is obvious. There are now fewer acute hospitals, and more care is required in the community for the very young, the elderly and those with problems for which there is no immediate cure, such as drug abuse, AIDS and other chronic conditions.

Recruitment and manpower. The predictions were that, in the mid-1990s, there would be fewer 18-year-olds leaving school. This group of school leavers (particularly females) has always been the main source of recruitment into nursing. There are also many more attractive careers, other than nursing, for women than there were 20 years ago.

Education. Nursing training had always been of the apprenticeship type and had low academic status, owing to the small amount of time spent in a formal educational setting. In addition to this, changing shift patterns, increased hours of work and a higher turnover of patients led to a reduction of supervision and teaching for students on the wards. Moreover, students were counted as part of the nursing establishment: wards and departments relied heavily on them to take responsibility for giving nursing care. New groups of students were re-orientated to practice settings at frequent intervals (sometimes every 8 weeks), and staffing levels were seriously reduced if students were not recruited or if they dropped out. Research showed that 70–80% of care was given by unqualified staff (i.e. mainly by students and care assistants). This meant that students were often left unsupervised and were expected to take on responsibilities for which they had not been prepared.

Outside the profession, the previous qualification of Registered Nurse had little more value than an A-level, making further academic advancement difficult. Student nurses did not have the time to explore in greater depth curriculum

Box 11.3 Fitness for practice (the Peach Report) (UKCC 1999)

Abridged recommendations from the Summary, September 1999

1. Careers services should offer a breadth of advice, encouraging access for all.
2. Recruitment and selection should be a joint responsibility between health care providers and Higher Education Institutions (HEIs).
3. The good practice of organisations cooperating in providing entry through Access programmes to pre-registration programmes should be extended.
4. The use of Assessment of Prior (Educational) Learning (AP(E)L) should be introduced within the Common Foundation Programme (CFP).
5. The CFP should be reduced to 1 year and should enable the achievement of a common level of competence. It should be taught in the context of, and enable integration with, the branch programmes and should introduce clinical skills and practice placements early in the programme.
6. Students who leave having successfully completed at least Year 1 of the CFP should be able to benefit by mapping their academic and practice credit against other credit frameworks.
7. More flexibility should be introduced concerning the timing of branch programme selection.
8. There should be an expansion of graduate preparation.
9. A common definition of attrition and a required minimum data set should be agreed.
10. The standards required for registration as a nurse should be constructed in terms of outcome competences, should make the practice component transparent and should specify consistent clinical supervision.
11. The benchmarking of subject-specific standards should address outcomes, which are core, and specific to nursing and to midwifery, are transferable, and are consistent with the Quality Assurance Agency's threshold for degrees and diplomas.
12. Consideration should be given as to whether pre-registration midwifery education should move to a competency-based approach.
13. Students, assessors and mentors should know what is expected of them through specified outcomes and competences which form part of a formal learning contract, give direction to clinical placements and are jointly negotiated between the health care providers and the HEIs.
14. The use of a portfolio of practice experience should demonstrate a student's fitness to practise and evidence of rational decision-making and clinical judgement.
15. The portfolio should be assessed through rigorous practice assessment tools.
16. The sequencing and balance between theory and practice should promote an integration of knowledge, attitudes and skills.
17. The current programme model of four branches of nursing should be reviewed in the light of changing health care needs.
18. Practice placements should achieve agreed outcomes, which benefit student learning and provide experience of the full 24-hour day and 7 day per week nature of health needs.
19. Interpersonal and practice skills should be fostered by the use of experiential and problem-based learning, increased use of stimulation laboratories and access to information technology, particularly in clinical practice.
20. There should be a period of supervised clinical practice of at least 3 months' duration towards the end of the pre-registration programme.
21. All newly qualified registrants should receive a properly supported period of induction and preceptorship when they begin their employment.
22. Programme changes should be systematically evaluated in respect of achieving fitness for practice.
23. Health care providers and HEIs should continue to develop partnerships to support students, curriculum development, implementation and evaluation, joint awareness and the development of service and education issues, and delivery and monitoring of learning in practice.
24. An accountable individual should be appointed by education purchasers to liase with health care providers and HEIs to support the provision of sufficient suitable placements, staff and students during placements, the development of standards and specified outcomes for placements, the delivery and effective monitoring of the contract.
25. Health care providers and HEIs should work together to develop diverse teams of clinical and academic staff offering expertise in clinical practice, management, assessment, mentoring and research.
26. Health care providers and HEIs should support time in education and practice for clinical and education staff respectively to enable competence and confidence.
27. Formalised arrangements for access to practice and education should be adopted by health care providers and HEIs
28. Health care providers and HEIs should formalise the preparation, support and feedback to mentors and preceptors.
29. Funding to support learning in practice should take account of the cost of mentoring, assessment by clinical staff, and lecturers having regular contact with practice.
30. To improve workforce planning for nursing, NHS requirements should increasingly be informed by comprehensive information from the private and independent sector.
31. The government departments concerned with health, social care and social services, education and employment should work collaboratively to ensure that the preparation of health and social care assistants is based upon common standards of practice values.
32. The health care professions should actively be encouraged to learn with and from one another.
33. Consideration should be given to the most appropriate method of funding students of nursing and midwifery in the future.

subjects such as sociology, psychology and physiology. A case was made for major reform of nurse education. Known as Project 2000, it was implemented in the early 1990s. Students were to be educated to diploma level and followed a 3-year full-time programme of 50% theory and 50% practice. The separate teaching of mental health, learning disability, sick children's and general nursing occurred only after all students undertook an 18-month common foundation programme. At a time of major curricular change, nurse education was also moving out of the NHS schools and colleges of nursing and into the university sector. This transition was completed in 1996/7. The combination of changed courses and the migration of nurse education into universities was not without its critics, particularly in relation to a perceived theory–practice gap in which newly qualified nurses were seen as less capable practically despite achieving a higher level initial qualification than most of their predecessors. The NHS became highly critical of the university sector, and so the UKCC established a commission to examine the future direction of pre-registration nursing and midwifery training. The commission chairman was Sir Leonard Peach and the report, *Fitness for Practice*, was published in 1999 (UKCC 1999). The main recommendations of this report are summarised in Box 11.3. As a result of the report and the Department of Health's directive to change the future of all nurse education by 2002, *Making a Difference* (DoH 1999), the nursing workforce will be expanded, access will be widened and entry to the Register will be more flexible with fast tracking for some students. The common foundation programme is now reduced to 1 year.

Meeting EC guidelines

Planning health care for the future involves bringing educational standards into line with European Community directives. Already, all students have to undertake particular experiences (maternity, mental health and community nursing) to be permitted to practise in Europe. Minimum hours of theory and practice in the nursing curriculum are also set by the EC.

Admission conditions

The UKCC set up a 'live' Register for first- and second-level nurses (Box 11.4), and is responsible for determining what theoretical and practical preparation is required. Second-level nurse training or enrolled nurse training has now been phased out and generally replaced by health care assistants studying NVQs (National Vocational Qualifications) in health care to level 4. It is the role of the National Boards to translate these standards into more detailed course regulations and curriculum guidelines. First-level and second-level nurses can all use the title of Registered Nurse (RN). The level and branch of practice will be indicated elsewhere, for example in a curriculum vitae. Nurses applying for registration from overseas must demonstrate that their

---

Box 11.4 **Qualifications included in the UKCC Register: parts of the UKCC Professional Register**

Part 1 First-level nurses trained in general nursing
Part 2 Second-level nurses trained in general nursing (England and Wales)
Part 3 First-level nurses trained in the nursing of persons suffering from mental illness
Part 4 Second-level nurses trained in the nursing of persons suffering from mental illness (England and Wales)
Part 5 First-level nurses trained in the nursing of persons suffering from mental handicap
Part 6 Second-level nurses trained in the nursing of persons suffering from mental handicap (England and Wales)
Part 7 Second-level nurses (Scotland and Northern Ireland)
Part 8 Nurses trained in the nursing of sick children
Part 9 Nurses trained in the nursing of persons suffering from fever
Part 10 Midwives
Part 11 Health visitors
Part 12 First-level nurses trained in adult nursing*
Part 13 First-level nurses trained in mental health nursing*
Part 14 First-level nurses trained in mental handicap nursing*
Part 15 First-level nurses trained in children's nursing*

*Diploma in Higher Education in Nursing (Project 2000)
First-level nurses (3 years preparation)
Second-level nurses (2 years preparation)

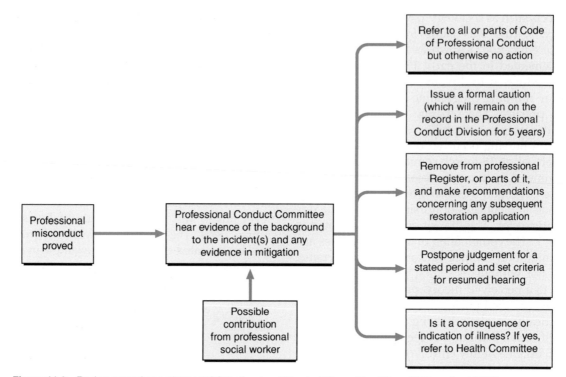

Figure 11.2 Review procedures of the UKCC Professional Conduct Committee (Pyne 1984, revised 1993).

programmes of preparation meet the same criteria. There is often variation in nursing programmes; if this is so, applicants are required to undertake a satisfactory period of adaptation before applying for registration. Length of experience since qualifying and other criteria may be considered for admission to courses leading to qualification beyond first or second level.

Further training

The need for continuing education has been discussed under 'Clause 3: professional development' and this has been introduced by the UKCC through their post-registration education and practice (PREP) requirements.

Standards of professional conduct

The question of standards puts a great responsibility on the UKCC, which ensures that standards are met and maintained through its Professional

Conduct Committee, composed of Council members. How the Committee functions is outlined in Figure 11.2. The UKCC issued guidelines in 1993 regarding complaints about professional conduct and the work of the committee (UKCC 1993b).

Minority groups within the profession

With the majority being registered general nurses, smaller groups such as occupational health nurses are sometimes forgotten. Regulations concerning the election of members of the profession to the statutory bodies and the required numbers from each of the specialisms are aimed at assisting the UKCC to ensure that all subgroups within the profession are adequately represented.

THE NATIONAL BOARDS

The Nurses, Midwives and Health Visitors Act 1979 and 1992 requires that England, Wales,

Scotland and Northern Ireland shall each have a National Board for nursing, midwifery and health visiting. These are corporate bodies with the following functions:

- to provide or arrange for others to provide, at institutions approved by the Board, courses of training with a view to enabling persons to qualify for registration as nurses, midwives or health visitors or for the recording of additional qualifications
- to ensure that such courses meet the requirements of the Central Council (UKCC) as to their content and standard
- to hold or arrange for others to hold such examinations as are necessary to enable persons to satisfy requirements for registration or to obtain additional qualifications
- to discharge their functions subject to and in accordance with any applicable role of the Council and have proper regard for the interests of all groups within the profession, including those with minority representation.

The National Boards, therefore, have a major executive function with respect to all that is involved in education, training and examinations. The National Boards no longer handle the funds for education. Funds for nurse education are held by the NHS regional offices who contract with higher education institutions to provide nursing and midwifery education according to local needs.

The UKCC and the National Boards

With the 1992 Nurses, Midwives and Health Visitors Act, the UKCC became the elected body and the National Boards much smaller in membership, the majority of members being appointed by government ministers. In 1997, a review of the UKCC and the four National Boards was undertaken and in 1999 the government accepted the recommendation that the five statutory bodies would be replaced by a single Nursing and Midwifery Council. The National Boards will maintain their current responsibilities until September 2001 and work is underway identifying the key changes to be made for the

transfer to the new UK-wide regulatory body for nursing, midwifery and health visiting. With the transfer of nursing and midwifery education into higher education there is a need to maintain a professional, statutory input into all education programmes, but the monitoring of these involves input from higher education, NHS Trusts and others purchasing education as well as the professional bodies.

PROFESSIONAL ORGANISATIONS AND TRADE UNIONS

Of the many professional organisations and trade unions that represent NHS employees only two will be mentioned here:

- the Royal College of Nursing (RCN)
- Unison: previously the Confederation of Health Service Employees (COHSE), the National Union of Public Employees (NUPE) and the National Association of Local Government Officers (NALGO).

THE ROYAL COLLEGE OF NURSING
Developments since 1916

The RCN was founded in 1916 and, initially, pressed for registration of all nurses. Its aims are, as at the beginning, to promote the science and art of nursing and to advance nursing as a profession. Membership is open only to nurses and students, and men were not admitted until 1960. The RCN balloted members on issues of affiliation with the Trades Union Congress (TUC), but the majority voted against; thus it became a non-affiliated trade union in 1977.

Benefits of membership

In the past 20 years, the RCN has become more proactive in matters of pay, conditions and standards in the NHS as well as nursing issues. Membership, now at 320 000, provides a comprehensive indemnity insurance scheme which helps members if found guilty of professional negligence. This is particularly attractive to members in view of the movement within the profession for nurses to extend their roles and take on more responsibility, and for those practising independently.

Other activities

The RCN Institute was formed in 1995 as a result of a merger between the RCN Institute of Advanced Nursing Education, the National Institute for Nursing, based at Oxford, and the RCN Daphne Heald Research Unit. It has one of the most extensive nursing libraries in Europe with online access. As a designated higher education institution, the RCN Institute offers a variety of post-registration degrees and postgraduate research opportunities and a range of continuing professional development opportunities. The RCN Institute offers flexible learning programmes and has centres in Belfast, Cardiff, Edinburgh, Leeds, Oxford and London. The RCN also provides the opportunity for nurse members to share their knowledge and experience through official forums and committees related to their specialism.

UNISON

In July 1993, as indicated above, three former unions (COHSE, NUPE and NALGO) combined to form Unison, making it the largest union in the TUC, with over 1.4 million members. Of these, over 455 000 are health workers, and there is a special nursing section. Unison recruits and represents all types of nursing staff, and all nurse members are protected by indemnity insurance. It is also expanding its specialist advisory groups (SAGs) to reflect fully the scope of expertise within the membership, for example in HIV/AIDS and the care of older people and those with learning disabilities.

JOINING AN ORGANISATION

Students and qualified staff should seek information regarding these and other organisations before deciding to join a particular group. Such a decision should take into account the individual's priorities and should include an assessment of which organisation may be able to offer more than another. Issues to consider are whether or not a branch of the organisation is well represented in the working area, its track record for negotiating better pay and conditions of service, and its support for individual members over grievances, professional issues, standards in the NHS.

THE INTERNATIONAL SETTING

THE EUROPEAN COMMUNITY

Legislation within nursing in the UK has been required to change in line with EC policy. The UKCC has a representative from its Council on the Advisory Committee on Training of Nurses in the European Community. It also has a representative on the comparable committee for midwifery. Discussion has been taking place with the EC for some time on 'sectional directives' for psychiatric nurses and, more recently, paediatric nurses, as many countries in the EC do not have specific training in these areas.

THE INTERNATIONAL COUNCIL OF NURSES (ICN)

The ICN was founded in 1900 by Mrs Bedford Fenwick, who was at that time Matron of St Bartholomew's Hospital in London (Hector 1973). The Council has gone from strength to strength, particularly in the last 30 years. Every member country provides from its national organisation (in the UK this is the RCN) a nurse (usually its president) to serve on the Council of National Representatives, which determines the policies of the International Council of Nurses. The headquarters of the ICN are in Geneva. Here it links with the World Health Organization and publishes the *International Nursing Review*. The ICN Congress is now held every 4 years, attended by thousands of nurses from all over the world. Recent congresses have been held in Korea, Spain and, in 1997, London. The next is in Denmark.

CONCLUSION

This chapter began by considering what exactly a profession *is*, and how nursing is changing to take on a new professionalism for the 21st century. Accountability is seen as one of the key issues of professionalism and we have seen how the UKCC Code of Conduct assists nurses in fulfilling this and other aspects of their role. The UKCC's other functions, such as the standards for admission to the Register and regulating standards of conduct, have also been considered. The professionalisation of nursing in the UK is an exciting arena and the effect of recent political events and the future role of nurses within the health care setting will undoubtedly contribute to its continuing future development.

REFERENCES

Abbott P, Meerabeau L 1998 The sociology of the caring professions, 2nd edn. UCL Press, London

Abortion Act 1967 HMSO, London

Access Modification (Health) Order 1987 HMSO, London

Access to Health Records Act 1990 HMSO, London

Benson 1992 Cited in: Pyne R 1998 Professional discipline in nursing. Blackwell Scientific, Oxford

Burnard P, Chapman C 1999 Professional and ethical issues in nursing, the code of professional conduct, 2nd edn. Harcourt, London

Clay T 1987 Nurses: power and politics. Heinemann, London

Clothier Report 1994 The Allitt inquiry: independent inquiry relating to death and injuries on the children's ward at Grantham and Kesteven General Hospital during the period Feb to March 1991. HMSO, London

Cohen P 1994 Stately union. Nursing Times 90(9):43

Crow R 1983 Professional responsibility. Nursing Times 79(1):19–21

Darley M 1996 Right for the job: accountability in the extended role. Nursing Times 92(30):28–29

Data Protection Act 1984 HMSO, London

Davies C 1995 Gender and the professional predicament in nursing. Open University Press, Buckingham

Davies C 1996a A new vision of professionalism. Nursing Times 92(46):54–56

Davies C 1996b Cloaked in tattered illusion. Nursing Times 92(45):44–46

Department of Health 1999 Making a difference: strengthening the nursing, midwifery and health visiting contribution to health and health care. Department of Health, London

Department of Health 2000 The NHS plan – a plan for investment, a plan for reform. Department of Health, London

Department of Health and Social Security 1986 Neighbourhood nursing: a focus for care. Report on the Community Nursing Review (the Cumberlege Report). HMSO, London

Department of Health and Social Security and Scottish Home and Health Department 1972 The report of the Committee on Nursing (the Briggs Report). HMSO, London

English National Board 1997 Specialist practitioner programme. ENB, London

Eraut M 1994 Developing professional knowledge and expertise. Falmer Press, London, ch 6

Faugier J, Butterworth T 1994 Clinical supervision: a position paper. School of Nursing Studies, University of Manchester, Manchester

Friend B 1996 Risky business: nurses' expanding role. Nursing Times 92(30):26–27

Gamarnikov E 1978 Sexual division of labour: the case in nursing. In: Kuhn A, Wople A M Feminism and materialism. Routledge and Kegan Paul, London

Greenhalgh Report 1994 The interface between junior doctors and nurses: a research study for the Department of Health. Greenhalgh and Co Ltd Management Consultant, Macclesfield, Cheshire

Harris A, Redshaw M 1998 Professional issues facing nurse practitioners and nursing. British Journal of Nursing 7(22):1381–1385

Hector W 1973 The work of Mrs Bedford Fenwick and the rise of professional nursing. Royal College of Nursing, London

Heywood Jones I 1999 The UKCC Code of professional conduct: a critical guide. NT Books, London

Human Fertilisation and Embryology Act 1990 HMSO, London

Mares P, Henley A, Baxter C 1985 Health care in multiracial Britain. London Health Education Council and National Extension College Trust, Cambridge

Nurses, Midwives and Health Visitors Act 1979 HMSO, London

Nurses, Midwives and Health Visitors Act 1992 HMSO, London

Parkin P 1995 Nursing the future: a re-examination of the professionalisation thesis in the light of some recent developments. Journal of Advanced Nursing 21: 561–567

Public Interest Disclosure Act 1998 HSC 1999/198 27 Aug 1999 The Public Interest Disclosure Act 1998 Whistleblowing in the NHS

Pyne R 1984 Managing the profession. In: Rowden R (ed) Managing nursing. Baillière Tindall, London

Pyne R 1998 Professional discipline in nursing. Blackwell Scientific, Oxford

Roach M S 1982 Caring: a framework for nursing ethics. Programme and abstracts, First International Congress on Nursing Law and Ethics, Jerusalem

Schon D 1983 The reflective practitioner: how professionals think in action. Basic Books, HarperCollins, New York

Taylor D 1996 Quality and professionalism in health care: a review of current initiatives in the NHS. British Medical Journal 312: 626–629

UKCC 1986 Project 2000: a new preparation for practice. UKCC, London

UKCC 1989 Exercising accountability: a framework to assist nurses, midwives and health visitors to consider ethical aspects of professional practice. UKCC, London

UKCC 1992a Code of Professional Conduct, 3rd edn. UKCC, London

UKCC 1992b The scope of professional practice. UKCC, London

UKCC 1992c Confidentiality and use of computers. UKCC, London

UKCC 1993a Standards for records and record keeping. UKCC, London

UKCC 1993b Complaints about professional conduct. UKCC, London

UKCC 1996 Guidelines for professional practice. UKCC, London

UKCC 1998a A guide for students of nursing and midwifery. UKCC, London

UKCC 1998b Guidelines for records and record keeping. UKCC, London

UKCC 1999 Fitness for practice: the UKCC Commission for Nursing and Midwifery Education (chair Sir Leonard Peach). UKCC, London

UKCC 2001 The PREP handbook. UKCC, London

Vousden M 1999 Appendix 2: The sixteen commandments: a modest proposal. In: Heywood Jones I (ed.) The UKCC code of professional conduct: a critical guide. NT Books, London

FURTHER READING

Casteldine G 1998 An update on the UKCC's work into higher level practice. British Journal of Nursing 7(22):1378–1380
Gives an overview of the responses to the consultation exercise and outlines what a higher level of practice will mean for the nursing profession.

Diamond B 1995 Legal aspects of nursing, 2nd edn. Prentice Hall, London
A good introduction to legal situations likely to be faced by nurses.

Henry C 1995 Professional ethics and organisational change in education and health. Edward Arnold, London
This book is developed from an Ethics and Values Audit carried out in 1992 and how this related to the development of mission statements, charters and codes. The content includes an introduction to the concept of professional ethics, aspects of equal opportunities, charterships for patients, the management of change and the implementation of policy.

Graham I 1995 Reflective practice – using the action learning group mechanism. Nurse Education Today 15:28–32
A practical approach to helping students to use reflection in and on practice as part of their learning.

Marks-Maran D 1993 Accountability. In: Tschudin V (ed) Ethics, nurses and patients. Scutari Press, London, pp. 121–134
Some more aspects of accountability.

Murphy K, Macleod Clark J 1993 Nurses' experiences of caring for ethnic minority clients. Journal of Advanced Nursing 18:442–450
One of the first research papers exploring this important area.

Nurses, Midwives and Health Visitors Act 1979 HMO, London

Salvage J 1997 Professionalisation – or struggle for survival: a consideration of changing nursing: changing times. Nursing Times 93(5):25–26
One of a number of short papers looking at nurse power and predicting a brighter future as long as nurses can express their values, skills and knowledge in ways that help patients and clients.

Thompson J, Melia K, Boyd K 1994 Nursing ethics. Churchill Livingstone, Edinburgh
A useful book for the student, that gives practical guidance and discussion to ethical dilemmas.

UKCC 1998 Guidelines for mental health and learning disabilities nursing. UKCC, London

UKCC 1999 Practitioner–client relationships and the prevention of abuse. UKCC, London

12

Evidence-based practice

Benjamin Gray   Pam Smith

CHAPTER CONTENTS

Nursing research   332
Historical perspective   332
What is nursing research?   334
Nursing stereotypes   334

Types of research   335
Scientific deductive research   335
Naturalistic inductive research   336
Action research   338
Triangulation   338

The research process   338
Stage 1: identifying the research topic   339
Relationship between research topic
and literature search   340
Formulating objectives, questions
and hypotheses   341
Stage 2: selecting an appropriate research
approach   342
Influencing factors   342
Stage 3: designing the study   343
Quantitative research   343
Qualitative research   345
Stage 4: developing data-collection methods
and instruments   347
Quantitative research   347
Qualitative research   349
Stage 5: collecting and recording the
data   351
Quantitative research   351
Qualitative research   352
Stage 6: analysing and interpreting
the data   353
Quantitative research   353
Using computers   353

Qualitative research   355
Stage 7: presenting the research
findings   356

Ethical issues   357

**Research as part of nursing knowledge
and practice   358**
Education   358
Practice   358
Nursing research   359
Being research minded   360

Conclusion   360

Acknowledgements   360

References   361

Further reading   363

Internet   363

Nursing research is vital both in understanding the complex factors associated with health, disease and illness and in devising and evaluating treatment and care. This chapter aims to:

- **discuss the concept of research mindedness**
- **explore the relevance of research to nursing knowledge and nursing practice**
- **outline different types of research**
- **describe the stages of the research process, as a basis for their practical application**
- **illustrate the importance of research in caring for adults, children and those with mental health problems or with learning disabilities.**

NURSING RESEARCH

The purpose of learning about research as a nursing student is to become 'research aware', rather than to turn into a fully-fledged researcher. Becoming 'research aware' is an important part of becoming 'research minded' and means:

- developing the confidence to have ideas and ask questions about nursing
- becoming familiar with research literature, methods and techniques
- being able critically to assess research reports
- being able to incorporate research methods and findings into knowledge and practice.

The Royal College of Nursing (1982) states that research mindedness 'implies a critical and questioning approach to one's work, the desire and ability to find out about the latest research in the area and apply it as appropriate'. Modern nursing is based on the principle that nurses must have a flexible and conceptually driven education. This should enable nurses to work in a variety of clinical and non-clinical settings in a rapidly changing NHS, to which nursing must respond.

Through education nurses must become research minded in order to be able to monitor, reflect upon and assess their everyday nursing practice. This chapter is designed to meet the

UKCC's new competencies, ensuring that current research and other findings are incorporated into practice (UKCC 2000). Other recent documents, *Fitness for Practice* (UKCC 1999a), *Nursing Competencies* (UKCC 1999b) and *Making a Difference* (DoH 1999a), all called for a more evidence-based approach to education and practice, together with the continued expansion and development of the nursing role (DoH 1999a, p. 5).

An evidence-based approach to practice means using information from research that will help nurses make the right decision regarding practice, be it in the ward or in the community. Nurses who are research minded collect information or evidence and reflect on their day-to-day practice so that they can improve their work and the quality of care they give to patients. These approaches are also in line with the government's clinical governance agenda which emphasises quality, professional accountability and standards of excellence underpinned by partnership, team work, audit and evidence-based practice (DoH 1998, 1999b).

A recent conversation with a district nurse, recounted in Case example 12.1, provides a current illustration of the efficacy of these approaches.

Historical perspective

Research is not new to nursing. Florence Nightingale was a tireless researcher and passionate statistician who stressed the importance of accurate observation and skilful questioning in the collection of patient information. Leading questions, she observed, always elicited inaccurate information (Nightingale 1990):

A want of the habit of observing conditions and an inveterate habit of taking averages are each of them equally misleading. There is no more silly or universal question scarcely asked than this, 'Is he better?' Who can have any opinion of any value as to whether the patient is better or worse, excepting the constant medical attendant, or the really observing nurse.

Nightingale's advice to 19th-century nurses is still relevant to nursing practice and research today: 'The most important practical lesson that can be given to nurses is to teach them what to observe – how to observe – what symptoms indicate

Case example 12.1

A recent conversation with a district nurse touched on quality of care and the types of devices used for dispensing medication for people with asthma. The district nurse said she was having difficulties in prescribing more modern asthma cylinders and equipment. The doctor of the local practice disapproved of the more modern asthma devices because there was no research to show that they were better for patients medically. Also, the new devices cost twice as much as the old asthma equipment.

The district nurse suggested that patients favoured the more modern devices. Patients told her in the general practice that the more modern devices looked better, were less bulky and easier to dispense. Patients therefore had social, personal and consumer values attached to the more modern types of devices. The values and choices that patients attached to modern devices increased the dispensing and continued use of asthma medication. Because patients favoured the more modern devices and continued to use them, the nurse told the researcher, they were better and more successful in medical terms.

Conversation then turned to a research paper in which the quality of life of patients with asthma had been linked to social, personal and subjective factors. Subjective feelings had been shown in the research to better the quality of life of the patient. Research showed that the patient's personal views – including views of health staff and methods of treatment – would significantly influence quality of life. Personal, aesthetic and consumer choices therefore play a substantial part in the dispensing of asthmatic medication and the quality of the patient's care (Drummond 2000).

The district nurse was able to bring the research paper to the attention of the doctor. The research was evidence that the nurse's suspicions were well founded and could be applied to general practice. The nurse had shown that patients' subjective and consumer views influenced their quality of life and their continued use of asthma medication. The nurse and the doctor had research evidence that the more modern asthma devices would be better in improving quality of life. The research mindedness of the nurse had influenced health practice and improved quality of care in the general surgery's running of asthma clinics.

investigated problems associated with nursing elderly people and critically examined their care. One important consequence of the study was a revolution in the prevention and treatment of pressure sores. The application of potions such as alcohol, iodine and egg white was replaced by the relief of pressure and the use of a risk assessment 'scale' to identify vulnerable patients.

Another landmark for nursing research was the inquiry entitled 'The Proper Study of the Nurse', undertaken by the Royal College of Nursing (RCN). This study, which in fact comprised a number of projects, was an example of systematic research undertaken to investigate various aspects of nursing care (McFarlane 1970, Inman 1975). Spencer (1983) has criticised this research as being dominated by a 'medical' approach, yielding statistical, 'objective' results rather than the subjective, 'qualitative' findings more appropriate, in his view, to nursing. However, despite its limitations, the RCN research provided nurses with their first large-scale opportunity to investigate their practice.

In 1972, the Briggs Report (DHSS 1972) made a major impact on the development of nursing research, with the recommendations that nursing should become a research-based profession and that 'a sense of the need for research should become part of the mental equipment of every practising nurse or midwife'. These recommendations were made in the light of evidence that insufficient attention was paid by nursing and midwifery education to research as 'a continuing activity' and a 'prelude to innovation'.

More recently, a taskforce was set up as part of the Department of Health Research and Development Strategy (DoH 1993). The importance of research to nursing was reaffirmed, and the contribution of small-scale projects undertaken as part of educational studies recognised. However, the taskforce saw these studies as no 'substitute for the generalisable and cumulative research which we would place at the heart of a strategy for advancing research in nursing'. Becoming research aware and research minded will therefore give you insights not only into what makes research 'generalisable and cumulative', but also into how it may fit into your own career plans.

improvement, what the reverse – which are of importance – which are of none – which are the evidence of neglect – and of what kind of neglect?'.

A study undertaken by Doreen Norton, first published in 1962 (Norton et al 1975), has since been recognised as an important landmark in the development of nursing research. Norton's study

Certainly, a vital part of any nurse's career is keeping informed about the latest research.

Modern nursing is about caring for the patient and reflecting on ways in which quality of care and improvements may be made. Nurses do this from day to day in their interactions with patients, visitors and other staff. A nurse may think of an event or situation that went awry and that could have been dealt with differently. Reflecting on an event with a patient during the day is very much like focusing on a research question that involves nurse–patient contact. For example, a nurse in routine work with a patient might ask and reflect upon the following questions:

- How could I have responded to the patient better?
- What interferences were there to my nursing?
- How did my colleagues help me complete my task with the patient?

Researchers will ask similar questions and try to come up with a number of answers.

Being research minded is therefore not a magic formula or an impossibility for nurses. Being research minded is formalising and making clear the knowledge that nurses already have. Research mindedness means being able to ask questions that nurses already raise from day to day (such as the questions that the nurse asks above) and then applying these questions to improve nurse practice. Research assists in forming a clear understanding of pertinent issues in nursing that are then applied to advance nursing knowledge and practice.

What is nursing research?

In common with other disciplines, nursing requires research to support both theory and practice. Research expands the profession's knowledge base and supports the development of new techniques. It contributes to the description and explanation of phenomena and provides a forum in which to generate and test ideas. 'Good' research comes from 'good' ideas, rather than from just perfecting one's research techniques (Open University 1979). Research is creative. It demands imagination and constant questioning

of the world about us. Nurses should be alert to the unique opportunities for questioning the experiences that are presented to them by their professional circumstances. A researcher in a Boston hospital once spoke of how one of her projects had arisen (Rempusheski 1987). She was a specialist nurse in the care of the elderly, but, by chance, her office was situated close to the maternity unit. She found that distressed elderly relatives often found their way into her office as they waited anxiously for news of the progress of their premature grandchildren in the special care baby unit. In the 'foreign land' of obstetrics, Rempusheski found a research project about the elderly. There was little in the literature about the involvement of grandparents in family care, especially of their pre-term grandchildren. Rempusheski submitted a research proposal and obtained funding, so that now 'the unknown is in the process of becoming known'. McHaffie (1991) has since published on the topic in the UK.

Hockey (1985) defines nursing research as research into activities that are 'predominantly and appropriately the concern and responsibility of nurses' (Cormack 1991). McFarlane (1980), with other nursing theorists such as Parse (1989) and Watson (1985), sees nursing as both an art and a science, and argues that nursing research cannot be limited to the quantitative approaches adopted by many doctors and criticised by Spencer (1983). Research in nursing is arguably improved if supplemented with social, psychological and sense-making accounts that draw upon the views of patients and nurses (Smith 1992, Ellis & Bochner 1999).

Nursing stereotypes

As part of becoming 'research minded', it is important to begin exploring some of the conflicting stereotypes relating to nursing and research. The popular conception of the nurse as engaged in 'women's work', which involves physical rather than mental labour, is hardly compatible with the notion of research as a 'scientific' and 'objective' – and thus somehow a more masculine – endeavour. In the stereotype, nurses are merely a pair of hands as well as the heart to the doctor's mind and guiding thoughts on illness. Although Salvage began to explode some of these gender stereotypes in nursing during the mid-1980s (Salvage 1985), there remains a persistent view within the medical and nursing hierarchy of the questioning nurse as an anomaly. Questioning still sometimes elicits the response 'You are not here to think, Nurse, but to do' (Hockey 1985).

Hockey (1985) writes that even as a young student nurse she kept a notebook in which she jotted down her ideas:

My first note dated September 1940 relates the elements of a discussion between a ward sister and myself, then a very junior probationer nurse. I was concerned about some patients getting bedsores (the notion of pressure sores was still many light years away) and why others did not: 'It could be the bed linen – it feels like boards but that is the same for all patients'. The ward sister did not seem too pleased. She informed me that I was here to heal the sores not to ask questions about them, and that we were far too busy, and in any case, if we knew the answer there wouldn't be any sores. I wrote: 'We don't know the answer, but shouldn't we?'

Hockey also describes nursing in a fever hospital during the Blitz. Because of the risk of shattering, glass partitions were removed. Surprisingly, there was no subsequent increase in the rate of cross-infection. Hockey asked the sister why this was so, given that the partitions had been seen as vital in preventing the spread of infection. What, therefore, was preventing it now? The reply came that she was tempting providence. 'Keep washing your hands,' Hockey was told, 'Watch and pray. We don't know why not, but we are thankful.' Hockey again notes in her diary: 'We don't know why not, but shouldn't we?' (Hockey 1985).

TYPES OF RESEARCH

SCIENTIFIC DEDUCTIVE RESEARCH

Research has traditionally been seen to be removed from practical matters, such as those described in Hockey's diary. It has been associated with intellectuals and academics, whose pursuit of objective truth is conducted systematically and scientifically under experimental conditions.

It is assumed that men are best suited to such endeavours of knowledge, because women will confound the truth with their subjectivity, emotion and intuition (Roberts 1981).

According to Chalmers (1982), many self-styled 'scientific' researchers mistakenly believe that, in order to undertake reliable research, it is necessary to adopt the 'pure' scientific methods used by physicists. These methods, said to be based on positivism, consist of careful observation and experiment and are used to collect 'facts', study their relationships and derive laws and theories from them. This scientific style of research, which is used to test hypotheses and theories, is also referred to as *quantitative* or *deductive* research, which follows set rules to deduce conclusions from a set of premises.

Because physics so closely matches the popular idea of a pure science, its theories and associated research methods hold high status as dealing in 'hard' facts. Ironically, many discoveries in the sciences are fortuitous, an example being Roentgen's discovery of X-rays in 1895. Further, physicists do not take their theories as fixed and unchangeable. Einstein, for example, was trying to prove all his life that his original theories were wrong – a process that the philosopher Karl Popper called the 'falsification' of science. The spirit of scientific research is to falsify results by retesting them.

Modern advances in biology illustrate that the knowledge and techniques used in scientific research are not necessarily 'pure', nor do they produce 'hard' facts. DNA, for example, was only discovered using new techniques from physics, the electron microscope showing that original theories on molecules were wrong. These findings were very important for the advancement of molecular biology. In his book *The Double Helix*, Watson (1980), one of the scientists involved in these discoveries, describes the excitement and competition they felt as they pushed back the frontiers of knowledge.

More recently, a spirit of ruthless scientific competition was demonstrated by US medical researchers towards their French counterparts in their bid to be the first to isolate the human immunodeficiency (HIV) virus. More recently still, the race to be the first to map the human genome (and to patent the genome for its commercial use or to keep that information free for everyone) has been very much in evidence in the new millennium. This kind of behaviour is a salutary reminder that scientists may sometimes be motivated as much by self-interest or financial gain as by altruism and the milk of human kindness. The AIDS story, as told by Shilts in *And the Band Played On* (Shilts 1987), is a powerful account of the interplay between politics and societal values in setting research agendas.

NATURALISTIC INDUCTIVE RESEARCH

The assumptions underlying research in the so-called pure sciences are not necessarily appropriate to research associated with the social sciences. Nor are the methods of the natural sciences (chemistry, biology, physics) necessarily to be extended to the social sciences (sociology, psychology, anthropology). In social settings, people have meanings and feelings (Schutz 1972). In order to take the human element into account, ethnographic methods of participant observation and interviews are used by anthropologists and sociologists. Ethnographic literally means 'drawing people' – describing their interactions with each other and depicting their lives in society for all to see. Ethnographic methods produce detailed accounts of social interactions and their associated meanings for different groups of people in their 'natural' settings. This naturalistic research style is referred to as *qualitative* or *inductive* research. Moving from particular observations to generalisations, the inductive researcher develops rather than tests theories based on interpretations from the data.

Inductive research is grounded in practice. McFarlane (1977) discusses this notion in the context of nursing as a practice discipline, and in response to the introduction of the nursing process in the UK. The nursing process, in McFarlane's view, provides a means of systematising, recording and analysing nursing practice as a basis for research. The stages of assessment, planning and identification of outcomes constitute 'a form of research to which every nursing practitioner can contribute and only the practitioner can

Box 12.1 **Inductive reasoning** (reproduced with kind permission from Benner 1984)

Expert nurse
In the beginning, I was writing down all the times the blood pressures were to be taken, and then I thought 'Hey, wait a minute, let me think about this and decide whether I need to take them or not. After all, it's not just something I'm supposed to do to make me feel better.' So I stop and think, what if I know what someone's blood pressure is? What does that tell me? Do I really need to know it? Especially with some of the postoperative eye patients who have been postop for a couple of days. We are expected to use our judgement as to when to discontinue the vital signs at night. So we carefully study the trends and the patient. Sometimes I substitute close observations so the patient can sleep.

Benner's commentary
In this example the nurse makes a judgement about the relative merits of rest and comfort over the prescribed therapy at a particular time in the patient's illness. There can never be precise scientific guidelines for these decisions because there could never be enough research done to capture the particulars of all situations. The nurse will always need to be able to weigh the important against the unimportant and, given the particular situation, risk choosing in the best interests of the patient.

identify the cognitive process by which she arrived at certain actions' (McFarlane 1977).

Benner's (1984) research describes these cognitive processes through exemplars, which describe how nurses learn, through practice, to become experts able to make highly skilled clinical judgements about their patients. The exemplar and commentary given in Box 12.1 illustrates nursing knowledge as derived from and grounded in practice.

Although there is a growing change towards the social and psychological aspects of patient care (Bingold 1995), an important gap in understanding comes from a lack of research by nurses on the types of care that are provided to patients. Nurses are at the cutting-edge of dealing with patients in practice and it is therefore plain that nurses must make a contribution to future debates at the cutting-edge of health care. Nurse contributions may include research that is based in practice and contributes to the running of nursing services. Or it may be a process of becoming research minded

Case example 12.2

'You get attached to the patient and attached to the family. The last little boy I looked after was diagnosed as leukaemic, had chemotherapy and had bone marrow transplant. The transplant failed and by the time we met him he'd had lots of problems at school and also with his family. He was dying and his parents just wanted him to be an ordinary little boy. They were encouraged to do that by a specialist cancer centre. I think that's what all caring agencies promote, that's normal and maintained as much as possible. But I think towards the end of that child's life, it was taken to an extreme by health and social services and the parents. The boy was apparently having nightmares and could see ghosts, but because the boy's parents had been told to maintain normality they did not know when to step away and show their emotions. The doctors and parents had, in a sense, stopped listening. I said that it would be good to move the boy in with the parents, into their bedroom in the last week, but nobody wanted to take on board the fact that the little boy was so poorly and needed to be closer to everyone' (Smith & Gray 2000, pp. 66–67; see also Kelly et al 2000).

and influencing how nurses interact with patients by keeping up with the latest research.

An example of how a nurse reflects on her experiences in a children's oncology and bone marrow transplant setting – and why it is important to include this in research findings – is shown in Case example 12.2. The nurse's experiences are grounded in children's oncology practice and illustrate the importance of research in improving quality of care. In the children's oncology setting, nurses have to deal with issues of dying, death and bereavement. The case example suggests that we need to focus more explicitly on systems of social and emotional care as well as levels of attachment to the patient. Children's oncology is a protracted and painful event for all those involved. Nurses, patients and relatives are engaged in reflections on how to manage medical, social and emotional demands. 'Cancer', as James says, 'is hard to hide' (James 1993, p. 97). This means that all involved have, at some level, to manage their responses and feelings. In some cases, this means having to work at maintaining the belief that everything is normal in the patient's life and in other cases it means being faced with the uncomfortable task of disclosure (James 1993).

Another similar example in learning disability is useful in illustrating the importance of research that is grounded in practice. In a study of Down's syndrome in an Australian paediatric cardiology clinic, Silverman (1981) looked at techniques and levels of disclosure to parents and children. In Silverman's research, the level of disclosure and intervention was based on the model of childhood that was held by health professionals. Invasive medical techniques with children with Down's syndrome were found to be discouraged both by health professionals and by some parents in order to preserve a model of the innocence of childhood. The children were also seen as medically flawed (with a hole in the heart) and the children's lifespan (taken from statistical and medical sources of information) was deemed to be too short to warrant invasive surgery. Medical intervention was seen to interfere with the quality of life of a child with Down's syndrome and with that child's essential innocence. Silverman found that there were assumptions being made about learning disability and childhood that might decrease the lifespan of children with Down's syndrome and also limit levels of disclosure and full consultation. Silverman found that the medical professionals involved saw learning disabled children as biologically damaged and impaired. These medical judgements, and perhaps prejudices, reduced treatment options which impacted on life expectancy. Reports in the UK press have highlighted these issues over the last few years in relation to Down's syndrome cardiology.

Both of these examples of research are grounded in nursing and health practice. The examples lend support to the view that the task in nursing research is to assess the social, psychological and emotional methods that are available in the everyday practice of nurses. Good nursing research looks at the ways in which nurses and patients are involved with each other and it looks at the ways in which nurses and patients deal with issues in nursing practice – in other words, the ways in which nurses and patients come to terms with very difficult processes. These may include levels of disclosure in children's oncology, levels of consultation in children's Down's syndrome cardiology and settings in which death, dying and bereavement are constantly present.

An awareness of the issues and findings of research is helpful in everyday practice. Nurses may draw on research in their actions with patients and may be better in providing consistent care. Medical operations, if deemed suitable, may increase with children with Down's syndrome, or at least a debate might be raised that might draw on public consultation. Nurses might look at children's oncology and see how their experiences match those of the nurse in the example. This would act as a support, in so far as experiences would be shared, and also show that there are various ways of interacting with patients at particular moments in that patient's treatment. After all, the nurse notes in the example that sometimes it is better to create distance with the patient and sometimes attachment is better in the nurse–patient relationship.

ACTION RESEARCH

Action research is a good example of research that integrates a variety of methods and which is particularly popular among nurses, social workers and teachers. In this approach, the researcher is an active participant, working closely with the subjects – identifying problems, implementing solutions and evaluating their effectiveness as part of a cyclical process. Bell (1999) concludes: 'The essentially practical, problem-solving nature of action research makes this approach attractive to practitioner–researchers who have identified a problem during the course of their work, see the merits of investigating it and, if possible, of improving practice.' Action and participatory research balances generalisable knowledge and benefits the community that is being researched. It does this primarily by collaborating with the community as experts and as equals in the research process (Macaulay et al 1999, p. 774).

TRIANGULATION

'Triangulation' is the term used to describe the use of a multi-method approach and/or data source to study a given research problem.

'Investigator triangulation' refers to the collection of data by more than one researcher in the same setting. The researcher can be more confident in the findings of a study if the same conclusions are reached by more than one method or investigator and/or through more than one data source. Corner (1991), a nurse researcher, confirms this view. She states that 'the use of triangulation of different methods and types of data in a simple study provides a richer and deeper understanding of the area under investigation than would otherwise be possible'.

THE RESEARCH PROCESS

We have already met the term 'process' in connection with McFarlane's (1977) discussion of the nursing process. The notion of process as a movement forward is easily demonstrated in the four stages of the nursing process:

1. assessment
2. care planning
3. implementation
4. evaluation.

In rethinking the nursing process for the 1990s, Marks-Maran (1992) stresses the need for nurses to go beyond the method to define what underpins it. She suggests that nursing's value systems, including holism and the centrality of nurse–patient relationships, are the key. Naturalistic research is closely associated with such values, especially the importance of the relationship between the researcher and the researched.

The term 'process' is also used in the quality assurance literature, where it appears as one of the categories within which quality of care may be evaluated. The American physician Donabedian wrote a paper in the mid-1960s that has since become very influential. He suggested that quality may be evaluated according to the 'structure', 'process' and 'outcomes' of care. By 'process', Donabedian meant the actual content and methods of work used by physicians while in contact with patients (Donabedian 1966).

The research process refers to the different steps involved in undertaking a research project. Like any process, its various stages may overlap. The process consists of identifying a topic, specifying underlying theories, formulating questions, selecting a suitable approach or style, specifying methods and devising a plan to take the study forward.

An important part of the research plan includes the careful consideration of time and financial budgeting, secretarial support and ethical clearance. Time spent resolving organisational, political and ethical issues repays itself with interest over the rest of the study.

The research process can be divided into the following stages:

- Stage 1: identifying the research topic
- Stage 2: selecting an appropriate research approach
- Stage 3: designing the study
- Stage 4: developing data-collection methods and instruments
- Stage 5: collecting and recording the data
- Stage 6: analysing and interpreting the data
- Stage 7: presenting the research findings.

The following sections outline these stages in the research process in some detail. Boxes within each section suggest questions that students might pose with respect to each stage when critically evaluating their own and others' research.

STAGE 1: IDENTIFYING THE RESEARCH TOPIC

Ideas for research can derive from everyday experience. When researchers embark on a new project they usually have a broad idea of what they want to study. They may discuss their idea with colleagues in order to compile a 'first thoughts' list of questions to help focus the research (Bell 1999). They will also search the literature, to find out what has already been written on the subject. The library is the best place to start: bibliographies, abstracts and indexes help to identify appropriate information quickly. Obtaining this information is referred to as 'information retrieval'.

Ogier (1989) gives some sound advice on searching the literature. First, she suggests clarifying the topic by identifying and listing key words associated with it. For example, when Ogier wanted to find out how the ward sister affected the learning environment for student nurses, she made a list of key words associated with her main research question in the following way (Ogier 1982):

- Sister: charge nurse, head nurse
- Learning: studying, teaching, understanding.

You can compile key words that are taken from research interviews, focus groups, and meetings with people such as tutors or your friends at nursing college. It may even be helpful to start at a very basic level. Perhaps you might just want to start by watching a favourite television programme. You can combine watching television or reading a newspaper with noting interesting points and key words on your note-pad. Always try to look at key words in terms of pros and cons. See how the ideas and key words relate to each other. For example, images of the nurse as an angel or as a maternal figure may be thought about as relating to stereotypes in society that portray women as natural care givers (Oakley 1974, Smith 1992). Always try to look at alternative perspectives, different arguments (for and against) and several explanations of the events you are researching. Never jump to an immediate conclusion but try to mull things over for as long as you can. This will help you to consider most of what is relevant, especially the relevance of your research to nurses, patients and other important groups. Taking your time will give you time to trawl through most of the relevant literature.

Making a list also helps to give the researcher some idea of where to start when visiting a library and beginning to look through abstracts, indexes and computerised information. It also makes it easier for the librarian to assist in selecting material. It is helpful to have a cut-off date for searching the literature. Depending on the topic and the amount of information available, this could be as little as 5 or as many as 40 years.

The organised researcher immediately records the details of what she is reading on index cards or in a designated exercise book. The most common

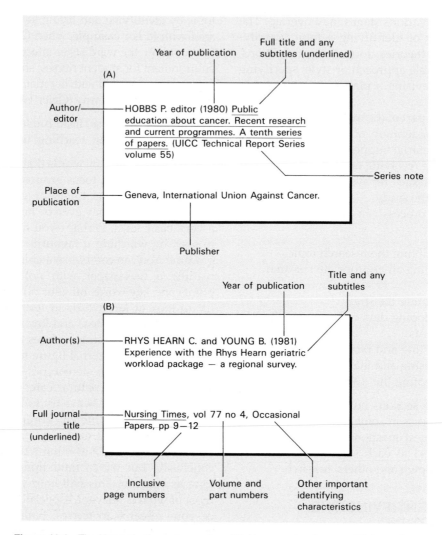

Figure 12.1 The Harvard referencing system. (A) Monograph reference. (B) Journal reference. (Reproduced from Cormack (1984) with the kind permission of Blackwell Scientific Publications Ltd.)

referencing systems are the Harvard (Fig. 12.1) and Vancouver (numerical) systems, used in both books and articles, depending on the house-style of the publisher.

Relationship between research topic and literature search

The researcher goes back and forth between the literature and the research topic in order to formulate research objectives, questions or hypotheses and select a suitable approach, style and method. The relationship between the research topic, the developing question and the literature search as described by Cormack (1991) is illustrated in Figure 12.2.

The formulation of the research question and approach should be summarised in a literature review at the beginning of a research report or article; this review should be comprehensive, up-to-date and relevant to the study (Box 12.2).

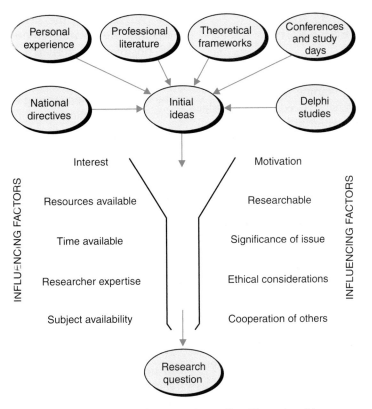

Figure 12.2 Development of a research question. (Reproduced from Cormack (1991) with the kind permission of Blackwell Scientific Publications Ltd.)

Box 12.2 **Critical assessment of research: Stage 1**

At the beginning of a research report or article, the research objectives/hypotheses and approach are summarised in a literature review; you will need to assess whether this review is comprehensive, recent and relevant to the study.

Questions to ask are:

• Does the literature review give evidence that the researcher knows their subject?
• Is the literature critically evaluated?
• Is the research problem stated as a hypothesis, as study objectives or as a general area of interest?

Formulating objectives, questions and hypotheses

The decision to set up objectives, questions or hypotheses will depend not only on the topic but also on the researcher's favoured research approach. Most experimental studies are geared towards testing a hypothesis. Some qualitative studies begin with neither hypotheses nor objectives but with the researchers having a general idea about what they want to investigate; hypotheses are developed as the research progresses. Bell (1999) cautions the inexperienced researcher against this unstructured approach and advises, at the very least, 'a precise statement of objectives'.

James, a nurse sociologist, illustrates these difficulties at the beginning of her qualitative research on nursing the dying. Among her fieldwork notes is the comment, 'One of the problems all during today has been the vast input of possible information and not knowing how to select it'. It was not until James had time to withdraw and reflect on her nursing fieldwork 'that what had been written during it looked as though it had any purpose or explanatory use' (James 1984).

STAGE 2: SELECTING AN APPROPRIATE RESEARCH APPROACH

Bell (1999) suggests that 'before considering the various stages of planning and conducting investigations, researchers need to consider the main features of well-established and well reported styles of research'. These (as discussed in 'Types of research', above) may be classified as either quantitative or qualitative research styles, and depend to some extent on the different disciplines with which they are associated.

In the past, nurse researchers were more likely to adopt quantitative research approaches, possibly because, as Spencer (1983) suggests, these styles were more in keeping with the work of their medical colleagues. However, over the past decade or so nurse researchers have also begun to embrace qualitative approaches, preferring to see the so-called 'divide' between the two approaches as more of a continuum in which, as Bell (1999) suggests, 'no approach prescribes nor automatically rejects any particular method'. Similarly, Haase & Myers (1988) note that some nurse researchers, dissatisfied with a forced choice between approaches, have advocated combining qualitative and quantitative methods.

Influencing factors

In the end, a researcher's decision to select a particular research approach depends on a number of factors. It may be that one approach is more suitable to a particular research topic than another, or that the resources available to the researcher, including their own experience and preferences, the availability of a research supervisor (also with particular preferences), time, secretarial support and money all contribute to the final decision.

Take the example of one of the present authors' own pieces of research (Smith 1987). This research began with the aim of studying the relationship between the quality of the nursing care received by patients and the quality of the ward as a learning environment for student nurses. At first, the research set out with a quantitative view, which wanted to test the hypothesis that the quality of the nursing on the ward would determine whether the learning environment was negative or positive. In research language, what the research was trying to 'prove' was that the quality of nursing on a ward was directly related to the quality of the learning environment. In other words, the learning environment was dependent on the quality of nursing. This way of posing a research hypothesis is very much in the deductive or quantitative tradition of experimental research, in which hypotheses are 'tested' on the basis of an underlying theory.

However, once in the research setting, it was quickly realised that it would be impossible to define the relationship between the quality of nursing and the learning environment in this way. It was decided, therefore, to disregard the original strategy in favour of qualitative inductive research. The reason for changing to a qualitative approach was because it was more appropriate to exploring with nurses and patients what quality of nursing and the learning environment meant to them and how they saw the two relating to each other. This approach was very time-consuming, because the researcher needed to work on a variety of shifts and wards in order to talk to nurses and patients. Talking to nurses and patients was therefore background data that helped generate the research questions. Research questions were generated inductively with nurses and patients and shaped the direction of the research. Rather than fitting everything into a ready-made hypothesis that the researcher already had in mind, a range of opinions was gathered from nurses and patients. This allowed the consultation of different views and generated a number of alternative research questions from background data (Glaser & Strauss 1967). In other words, research was grounded in the practice of nurses and the experiences of patients. This allowed research to be directly pertinent to health services and to consider what was going on and important to people there and then.

Quantitative methods are useful in research when looking for a large amount of generalisation, reproducibility and a wide sample. Qualitative methods are particularly good at looking at the details of clinical and non-clinical

Box 12.3 **Critical assessment of research:**
Stage 2

Questions to ask are:

- Does the researcher declare their particular research approach?
- Is it appropriate to the research topic under study?
- Are any other factors evident, for example available time, money or expertise, for why the researcher has chosen the particular research approach?
- Does the researcher make clear a particular theoretical framework underlying the approach?

settings, the local implementation of social and health policy, social interactions between people, the meanings that people have and express to each other, and the use of language (whether in speech or written words).

Box 12.3 outlines several questions to be asked during the critical assessment of Stage 2 of the research process.

STAGE 3: DESIGNING THE STUDY

The design of a research study depends largely on whether the researcher adopts a quantitative, deductive research approach or a qualitative, inductive one. The most common types of study design are experimental and descriptive. The notion of study design is more applicable to quantitative than to qualitative research.

Quantitative research

Experimental designs

Experimental designs range from the very simple to the very complex. A simple design would be to test the effects of one single variable on another one. In the experimental context, variables are studied in pairs. Each of the paired variables has a separate name: the 'independent' (or 'causal') variable and the 'dependent' variable, which alters as a consequence of the independent variable.

Randomised controlled trials (RCTs) are the most common examples of experiments used by doctors and familiar to many nurses in the context of drug and product (i.e. clinical) trials. The Department of Health's research and development strategy identifies the RCT as one of the most important ways of finding out whether or not treatments are effective. The Cochrane Centre in Oxford has been set up to review trial findings and disseminate them to clinicians and purchasers. In the context of the new market-led health service, this is seen as important in encouraging the use and purchase of 'tried and tested' health care. Nursing treatments have also been reviewed in this way. For example, Cullum, a nurse researcher, undertook a review of the community nursing management of leg ulcers and found the need for more trials to be undertaken to demonstrate their effectiveness (Cullum 1994). Sapsford & Abbott (1998) also point out that 'the logic of experimental design underlies all serious attempts to evaluate policy or practice'.

In order to set up an experiment or trial, the researcher decides, on the basis of logic, which variable is to be independent or dependent within a given experiment. For instance, if the researcher wants to test whether a particular intervention (i.e. the independent variable – for example the introduction of a new drug, a leg ulcer treatment or a counselling session) has affected the patient's recovery (i.e. the dependent variable), she would choose an experimental design for the study, involving a control group and an experimental group. The experimental group is a group of people to whom the experimental treatment (drug or counselling session) is given. The experimental group is compared with the control group, to whom no experimental treatment is given. The researcher studies the effects that each variable has on the other in two randomly selected experimental and control groups. In cross-over designs, the study subjects may also be used as their own controls, receiving different types of interventions at different stages of the study, using a 'cross-over' design. The logic behind this type of design is that more precise results may be obtained by comparing interventions in the same individual rather than across different groups.

The principles of **random selection and matching** are applied to the study's subjects. In random selection, all members of the population under study have an equal chance of being included in the study. 'Matching' refers to ensuring that subjects in the experimental and control groups are as similar as possible on characteristics (e.g. race, age, gender, class and occupation) that one might judge to be important. Any differences observed following the intervention could therefore be deemed to be attributable to the intervention rather than to differences between the two groups. Thus, random selection and matching allows causal inferences to be drawn from the results or outcomes of the intervention (e.g. the speed of recovery).

Webb & Wilson-Barnett chose an experimental design for their study of the relationship between counselling and women undergoing hysterectomy (Webb & Wilson-Barnett 1983). The design of the study is presented in Figure 12.5.

Webb & Wilson-Barnett (1983) added a third or 'placebo' group to their study design. Rather than receiving no intervention at all, as in the case of the control group, the placebo group was involved in a 20-minute conversation. This conversation avoided the topic of recovery, whereas the experimental group received a 20-minute counselling session offering them information and advice to promote recovery.

The reason for introducing a placebo group into a study is two-fold. First, it may help to discount any bias on the part of researcher or patient in their judgement (whether favourable or otherwise) with regard to the experimental intervention. Second, it provides a control for the frequency of spontaneous changes that may occur in the patient independent of the intervention under study. That spontaneous changes can occur during the experimental process is referred to as the Hawthorne effect, because it was first described by researchers undertaking studies in a factory of that name. If, however, differences only occur in the experimental group when compared with both the placebo and the control groups, researchers are more able to claim that the differences are attributable to the intervention under study (Sapsford & Abbott 1998).

Webb & Wilson-Barnett (1983) also designed their study in such a way as to reduce the risk of the researcher having an effect and so biasing the outcome of the study. Two researchers were involved. One researcher randomly allocated the patients to one of the three study groups and carried out the intervention (phase 2), while another researcher carried out the data collection visits (phases 1 and 3; see Fig. 12.5). Roles were regularly changed so that the researchers were unaware of the group to which the patient had been assigned.

It should be noted that structured interview schedules were used. Scales included a depression inventory, a mood adjective checklist and a self-concept scale.

In this way, the researchers did not have any expectations based on any prior knowledge of the three groups to which the patients were assigned; if they had, this might have influenced the outcome of the interviews and rating scales. For example, had the researchers known that the patients had received the experimental intervention, they might unconsciously have behaved in particular ways (e.g. using an encouraging tone of voice), which might have influenced the results obtained from the interviews and scales. Designing the study in this way helped to reduce the effects of researcher bias.

Trials are said to be 'double blind' when neither researcher nor subject knows which group the subject has been allocated to. Thus, as both parties are 'blind' to the particular treatment being given to particular patients, it is hoped to reduce what have been described as 'expectancy effects'.

Descriptive study design

The survey is an example of a descriptive study design and is also in the quantitative tradition. The aim of a survey is to obtain information that can be analysed and from which patterns can be extracted (Bell 1999). Information can be gathered in a survey in a variety of ways, including questionnaires, schedules and checklists. It is very important that all the respondents are asked the same questions in the same way. Rating scales of the type used by Webb & Wilson-Barnett (1983) may be devised in order to measure attitudes, beliefs or motivation. The survey primarily aims to collect facts in response to the questions

'What?', 'Where?', 'When?' and 'How?' (Bell 1999). Explanatory surveys that ask the question 'Why?' are sometimes conducted to follow up the information obtained from descriptive surveys.

If the study population is too big for everyone to be included in the survey, respondents will be randomly selected, as in an experimental study. This will help to ensure that the results are representative of the population from which they are drawn.

Study design depends largely on whether the researcher adopts a qualitative or quantitative research approach. For example, if research wanted to test whether a particular intervention (e.g. the introduction of specialised tutorials) had affected the relationship between the quality of nursing and the ward learning environment (Smith 1987), an experimental design would have been chosen for the study. The research would have required a control group (ward 1) and an experimental group (ward 2). Each ward population – i.e. patients and nurses – would have had to be randomly selected and then matched so that causal inferences could be drawn from the outcome measures (e.g. quality of nursing and ward learning) that had been chosen.

Qualitative research

Since qualitative research is concerned with subjective meanings for the participants in naturalistic settings, the principles applied to quantitative research in order to control the research environment are inappropriate. Differences in sampling technique illustrate this point.

Sampling is purposive and theoretical. Qualitative researchers do not seek 'representative' samples, but rather select those individuals with special knowledge or characteristics that will increase their understanding of the study phenomena. The next step is to develop theory from their findings and, where necessary, to collect additional information, through further theoretical sampling of groups and settings.

James (1984) and Melia (1982) both used purposive, or theoretical, sampling to establish their study subjects and settings. James worked on hospital wards and in a hospice in order to study the different ways in which dying patients were nursed. Melia asked for student nurse volunteers from a school of nursing in order to find out about their experiences of nurse training. In quantitative research traditions it would not have been acceptable to ask for volunteers to take part in the study: only random sampling would be seen to guarantee that the study sample was representative of the target population. However, for qualitative researchers who want to increase their understanding of the research setting, purposive or theoretical sampling is the method of choice. They also believe in declaring their personal opinions and acknowledging their own part in the research setting from the outset. Melia, for example, declares that by actively involving herself with the people she was studying she was in a much better position to present an 'account of how the participants see the situation or phenomenon in question; the analysis then goes beyond this point when analytical concepts which transcend the meanings of actors are developed' (Melia 1982).

In qualitative research, the steps of the research process are much less distinct than in quantitative research. Study design, development of hypotheses and methods, collection and analysis of data are closely integrated, and for this reason are not described separately.

Feminist perspectives

Qualitative research permits researchers to write themselves into the research and declare their personal opinions. In recent years, feminist researchers have drawn attention to this important issue, particularly in relation to gender.

Many feminists favour qualitative research. Oakley (1981) criticises quantitative research for the way in which it mystifies 'the researcher and the researched as objective instruments of data production' and condemns 'personal involvement as dangerous bias'. For Oakley, who has studied various aspects of women's lives, ranging from housework to childbirth, the use of subjectivity in research is essential to both the collection and production of data (Oakley 1974, 1981). Oakley's favoured method of data collection is in-depth interviewing, which allows her to develop rapport, and in some instances friendships, with the women studied. Oakley's personal concerns, commitment to feminism and opinions would seem relevant if consideration is given to the lack of focus on nurses, who are predominantly perceived as being a female stereotype of the natural care giver. Women and nurses are often treated as little more than an invisible workforce (and sometimes remain unseen even in good research). Oakley writes: 'In a fifteen year career as a sociologist studying medical services, I confess that I have been particularly blind to the contribution made by nurses to health care. Indeed, over a period of some months spent observing in a large London hospital I hardly noticed nurses at all' (Oakley 1984, p. 26).

The feminist researchers Stanley & Wise (1983) drew attention to the potential power of the researcher over the researched, as information is extracted without reciprocity or responsibility. These observations are particularly relevant to nursing and health care research, in which nurses and patients can be especially vulnerable to external authority structures. James, for example, was concerned that because she was a participant observer, the nurses would become so used to her being around that they might forget they were the subjects of her research. She decided, therefore, periodically to make outrageous statements to remind people that there was a researcher in their midst (James 1984).

A constant struggle in research is between being 'in-group' and being 'out-group'. There is nearly always a tension between fully participating with people in the research to the extent that you become seen as a member of the group, or, alternatively, maintaining social and critical distance, in which case you are 'out' of the group and treated differently (sometimes even with suspicion). A good half-way house is to take time to cultivate personal relations with people in the research, while making sure to critically attend to what people are saying to you. There are no specific maxims for good research, but in general the researcher must be:

- open to new ideas
- attentive to the views of individuals and groups in the research

- flexible to change and other people's needs
- critical of their own and others' assumptions.

This helps research to be relevant, since the researcher is listening to what people have to say and discussing their views with them by probing and developing issues. The feminist maxim states that 'the personal is political'. Personal and political awareness is helpful in the nurse researcher's reflection on gender in health. It is helpful in understanding the relationship that the nurse researcher has with families, staff, patients and research participants. It is central in ensuring equality of opportunity.

Webb has explicitly introduced feminist perspectives into nursing research. She describes feminist research (Webb 1984) as a 'critique' that: 'aims specifically to work towards defining alternatives and understanding everyday experience in order to bring about change. Analysis and critique of research methods leads on to analysis and critique in the research context through consciousness raising both for researcher and researched.'

In her 1993 update, Webb suggests that 'a short-hand definition [of feminist research] perhaps could be phrased as "research *on* women, *by* women, *for* women". What is distinctive about feminist methodology is its engagement with issues of concern particularly to women and its acceptance of a variety of methods'.

The contribution of feminist perspectives to nursing research is particularly pertinent, given that nursing is a predominantly female occupation, and nurses are involved in traditionally female roles and work activities prescribed by the predominantly male medical profession. Feminist perspectives are committed to making gender and power relations visible in the world about us and in the relationships between researcher and researched.

Until recently, feminist research almost exclusively embraced qualitative approaches. Oakley (1989), in an apparent break with tradition, brought a feminist perspective to the seemingly most explicit of quantitative research approaches, the randomised controlled trial (RCT), in order to study social support in the antenatal care of 'at-risk' mothers. In a detailed article, she demonstrated how the best of the two approaches could be combined to address sampling accuracy, the selection of appropriate methods, the informed consent of subjects, the formulation of research questions, and the analysis and use of findings from women's perspectives rather than from the dominant male medico-scientific, professional view of the world.

The following example gives an unexpected perspective on sampling accuracy. Citing the case of random allocation of subjects to experimental and control groups, Oakley showed how midwives' intuitive judgements were sometimes in conflict with objective sampling techniques. She put this down to health professionals' ideology, which previous researchers had shown led 'to discriminatory stereotyping of women, based on such characteristics as working class or ethnic minority'. This example is a further illustration of how a feminist approach differed from the more usual 'hands-off' conduct of RCTs. Midwives were responsible for recruiting and randomly sampling the women who attended antenatal clinic. It was only because Oakley chose to keep in close contact with the midwives that she was able to discuss how they felt about random sampling. In the end, she probably obtained a more accurate sample than she might have done had she not engaged with them.

Box 12.4 outlines questions to be asked in Stage 3 of the research process.

Box 12.4 Critical assessment of research: Stage 3

The questions you ask here will depend very much on the underlying approach adopted by the researcher and how it has influenced the study design:

- What is the sample size? How was it selected, and is it representative of the population under study?
- Was there a control group and an experimental group?
- (In qualitative studies) Are the unique issues of sampling of the qualitative study addressed, and are the characteristics of the population outlined?
- Does the researcher write themselves into the study and declare their biases?
- Is the statement of the research problem, as hypotheses or objectives, appropriate to the study design and the topic for investigation?

STAGE 4: DEVELOPING DATA-COLLECTION METHODS AND INSTRUMENTS

Quantitative research

The pilot study

In the quantitative research tradition, a pilot study is likely to be conducted when data collection methods and techniques are developed as a prelude to the main study. Common tools include questionnaires and non-participant observation schedules.

One of the reasons for conducting a pilot study is to develop research tools that are reliable (i.e. whose results can be replicated under a variety of conditions) and valid (i.e. they measure what they purport to). This emphasis is seen to be a vital component of pursuing objective scientific proof.

Developing the questionnaire

A common questionnaire design is the Likert scale, in which respondents are asked to rate their responses on a scale of 1 to 4, 5 or 6. One such example is Fretwell's Ward Learning Environment Rating Questionnaire (Fretwell 1985) (Fig. 12.3). This 36-item questionnaire covers different aspects of the learning environment, including ward atmosphere and staff relations, ward teaching, provision of learning opportunities, patient care, anxiety and stress. Nursing students and staff were asked to rate each item as a factor in the ward learning environment on a scale of 1 (strongly disagree) to 5 (strongly agree). The scores were then added together and an average mean score obtained for each aspect of the learning environment and for the ward overall. This questionnaire was devised in the early 1980s and if it were going to be considered for use in contemporary research, it would be advisable for the researcher to check that the language and terminology are still current.

Entire textbooks have been written on questionnaire design. The student may find Oppenheim (1992) and Moser & Kalton (1985) especially helpful. However, there are a few basic rules to observe

PRIVATE AND CONFIDENTIAL

WARD LEARNING ENVIRONMENT RATING QUESTIONNAIRE

Ward.. Student ☐   Pupil ☐   Trained nurse ☐

(Please tick)

The following statements are concerned with nurse training in the ward. For each statement please indicate your opinion by placing a tick (✓) in one of the five boxes. There are no right or wrong answers, but please try to avoid the 'uncertain' column unless you really cannot agree or disagree. If you want to clarify or explain your choice, make your comments in the box provided.

Note: The term 'learner' is intended to include both student and pupil nurses. 'Sister' applies equally to charge nurses.

SECTION A (Questions 1 to 3 to be answered by student and pupil nurses only.)	Strongly agree	Agree	Uncertain	Disagree	Strongly disagree	Comments
1. This was a good ward for student/ pupil learning.						
2. I am happy with the experience I have had on this ward.						
3. I learnt very much on this ward.						

(Remaining questions to be answered by everyone.)

	Strongly agree	Agree	Uncertain	Disagree	Strongly disagree	Comments
4. The number of staff is adequate for the workload.						
5. There is very much to learn on this ward.						
6. There are enough trained nurses in relation to learners and auxiliaries.						
7. The workload does not interfere with teaching or learning.						

Figure 12.3 Extract from Ward Learning Environment Rating Questionnaire. (Reproduced with kind permission from Fretwell 1985.)

in designing a questionnaire, such as constructing questions that use language familiar to the respondents (see the point made above about using the Fretwell questionnaire in contemporary research) and that are free of in-built biases (thus avoiding the 'leading questions' that Florence Nightingale warned against). Cicourel believes that research instruments such as questionnaires allow researchers to devise coding rules and scaling devices to 'transform the structure of social action into quantifiable elements', from their own but not necessarily the respondents' point of view. He gives important advice when he says (Cicourel 1964): 'Operational definitions of sociological concepts [e.g. nursing, quality of care, learning environment] need to be constructed in such a way in order that everyday life experience and conduct is reflected in them.'

Non-participant observation schedules

Similarly, the same basic rules should be followed in constructing observation schedules, such as those for observing quality of nursing (Wandelt & Ager 1974), ward sister activity (Pembrey 1980), ward reporting systems (Lelean 1975) and paediatric ward organisation (Hawthorne 1974). An extract from Wandelt & Ager's Quality Patient Care Scale is given in Figure 12.4. As this tool was originally developed for use in the USA, it is important that its design and language are assessed for their relevance to British research and evaluation.

Qualitative research

Qualitative research approaches are inductive, in that theoretical concepts are developed from the data as they are collected and analysed as the study progresses. We can see that this approach differs from quantitative, deductive research, in which all the data are collected before analysing them in order to test existing concepts and theories. The qualitative researcher regularly leaves the field to code, reflect on what is observed and make inferences from the data to guide future fieldwork.

Grounded theory is an example of an integrated, qualitative research approach popular among nurse researchers (Glaser & Strauss 1967). The approach provides a flexible framework for inductive research. Data are collected, coded and analysed in order to develop conceptual categories and formulate hypotheses to guide ongoing data collection. Grounded theory shares features with other qualitative approaches in that data analysis is part and parcel of the research process and begins early on in the study. More recent texts on using grounded theory as a research approach are now available (Strauss & Corbin 1994), but the basic framework remains the same.

Ethnography and phenomenology are other examples of qualitative research approaches that have gained in popularity among nurse researchers over the last decade. Ethnography is seen by many nurses as being eminently suitable to the detailed study of small groups within health care settings, because of its attention to culture and meaning. The key method of ethnography is participant observation, through which in-depth descriptive accounts are developed from detailed field notes. Some ethnographers go beyond descriptions to compare their findings with existing social theories (e.g. 'deviance') and also to reflect on how one in-depth study may also reflect what is going on in the outside world. For example, a detailed study of health care reforms among district nurses in one health care setting reflected the wider policy issues taking place at government level (Smith et al 1993). Critical ethnographers give back their accounts to the people they have observed to challenge their perspectives and incorporate the participants' views into their findings (Street 1992).

Ethnomethodology, meaning people's methods or ways of interacting with each other, looks at practical reasoning and purposefully orientated action in social life (Garfinkel 1967). In particular, ethnomethodology concentrates on people's commonsense accounts of the social world – in other words, how people make sense of the social and historical circumstances in which they find themselves. Ethnomethodology investigates the taken-for-granted and commonsense reasoning of people (termed 'actors' or 'members') in different settings. Accounts of the social world are termed 'members' meanings'. The person or member will purposefully orientate their action not only to a perceived end but also according to their immediate setting. Ethnomethodology looks at how people understand the world in which they live. For example, the meaning and appropriate type of emotional disclosure that nurses and patients make to each other will vary according to different clinical settings. The nurse organises the type of

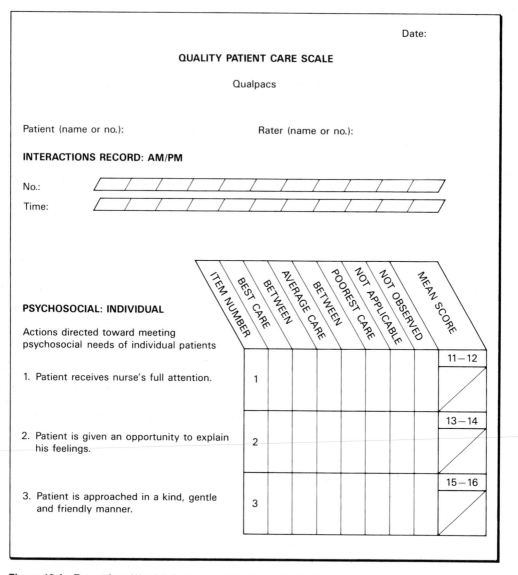

Figure 12.4 Extract from Wandelt & Ager (1974) 68-item Quality Patient Care Scale. (Reproduced with kind permission of Appleton & Lange.)

emotional contact that is required according to the clinical setting, the needs and views of other people present, interactions with staff and patients and the immediate circumstances of work. Obviously, the emotional disclosure and attachment with the patient will vary in clinical settings such as children's oncology, blood tests in haematology, baby clinics, or informing a relative of a patient's bereavement. Nurses orientate their action not only to a perceived end with the patient but also to the emotional and interpersonal setting (see James 1989, Smith 1992, Smith & Gray 2000). Ethnomethodology makes these social interactions explicit rather than taken-for-granted.

Benner has popularised **phenomenology** through her writings, including *From Novice to Expert* (Benner 1984) referred to in Box 12.1. Benner gives credence to the unique nature of the individual and the importance of the 'lived experience'. Phenomenologists use in-depth interviewing and detailed analysis and commentary of the content. In her research on nursing as critical companionship, Titchen (1998) draws on sociological phenomenology (Schutz 1972) to look at nurse–patient relationships. She develops notions of skilled and critical companionship that draw on a variety of traditions in humanistic social science and philosophy. Certainly, at one level, models of companionship are central in looking at the existential and emotional closeness of practitioner and patient. At another level, Titchen divides critical companionship into several domains (the relationship domain; the rationality-intuitive domain; the facilitative use of self domain) that are helpful in facilitating the acquisition and development of craft knowledge (the know how, spontaneous and practical knowledge that is involved in the routine of nursing). Titchen's study shows that the use of experiential learning and guided reflection are central in developing supportive relationships at work with colleagues and patients. The development of skilled and critical companionship informs educational methods and essential qualities of nurse leadership. This research makes explicit the nursing qualities of mutuality, reciprocity, self-reflection, critique, consciousness raising, and articulation of craft or working knowledge which are important in nursing and nurse leadership.

Each of the above approaches is informed by the social sciences. Grounded theory, for example, was first developed by sociologists, ethnography by anthropologists and phenomenology by philosophers (Thorne 1991). They were formulated by social scientists who were reacting to what they saw as the 'rigidity' of the 'scientific' quantitative approach to research.

Validity and reliability

The validity and reliability of data are integral to qualitative research approaches. Validity is implicit when data are simultaneously collected, handled and analysed to shape ongoing data collection and to develop and confirm evolving

---

Box 12.5 Critical assessment of research: Stage 4

The questions you ask here will depend very much on the underlying approach adopted by the researcher:

- (In quantitative studies) Was a pilot study carried out? If so, what changes were made to the main study as a result of the pilot?
- Were issues of validity and reliability (including adequacy and dependability) addressed from each perspective?
- (In qualitative studies) Does the researcher present hypotheses, concepts and theories derived from the data?

---

theories and concepts. Hall & Stevens (1991) prefer to use the term 'adequacy' rather than validity to evaluate the whole research process from formulation of questions, selection of methods to outcomes that incorporate the participants' perspectives. Reliability (which Hall & Stevens call 'dependability') is ascertained by means of the researcher's in-depth involvement in the field over time and with increasing familiarity, which means s/he is able to check the accuracy and recurrence of the data in a number of settings and from a number of participants (Morse & Field 1996).

Questions concerning validity and reliability are among those to be asked in Stage 4 of the research process (Box 12.5).

STAGE 5: COLLECTING AND RECORDING THE DATA

Quantitative research

The most common quantitative means of data collection are questionnaires, semi-structured interviews and non-participant observation; these are developed during the pilot phase of the study. Webb & Wilson-Barnett (1983) (see above), for example, used a variety of these methods, including structured interview schedules, a depression inventory scale, a mood adjective checklist and a self-concept scale (Fig. 12.5). The process of developing such data collection tools is described in the preceding section.

	Phase 1 5–6 days postoperatively	Phase 2 6–7 days postoperatively	Phase 3 4 months postoperatively
Experimental group	Interview and scales	20-minute advice and information session	Interview and scales
Placebo group	Interview and scales	20-minute conversation	Interview and scales
Control group	Interview and scales	No intervention	Interview and scales
Note: Structured interview schedules were used. Scales included a depression inventory, a mood adjective check-list and a self-concept scale.			

Figure 12.5   Diagram of a study by Webb & Wilson-Barnett on the relationship between counselling and recovery from hysterectomy. (Reproduced by kind permission of *Nursing Times*, where this article first appeared on 23 November 1983.)

In order for researchers to retrieve their data easily and accurately for analysis and interpretation, it is important that, during data collection, they develop systems to ensure this. In quantitative studies, it is likely that the data are collected and recorded on standardised forms, for example self-administered questionnaires and structured interview schedules.

Qualitative research

As noted above, the most common qualitative research methods include participant observation and in-depth interviewing, to study complex phenomena such as care of the dying and student nurse socialisation.

Participant observation

The classification of the participant observer role is well documented in the literature. The observer's participant role can be seen on a continuum from complete (even covert), in which the subjects are unaware that they are being studied, to non-participant, in which the observer records data from the sidelines. A common compromise is for the researcher to adopt the role of observer-as-participant, in which they are known to be conducting research but participate in the everyday activities of the research setting.

Collins (1984) suggests that full participation is essential if the researcher is to understand the subjects and settings under study. He calls this understanding 'participant comprehension'.

> **Box 12.6 Critical assessment of research: Stage 5**
>
> The questions you ask here will depend very much on the underlying approach adopted by the researcher and how it has influenced the choice of method. For both qualitative and quantitative studies:
>
> - What research methods were used?
> - Were they justified and explained according to the approach adopted?
> - Were they appropriate?
> - Were copies of questionnaires, and of interview and observation schedules, available in the report?
> - Were methods of recording and retrieving data clearly described?

One of the authors of this chapter conducted her own pieces of research (Smith 1987, 1992), which aimed to emulate Collins's approach during participant observation on the wards. When observing classroom activities, the researcher was a complete observer, sitting at the back of the room trying to be a 'fly on the wall'.

Melia (1982) applies the participant observer concept to in-depth interviewing. She contends that 'the close involvement of the researcher in the production of the data is as true of the informal interview method of data production as it is of participant observation'. Not only was Melia familiar with the setting from which her subjects came, being a nurse herself, but she also used the interview as a forum through which to interact with them in the production of data.

In qualitative studies, the researcher has to develop ways of recording fieldwork notes during participant observation, such as by keeping index cards to record observations as events take place, for example mealtimes in a day nursery. Interviews are (with the participants' permission) most often tape-recorded. The tapes are then transcribed into typescript form to facilitate analysis of the interview contents.

Box 12.6 outlines questions for Stage 5.

STAGE 6: ANALYSING AND INTERPRETING THE DATA

Data analysis and interpretation is often the most time-consuming phase of the research process. In planning a research project, it is wise to allocate twice as much time for analysis and interpretation as for data collection: if it takes 2 months to collect data, it is likely to take 4 months to analyse and interpret them. Processed data are referred to as 'findings' or 'results'. Methods of data analysis vary according to the underlying research approach.

Quantitative research

In quantitative research, data are analysed numerically once they have been collected. Large-scale surveys and experimental studies require statistical testing of hypotheses. Statistical associations and differences between variables are established, and causal inferences may be made. Tests are used to establish the statistical significance of these associations and differences.

Statistical tests are based on probability theory, and the researcher will need to consult a statistician in order to choose the appropriate test given the size of sample, type of data and questions being asked. Most statistics textbooks include a chart that helps the researcher to select the appropriate tests. In short, the data are manipulated statistically in order to ensure that the results have not occurred by chance. You will usually see this written as '$p < 0.05$' or '$p < 0.01$' beside the results. The p values mean that the probability of the results having occurred by chance is less than 5% or 1% respectively. When the probability of results occurring by chance is greater than

5%, they are usually considered to be 'not significant' (NS).

The importance of logic in interpreting results cannot be underestimated. Just because a significant result seems to have been obtained, it does not mean that cause and effect are automatically established. A number of conditions need to be met if causality between variables is to be demonstrated. First and foremost, the researcher must make sure that an accidental link does not bind independent and dependent variables together in a spurious relationship. The sociologist Rosenberg (1968) gives a familiar example to illustrate this point. In Sweden, a relationship was found between the number of storks and the number of children born in a given area. This finding could be interpreted as meaning that in some way the storks were a causal factor in the number of babies being born. Rosenberg explains: 'The reason for the relationship between number of storks and number of babies is urban–rural location. Most storks are found in rural areas and the rural birth rate is higher than the urban birth rate. … Unless one guards against such accidental associations, one is in danger of reaching erroneous and misleading conclusions.'

Using computers

In large-sample surveys, it is likely that the researcher will store data in a computer. This will potentially ease and speed up data analysis. If the sample is small, however, it may be quicker to analyse the data by hand. Data, it should be remembered, are only as good as the operator who enters them into the computer and the logic that inspires decisions about statistical tests. Preparing data for analysis may also be very time-consuming. First, crude data are taken from the questionnaire or interview schedule and coded, ready to be 'punched' into the computer. The data will ideally be inserted into a ready-made spreadsheet to create a database. The database can then be used in conjunction with a statistical programme such as SPSS (Statistical Package for the Social Sciences) to analyse the data using summary statistics (e.g. frequencies and average – mean, median and modes) and appropriate statistical significance tests (Jolley 1991).

Truman (1992) defines information technology (IT) as 'the generic term used to describe the processing of information using micro-processor-based electronic equipment' (i.e. computers). The 1970s marked the advent of the computer age, and intensive research and development has ensured a rapidly changing technology. Because of this, computers are constantly being updated. The development of the microchip has meant not only that their design has become much more compact, but that computer 'memory' – i.e. the amount of information computers are able to store on their hard disk at any one time, and the speed with which they can process it – has also increased.

The computer's nerve centre is the central processing unit (CPU), which responds to instructions contained in specially designed programmes (software). A computer system is made up of a number of components, known as hardware, represented diagrammatically in Figure 12.6. These include input devices, such as the keyboard, mouse and modem, output devices, including the printer, monitor or visual display unit (VDU) and modem, and data storage systems, such as hard disk, floppy disk, laser disk or CD-ROM (compact disc-read only memory).

The most common applications of IT to research, including some of the examples referred to elsewhere, are:

- word processing
- spreadsheets
- databases, including CD-ROMs of references and other library information
- statistical analysis, using, for example, SPSS
- textual analysis, for example the Nudist and Ethnograph programs.

There are many different programs available for each of these applications, and (like computer hardware) they are constantly being updated and developed.

Since large amounts of personal information can be stored on databases, the Data Protection Act was introduced in 1983 to ensure the accuracy and security of the data being stored. Anyone undertaking research using personal records is required to register under the Act with a local data protection officer. This measure helps to ensure that the data are being used for the purposes stated, and to maintain confidentiality and security of the system.

The internet or World Wide Web (www)

In recent years, the World Wide Web (www) and the revolution in computer technology has

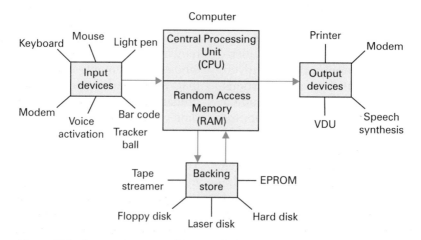

Figure 12.6   A computer system (Truman 1992).

influenced the ways in which research is conducted and disseminated to audiences. There are now many research journals available online and search engines that allow you to type in key words and then produce lists of results. Information technology and the net are useful in gathering and sharing information on web pages, by email, in forum discussions and newsgroups. The virtual reality of the web makes surfing the net a very quick way of gathering information. Information on research, nursing, and just about anything else you care to imagine, can be retrieved at the touch of a button.

Some useful places to start searching are shown in alphabetical order at the end of the chapter, after the Further reading list (p. 363).

Hardey's paper on the internet (Hardey 1999) says that the internet poses problems for the medical profession in terms of notions of expertise. He writes:

The Internet is an inherently interactive environment that transcends established national boundaries, regulations and distinctions between professions and expertise. It is shown that it is the users of Internet information rather than authors or professional experts who decided what and how material is accessed and used. It is concluded that the Internet forms the site of a new struggle over expertise in health that will transform the relationship between the health professions and their clients. (Hardey 1999, p. 820)

There are professional, ethical and information sharing issues that are associated with research on the net. At present, it is extremely difficult to regulate the internet or hold individuals or companies responsible for unethical research practices. Copyright on the net is ambiguous, meaning not only that most information is free and transcends boundaries, but that individuals and companies are not accountable for the bad press of individuals, libellous remarks or improper research and ethical practices. Web service providers say that they are unable to regulate what goes on their notice boards or is discussed in forums.

This means that the internet, as well as having a great potential for freedom of information in research, may be abused for propaganda purposes or for slurring individuals. It has come to the attention of the terrestrial media that right-wing and extremist organisations use the internet for displaying their prejudiced opinions. False research saying that the holocaust never happened has been transmitted on the net for many years. Recently, the holocaust denial of historian David Irving was overturned in a test case that established the genocide that went on in concentration camps.

The main message to be taken from this for potential researchers is to be very prudent about the information you receive and transmit via the internet. Although research expertise and forms of health consultation are challenged by the web, it should be recognised that there are experts in computers and encryption. Hackers can enter accounts and unofficial web pages and false information can be quickly transferred to mirror sites once discovered.

The internet revolution is in a stage at the moment that is very much like the point at which the commercial printing of paper became affordable and popular some 200 years ago. The popularity of the printing press in the late eighteenth century allowed dissent to become widespread and is sometimes credited by historians for augmenting the French revolution.

At the present time, the internet offers a large amount of information and both positive and negative uses of the internet must be considered. The web is certainly a revolution in technological information sharing that may offer the possibility of future social and health revolutions. For example, the web has allowed consultation with 'open government', easy access to information for all those who can get to a computer terminal, and has started to potentially change relationships in health services such as is the recent case (June 2000) of the public consultation on changes in the NHS (www.nhs.uk/nationalplan).

Qualitative research

In qualitative research, analysis takes place alongside data collection. Data are collected, coded and analysed in order that the researcher can decide what future data should be collected, and from where and from whom they should be obtained. The process of coding and analysis continues in order to generate in-depth descriptions, interpretations and theoretical perspectives. Thus, in qualitative research, data analysis is part and parcel of the research process. Open-ended questionnaire comments can be treated in a similar way.

In qualitative analysis, themes, concepts and theoretical propositions are derived from the data as the study progresses in order to describe phenomena through narratives and accounts as a way of understanding, explaining and making inferences. This integrated research approach is the hallmark of the qualitative research process.

We have seen how Melia (1982), using grounded theory, approached the study of student nurse socialisation and involved herself in the research process and in data production. But how did she produce her findings? The following gives an example of how she derived categories from her data in order to explain the way in which student nurses constructed their world.

Analysis of the interviews yielded six conceptual categories, which Melia used as a framework for presenting substantive issues raised by the students in her study. The categories were as follows: 'learning and working', 'getting the work done', 'learning the rules', 'nursing in the dark', 'just passing through', 'doing nursing' and 'being professional'. From 'nursing in the dark', for example, she derived further categories, which she labelled 'coping with the dark', 'fobbing off the patient' and 'awareness contexts'. 'Awareness contexts' related to confusion about who knew what about patients' diagnoses and treatments, and was a concept first developed by Glaser & Strauss (1965) in a study of dying patients.

Melia illustrated her findings with interview data. She also illustrated the way in which qualitative researchers use concepts described in previous studies to interpret and confirm their findings. Rather than fitting in her data to the exact categories derived by Glaser & Strauss, Melia used their work to 'highlight the uncertainty which surrounds the whole business of student nurses talking with patients. The uncertainty both of their own knowledge and that of

the patient seemed to be the crux of the problem facing the students'.

As stated above, there are a number of computer software programmes, such as Ethnograph and Nudist, for analysing qualitative data as text, but the development of ideas and findings still depends on the hard work of the researcher.

The questions to assess Stage 6 of the research process are given in Box 12.7.

STAGE 7: PRESENTING THE RESEARCH FINDINGS

In our discussion of data analysis and interpretation (above), we saw some of the ways in which research findings and results can be presented: qualitative research is presented through words and narratives, quantitative research through numbers and statistical manipulations and perhaps also in tables and graphs.

Researchers may change their style of presentation according to their audience. Melia wrote up her research for two journals: the *Journal of Advanced Nursing* (Melia 1982) and *Nursing Times* (Melia 1983). To the non-researcher, the article in the first journal may appear 'jargonistic', using language that is difficult to understand. In the *Nursing Times* article, the language is much more

---

Box 12.7 Critical assessment of research: Stage 6

Questions to ask are:
- Does the researcher outline a plan for keeping data organised and retrievable from fieldwork observation and interviews?
- Does the researcher clearly explain how the data were prepared for analysis and how they were analysed?
- (In quantitative research) Are the reasons for choosing particular statistical tests given?
- (In quantitative research) Does the researcher include the statistical significance of the results?
- (In qualitative research) Do the findings contribute to theory building?
- Do the results/findings relate to the original research questions, and does the researcher show evidence of having drawn logical conclusions from the data?

Box 12.8 **Critical assessment of research: Stage 7**

Questions to ask are:
- Is the research clearly presented, both visually and verbally?
- Do the recommendations and applications to practice follow logically from the preceding sections of the report?

accessible and easier for the field-level nurse to understand.

The issue of whether the researcher should write in the first or third person is discussed by Webb (1992). The convention in quantitative research has been to maintain objectivity by writing in the third person. In this way, the researcher is seen to be authoritative. Qualitative, and particularly feminist, researchers have preferred to write in the first person. In this way they are able to write themselves into their research accounts and make their methods and findings more accessible to the reader.

Researchers have a responsibility to disseminate their findings and demonstrate their application to practice. Norton and colleagues' 1962 research on pressure area care (Norton et al 1975) is a case in point (see 'Historical perspectives', above).

Box 12.8 identifies questions for Stage 7.

ETHICAL ISSUES

Research must always be scrutinised for its ethical implications. In order to protect both subjects and researchers, health authorities are required to set up local ethics committees. Ethics committees are also found in NHS Trusts and universities. Professional bodies such as the Royal College of Physicians and the Royal College of Nursing produce guidelines to assist researchers to consider the ethical dimensions of their research proposals (RCN 1993). *Nursing Ethics* is an international journal which publishes widely on a range of topics and helps to raise the profile of debates around the ethics of both research and practice.

Unexpected ethical consequences can result from seemingly neutral theoretical science; for example, the application of theoretical physics to the development of the atom bomb did untold harm and formed no part of Einstein's original intentions. Similarly, Darwin's theory of evolution was used by many Victorian biologists to advance pejorative racial stereotypes. This was especially true in Australia during the nineteenth century, when social Darwinism, as it was known, put forward racist stereotypes of Aboriginal inferiority that tried to establish European cultural dominance.

Unlike obviously intrusive clinical trials and research practices such as giving placebos rather than treatment or testing drugs with unknown side-effects, qualitative research is often seen as exempt from the need to be scrutinised by an ethics committee. However, the ethical implications of covert research – i.e. research undertaken without the subjects' knowledge – are apparent when findings are reported without the subjects ever having known they were being observed.

Consider, too, the ethical implications of interviews about feelings and emotions, such as those conducted during Brown & Harris's study (1978) of the social origins of women's depression. Other more recent examples of considering the participant's view may be considered with respect to research on women involving cervical screening (Howson 1999) or young women's experiences of abortion (Harden & Ogden 1999). Such interviews need to be carefully managed so as not to distress the interviewee.

Ethics committees require researchers to prepare a written consent form, to be signed by the subjects, following a full explanation of events, before the research commences. This is known as informed consent. Any nurse is within their rights to ask to see the consent form before allowing researchers access to patients (see Ch. 3).

Research on people with mental health problems, those with a learning disability or children is problematic. This is because these groups are vulnerable to improper research practices. There is the issue of whether children, those with a learning disability and mental health service users can make informed decisions and give their full consent (or whether someone can consent on their behalf). This is particularly problematic if one considers the capacities of these groups to give informed and free consent as is required in law. Whether these groups have a full understanding of what you tell them and the implications of being in a research project is of paramount importance in ethical terms.

RESEARCH AS PART OF NURSING KNOWLEDGE AND PRACTICE

EDUCATION

Most students in institutes of higher education would take it for granted that the knowledge being imparted was research based. However, as we have seen, nursing is a relative newcomer to the world of research. What, then, is research likely to mean for student nurses? In class, teachers may refer to the latest research findings. They will also expect students to undertake a literature review on a given topic as part of written assignments, whether projects or essays. In clinical areas, students may find that trained staff apply research to practice or use it to evaluate care.

There is still some controversy on whether or not there is a discrete body of knowledge that constitutes nursing theory. Some educators and researchers prefer to see nursing as a multidisciplinary field, drawing on a variety of areas such as psychology, biology and sociology for its theoretical underpinning.

Recent policy initiatives in education (UKCC 1999a, 1999b; DoH 1999a) attempt to redefine nursing knowledge in terms of the 'new nursing'. According to Salvage (1990), the new nursing dates back to the 1970s and is linked to an interest in nursing theory associated with the growth of academic nursing, the women's movement challenging male (i.e. doctor) domination and the redefinition of the nurse's unique contribution to healing. Salvage summarises an important element of the new nursing ideology and practice as 'transforming relationships with patients – away

from the biomedical model which views medical intervention as the solution to health problems, towards a holistic approach promoting the patient's active participation in care'.

Others, particularly feminists, prefer to see knowledge redefined in nursing's and women's own terms.

PRACTICE

Research is learned by doing as well as by reading what researchers have chosen to record about their methods and results. Physics and psychology students learn research techniques in the laboratory. Nurses learn them in the wards as they observe, measure and question. Thus, as Bond said, 'measurement in nursing is not only the province of those whose orientation leans towards research' (cited in Tierney et al 1988).

As Hockey (1985) and Rempusheski (1987) show us, some of the best research ideas come from everyday practice. Nurses now have a body of knowledge to which they can refer, unlike Hockey, who could only speculate on the cause of pressure sores and the spread of infection.

The advent of the new nursing has been associated with a number of innovations, including primary nursing and the setting up of nursing development units (NDUs). Such units are ideally suited to the development of research and research-based practice. For example, one NDU known to one of the authors, during its 3-year history undertook a number of research-based initiatives, such as evaluating the quality of nursing following the introduction of primary nursing and a study of the effect on patients and staff when nurses came out of uniform (Bamford & Sparrow 1990, Bamford et al 1990). The reasons for the rise and fall of the unit are discussed elsewhere (Jones & Bamford 1998). More recently, a study was undertaken to identify the factors influencing the progress of NDUs in six different settings (Gerrish & Ferguson 2000). A combination of clinical leadership, organisational factors and external support were identified.

Rees (1992), citing Schön, suggests that research skills are closely associated with developing the skills of reflective practice and promoting new ways of seeing, thinking, doing and knowing required to develop nursing and patient care.

In mental health, Harper (1994) says that research helps professionals to realise that their ideas of mental health and illness shape processes of referral, assessment and intervention. Understanding the importance of research can be incorporated into training and aid professionals in daily practices. Harper says that his research helps in several ways:

- it aids the appreciation of sometimes conflicting demands made upon mental health professionals
- it portrays the various stances that may be taken in the mental health services and the different terms and languages that are available
- it shows the positions that professionals may be guided into and influence others towards
- and it shows the social and personal dimensions of working in the health services (Harper 1994).

Cowan's (1994) and Jodelet's (1991) studies on images of mental health and illness show that community attitudes are vital in research on the reception and setting up of local mental health projects. Negative images of physical and sexual abuse by mental health service users are raised by residents who obstruct the setting up and running of community mental health schemes. Such negative images require a positive response by nurses in order to allay public fears. The public needs to be consulted. Consultation may include evidence-based research that the nurse can draw upon and which shows the success of other local projects in the UK. Another path of consultation is meetings between the public and service users, so that both groups can articulate their points of view. Health professionals may act as intermediaries between the groups and make suggestions at consultation that are research and evidence-based (see Cowan 1994 and HMSO 1999).

Research is vital in elaborating the relationships that nurses have with patients and other groups of people. Research of these relationships may involve the contact of nursing groups with each other in different settings (the hospital, community, educational establishment, clinical contexts, etc). Alternatively, research on relationships

that nurses have with other professions which involves looking at divisions of labour may prove useful (Daykin & Clarke 2000). Research on nurses' relationships with patients and relatives may scrutinise the many roles that nurses have to play in the provision of care (Smith 1992, Allen 2000, Smith & Gray 2000). Studies of caring relationships between nurses and patients work as exemplary models for other nurses to build upon their practices with patients and therefore how nurses can improve care (Smith 1992, Smith & Gray 2000).

NURSING RESEARCH

Nursing research takes place at a number of different levels. There are those nurses who have studied for higher degrees such as masters and doctoral degrees. Many of the resulting dissertations and theses can be found in the Steinberg Collection of the Royal College of Nursing library in London. This collection bears witness to the vast range of nursing topics that have been researched over the years. In addition, many nurses have undertaken research-based projects as part of their pre- and post-registration nursing courses. Other nurses have decided that they would like to undertake a research project as part of their job. One of the authors of this chapter knew a clinical nurse specialist who cared for children with long-term tracheotomies. She felt that these families' needs were so special that she wanted to find out more in order to evaluate and perhaps improve the children's care. She did this by interviewing the children's mothers. Her findings helped her to prepare discharge guidelines for the children, which included the allocation of a primary nurse to promote continuity of care, planned home visits prior to discharge, improved community liaison and the preparation of as many people associated with the child as possible to undertake tracheotomy care, rather than relying solely on the mother (Jennings 1989). This study is a good example of applied research undertaken to evaluate and improve practice.

Many nurses still acquire their research experience through working as data collectors with doctors. It is not unusual for them to feel frustrated if they find that nursing and medical values come into conflict. One research nurse, an experienced ward sister, was involved in a two-centre study to investigate palliative treatments of oesophageal cancer. She found herself unable 'objectively' to fill in quality of life scales with the patients. As the patients came back for repeat treatments and clinic attendances, the research nurse got to know them, and a rapport was established. Some patients visibly brightened when they saw her, and she was aware that this, in turn, improved their quality of life scores. In other words, her presence biased the scores of some patients for the better. The doctors found great difficulty in accepting her 'subjective' observations (Grigg & Smith 1989). However, medical research can often be an important starting point for a career as a nurse researcher. Students should watch for medical research being undertaken on their ward; it could be that the person collecting the data is a nurse.

Being research minded

The content of this chapter has been designed to make nursing students 'research minded', so that they are confident to ask questions and seek information about the clinical and educational world about them. Choosing a user-friendly textbook is a good starting point and now, with access to the internet, the range of materials and speed with which they can be accessed has greatly increased. Whether we read research reports in text form or on screen we must be able to evaluate them critically as part of research mindedness, since we need to be confident that we can apply research findings to practice.

Local university faculties of health and nursing or NHS Trusts may employ nurse researchers and run research interest groups or journal clubs as part of a research network. The library is always a good place to begin networking. Since nurse education has been sited in universities, research mindedness has taken on a new meaning. The Research Assessment Exercise (RAE) which began over a decade ago has meant that nurse educators need to be involved in undertaking research as well as ensuring that their teaching is research based. Their performance is measured in the number of funded research projects undertaken within the institution and the publication of papers in academic journals. This means juggling the competing demands of teaching, supervising students in the field with research associated activities (Traynor & Rafferty 1999). Nursing research has certainly progressed from the days when Hockey, as an inquiring probationer nurse, was told to 'watch and pray'. After nearly 50 years, there are a few more answers to our questions but many more remain.

CONCLUSION

Until the 1960s, research played only a minor role in the development of nursing practice, education, management and leadership. In the new century, however, it is realised that high-quality care cannot be achieved without challenging previously held beliefs and practices, and formulating innovative approaches to nursing, teaching and managing. Consequently research now enjoys a higher profile in nursing and is applied as an evidence base to nursing education and practice.

There are many approaches and methods of research. This chapter has outlined some of them and clarified the stages of the research process, with examples from literature and branches of nursing. Principles to ensure the valid collection, analysis and interpretation of data have been highlighted.

Having worked through the chapter, students will be able to contribute to and criticise research studies, incorporating the results into their own practice. The ultimate goal of the research minded practitioner is to apply research evidence that improves the quality of patient care.

ACKNOWLEDGEMENTS

To students, friends and colleagues – past and present – who have responded to and challenged our research assumptions and teaching methods over the years.

REFERENCES

Allen D 2000 Negotiating the role of expert carers on an adult hospital ward. Sociology of Health and Illness (22)2:149–171

Bamford O, Sparrow S 1990 Nursing development units: a virtue in uniformity? Nursing Times 86(41):46–48

Bamford O, Dinean L, Pritchard B, Smith P 1990 Change for the better. Nursing Times 86(23):28–33

Bell J 1999 Doing your research project: a guide for first time researchers in education and social science, 2nd edn. Open University Press, Buckingham

Benner P 1984 From novice to expert: excellence and power in clinical nursing practice. Addison Wesley, Menlo Park, CA

Bingold S 1995 Befriending the family: an exploration of the nurse–client relationship. Health and Social Care in the Community 3:173–180

Brown G, Harris T 1978 The social origins of depression in women. Tavistock, London

Chalmers A F 1982 What is this thing called science?, 2nd edn. Open University Press, Milton Keynes

Cicourel A 1964 Fixed choice questionnaires: method and measurement in sociology. Free Press, New York

Collins H M 1984 Researching spoonbending: concepts and practice of participatory fieldwork. In: Bell C, Roberts H (eds) Social researching: politics, problems, practice. Routledge and Kegan Paul, London, pp 54–69

Cormack D F S (ed) 1984 The research process in nursing. Blackwell Scientific, Oxford

Cormack D F S (ed) 1991 The research process in nursing, 2nd edn. Blackwell Scientific, Oxford

Corner J 1991 In search of more complete answers to research questions. Quantitative versus qualitative research methods: is there a way forward? Journal of Advanced Nursing 16(3):718–727

Cowan S 1994 Community attitudes towards people with mental health problems. Journal of Psychiatric and Mental Health Nursing (1):15–22

Cullum N 1994 Leg ulcer treatments: a critical review, parts 1 and 2. Nursing Standard 9(1):29–33; 9(2):32–36

Daykin N, Clarke B 2000 'They'll get the bodily care'. Discourses of care and relationships between nurses and health care assistants in the NHS. Sociology of Health and Illness 22(3):349–363

Department of Health 1993 Report of the taskforce on the strategy in nursing, midwifery and health visiting. HMSO, London

Department of Health 1998 A first class service: quality in the new NHS. HMSO, London

Department of Health 1999a Making a difference. HMSO, London

Department of Health 1999b Clinical governance: quality in the new NHS. HMSO, London

Department of Health and Social Security 1972 Report of the Committee on Nursing (the Briggs Report). HMSO, London

Donabedian A 1966 Evaluating the quality of medical care. Millbank Memorial Fund Quarterly 44:166–206

Drummond N 2000 Quality of life with asthma: the existential and aesthetic. Sociology of Health and Illness 22(2):235–253

Ellis C, Bochner A 1999 Bringing emotion and personal narrative into medical social science. Health: An Interdisciplinary Journal 3(2):229–237

Fretwell J 1985 Freedom to change. RCN, London

Garfinkel H 1967 Studies in ethnomethodology. Prentice Hall, New Jersey

Gerrish K, Ferguson A 2000 Nursing development units: factors influencing their progress. British Journal of Nursing 9(10):626–630

Glaser B G, Strauss A L 1965 Awareness of dying. Aldine, Chicago

Glaser B G, Strauss A L 1967 The discovery of grounded theory. Weidenfeld and Nicolson, London

Grigg D, Smith P 1989 Emotional labour, nursing worth and the research process: measuring the quality of life. Paper presented at Royal College of Nursing Research Society Conference, Swansea University, 14–16 April

Haase J E, Myers S T 1988 Reconciling paradigm assumptions of qualitative and quantitative research. Western Journal of Nursing Research 10(2):128–137

Hall J M, Stevens P E 1991 Rigor in feminist research. Advances in Nursing Science 13(3):16–29

Harden A, Ogden J 1999 Young women's experiences of arranging and having abortions. Sociology of Health and Illness 21(4):426–444

Hardey M 1999 Doctor in the house: the internet as a source of lay health knowledge and the challenge to expertise. Sociology of Health and Illness 21(6):820–835

Harper D 1994 The professional construction of 'paranoia' and the discursive use of diagnostic criteria. British Journal of Medical Psychology 67:131–143

Hawthorne P 1974 Nurse, I want my mummy! RCN, London

HMSO 1999 Reform of the Mental Health Act 1983. Proposals for consultation. HMSO: London (http://www.official-documents.co.uk/document/cm44/4480/4480.htm)

Hockey L 1985 Nursing research: mistakes and misconceptions. Churchill Livingstone, Edinburgh

Howson A 1999 Cervical screening, compliance and moral obligation. Sociology of Health and Illness 21(4):401–425

Inman U 1975 Towards a theory of nursing care. RCN, London

James N 1984 A postscript to nursing. In: Bell C, Roberts H (eds) Social researching: politics, problems, practice. Routledge and Kegan Paul, London, p 137

James N 1989 Emotional labour: skill and work in the social regulation of feelings. Sociological Review 37(1):15–42

James N 1993 Divisions of emotional labour: disclosure and cancer. In: Fineman S Emotion in organizations. Sage, London

Jennings P 1989 Tracheostomy care: learning to cope at home. Paediatric Nursing 7(1):13–15

Jodelet D 1991 Madness and social representations. Harvester, London

Jolley J 1991 Using statistics. Computing in Practice: Information Management and Technology Series. Nursing Times 87(25):57–59

Jones A, Bamford O 1998 Nursing development units: perspectives and prospects for research and practice. In: Smith P (ed) Nursing research: setting new agendas. Hodder Headline, London, ch 9

Kelly D, Ross S, Smith P, Gray B 2000 Death, dying and emotional labour: problematic dimensions of the bone marrow transplant nursing role? Journal of Advanced Nursing 32(4): 952–960

Lelean S R 1975 Ready for report, nurse? RCN, London

Macaulay A, Commanda L, Freeman W, Gibson N, McCabe M, Robbins C, Twohig P 1999 Participatory research maximises community and lay involvement. British Medical Journal 319:774–778

McFarlane J K 1970 The proper study of the nurse. RCN, London

McFarlane J K 1977 Developing a theory of nursing: the relation of theory to practice, education and research. Journal of Advanced Nursing 2:261–270

McFarlane J K 1980 Nursing as a research-based profession. Nursing Times Occasional Paper 76(13):57–60

McHaffie H E 1991 Neonatal intensive care units: visiting policies for grandparents. Midwifery 7(3):122–123; 7(4):193–203

Marks-Maran D 1992 Rethinking the nursing process. In: Jolley M, Brykczynska G (eds) Nursing care: the challenge to change. Edward Arnold, London, pp 92–95

Melia K 1982 'Tell it as it is': qualitative methodology and nursing research: understanding the student nurse's world. Journal of Advanced Nursing 7:327–335

Melia K 1983 Students' view of nursing: discussion of method. Nursing Times 79(20):24–25

Morse J M, Field P A 1996 Nursing research: the application of qualitative approaches, 2nd edn. Chapman and Hall, London

Moser C A, Kalton G 1985 Survey methods in social investigations, 2nd edn. Gower, Aldershot

Nightingale F 1990 (first published 1859) Notes on nursing. Churchill Livingstone, Edinburgh

Norton D, McLaren R, Exton-Smith A N 1975 (first published 1962) Investigation of geriatric nursing problems in hospitals. Churchill Livingstone, Edinburgh

Oakley A 1974 The sociology of housework. Martin Robertson, London

Oakley A 1981 Interviewing women: a contradiction in terms. In: Roberts H (ed) Doing feminist research. Routledge and Kegan Paul, London, p 581

Oakley A 1984 What price professionalism? The importance of being a nurse. Nursing Times 80(50):24–27

Oakley A 1989 Who's afraid of the RCT? Some dilemmas of the sample method and 'good research practice'. Women and Health 15(4):25–59

Ogier M 1982 An ideal sister. RCN, London

Ogier M 1989 Reading research. Scutari Press, London

Open University (Course Team DE304) 1979 Block 1. Variety in social science research. Introduction to the course and block 1. In: Research methods in education and the social sciences. Open University Press, Milton Keynes, p 3

Oppenheim A N 1992 Questionnaire design and attitude measurement. Heinemann, London

Parse R R 1989 Essentials for practising the art of nursing. Nursing Science Quarterly 2(3):111

Pembrey S E M 1980 The ward sister: key to nursing. RCN, London

Rees C 1992 Practising research based teaching. Nursing Times 88(2):55–57

Rempusheski V 1987 Making lemonade out of lemons. Alpha Chi News 10(2):3

Roberts H (ed) 1981 Doing feminist research. Routledge and Kegan Paul, London

Rosenberg M 1968 The logic of survey analysis. Basic Books, New York

Royal College of Nursing 1982 Promoting research mindedness. RCN, London

Royal College of Nursing 1993 Ethics related to research in nursing. RCN, London

Salvage J 1985 The politics of nursing. Heinemann, London

Salvage J 1990 The theory and practice of the 'new nursing'. Nursing Times Occasional Paper 86(4):42–45

Sapsford R, Abbott P 1998 Research methods for nurses and the caring professions. Open University Press, Milton Keynes

Schutz A 1972 The phenomenology of the social world. Martinus Nijhoff, The Hague

Shilts R 1987 And the band played on: people, politics and the AIDS epidemic. Viking, New York

Silverman D 1981 The child as social object: Down's syndrome children in a paediatric cardiology clinic. Sociology of Health and Illness 3(3):254–274

Smith P 1987 The relationship between quality of nursing care and the ward as a learning environment: developing a methodology. Journal of Advanced Nursing 12:413–420

Smith P 1992 The emotional labour of nursing: how nurses care. Methodological Appendix. Macmillan, Basingstoke

Smith P, Gray B 2000 The emotional labour of nursing: how student and qualified nurses learn to care. A report on nurse education, nursing practice and emotional labour in the contemporary NHS. South Bank University, London http://www.health-fc.sbu.ac.uk/emlab

Smith P, Mackintosh M, Towers B 1993 Implications of the new NHS contracting system for the district nursing service in one health authority: a pilot study. Journal of Interprofessional Care 7(2):115–124

Spencer J 1983 Research with a human touch. Nursing Times 79(12):24–27

Stanley L, Wise S 1983 Breaking out: feminist consciousness and feminist research. Routledge and Kegan Paul, London

Strauss A, Corbin J 1994 Grounded theory methodology: an overview. In: Denzin N K, Lincoln Y S (eds) Handbook of qualitative research. Sage, Thousand Oaks, California, pp 273–285

Street A F 1992 Inside nursing: a critical ethnography of clinical nursing practice. SUNY, New York

Thorne S E 1991 Methodological orthodoxy in qualitative nursing research: analysis of the issues. Qualitative Health Research 1(2):178–199

Tierney A, Closs J, Atkinson I et al 1988 On measurement and nursing research. Nursing Times Occasional Paper 84(12):55–58

Titchen A 1998 A conceptual framework for facilitating learning in clinical practice. Occasional Paper No 2. Centre for Professional and Education Advancement, Australia

Traynor M, Rafferty A M 1999 Nursing and the Research Assessment Exercise: past, present and future. Journal of Advanced Nursing Education 30(1):186–192

Truman A 1992 Information systems in modern nursing. In: Jolley M, Brykczynska G (eds) Nursing care: the challenge to change. Edward Arnold, London, p 140

UKCC 1999a Fitness for practice. UKCC, London

UKCC 1999b Nursing competencies (ncomp). UKCC, London

UKCC 2000 Requirements for pre-registration nursing programme. UKCC, London

Wandelt M A, Ager J 1974 Quality patient care scale. Appleton Century Crofts, Norwalk, Connecticut

Watson J 1985 Nursing: the philosophy and science of caring. Little, Brown, Boston

Watson J D 1980 The double helix: a personal account of the discovery of the structure of DNA. Atheneum, New York

Webb C 1984 Feminist methodology in nursing research. Journal of Advanced Nursing 9:249–250

Webb C 1992 The use of the first person in academic writing: objectivity, language and gatekeeping. Journal of Advanced Nursing 17:747–752

Webb C 1993 Feminist research: definitions, methodology, methods and evaluation. Journal of Advanced Nursing 18:416–423

Webb C, Wilson-Barnett J 1983 Hysterectomy: dispelling the myths: 1 and 2. Nursing Times Occasional Paper 79(30):52–54; 79(31):44–46

http://www.nhs.uk/nationalplan (June 2000)

FURTHER READING

The following title has been selected for its classic status from one of the pioneers of nursing research. It refers to issues which are not often discussed in the public domain.

Hockey L 1985 Nursing research: mistakes and misconceptions. Churchill Livingstone, Edinburgh

The following titles have been selected because they pay particular attention to some of the issues associated with reviewing and undertaking qualitative research:

Popay J, Rogers A, Williams G 1998 Rationale and standards from the systematic review of qualitative literature in health services research. Qualitative Health Research, 8(3):341–351

Silverman D 1985 Qualitative methodology and sociology: describing the social world. Gower, Aldershot

Silverman D 1993 Interpreting qualitative data: methods for analysing talk, text and interaction. Sage, London

Silverman D (ed) 1997 Qualitative research: theory, method and practice. Sage, London

The following titles were edited by one of the authors and have been selected for their complementary approaches to nursing and health care research:

Smith P (ed) 1997 Research mindedness for practice. Churchill Livingstone, Edinburgh

Smith P (ed) 1998 Nursing research: setting new agendas. Arnold, London.

INTERNET

Some useful places to start searching are shown below. It should be noted that web-sites are subject to change and therefore some amount of searching is necessary. Sometimes pages will expire or be moved to other internet addresses (or, if illegal, web pages may jump to mirror sites). Search engines are usually good for identification and location of relevant web-sites on research.

Cochrane database

http://www.update-software.com/ccweb/cochrane/revabstr/ccabout.htm

Department of Health

http://www.doh.gov.uk/dhhome.htm

Harcourt International, Journals

http://www.harcourt-international.com/journals/default.cfm

Links Page

http://www.sciencekomm.at/journals/medicine/nurse.html

Nursing Standard

http://www.nursing-standard.co.uk

Royal College of Nursing

http://www.rcn.org.uk/

British Medical Journal

http://www.bmj.com

Journal of Advanced Nursing

http://www.blackwell-synergy.com/ issuelist.asp?journal=jan

Nursing Times

http://www.nursingtimes.net/

Sociology of Health and Illness

http://www.blackwellpublishers.co.uk/journals/SHIL/

York Centre for Systematic Reviews and Dissemination

http://www.york.ac.uk/inst/crd

UKCC

http://www.ukcc.org.uk/

13 Nursing theory and nursing care

Pat A. Downer

CHAPTER CONTENTS

Introduction 365

How and where does care take place? 366

Concepts, theories, models and care pathways 367
    Concepts 368
    Theories 368
    Models and the nursing process 369
        Assessing 370
        Diagnosing 371
        Planning 371
        Implementing 371
        Evaluating 372
    Biomedical model of care 372
    Roper, Logan and Tierney 372
    Roy's Adaptation model of nursing 374
    Orem's Self-care model 375
    Casey's model 380
    Integrated care pathways 381
        Definitions of an integrated care pathway 382

Record keeping 384
    Types of records kept 384
    Guidelines for good record keeping 386

Conclusion 388

References 389

Further reading 390

Essential reading 390

This chapter will enable you to explore the theories behind the practice that you will see in a variety of settings throughout your foundation studies and your nurse training. It will explore some of the issues of nursing that underpin the outcomes that are to be achieved for entry to the branch programmes. It will also form the basis of the competencies under care delivery for entry to the register (UKCC 2000a). To achieve this, the chapter will:

- examine concepts, theories and models of nursing
- explore nursing theory
- discuss the process of nursing
- consider how individuals may be cared for in a variety of settings
- examine the requirements for patient record keeping
- give opportunities for activities and reflections in a learning diary and/or profile.

INTRODUCTION

As a student nurse you will have the opportunity of caring for people with very different needs in a variety of locations and so it is important that you have an understanding of some of the evidence that underpins the practice that you will participate in. Nursing is constantly changing and our patients are now more informed about their condition and are encouraged to take an active part in their own care. To help achieve this empowerment for your patients you must be able to adapt the theories to your patients' needs and truly achieve individualised care. This chapter will give you some frameworks to consider when delivering nursing care.

HOW AND WHERE DOES CARE TAKE PLACE?

First, consider where and with whom you might be delivering nursing care to enable you to set the scene for understanding the theories and practice of nursing. Imagine a young boy having a road traffic accident and breaking a leg. The following paragraph will plot the journey of this child during his care.

The first contact with health care for the child will be a first-aider at the scene of the accident. On the arrival of an ambulance, the first-aider will hand over the care of the child to the ambulance crew who will be able to assess the injury to the child and start treatment which could be in the form of immobilising the leg and relieving the pain. The crew is trained to intubate and commence intravenous infusions if necessary. A record of the accident will be made and biographical details will be noted. On arrival at the accident and emergency department, nurses, doctors, radiographers and possibly a health care assistant will care for the child. The child will then discover how doctors specialise in different aspects of medicine, and will be introduced to the anaesthetist and the operating department nurses while in theatre. On arrival on the ward a new set of nurses will meet and care for the needs of the child and the team might also include a play leader and a physiotherapist. At every hand-over of the child's care the documentation will be passed on and a plan of care will emerge. From this the various locations and the diversity of the teams in which care is given to this child can be appreciated. The student nurse will need to adapt to these clinical placements and have an understanding of the way in which care is delivered in each area. This chapter will help the student to understand the different ways in which care is delivered.

From the scenarios in Activity 13.1 you can appreciate the move to treating patients in the community rather than in hospital. This is in line with the recommendations of the 1989 Community Care: an Agenda for Action, Act. The nurse can also be seen as playing a central role in coordinating care for each patient.

Having an appreciation of where care is delivered, and by whom, we must reach an understanding of the words 'concepts', 'theories' and 'models', as these areas are the building blocks on which nursing is developed. However, the term 'nursing' is itself a difficult word to define. The difference in the care given to a young motorcyclist attending an accident and emergency

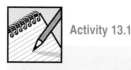

Activity 13.1

Consider three other patients and try to identify where they might receive their care and by whom it might be given:
Patient 1: a 77-year-old lady who develops a chronic chest infection
Patient 2: a 34-year-old man with severe learning disabilities
Patient 3: a 53-year-old man with acute depression.

Scenarios
Patient 1. This lady would have initially been seen by her general practitioner at the GP surgery. The practice nurse and health visitor for the elderly might also have seen her, and the district nurse too if care was needed in her home. This condition is usually treated at home. The patient would also have seen the local pharmacist to obtain her medication. If the condition had worsened, then her GP would have referred her to the local district hospital where she would have been admitted and cared for by another team.

Patient 2. This patient may live in a small home with other people with learning disabilities and would be cared for by the team managing this home. The team could include a registered nurse (learning disabilities), a care assistant and a social worker. The patient may attend a day centre run by social services. He would be registered with a local GP and entitled to the same care as all other people living in the community.

Patient 3. This patient may have had his problem first identified at work and so the occupational health nurse may have been involved. The patient's GP and a community psychiatric nurse (CPN) would have cared for him and together they might have arranged for him to attend a day hospital for further care.

department following a road traffic accident and the care given to a middle-aged woman with a severe learning disability living in a community home is enormous, and yet both types of care are described as nursing. Thus, nursing is not just about practice it is about how we utilise the knowledge and skills in the delivery of care. It is also about working with others in uni- or multi-disciplinary teams wherever the care is needed, as no one person can be totally responsible for the care of a patient.

Historically, nursing generally took place in hospital wards, but more recently government initiatives have encouraged people to remain in their homes for their care. This is indeed to be encouraged, particularly with children, for whom hospitalisation should only be considered if care cannot be provided at home. There has also been a move to close the large institutions for people with mental illness and now care may be delivered in the more appropriate setting of a group home or the patient's own home, with the opportunity to attend a day hospital for specialised care (DoH 1989a).

'Nursing' now needs to be explored a little further (Activity 13.2). Your reflections for Activity 13.2 will probably focus on groups of activities, for example:

- 'Doing' activities, e.g. measuring blood pressures, talking with patients, undertaking personal hygiene and administering medicines. These are known as psychomotor activities.
- Knowledge (the nurse understanding why the activity is undertaken). The reasons behind measuring a blood pressure or giving a particular medicine. These are known as cognitive activities.

Activity 13.2

While in practice, observe a nurse undertaking nursing care, reflect on this in your diary or profile and then repeat the exercise while in the four branch settings. Compare all reflections and then try to define nursing.

Activity 13.3

Visit the web-site for the UKCC (www.ukcc.org.uk) and read the Code of Practice.

- The way in which these activities are undertaken, e.g. the encouragement given to a patient to self-administer medication or empathy to a family when caring for a terminally ill relative. These are known as 'affective activities'.

The debate on whether nursing is a science or an art has continued since the times of Florence Nightingale and will go on as nursing continues to change. What is important, however, is that student nurses are aware of what they are doing and why they are doing it, and that they are working within the Code of Professional Conduct as set down by the United Kingdom Central Council for Nursing, Midwifery and Health Visiting (UKCC 1992) (see Ch. 1 and Activity 13.3). The purpose of the Council is to protect the public through professional standards and the delivery of care must adhere to these standards.

CONCEPTS, THEORIES, MODELS AND CARE PATHWAYS

In this section of the chapter we will explore the important developments that have occurred in nursing, specifically concentrating on various models of nursing and the subsequent development of care pathways. It will start with discussing concepts and theories and proceed to examine the nursing process. It then looks in detail at the models suggested by Roper, Logan & Tierney (1996), Roy (1976), Orem (1985) and Casey (1988). These are four of the most widely-used models of nursing currently employed in practice. The section will conclude with a discussion on care pathways and their application for patient care.

Concepts

'Concept' is a word that describes objects, feelings and ideas. Nursing is made up of many concepts and some were explored in Activity 13.2.

The themes you find in Activity 13.4 are your concepts about nursing and should be common to those with whom the nurse is working. Concepts are our beliefs and help us make sense of what is happening around us. These concepts are sometimes expressed as a philosophy of care and while in practice the student nurse should ask if the placement has a philosophy and where it is displayed for staff and patients to see. The four themes identified in Activity 13.4 are the basis on which models of nursing are often explained.

As a student nurse you might not have had experience of working with mentally ill or terminally ill patients before commencing your training. However, when you have this opportunity you will be able to make sense of what is happening. When you recognise common objects such as armchairs and televisions, beds and lockers, you know whether you are working in someone's home or in a hospital ward. From your reflections you may also notice that concepts apply not only to physical items but also to areas such as pain, empathy and mental health. These concepts help us to understand what is happening to the patients and thus help to improve our communication, both with our patients and with our colleagues. Good communication is the key to effective care, especially when patients themselves have problems with communication, for example a person with a severe learning disability or an unconscious patient.

We must also remember that our patients have concepts and these need exploring to ensure

Activity 13.4

Return to Activity 13.2 and now consider if you can find, in your reflections, any common themes relating to beliefs about:

- people
- society
- health
- nursing.

good communication and understanding. Consider the differences between the postoperative care we give now and that given some 30 years ago. Nowadays patients are encouraged to be mobile as soon as possible. However, if the last experience the patient had of surgery was 30 years ago, he will be expecting to stay in bed for several days postoperatively. The patient's concept of care will need revisiting and explained otherwise he will be unhappy with the care he receives when he is asked to be mobile within hours of his surgery. The patient might also be expecting to stay in hospital a lot longer than is considered necessary today.

You can see that concepts form the basis to all our theories. Fawcett (1989) suggests that models are constructed from concepts and subsequently theories may be formed from models, but that a conceptual framework is not a theory. However, Meleis (1997) takes a wider view of theory and suggests that they do include conceptual frameworks.

Theories

Florence Nightingale in 1859 produced *Notes on Nursing: What it is, and What it is Not* (Nightingale 1946). That title aptly describes the study of nursing theory in the 21st century, as it exactly describes what nursing is. It tells us what and why care should be given and thus excludes what should not be done. However, theory has developed over time and now there is a strong initiative to ensure that all practice is evidence based. Nurses must question the reason for doing rather than accepting that 'it' has always been done in a certain way.

Consider the changes in wound care. Historically, wounds were cleaned at each dressing change using a cleansing solution applied with cotton wool. Cotton wool is no longer used as it has been proved that the fibres stick to the wound surface and that cleansing in this way can remove the newly granulating tissue. Here we can consider two theories relating to the same area of practice. The first theory contains concepts of 'cleansing' to 'promote wound healing' whereas the second theory considers the same concept of 'wound healing' and yet dismisses the concept of 'cleansing using cotton wool'. Theories are the joining together of concepts. However, the most important thing to consider about a theory is 'Can it be tested?'.

There are two types of theories (Pearson & Vaughan 1994):

- deductive
- inductive.

Deductive theory is when someone comes up with a theory and suggests that it might be applicable to nursing practice. Consider the use of play and education in school. We now know that children learn by doing and by being involved and so this theory could be applied to nursing practice by involving children in their own care and thus enabling them to learn about their condition.

Inductive theory, however, comes out of practice. A community nurse may recognise that when a group of patients suffering from venous ulcers attend the surgery for their care (as opposed to the district nurse attending them at home), they have a better response rate. The theory that this could be due to group support could be tested and lead to a variation in the delivery of care. The theory would have come out of practice and would therefore be inductive.

Models of care, which come from practice, are inductive.

MODELS AND THE NURSING PROCESS

Models are used regularly throughout everyday life and give us the information we require about a subject in a representative way (Activity 13.5).

For Activity 13.5 you may have considered maps, plans and models. All of these may have been useful in getting you to the right place and the right room in a complex building. They have had no real relationship to the actual size of the area you were negotiating and yet they have been

a useful guide for you. In the same way, you may have looked at a model of a hip joint – you know that this particular model could not work in the body and yet it was representative of that joint. You can see that such models are useful as a guide or framework for our lives. This type of model is known as a physical model. Similarly, in nursing, models are very useful to help us with the delivery of care. Nursing models, however, are not physical models but conceptual models and are made up of concepts and theories. These models were produced to help guide nurses in their patient care and to achieve uniformity of care within a practice setting.

As nursing changes rapidly, debates continue on the usefulness of models in nursing practice. Reed (1995) suggests that nursing has developed beyond frameworks. Tierney (1998) self-examines the question 'Nursing models: extant or extinct?' in relation to the model she helped develop in 1980 (Roper et al 1980) and concludes that there is still a place for them. Theorists will continue to debate their usefulness but in practice models are still a useful tool to aid nursing practice. Many areas you will work on will have taken the essence of a model and then adapted it for their particular area and this is to be encouraged. The student nurse's responsibility on each placement will be to identify whether a model is being used, if so, to determine which one, and then to learn about the model to enable the nurse to deliver care in the same way as the team she is working with.

It is important at this stage of your training to realise why frameworks are required for patient or client care.

Imagine that you are about to set off on a journey and all you are told is that you will be taken from A to B. How you get there is a mystery – you are not in control of the situation nor are you given any choice. If, however, you are told that you can:

- use the motorway and get there quickly, or
- go the scenic route and stop off to visit a place of interest, or
- travel on a direct, non-motorway route which will only take a little longer than the first

Activity 13.5

What models have you used in daily life in the last week?

option but will give you time to see the countryside

you can now make a choice. This knowledge should empower you about the decision and take away some, if not all, the uncertainty of the journey. Of course there might be unexpected occurrences, for example traffic queues along the way, but these can be dealt with at the time.

Now compare the above scenario with being admitted to hospital. Imagine you are told by your general practitioner that you are to go to hospital for surgery as you are complaining of a pain in your left side. On arrival you are put into a bed and told that you will only be in for a few days, but told nothing else. Immediately the situation is out of your control – you do not know what is expected of you and you probably become very anxious. If, however, the nurse were to describe your care and what you were expected to achieve during these few days you would be better informed and able then to cope with all eventualities, for example an infection, or going home earlier than expected.

Thus frameworks of care can help nurses in planning care with patients or clients to ensure that they understand what is happening and what is expected of them. It will also help inform any carers about the situation. This type of delivery could also be audited to see if the care was delivered in a satisfactory way.

Before exploring various different nursing models, let us consider how models are used in nursing, as it is important to remember that they cannot be used in isolation. They are commonly used in what is described as the nursing process. This process is an adaptation of a problem-solving circle and applied to nursing, hence it could be described as a deductive theory (Fig. 13.1).

This is a circular process that can be left as each problem is solved. Let us consider the stages of the process before applying them to a case example.

Assessing

This will enable the nurse to undertake a holistic assessment of the patient considering all of the

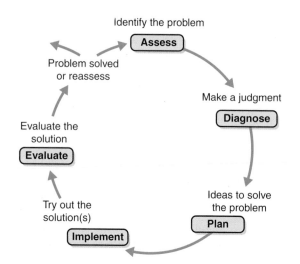

Figure 13.1 A problem-solving circle compared to the nursing process.

patient's individual needs in order to identify his problems. It is at this stage that a model of assessment can be used. Needs or problems might be expressed as 'actual' or 'potential'. With experience and knowledge you will become more expert in identifying potential problems – these are the problems that are not apparent at present but that, if preventative steps are not taken, may become problems in the future. A good example of this is a person who is normally mobile and then becomes immobile, for example following an accident. The patient may then be at risk of developing pressure sores as he is unable to shift his weight. In recognising this, the nurse could ensure that a suitable pressure relieving mattress was put on the patient's bed and thus prevent a sore (see Case example 13.1).

A model will be based on certain beliefs and so the actions taken to implement the care will be based on these beliefs and hence it is important to select the correct model. For example, you might wish to use a model that encourages the person to be self-caring, in which case you might choose Orem (1985) or a model based on activities of living (Roper et al 1980). It is, however, important to remember that a nurse cannot work in isolation and so you will find that the setting in which you are working will have an agreed model of care.

This will ensure that the care is effective as every team member is delivering care based on common beliefs. Some areas will have adapted some of the elements of a model and then produced their own specific model to meet the needs of their patients (Activity 13.6). Other areas have moved away from care plans derived from a model of care and have introduced care pathways. These are plans of care for groups of patients all with the same condition and then individualised for the specific patient or client (these will be discussed later in the chapter).

Diagnosing

Some practitioners, to clarify the patient's problems before moving on to the planning stage, add this stage into a model. There continues to be debate within the nursing profession around the issue of nurses making diagnoses; however, without a decision being made it would be impossible for the nurse to proceed with constructing a plan of action. It is to be remembered that this is a nursing diagnosis and not a medical one and so enables the nurse to prescribe care for the patient.

Planning

This is the stage of the process that the nurse, in conjunction with the patient and, if appropriate, the carers, sets achievable goals and plans how they can best be achieved. The goals may be short term, for example nothing by mouth prior to surgery, or long term, for example prepare and cook own food for a client with a learning disability. It is vital that the patient's individual needs are

recognised at this point because if you are aiming for concordance with your patient, he must be involved in the negotiations. Patients should be encouraged to participate in setting their own goals as everyone views their condition differently: a newly diagnosed diabetic, for example, might want to take immediate control of his care, whereas others might need a little time to take on this new role. It is also important that the goals set are achievable for the patient and so avoid disappointment if a goal is not achieved. Discussion with the patient at this stage is essential.

Having agreed the goals with the patient you can move on to the next stage – how the goals will be achieved.

Implementing

This is the stage of the process when clear direction is given about what is to be done, when it is to be done, and by whom. The clarity in this part of the plan aids communication between all concerned with the care. It will also give the client or patient a clear picture of the course of the care and may encourage them to participate in the plan.

Written plans need to be explicit and written in such a way that the patient can understand them. Plans are for carers and patients and they are entitled to read them (discussed later in the chapter, under Record keeping). The plan must give very clear instructions as to who is to do what and when. Here are a few examples:

- 'The mother will feed the baby, using prepared bottles of milk, every 3 hours.'
- 'The client will get up each morning at 7.30 a.m., wash and dress himself before breakfast at 8.30 a.m.'
- 'The health care assistant will help with personal hygiene needs until the patient is able to do it unaided.'
- 'The nurse will prepare the patient for theatre using the preoperative check list.'

Some clinical areas will have printed plans of care that are common within that area, for example preoperative check lists and discharge forms.

Evaluating

This is the most important step of the process as it informs both the carer and the patient whether goals have been achieved or are being achieved. It is the signpost for future action, either to note success or to reassess the situation and plan new goals. It is thus important to set achievable goals so that the patient/client will be encouraged rather than discouraged. It is possible to set short positive goals to note progress rather than regression, for example a terminally ill patient in pain may have a goal of being pain free for 1 hour whereas a patient with chronic arthritis may have a goal of being pain free for 6 hours. Measurable goals are beneficial in enabling evaluation to be performed.

At this stage of the process some problems will be solved but other problems may be noted, and so the cycle must start again with assessment.

For the process to commence, a model of assessment is utilised. The following section of the chapter will explore the common models in practice.

BIOMEDICAL MODEL OF CARE

This is probably the first documented model of practice and, although one that is rarely used in nursing today, some medical schools still use the concepts within the model in the preparation of doctors. Hence, it is important to have an insight into the beliefs of this model of care as doctors within the team may be using it. The concepts of the model are beliefs and values, the goals of care and the knowledge required to achieve the outcomes. The beliefs and values are that all humans are made up of biological components and that all interact together to achieve a balance, homeostasis. An imbalance in this homeostasis is regarded as the 'problem' or 'disease' with little or no consideration being given to psychosocial problems. The goals of this model are to cure or treat the imbalance and so the knowledge required to achieve this is centred on such subjects as microbiology, anatomy and physiology, pathology and pharmacology.

This type of model worked well with routine, traditional physical care but made no allowances for the individuality of the person. Hence nurses who recognised that their patients were all different needed to develop models to encompass these individual needs, building on the physiological, social, behavioural and spiritual aspects as discussed in Chapters 6–8.

ROPER, LOGAN AND TIERNEY

This model was developed in 1980 from a model of living first discussed by Roper in 1976. It was then progressed to a conceptual model for nursing and is probably the model most commonly used in the UK, particularly in adult nursing. It is based on a concept of nursing proposed by Henderson (1966). Henderson suggested 14 'activities of daily living' and from these Roper and colleagues (1980) developed the 12 activities which 'people engage in to live'. These activities are:

- maintaining a safe environment
- communicating
- breathing
- eating and drinking
- eliminating
- personal cleansing and dressing
- controlling body temperature
- mobilising
- working and playing
- expressing sexuality
- sleeping
- dying.

These activities of living are then set against a lifespan continuum where conception to death is aligned to a continuum from total dependency to independence to dependency. The activities of living can be plotted on the continuum to assess the patient or client's needs and to plan to which stage of the continuum they are trying to return. Take, as an example, an adult who is, ordinarily, independent for the activity of elimination. The patient has to have a temporary colostomy formed to aid recovery from major bowel surgery. The patient at this time will be dependent for care of the colostomy until taught how to care for it himself and then, long term, independent again when the colostomy is closed and reversed to enable normal bowel actions to resume. In addition to

Case example 13.1

Mrs Bartlet, aged 77 years, lives in a 'granny annexe' at her daughter's home. She is admitted to the ward via the accident and emergency unit following a fall that morning. She is diagnosed with a fracture of the neck of her left femur.

Assessment using 12 activities of living (Roper et al 1980) was as follows:

- *Maintaining a safe environment*
  Mrs Bartlet fell on the stairs and will need a handrail fitted before discharge. Has lived alone safely since her husband died 4 years ago.
- *Communication*
  Mrs Bartlet is able to explain how she fell. She wears glasses for reading and watching the television but not when moving around the house. She has no problems with hearing. Her body language shows that she is in discomfort from her injury. Mrs Bartlet is aware of the name of the ward to which she has been admitted.
- *Breathing*
  Mrs Bartlet has no problems with her breathing. Her respiration rate is 20.
- *Eating and drinking*
  Mrs Bartlet prepares her own breakfast and snack at lunchtime. She has her main meal with her daughter and her family at 6 p.m. She has a cup of tea with her breakfast, coffee at midmorning and after lunch. A small cold drink is taken with her evening meal. At present she is nil by mouth in preparation for her operation.
- *Eliminating*
  Mrs Bartlet normally has her bowels open once a day. She needs to get out of bed at least once during the night to pass urine but has no incontinence. At present she is unable to get out of bed and so will need to use a bedpan.
- *Personal cleansing and dressing*
  Prior to her accident, Mrs Bartlet was self-caring. She has a shower every morning but admits that she preferred it when she could get into a bath. She will need assistance with this at present.
- *Controlling body temperature*
  Mrs Bartlet says that she enjoys the central heating in her home and was appropriately dressed for the time of year. Temperature 36°C.
- *Mobilising*
  Mrs Bartlet is now immobile. Prior to this accident she says that, although a little slow, she is able to get around her home and, when her daughter takes her there, is able to walk around the shops. She uses no aids. Waterlow assessment will be undertaken to assess her risk of pressure sores.
- *Working and playing*
  Mrs Bartlet has not worked since having her two children (55 and 53 years old). Her husband was an accountant. She has many hobbies including reading, television, attending church and spending time with her grandchildren.

- *Expressing sexuality*
  Mrs Bartlet enjoys shopping for clothes. A local hairdresser comes to her house every 2 weeks to wash and dry her hair and cut it when necessary.
- *Sleeping*
  Her normal pattern of sleep is 10.30 p.m. until 6 a.m. and she says she often has a little nap after lunch.
- *Dying*
  Mrs Bartlet was able to discuss the risks of a general anaesthetic at her age but said 'I have had a good life'.

This example highlights how an elderly person can become dependent on carers following an accident but, despite her age, following successful surgery, she could return home and continue living almost independently. You may also notice that although the activities of living cover a broad spectrum, other assessments and measurements will need to be undertaken (e.g. Waterlow risk assessment, temperature and respiration rate). From the assessment, the following actual problems can be identified:

- pain
- immobility
- personal hygiene: needs help at present
- elimination: needs help at present
- eating and drinking: nil by mouth prior to surgery.

The potential problems for this lady are:

- pressure sores from immobility
- thrombosis from immobility
- dehydration from surgery preparation.

Hence, from using a model, the nurse can obtain a clear picture of the patient and the patient's needs and plan the appropriate care.

the continuum, the following were identified as influencing activities of living:

- biological factors
- psychological factors
- sociocultural factors
- environmental factors
- politicoeconomic factors.

Case example 13.1 shows an assessment of a patient using the activities of living model.

Once the care is decided a care plan can be written, clearly explaining when, and by whom, the care is to be delivered. If clear plans are written they will be easy to follow by all carers. Explicit instructions and goals also aid evaluation as the carer can easily identify what everyone is trying to achieve.

However, one of the criticisms of this model is that it can concentrate on the physical aspects of care rather than on other areas. Murphy et al (2000) suggest that from a small research study undertaken in Ireland, it was found not to be suitable for psychiatric nursing. It was as a result of this type of criticism that a plethora of conceptual models developed, despite the view of Riehl & Roy (1980) that a universal model of nursing might have emerged. The diversity of models also encompassed the multidisciplinary approach to care that is now being encouraged.

ROY'S ADAPTATION MODEL OF NURSING

This model of nursing was described by Sister Callista Roy in the 1960s and first used in the USA in 1970. Subsequently it has been adopted in the UK and has been used more widely in the field of psychiatric nursing. The framework suggests that a person, as a whole being, responds or adapts to changes, described as 'stimuli'. These stimuli can be within the body or in the surrounding environment. It is suggested that using this model can enhance patient-centred care and accountability of nursing as a scientific discipline.

Roy strongly believes that everyone is an individual and the way everyone reacts to the environment is central to this model. Rambo (1984) described these assumptions as follows:

- Each person, as an integrated whole, comprises biological, psychological and social parts, and these interact with the environment.
- People adapt to changes that occur to maintain homeostasis.
- The stimuli to which people respond are of three types
  (a) focal – these are things that are present within the person, for example a headache, a bereavement
  (b) contextual – these are the stimuli in the environment that might give a negative response, for example pollution, poor social circumstances
  (c) residual – these are the person's past learning and responses to that learning, for example one woman might tolerate pain during childbirth as she accepts that it is part of the process,

whereas another might expect labour to be pain free and therefore expect analgesia.

Everyone is an individual and will therefore adapt to situations differently. Providing that stimuli are within the coping adaptations of that person, homeostasis will be maintained. If, however, the stimuli are too great, the responses made will not be adequate to balance – this is known as a maladaptive or negative response. For example, following the loss of a job, one person might respond by thinking of it as another opportunity in life and cope well; that would be a positive adaptation. Another person so affected might respond with anger, sleeplessness and poor appetite; that would be a negative adaptation response.

Roy suggests that there are four adaptive modes used to respond to stimuli to maintain integrity:

1. physiological
2. self-concept
3. role function
4. interdependence.

Physiological. As the name suggests, this is associated with the structure and function of the body and in particular how the body reacts to exercise, rest, nutrition, elimination, fluids and electrolytes, oxygen and circulation, regulation of temperature, senses and endocrine activities.

Self-concept. This focuses on the way the person perceives himself both physically and mentally – for example does the person perceive himself to be fat or thin, happy or sad?

Role function. The focus here is on social integrity and the roles one plays within it. These roles can be primary, secondary or tertiary and hence illness can impact on these roles. One's adaptation to illness in a tertiary role might be minimal as compared to a primary role, where illness could cause an imbalance to the homeostasis.

Interdependence. This focuses on social integrity and the ability to maintain a balance between independence and dependency on others. For example, an elderly person living alone may be able to be independent in cooking meals for himself but dependent on others for shopping and providing the food to be cooked as he is unable to get to the shops.

The person must make positive adaptations to stimuli to remain healthy and this is dependent on having the ability and energy to do this. Illness occurs when the adaptations needed are too great for the individual to make a positive response.

The goals for nursing in this model must therefore be in supporting the patient's adaptation to these stimuli. This can be achieved by:

- assessment of behaviour
- assessment of factors influencing the responses
- identifying problems
- setting achievable goals
- selecting appropriate interventions
- evaluation.

Case example 13. 2 shows an assessment using Roy's model (see also Activity 13.7). Some of the problems you should have identified in Activity 13.7 are:

- anxiety due to: fear of failure, family expectations and job prospects
- electrolyte imbalance due to overdose and vomiting
- tiredness due to anxiety
- poor nutrition due to unbalanced diet.

The outcomes for these problems could be achieved by referral to a community psychiatric nurse for management of the anxiety and to John's tutor for extra support or for an extension for the examination.

Following investigation for electrolyte imbalance, this could be corrected. Advice on the correct fluid intake, particularly water, and perhaps a recommendation to reduce the quantity of alcohol consumed could be offered. John's tiredness may be overcome if his anxiety is reduced or relaxation techniques could be investigated with him. His

poor nutritional status could be discussed at a later stage and so prevent any long-term problems. Following this assessment a plan of care could be agreed with John, implemented and then evaluated.

Using Roy's model of adaptation you can see how John reacted to various stimuli in a negative way to cause him problems in comparison to his friends who had similar stimuli and yet who were able to adapt in a positive way. You will also be aware that this patient was seen in an acute setting for general nursing and yet could be seen as a patient with a mental health problem. This is an opportunity for adult branch students to gain experience of mental health nursing. Roy's Adaptation model is a useful framework to use for patients as it considers them as individuals within the larger environmental setting.

Case example 13.3 illustrates an assessment using Roy's Adaptation model within the mental health branch of nursing.

OREM'S SELF-CARE MODEL

Dorothea Orem developed her own model of nursing and first published it in 1980. It is based on the philosophy that all individuals wish to care for themselves. This understanding links well to the theories of health education and promotion discussed in Chapter 10. Although one of the earliest models of nursing, Orem's model has remained a favourite with nurses particularly in the fields of rehabilitation and community care and hence fits well with recent government initiatives. If all care were delivered by the patient there would be no need for carers, but the scenario is not as simple as that. Consider a baby. It is impossible for a baby to be self-caring and so the self-care agent is the parent or guardian who will gradually teach the youngster to be self-caring within the developmental stages of life. Indeed, the health visitor, to ensure these stages are being reached, checks them at specific milestones. If they are not achieved then referral to other agencies for specific help is requested. This continuum of life was also a key element of the Roper et al (1996) model of nursing.

 Activity 13.7

Read the account of John in Case example 13.2. Try to assess his problems and identify the desired outcomes and the nursing actions that could be taken.

Case example 13.2

John, aged 21 years and a university student, is brought to the accident and emergency department by ambulance. His flatmate David had called the ambulance when he returned home and found John semi-conscious. There was a bottle of pills by his side. On arrival at hospital he was conscious.

Biographical details were taken and recorded but as the format for these is universal to all models they have been omitted to focus on the model of care. The format is one commonly adopted and as suggested by Roy.

	Behaviour	Focal stimuli	Contextual stimuli	Residual stimuli
Physiological				
Oxygen and circulation	Is breathing by himself but drowsy at times	Smoking is an irritant to breathing	Impacting on conscious state	All four people in flat smoke
	Smokes 20 cigarettes a day			
Fluid and electrolytes	Has drunk three pints of beer	Electrolyte imbalance		
	Has vomited			
Elimination	Urine specimen required for testing			
	No problems with micturition normally			
	Bowels opened daily			
Nutrition	Eats 'instant' foods mainly hamburgers, chips and curries	This is not a nutritious diet Poor knowledge of what he should be eating	This is the type of food readily available on campus and near to flat	All flatmates on restricted budget
Rest/activity	Not sleeping at present	Anxious about final examination and took a few tablets to help him sleep	Friends all coping with study	Will not get degree and therefore no job
Regulation	Temperature and pulse within normal limits			
	B/P 130/70			
Self-concept				
Physical self	John likes to buy fashionable clothes		Dresses like his peers	Parents disapprove of hairstyle
	Likes his shaven head			
Personal self	John says that he can't face his exams	He is aware other siblings have all achieved well and he is struggling	All his friends appear to be coping	He doesn't know anyone who has failed
Role function				
Primary	Young male	Enjoying life		
Secondary	Student	Anxious that he will fail his final exams	No job offers	All friends have jobs to go to
Tertiary	Youngest child of four	Thinks he is not as clever as others	All attended university	All siblings achieved a first degree
Interdependence				
	In hospital at present	Voluntary patient	Not sectioned under Mental Health Act	Does not like being in hospital
	Plans to return to flat with friends	Will need help	Friends are happy to support John	Father is in army and expects him to succeed
	Does not want to tell parents about this episode			

Case example 13.3

Tom is 35 years old and unmarried and lives in a housing association flat. He has been in contact with the mental health services since the age of 22 when he was diagnosed with schizophrenia. The community psychiatric nurse who administers injections of antipsychotic drugs every 3 weeks maintains his condition. Tom will not admit that he is ill but agrees to the medication.

Tom's sleep is disturbed at times and he is regularly heard talking to himself. He is self-caring but a heavy smoker. He is unemployed with few social contacts except for the friends he meets at the day centre. He has little contact with his parents.

	Behaviour	Focal	Contextual	Residual
Physiological				
Oxygen and circulation	Tom smokes 30 cigarettes a day and is often breathless when walking	Smoking is an irritant	Poor social conditions	Most of his social contacts smoke
Fluids and electrolytes	Tom enjoys making and drinking tea			
Elimination	No problems with micturition and elimination			
Nutrition	Tom eats instant/ready prepared meals. He does not enjoy shopping for food	Poor nutritional status	Can buy burgers and chips readily from nearby shop	Tom thinks cooking is a woman's job
Rest/activity	Tom is unemployed and has little interest in doing anything. He attends the day centre 3 days a week	Unemployment causes financial restraints	Few opportunities for employment	Other social contacts are unemployed
Regulation	Respirations are a little rapid Temperature and pulse within normal limits	Smoking affects Tom's breathing		
Self-concept				
Physical self	Tom is not interested in how he dresses or looks	Tom thinks he is appropriately dressed	Little money available for clothes	Dresses similar to friends
Personal self	Tom does not accept that he is ill	Tom accepts his medication to help the voices he hears		Has always talked to the voices in his head
Role function				
Primary	Single male	Tom is happy by himself	Difficult to find a partner	
Secondary	Unemployed	Does not want to go to work	Very little money to spend	Other friends are unemployed
Tertiary	Son	Tom has little contact with his parents		Parents could not accept/understand Tom's behaviour
Independence				
	Lives alone in housing association flat	Independent	Poor social conditions	
	Needs medication	Dependent on community psychiatric nurse	Nurse encourages Tom with social skills	Improvement from institutional care

In the same way, a nurse may become the self-care agent when a person becomes ill and is unable to care for himself. The goal of nursing for this model is to return the patient to being self-caring. If, however, this is impossible, for example in the case of a client with a severe learning disability and mental illness, then a self-care agent will undertake those functions that the client is unable to achieve. Such functions are known as self-care deficits. These deficits can be compensated in three ways:

1. Total compensation where the nurse or carer totally undertakes the actions of the self-care deficit, for example a terminally ill patient or an unconscious patient.

2. Partial compensation where the carer works with the patient to meet his self-care needs. In this way the patient is able to feel in control of his care with the support of a carer. For example, a patient discharged home from hospital following surgery for a hip replacement may require help with shopping and personal hygiene but otherwise be independent.

3. Educative/supportive compensation. In this case the nurse is required to teach patients or carers how to deliver care themselves, for example a patient with a newly formed colostomy. This patient has the potential to be self-caring but needs to be taught how to undertake this new care. Similarly, in the case of a child with a colostomy the parents or guardians might need to be taught how to do this to enable them to partially compensate for the child until he could be taught how to do it himself.

The assessment of the patient's needs is undertaken against the three compensatory zones. Orem (1985) describes the self-care requisites that she considers are common to all people for effective living. They are:

- *Air*. The ability to maintain a sufficient intake of air.
- *Water*. The ability to take in sufficient water to live.
- *Food*. The ability to maintain enough food intake for life.
- *Elimination*. Being in control of elimination and excretion processes.

- *Activity/rest*. Orem suggests that there should be a balance in life between rest and activity and that the person should be in control of this.
- *Solitude/social intervention*. The person should be able to participate in activities of social intervention and quietness and maintain a balance between them.
- *Prevention of hazards*. In self-care the person should be able to prevent hazards to themselves.
- *Promotion of normality*. The person should be able to interact in society and with chosen groups of friends.

Thus the plan of care and implementation of this care would be compensatory for the self-care deficits.

Case example 13.4 shows an assessment of Ben, a patient with Down's syndrome, using Orem's model of care. The plan of care for Ben would need to be detailed, for example dressing. This would need to be broken down into many stages; here are a few examples of the stages:

1. Ben chooses what clothes he will wear. Carer dresses Ben.
2. Ben puts on his underwear unaided. Carer does the rest.
3. Ben puts on his underwear and trousers. Carer does the rest.
4. Ben does up the zip and buttons on his trousers after putting them on. Carer does the rest.

The series would be continued as and if Ben was able to progress. This is a long process in comparison to the partial compensation required for a patient postoperatively or total compensation for an unconscious patient who regains consciousness following an anaesthetic.

When working with patients with learning disabilities you will need to enquire if a model is used and how it has been developed to adapt to the long-term problems. Some new outcome models are being developed in this field but are very specialised.

In conclusion Orem (1985) discusses developmental self-care requisites where the person needs help due to the developmental stage of life that he is at, and health deviation deficits.

Case example 13.4

Ben Smith, aged 42, has Down's syndrome and has recently been moved from a large institution to a 17-bedded nursing home for people with severe learning disabilities.

Ben was assessed on admission to the home and a care plan written for him. Ben's care plan will be very different from those you may have experienced in a hospital ward or the community as Ben's care will be for the rest of his life since he has no living relatives and needs constant care. The plan will be amended as he reaches his goal but it may take several months/years for him to achieve a goal. Hence, each goal will need to be broken into small achievable targets for Ben.

	Self-care	Total compensation	Partial compensation	Educative/supportive compensatory
Air	Ben has no problems with breathing			
Water	Ben is able to drink unaided		Drinks need to be supplied for Ben to drink with meals	To encourage Ben to get his own drinks when needed
Food	Ben is able to feed himself	Ben needs his food supplied	Ben likes to choose what he eats	To teach Ben to prepare some of his food. To encourage Ben to accompany a carer to do the shopping for food
Elimination	Ben is self-caring			
Activity/rest			Ben attends a day centre for activities. He is taken in the mini bus	To encourage Ben to make choices
Solitude/social intervention	Ben enjoys watching television and is able to switch this on and off	Ben does not like mixing with people he does not know. Carers need to take him out to socialise	Carers to accompany Ben on social outings that he has requested	To teach/support Ben in socialising
Prevention of hazards		Ben is unaware of any danger		To try to make Ben aware of dangers such as traffic
Promotion of normality	Ben mixes well within the nursing home	Ben needs help with socialising outside the home and with personal hygiene and dressing	Ben will wash himself if taken to the bathroom and given all the toiletries	To encourage Ben to wash and dress himself appropriately

Activity 13.8

When on a placement, record in your profile the details of a patient that you have met. (Remember to use pseudonyms and maintain your patient's confidentiality.) In light of these details, assess your patient's needs using Orem's model of nursing. Compare the outcomes of the assessment undertaken by the patient's named nurse with yours. With your mentor discuss the similarities and differences.

These are when the person requires a change in self-care due to illness, for example a newly diagnosed diabetic patient.

Activity 13.8 will enable you to practise an assessment and to compare it with a model of care being used. If Orem is the model of choice of this placement, you can compare how well you have assessed this patient. Do reflect on this exercise and discuss it with your mentor.

CASEY'S MODEL

When nursing children, either at home or in hospital, it is important to remember that consideration must also be given to the child's parents or guardians. This has been emphasised in many reports including the UK Children Act (DoH 1989b). This participation is referred to by a variety of terms:

- family-centred care
- partnership in care
- care by parents
- parent involvement.

Whatever term is used, it means that the parent or guardian is involved in the care of the child. This involvement must be negotiated with the nurse and the child, if old enough, and a clear plan written to ensure that all parties understand and accept their responsibilities.

A framework for this delivery of care is required and the one most commonly adopted is the Casey model (1988). Lee (1998) does not consider this to be a true conceptual model but Casey (1988) would defend the model as being based on concepts of the person, health, the environment and nursing. The 'person' concept is split into two parts: the family and the child. The child's needs are protection, sustenance, stimulation and love.

Casey (1988) describes a continuum starting at conception through to maturity. At the start of this the child is dependent on carers for all its needs but at the end is independent and self-caring. The process of functioning, growing and developing is based on the following aspects:

- physical
- emotional
- intellectual
- social
- spiritual.

When undertaking an assessment the nurse will need to explore the structure of the family and establish who normally undertakes the caring role. With more women in full-time employment some grandparents are assuming the role of main carer. Likewise, with a rise in divorce and remarriage the family structure is getting more complicated. It is essential for the nurse to have an understanding of the family structure to enable effective communication.

The process of assessment and care for the child will be between the child, the nurse and the family carer. Casey (1988) does not suggest a list of needs to be considered but takes an umbrella approach. Hence your assessment should be based on the following areas:

- what family care the child routinely receives
- the child's present condition, both physical and psychological
- what nursing care the child needs
- the ability and willingness of the child and/or family to participate.

Case example 13.5 illustrates the use of the Casey model with a child with asthma.

This simple framework can also be followed when a child is admitted to hospital. Most parents like to continue with the care of their child but the nurse does need to negotiate this care with the family so that they fully understand what is expected of them and to ensure that they are happy to participate in that care. You will observe some parents just wishing to continue to help

Case example 13.5

Emma is 5 years old and was diagnosed with asthma at the age of 3 when her mother brought her to see her general practitioner as she was waking at night with a cough. Since then she has been reviewed every 6 months by the practice nurse who is a specialist in the care of asthma. On this visit Emma is being reviewed prior to commencing school full time.

The care plan that was being reviewed was as follows:

Emma

- To use metered inhaler with spacer device
- To do a peak flow every morning and evening and watch mother record in book
- To tell an adult when she is short of breath or has a cough so she can use her inhaler.

Family

- To keep a symptom diary stating when Emma becomes short of breath, for example when playing, sleeping or running
- To record Emma's peak flow measurements
- To encourage Emma to use her inhaler
- To encourage Emma to participate in exercise, for example swimming
- To provide Emma with a balanced diet
- To visit school and talk with teachers and school nurse about medication.

Nurse

- To review Emma's peak flow recordings and symptom diary
- To check Emma's inhaler technique
- To weigh and measure Emma
- To educate family and child about asthma and in particular about use of different inhalers
- To encourage Emma to participate in all school activities.

This plan enabled all those involved to have clear guidelines for what was expected of them and to make evaluation easier by reviewing each step. You can see how the partnership between the child, family and nurse was established. Once at school, there will be a need to include the teachers within the plan so they understand which inhaler Emma should use. They will also need to discuss with the family the safekeeping of the inhaler while she is at school. Other children in the class might also be included in the care as they can help by telling the teacher if they notice Emma is coughing but unable to ask for help herself. Other children with asthma might also be introduced to Emma.

with personal care while others might be actively involved in administering oxygen or managing the care of their child's tracheotomy. The nurse needs to support the family in the giving of this care and this might be by teaching them or, once taught, by encouraging them to continue.

As you will have become aware, the nursing models discussed above are just a few of the models available. This chapter cannot give you the depth required to study each model in detail but rather aims to give an overview so that you have a broad picture of what is available. You will then need to read about the individual models as you use them on your placements. There are many texts available which will give you more detail of these and a suggested reading list can be found at the end of this chapter to help you to develop your knowledge.

Nursing models have made a great impact on the way in which care is assessed and planned. However, nursing is dynamic and constantly changing to respond to patients' needs, government initiatives and research. Nursing models and the nursing process have indeed structured the way in which nursing care is delivered but Marks-Maran (1999) suggests that although it is a useful tool to record patient care, it does not encompass the reasoning behind the care given. At the same time there is a strong initiative to promote evidence-based care that is individualised to the patient but that can be easily audited. This has led to the development of care pathways. The Department of Health (1998), in its document *A First Class Service: Quality in the New NHS*, recognised the need for universal evidence-based programmes of care – care pathways meet this need.

INTEGRATED CARE PATHWAYS

This is a generic term describing the care that should be given to a patient with a specific condition. There does, however, still seem to be some confusion among nursing and health care professionals as to what to call these plans/frameworks. Commonly used terms to describe a framework of care are:

- integrated care pathways
- critical pathways
- care programmes
- care protocol.

These plans of care are based on the knowledge of nurses and research and describe the plan or pathway for the patient. The pathways are usually for use by all disciplines as opposed to just nurses and so reduce the complications of different parts of the care being recorded on different notes that are kept separately. It also enhances greater understanding within the multidisciplinary team by enabling them to deliver an agreed plan of care for the patient while everyone is aware of what other disciplines are doing. The patient also benefits from this by having a total picture of the care.

Naturally, all patients are individual and will have individual needs in addition to the 'common' needs. These needs are referred to as variances (Lowe 1998) and are added to the pathway. For example, if a patient following surgery for a hysterectomy develops a pyrexia, that patient would be following a common pathway for the hysterectomy and a variance for the pyrexia would be added to the pathway. Such variances can be analysed and if they become common to most patients on that pathway they can be added to it or investigated as to the reason why such a variance is occurring. This investigation is undertaken as an audit.

The aim of a care pathway is therefore to give a patient a guide to his care, based on evidence, and to achieve the best outcome of the treatment and care for that patient. The guide will ensure that the patient is aware of what is expected of him and what care he should expect.

Return to Activity 13.5 in which you considered models and frameworks and now consider their limitations. One of the limitations of some models is that they are used by only one set of carers. Each discipline has its preferred model and this may result in confusion for patient and carers, as they are not fully conversant with each other's model. These uni-disciplinary team's plans of care are often stored separately, which adds to the confusion for those attempting integrated care. This is why there has been a move towards multidisciplinary care and the recording of all care in just one programme.

Before proceeding to examine pathways further, multidisciplinary teams need to be explored.

Here again, many terms are used to describe the idea of people from different disciplines working together. Leathard (1994) tries to clarify the situation by correlating them into three groups, namely:

- concept based
- process based
- agency based.

She suggests that words such as 'interdisciplinary', 'multidisciplinary', 'holistic' and 'generic' are concept based, whereas 'joint planning', 'teamwork', 'liaison', 'synergy' and 'collaborative working' are process based. The agency-based division is 'inter-agency', 'healthy alliances', 'locality groups' and 'consortium'. While on placement you will need to find out how the multidisciplinary team is made up and how they prefer to be described.

What is important to remember is that each patient will have his own specific team made up of the carers pertaining to his individual needs (Case example 13.6 and Activity 13.9).

We should now consider the notes and records for the patient in Case example 13.6, and where they might be kept. The district nurse, for example, would have notes that Mrs Dark would keep in the flat, whereas the general practitioner would record notes at the surgery and these would probably be computer generated. Carers from social services may well have further notes. So you can see the complexity for the person trying to coordinate the care and for the patient herself. One set of notes used by all carers would be simpler and the way in which notes should be recorded will be discussed later. A further complexity in this case management would be carers using different models of care.

It was to overcome these complexities that care pathways were developed.

Definitions of an integrated care pathway

A care pathway is a plan of treatment and care that is agreed and written by the multidisciplinary team for a specific episode of care. This plan will be based on the best available evidence to achieve the best possible outcome. Hence, the

Case example 13.6

Mrs Dark is 84 years old and lives alone in a warden controlled flat. The block of flats is purpose-built for elderly residents and is owned by the local council. Mrs Dark has suffered from diabetes for 40 years and is now partially sighted. She enjoys socialising with the other residents and attending church every Sunday. She needs help to have a bath and to monitor her blood to ensure her diabetes is in control. She self-administers her insulin. Her main meal is taken with the other residents in a central dining room and she prepares other meals for herself. Her married daughter takes her shopping once a week.

The following list shows some of the carers in the team for Mrs Dark and the reason for their involvement. The list is in no specific order.

Carer	Reason for involvement
Warden	Providing meals and emergency cover via call bell system
Daughter	Takes mother shopping
District nurse	Coordinates care for diabetes and acts as team coordinator
Diabetic specialist nurse	Visits on request of district nurse. Advises on special equipment for the administering of insulin
Health visitor for the elderly	Visits to undertake over 75 year health check
Home care assistant	Helps Mrs Dark to have a bath
Social worker for the blind and partially sighted	Advises on benefits and adaptations for the home. May refer to an occupational therapist
Chiropodist	To care for Mrs Dark's feet
General practitioner	To prescribe insulin and care when Mrs Dark is unwell
Ophthalmic consultant or/and optician	To monitor Mrs Dark's sight and prescribe glasses
Vicar	To help with Mrs Dark's spiritual needs
Local pharmacist	Dispensing and delivering medication as required

This team is unique to Mrs Dark and the district nurse might well be the key player to coordinate the team. Her experience and knowledge will enable her to refer to other agencies as and when appropriate.

Activity 13.9

Look at the description of Mrs Dark, the patient in Case example 13.6. Map out a team that could be involved in her care.

methods of care and timetable for events will be evidence based.

A standardised care pathway should give the patient a clear plan of treatment and care that will be followed for a specific incident of care. This will enable patients to be better informed about their care and the progress that they are making. The plan will be pre-printed and so available to show patients and to help in explaining their plan of care to them. It will help them to feel empowered and involved in their care and will enable them to ask significant questions about it. It will also ensure that the care delivered is consistent with the plan, despite the fact that staff may change.

For the carers, pathways have many benefits and these can be summarised as follows:

• they enable standardised treatments for specific conditions, thus ensuring that there is parity of care
• carers are informed about the total package of care for the patient
• they are tools to monitor the patient's total progress
• they enable individuality by addition of variances
• they aid planning and bed management as the manager will be able accurately to calculate the expected hospital stay for individual conditions
• they reduce multiple notes and thus avoid duplication and time spent by each professional group completing their own set of notes.

As pathways are written for patients with similar conditions, rather than for a specific patient, let us explore a pathway for a patient who has suffered a stroke. It can then be individualised later.

First, the team who may be involved in the care of this patient needs to be identified. The team

Table 13.1 An admission assessment for a patient who has suffered a stroke

Carer	Action	Achieved	Variance
Nurse	Admitted within 4 hours Nursing assessment completed Base line observations recorded Fluid balance chart commenced Waterlow score completed Nutritional assessment Anti-embolism stockings applied		
Speech therapist	Dysphagia assessment		
Doctor	Medical assessment completed Medications reviewed Blood taken Chest X-ray ordered ECG performed		
Pharmacist	Medication confirmed and dispensed		
Multidisciplinary team	Manual handling assessment		

will consist of: nurses, doctors, speech therapists, physiotherapists, occupational therapists, dieticians, pharmacists and social workers. All these people would have their specific actions identified within the pathway. The pathway would then be arranged into specific time zones, namely: admission, day 1 to day 6 and then discharge/transfer. Discharge would be planned for throughout the admission but a summary completed on discharge.

Table 13.1 suggests the type of assessment and actions that would be documented for admission assessment. The person completing the action would sign the actions. If a variance was noted this would then be recorded, for example if a patient refused to wear the anti-embolism stockings. A plan for day 1 might include in its list such things as dysphagia reassessment, observations, nursing care, fluid balance charts, discharge planning and education. The total plan would give all concerned in the care a guide as to the plan of actions for this patient and so offer the best treatments for that patient at the optimum time.

This has been an overview of care pathways and a list of some further reading that will help your understanding can be found at the end of the chapter.

Whichever model of care or care pathway you learn about and use on your placements you will need to have a clear understanding of record keeping.

RECORD KEEPING

A most important part of nursing care is to keep accurate records. This section of the chapter will give an insight to the nurse's specific requirements as stated by UKCC (1998) and how these guidelines apply to the various ways in which nurses keep records.

The UKCC guidelines for record keeping (UKCC 1998, p. 7) state that: 'Record keeping is an integral part of nursing, midwifery and health visiting practice. It is a tool of professional practice and one which should help the care process. It is not separate from this process and it is not an optional extra to be fitted in if circumstances allow.' This statement clearly sets record keeping into the process of nursing, whatever model or framework is being used.

Types of records kept

There are many types of records and methods of completion in use in practice (Activity 13.10).

These will be considered before exploring in more depth what should be included.

The types of records that you might have seen are:

- *Patient held records*. These are normally used in community settings by, for example, district nurses, community psychiatric nurses and midwives. This encourages patients to read their records and be involved in them. They are also encouraged to add to the documentation.

- *Parent held records*. Either the midwife or the health visitor gives these to the parent or guardian. The parent/guardian is encouraged to bring the notes with them when the child is seen at the health centre or surgery to enable additions to be made to the records. This type of record is very useful if the person moves away and prevents the wait for notes to be posted on to the new carer. This record is a useful place to record the immunisations that the child has received.

- *Nursing notes*. The format of these will be dependent on the framework being used. They are either printed with the headings of the model being used or come in a printed standardised format for that condition. These are different from a care pathway as they are for each aspect of care, for example, one for preoperative surgery and another for postoperative care. These should be readily available for the patient to read and so are often kept on the patient's locker or bed. Some however are stored at the nurses' station to aid the nurse when caring for a group of patients.

- *Medical notes*. In the hospital it is common practice to store these separately from the nursing notes. However, they are, with consent, available for the nurse to read. Investigation results such as X-rays and blood results are commonly stored with the medical notes. The patient has specific rights of access to these notes.

- *Multidisciplinary notes*. These notes are a combination of the notes for all professional teams caring for the patient. They can appear very bulky and difficult to follow at first but are a useful aid to care. Notes, per profession, are often colour-coded to aid reading and completion. The advantage of this type is that any carer has access to the complete picture of care for the patient.

- *General practitioner notes*. These are notes kept by the patient's general practitioner and comprise notes made by the general practitioner and discharge letters following episodes of care in acute settings. These notes make up the total picture of care for the patient and are transferred to a new general practitioner if or when the patient moves. They should be a total record 'from cradle to grave'.

- *Integrated care pathway*. This is a printed plan of care for use by the multidisciplinary team. The care is prescribed on a daily basis and on each day there is a list of actions for the individuals to complete. The prescribed care is evidence based and therefore not a list of tasks to be undertaken.

- *Biographical details*. These are essential details of the patient and the content of these is common to all patients for whatever framework of care delivery is being used. Box 13.1 shows the type of biographical information that is required. This information can be completed by the patient, if well enough, and can be seen by the patient as a useful thing to do while waiting to be admitted. A criticism often heard by patients is that they repeatedly give the same details. Multidisciplinary notes can overcome this problem.

All the above notes can be written by hand or placed immediately on a computer. The majority of general practitioners' notes are now computerised and the government plans that all will be connected to the NHS highway to ensure speedy, efficient communications between the community and acute settings.

You will have noted from the UKCC guidelines (UKCC 1998) that record keeping is an integral part of nursing, and the reasons for – and importance of – record keeping needs to be fully understood.

Records can be seen as a focus for communication between carers. Full written or computerised

Box 13.1	**Typical biographical details required from a patient on admission to an acute setting**

- Full name
- Preferred name (the name by which the patient likes to be addressed)
- Address
- Telephone number
- Date of birth and age
- Preferred language
- Ethnicity
- Religion
- Next of kin or contact
- Address and telephone number of next of kin or contact
- Second contact name
- Address and telephone number of second contact person
- General practitioner, name address and telephone number
- Occupation
- Social circumstances. This is important information for discharge planning and may be included in the model assessment or in the biographical details. Does the patient live in a house or a bungalow? Does the patient live alone? Where is the bathroom? Are there steps in the house?
- Past medical history
- Diet requirements
- Allergies. This question is normally placed in a prominent position on the first page of the notes to alert carers to it.

information about the patient and the patient's condition will enable other carers to continue the planned care in the knowledge that they are fully informed of all relevant details. This is of particular importance for patients with communication problems, for example someone who speaks a different language, a person with a severe learning disability, a baby who cannot yet talk, or an unconscious patient. This record will aid communication within the multidisciplinary team, as it will be available to all within the team.

Continuity of care between carers will be ensured with the aid of a complete record of care and plans for that person. This plan, being based on the best available evidence, will lead to high standards of clinical care for the patient. With a complete picture of the care given, patient problems should be easily identified as soon as they occur. This in turn will lead to problem solving

and, again, a high standard of care (Smallman 1999).

In conclusion, records should be an accurate account of the total care planning, treatments and delivery for the patient. Unfortunately, there is no universal way in which records are kept. The UKCC (1998, p. 7) suggests the following as criteria for good records and in so doing enhances the impact upon practice (UKCC 2000b):

- The record is a product of local multidisciplinary discussion and the patient or client.
- It is evaluated and adapted in response to patient and client need.
- It enables nurses, midwives and health visitors to care for the patient or client in all environments at all stages of the care process.
- It promotes communication between all carers and the patient or client.

Although there is no one preferred model or framework for keeping records, there are recommendations for the content of the records and the way in which they are documented, known as the style. The following suggestions are all based on (but expanded upon) the guidelines of the UKCC (1998, p. 8) and will help when completing records. You should always ask your mentor to countersign your records, as she is accountable for the care given to the patient.

GUIDELINES FOR GOOD RECORD KEEPING

Records should:

'Be factual, consistent and accurate'
What is written in the notes must be an accurate record of what was done or observed. Consistency refers to the usual way that the records are recorded. If a care plan states what care is to be given and it is normal practice for the nurse to only record what has not been completed and the reason why, this is what would be expected. If, however, the custom is to record exactly what you did then this would be consistent with the usual way of recording for this practice. It is your responsibility to find out what is normal practice for the practice area you are working on.

Do check that all your documentation is accurate, especially, for example, when referring to left and right.

'Be written as soon as possible after an event has occurred, providing current information on the care and condition of the patient or client'

This clause suggests that at the completion of an episode of care the records for that episode should be completed. This will encourage the patient to be involved with the record keeping and will avoid having a bulky pile of notes to be recorded at the end of a shift. Completing the records as soon as possible after the event will encourage accurate record keeping. It is difficult to recall exactly what happened several hours previously and it is best practice to record things at the time they are done. This will also provide current information for all involved in the care.

'Be written clearly and in such a manner that the text cannot be erased'

As specified earlier in this section, notes are central to good communication and so need to be able to be read. This information is often required quickly and so ease of reading is also important. You may be able to read your handwriting but can others? (Activity 13.11).

You should write all your notes in permanent ink that cannot be erased. Remember you might be asked questions about what is recorded up to 7 years after the event and a complete set of records would be required and one that has not faded or been erased.

'Be written in such a manner that any alterations or additions are dated, timed and signed in such a way that the original entry can still be read clearly'

All alterations should be clearly visible. This means that correction fluids should *not* be used. A single line through the error and the new entry clearly written is the correct method to use. This correction should be *dated* and *signed*. Mistakes do happen when writing and so be open about them. This will ensure that your records are not altered in any way.

'Be accurately dated, timed and signed, with the signature printed alongside the first entry'

If the record is to be meaningful then the above conditions need to be met. Some documentation will have a page at the beginning where all people involved with the care of the patient will print their name, sign against it and add their initials. This will enable entries within that specific documentation to be initialled rather than have a full signature. All carers must make themselves aware of what is customary for that placement as regards the way in which records are signed.

'Not include abbreviations, jargon, meaningless phrases, irrelevant speculation and offensive subjective statements'

Health care, unfortunately, survives on abbreviations and jargon. Patients should be able to understand their own records and so have a right to have them written in a form that they can comprehend (Activity 13.12).

As you gain in experience it is useful to return to Activity 13.12 and realise just how quickly you pick up and use the jargon. Benner (1994) explores the concept of novice to expert. At the novice stage there is little understanding and this is developed as one progresses along the continuum. She also states that on changing jobs one reverts to being a novice and this can be caused by the lack of understanding caused by the jargon used. Throughout

Activity 13.11

Find a page in your diary or profile that has been hand-written. Ask two or three colleagues if they can read and understand what you have written. This is a good test as the piece of work has not been especially written for the exercise when you might be 'trying harder' with your writing.

Activity 13.12

Listen to a hand-over report between nurses and list all the abbreviations and jargon used. How many did you understand? Ask your mentor to explain those you did not understand.

Imagine you are the patient and consider how much of what was said you would have understood.

nurse training there is the opportunity to experience a number of very different clinical placements and each placement will potentially have its own jargon. It is the nurse's responsibility to ensure that she understands about the patient's care, so if you are unsure, ask. You might become the patient's advocate by asking, as the patient might have wanted to ask but not liked to in case it was something they should have known.

'Meaningless phrases' refers to such statements as 'slept well' and 'good night'. If, for example, you observed a patient who was restless at night it would be good practice to record 'the patient was restless at 2 a.m. and was complaining of pain' rather than 'the patient was restless' as this would not communicate the reason for the patient's restlessness and would be relatively meaningless. Subjective statements are, for example, 'noisy', 'quiet', 'fat' or 'interfering' when referring to a patient. These must be avoided, as they are offensive and written in a subjective way.

'Be readable on any photocopies'
This normally means writing in black ink but such things as allergies highlighted or written in another colour. Whatever colour is used, it must be readable on a photocopy.

'Be written, wherever possible, with the patient or client or their carer'
The records that are being made are about another person and that person has the right to know what is being written about them and to be involved in the decisions being made. Patient involvement was stressed when considering frameworks for care and so this is an extension of that role.

'Be written in terms that the patient can understand'
The explanation of this clause is the same as the one for abbreviations (above).

'Be consecutive'
All recordings should be in time and date order. This will aid communication between carers and help prevent mistakes being made, for example if a medication is given but not recorded until much later, it potentially could be given twice.

'Identify problems that have arisen and the action taken to rectify them'

This clause should be taken into consideration when plans for redesigning frameworks are being discussed to ensure that this is included.

'Provide clear evidence of the care planned, the decisions made, the care delivered and the information shared'
This final clause summarises the need for good records of nursing care and how that care is delivered. It reiterates that the patient is central to the notes by requiring the nurse to record the information given to the patient. This is important, especially when teaching patients new skills or when explaining their condition, as a record is needed of their understanding.

Adherence to the above guidelines will ensure that the nurse's records are a comprehensive report of the care given to the patient. Records may be used as evidence in a court of law, by the UKCC in a professional misconduct investigation, or by the health service commissioner as part of a local investigation. The law sees records as evidence of care given and therefore anything that is not recorded is viewed as not undertaken.

In areas such as mental health and child protection there are additional legislative practices to be followed. This knowledge should be expanded on while working in those particular placements to ensure that it is up to date.

All patients and clients have the right, under the Access to Health Records Act 1999, to view any manual health records written about them made after 1 November 1991. Computer-held records are secured under the Data Protection Act 1984 and protect the storage and information held on these records and the access to these records by the patient.

Records are confidential and you must ensure the confidentiality of your patients' and clients' records. This is an important factor to remember, especially when reflecting on care or being asked in your studies to consider examples from practice.

CONCLUSION

This chapter has explored some of the theories of nursing and the frameworks by which these theories are interpreted into practice. Nursing is a

Activity 13.13 End of chapter assignment

During your next clinical placement, observe a registered nurse admit a patient using a model of care. In your diary/profile reflect on this experience. Using this patient's information as your case study, use a different model of nursing and reassess the patient's needs. Compare your theoretical outcomes with those of the real assessment and decide which would have been the most helpful model for that patient and why.

dynamic profession and so evidence is changing rapidly. This in turn leads to the development of new theories and new ways of working. There is an ongoing debate between theorists and practitioners about the gap between theory and practice. Schon (1987) described this as the swamp between the hard evidence of the theory and the softer interface of practice. As has been seen from this chapter, theory underpins practice, and examples of this have been given. The challenge ahead is for theory and practice to work closer together and the student nurse is in an ideal position to ensure that this happens (Activity 13.13).

REFERENCES

Access to Health Records Act 1999 HMSO, London
Aggleton P, Chalmers H 1986 Nursing models and the nursing process. Macmillan, Basingstoke
Archibald G 2000 A post-modern nursing model. Nursing Standard 14(10):40–42
Benner P 1994 From novice to expert: power and excellence in nursing practice. Addison-Wesley, Menlo Park
Casey A 1988 A partnership with child and family. Senior Nurse 8(4):8–9
Data Protection Act 1984. HMSO, London
DoH 1989 Community care: an agenda for action. HMSO, London
DoH 1989 Children Act. HMSO, London
DoH 1995 Building bridges: a guide to arrangements for inter-agency working for the care and protection of severely mentally ill people. HMSO, London
DoH 1998 A first class service: quality in the new NHS. HMSO, London
Elliott-Cannon C 1990 Mental handicap and nursing models. In: Savage J, Kershaw B (eds) Models of nursing, 2nd edn. Scutari, Harrow
Fawcett J 1989 Analysis and evaluation of conceptual models of nursing, 2nd edn. Davis, Philadelphia

Fraser M 1996 Using conceptual nursing in practice: a research based approach, 2nd edn. Chapman and Hall, London
Hartwell D 1991 Dorothea Orem self-care deficit theory. Notes on Nursing Theory No 4. Sage, USA
Henderson V 1966 The nature of nursing. Macmillan, London
Herring L 1999 Critical pathways: an efficient way to manage care. Nursing Standard 13(47):36–37
Layton A, Moss F, Morgan G 1998 Mapping out the patient's journey: experiences of developing pathways of care. Quality in Health Care 7(supplement):S30–S36
Leathard A 1994 Going inter-professional: working together for health and welfare. Routledge, London
Lee P 1998 An analysis and evaluation of Casey's conceptual model. International Journal of Nursing Studies 35(4):204–209
Louette R 1991 Callista Roy: an adaptation model. Notes on Nursing Theory No 3. Sage, USA
Lowe C 1998 Care pathways: have they a place in the new NHS? Journal of Advanced Nursing Management 6(5):303–306
Marks-Maran D 1999 Reconstructing nursing: evidence, artistry and the curriculum. Nurse Education Today 19(1):3–11
Marriner-Tomey A 1994 Nursing theorists and their work, 3rd edn. Mosby, Missouri
Mckenna H 1993 The effects of nursing models on quality of care. Nursing Times 89:43–46
Meleis A I 1997 Theoretical nursing: development and progress, 3rd edn. Lippincott, Philadelphia
Miller J 1995 Nursing patients through pathways of care. Professional Nurse 10(12):759–762
Murphy M, Cooney A, Casey D, Connor M, O'Connor J, Dineen B 2000 The Roper, Logan and Tierney (1996) model: perceptions and operationalization of the model in psychiatric nursing within a health board in Ireland. Journal of Advanced Nursing 31(6):1333–1341
Nightingale F 1946 Notes on nursing: what it is, and what it is not. Lippincott, London
Nott A 2000 The care pathway approach in an acute mental health inpatient department. Nursing Times 96(11):44–45
Orem D 1985 Nursing concepts of practice, 3rd edn. McGraw-Hill, New York
Page M 1995 Tailoring nursing models to client's needs: using the Roper, Logan and Tierney model after discharge. Professional Nurse 19:284–288
Pearson A, Vaughan B 1994 Nursing models for practice. Butterworth-Heinemann, Oxford
Rambo B 1984 Adaptation nursing: assessment and intervention. W B Saunders, Philadelphia
Reed P G 1995 A treatise on nursing knowledge development in the 21st century: beyond postmodernism. Advances in Nursing Science 17(3):70–84
Reihl L, Roy C 1980 Conceptual models for nursing practice. Appleton, New York
Roberts D, Mackay G 1999 A nursing model of overdose assessment. Nursing Times 95(3):58–60
Roper N, Logan W, Tierney A 1980 The elements of nursing: a model for nursing based on a model of living. Churchill Livingstone, London
Roper N, Logan W, Tierney A 1996 The elements of nursing: a model for nursing based on a model of living, 4th edn. Churchill Livingstone, London

Roy C 1976 Introduction to nursing: an adaptive model. Prentice Hall, New Jersey

Schon D 1987 Educating the reflective practitioner. Jossey-Bass, San Francisco

Scott E, Cowen B 1997 Multi disciplinary collaborative care pathways. Nursing Standard 12(1):39–42

Smallman M 1999 Record keeping. Community Nurse 4(12):15–16

Tierney A J 1998 Nursing models: extant or extinct. Journal of Advanced Nursing 28(1):77–85

Walshe M 1998 Models and care pathways in clinical nursing: conceptual frameworks for care planning. Baillière Tindall, London

Wright S 1990 Building and using a model of nursing, 2nd edn. Edward Arnold, London

UKCC 1992 Code of professional conduct. UKCC, London

UKCC 1998 Guidelines for record keeping. UKCC, London

UKCC 2000a Requirements for pre-registration nursing programmes. UKCC, London

UKCC 2000b Perceptions of the scope of professional practice. UKCC, London

---

FURTHER READING

Concepts, theories and models

The following books and articles will give you a broader understanding of the use of concepts, theories and models in nursing. They will expand on the introduction to the subject gained from this chapter.

Aggleton P, Chalmers H 1986 Nursing models and the nursing process. Macmillan, Basingstoke

Fawcett J 1989 Analysis and evaluation of conceptual models of nursing, 2nd edn. Davis, Philadelphia

Fraser M 1996 Using conceptual nursing in practice: a research based approach, 2nd edn. Chapman and Hall, London

Page M 1995 Tailoring nursing models to clients' needs: using the Roper, Logan and Tierney model after discharge. Professional Nurse 19:284–288

Roper N, Logan W, Tierney A 1996 The elements of nursing: a model for nursing based on a model of living, 4th edn. Churchill Livingstone, London

Nursing models

Nursing models is a huge subject area and this chapter will have given you an introduction. To enhance your knowledge further, a selection of books and articles has been chosen to cover the models discussed within the chapter. They will be a useful reference for you whilst on clinical placement to learn more about the model in use in that area of practice.

Archibald G 2000 A post-modern nursing model. Nursing Standard 14(10):40–42

Coyne I 1996 Parent participation: a concept analysis. Journal of Advanced Nursing 23(4):733–740

Elliott-Cannon C 1990 Mental handicap and nursing models. In: Savage J, Kershaw B (eds) Models of nursing, 2nd edn. Scutari, Harrow

Hartwell D 1991 Dorothea Orem self-care deficit theory. Notes on Nursing Theory No 4. Sage, USA

Louette R 1991 Callista Roy: an adaptation model. Notes on Nursing Theory No 3. Sage, USA

Marriner-Tomey A 1994 Nursing theorists and their work, 3rd edn. Mosby, Missouri

Orem D 1985 Nursing concepts of practice, 3rd edn. McGraw-Hill, New York

Pearson A, Vaughan B 1994 Nursing models for practice. Butterworth-Heinemann, Oxford

Roberts D, Mackay G 1999 A nursing model of overdose assessment. Nursing Times 95(3):58–60

Roper N, Logan W W, Tierney A J 1996 The elements of nursing, 4th edn. Churchill Livingstone, Edinburgh

Tolson D 1996 The Roy Adaptation model: a consideration of its properties as a conceptual framework for an intervention study. Journal of Advanced Nursing 24(5):981–987

Walshe M 1998 Models and care pathways in clinical nursing: conceptual frameworks for care planning. Baillière Tindall, London

Wright S 1990 Building and using models of nursing, 2nd edn. Edward Arnold, London

Care pathways

This is a selection of further reading particularly related to the inter-agency and interprofessional care given to patients when a care pathway is used.

DoH 1995 Building bridges: a guide to arrangements for inter-agency working for the care and protection of severely mentally ill people. HMSO, London

Leathard A 1994 Going inter-professional: working together for health and welfare. Routledge, London

Lowe C 1998 Care pathways: have they a place in the new NHS? Journal of Advanced Nursing Management 6(5):303–306

Nott A 2000 The care pathway approach in an acute mental health inpatient department. Nursing Times 96(11):44–45

Herring L 1999 Critical pathways: an efficient way to manage care. Nursing Standard 13(47):36–37

Layton A, Moss F, Morgan G 1998 Mapping out the patient's journey: experiences of developing pathways of care. Quality in Health Care 7(supplement):S30–S36

Miller J 1995 Nursing patients through pathways of care. Professional Nurse 10(12):759–762

Scott E, Cowen B 1997 Multi disciplinary collaborative care pathways. Nursing Standard 12(1):39–42

Walsh M 1998 Models and critical pathways in clinical nursing, 2nd edn. Baillière Tindall, London

---

ESSENTIAL READING

UKCC 1998 Guidelines for records and record keeping. UKCC, London
OR *the summary of the above on*
http://www.ukcc.org.uk/NewStandards.htm

14

Safe nursing practice

Tracey Heath   Pam Taylor

CHAPTER CONTENTS

Introduction 392

Adopt a questioning approach 393
Getting started with reflection 393
Models for reflection 394

Inform your practice with up-to-date knowledge and evidence 398
Informed decision making 398
Policies, protocols and care pathways 399
Care pathways 400
Audit 401

Know your limitations 401
Professional self-regulation 402

Be aware of hazards in the environment 402
Health and safety for patients and staff 402
Infection control and the role of the nurse 403
What is infection? 403
Hospital infection 404
The infection control nurse and infection control policies 406
Policies and procedures in relation to infection control 407
Disposal of waste and equipment 407
Methicillin resistant *Staphylococcus aureus* (MRSA) 409
Food hygiene 410
Food regulations 410
Moving and handling 410
Safe administration of medicines 411
Storage 412
Prescribing 413
Administering 413
Self-administration 413
Receiving medicines 413
Practical skills of giving medication 414

Remember that prevention is the key 414
Nutrition 414
Assessing nutritional needs 415
Assisting patients with feeding 415
Hydration and fluid balance 416
Why is water so important? 416
Signs and causes of dehydration 417
Maintaining adequate hydration 417
Fluid balance charts 418
The importance of nursing observations 418
Routine clinical nursing observations and tests 419
Prevention of the complications of immobility 421
Deep vein thrombosis 421
Pressure sores 422
Helping patients and clients to wash and dress 423

Take prompt action in the case of an emergency 424
The process of cardiopulmonary resuscitation (CPR) 425
Possible causes of collapse 426

Communicate effectively 426
Informed consent for patients and clients 427
Obtaining consent 428
Documentation 429
Some principles of communicating well with patients and other personnel 429
Confidentiality 430

Report concerns 430

References 431

Further reading 432

Appendix 1 433

At the end of this chapter the student should be familiar with the essential principles of safe nursing practice and should:

- be aware of the value of reflecting on practice and the necessity for evidence-based practice
- understand the relevance of protocols and guidelines and the use of integrated care pathways
- know how to recognise one's own limitations and ask for guidance when needed
- be familiar with the most common hazards in the nursing environment and how to avoid danger to staff and patients
- be aware of the potential clinical problems that may result from actions or omissions by nurses in the course of their normal duties such as ensuring adequate nutrition and hydration and preventing the consequences of immobility
- know how to take prompt action to deal with emergencies such as sudden collapse and be familiar with the principles of cardiopulmonary resuscitation
- recognise the importance of good and effective communication, both verbal and written, in health care
- be aware of the need to maintain professional standards by promptly following the procedures and policies in place for reporting matters about which they may have concerns, for example non-accidental injury or suspected fraud.

INTRODUCTION

'The very first requirement in a hospital is that it should do the sick no harm'

Florence Nightingale
(Nightingale 1859, 2001)
((http:chatna.com/author/nightingale.htm))

The above often-quoted remark would appear no less appropriate today than when it was made by Florence Nightingale over a century ago. Furthermore, it is a sentiment that applies equally well to all sectors of health care and to all branches of nursing. Recent events would suggest, however, that we cannot take for granted the 'fact' that our practice causes 'no harm'; it is doubtful that we ever could.

During the 1990s, a number of prominent service failures in areas such as bone tumour diagnosis, paediatric cardiac surgery, cervical screening and wrong injection routes for powerful drugs have undoubtedly caused the public to revise their perception of the health care system and the people who work within it (Nicholls et al 2000). While the aforementioned examples may have made headline news, events in day-to-day practice frequently serve to remind us that we must constantly question our automatic assumption that health care does the patient no harm. For example, hospital acquired pressure sores, methicillin resistant *Staphylococcus aureus* (MRSA) and preoperative anxiety are all conditions that can have immensely detrimental physical, psychological and social consequences for the individual.

Perhaps today more than ever, given the complexity and pace of change within health care, we need to be clear and explicit in our attempts to assure both ourselves and the general public that our practices are safe and effective.

Clinical governance is a relatively new concept introduced into the British health care system by the Labour government in 1998. It is described as: 'a framework through which NHS organisations are accountable for continuously improving the quality of their services and safeguarding high standards of care by creating an environment in which excellence in clinical care will flourish' (DoH 1998).

Clinical governance encourages safe practice. Many of its central components are familiar to most health care professionals. Since the 1980s, quality has been high on the health care agenda. Concepts such as audit, clinical effectiveness, evidence-based practice and risk management are common currency. Clinical governance brings with it a greater emphasis on accountability and the need to be open and honest if errors are to be prevented and acted upon quickly when they do occur. Greater weight is also placed on patient or client and public involvement at all levels of service development.

Recent government policy changes will hopefully go some way towards increasing the public's confidence in the National Health Service and supporting nurses and other health care workers in their quest to deliver safe and effective care. Organisations such as the National Institute for Clinical Excellence (known as NICE) are already helping us to identify, through the development of national service frameworks and clinical guidelines, what good practice should look like. In this chapter we explore what these issues mean for the individual practitioner by considering the fundamental practice skills which nurses will undertake during their foundation year and beyond, and describing how nurses can ensure that their practice is safe, of high quality, and will 'do the patient no harm'.

The chapter is divided into eight themes which could be regarded as the eight essential principles of safe practice. They are:

- adopting a questioning approach
- informing your practice with up-to-date knowledge and evidence
- knowing your limitations
- being aware of hazards in the environment
- remembering that prevention is the key
- taking prompt action in the event of an emergency
- communicating effectively
- reporting concerns.

ADOPT A QUESTIONING APPROACH

The first principle of delivering safe and effective care is to adopt a questioning approach to your own practice and that of others. This involves not only being able to account for your actions – explaining why you are undertaking a particular activity and ensuring that you have the necessary knowledge and skill – but also reflecting on past situations and events to ensure that you maximise the learning available to you.

 Activity 14.1

Think for a moment of a time when you reflected. You may have quarrelled with someone, for example. When reflecting upon the incident, what did you do? What stages do you think we go through when we reflect?

Sometimes seemingly ordinary situations can teach us a great deal if we take the time to make sense of them. Reflection is a process many of us engage in outside our professional role when we are trying to make sense of an experience or situation we have been faced with (Activity 14.1).

When we reflect we describe, analyse and evaluate, and learn from our experience. That is, we recall the event and as many details as we can; we remember how we felt at the time, how we and others behaved and what influenced this; we make judgements about the positive and negative aspects of the incident; and we identify what we have learned, including how we might handle events differently next time (Case example 14.1).

GETTING STARTED WITH REFLECTION

Some people are naturally more reflective than others but everyone can learn these skills. The reflective process has its origins in experiential learning and is designed, as the term suggests, to help you to learn from your experiences. There is no one right way in which to reflect, or topic to reflect upon, but various models are available which may help to get you started. Activity 14.2 will help get you started on reflection in nursing practice.

The following are examples of issues upon which you may have decided to reflect:

- Why was I so eager to share with my friends the fact that I had undertaken my first injection?
- Why are students usually the ones asked to undertake the 'obs' (observations of patients' vital signs such as their temperature, pulse, respiration and blood pressure) on my current placement?

Case example 14.1

Sue had recently taken her friend to an expensive local restaurant as a birthday treat. When their chosen meal had arrived the friends noticed that the food was barely warm and that one of the side dishes was missing. Not wishing to complain, the girls ate the food, paid the bill (including the service charge) and set off for the cinema. Throughout the film Sue felt extremely angry, and hardly spoke a word to her friend during the walk home afterwards, except to complain about the restaurant.

Description
The following day Sue reflected upon the evening. She recalled the details of the event, how angry she had felt at the time and how sorry she now felt for 'spoiling' her friend's birthday treat. She also recalled how her friend had tried to engage her in conversation about the film and her forthcoming career move, but that she had not showed any real interest.

Analysis
Sue recognised that her anger had stemmed from the events in the restaurant. She was angry that the meal was not of an acceptable standard, especially as the venue had been highly recommended. Moreover she realised that she was angry with herself for not addressing the problem at the time, for paying the service charge and for letting the incident affect the rest of her evening.

Sue had wished to avoid confrontation but now realised that the staff were friendly and that there was no reason why the issue could not have been resolved amicably and quickly. She had not wished to make a 'fuss' or 'be trouble' but she recognised that she was within her rights to complain and that she had indirectly caused more 'fuss' by remaining angry all evening.

Evaluation
The event had been a negative experience on the whole, although she had realised what a good and patient friend she had.

Learning from the experience
Sue identified several things she would do next time. She would call the waiter over and explain the problem. If the issue was not resolved to her satisfaction she could explain that she would not be paying the service charge or visiting again in future. Furthermore, Sue recognised that should she not wish to say anything, that was her choice, but that nothing would be gained from continued anger. She would let the matter rest and enjoy the remainder of her evening.

• Why have I started to use abbreviations (such as TPR and BP, MSU) when I write or speak? What impact has this practice had on the patients I care for, and on myself?
• What makes my mentor a 'good' nurse?

 Activity 14.2

Think of a recent incident or issue from your nursing practice to reflect upon. You may choose:

• an incident which sticks in your mind and which you have replayed several times
• a time when you were particularly pleased with your practice
• a situation which you feel you did not handle too well
• an aspect of your own or someone else's behaviour that surprised you
• an activity which is carried out frequently and appears 'routine'
• something you heard in a lecture which made you think about your practice.

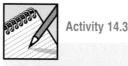 **Activity 14.3**

Try using Gibbs's (1988) cycle to reflect upon the incident or issue that you identified in Activity 14.2.

Now reflect on the same issue using Holm & Stephenson's (1994) framework or Johns's (1995) Model of Structured Reflection. Which did you find most helpful?

MODELS FOR REFLECTION

Some models are more complex and detailed than others. It is important to remember that they are tools to help you reflect, and that not all of the questions they contain will be relevant to every situation. As you become more experienced you may find the framework proposed by Gibbs (1988) provides sufficient guidance, or a more detailed framework may prove useful, such as that suggested by Holm & Stephenson (1994) or Johns (1995) (Fig. 14.1 and Activity 14.3).

Systematically reflecting upon an event may lead to learning that may have otherwise been missed. Writing down your reflections in a diary will provide evidence of your learning, a vital requirement throughout your career as a registered nurse. Case example 14.2 shows an example of reflection about an everyday activity in nursing and one with which many students will be familiar.

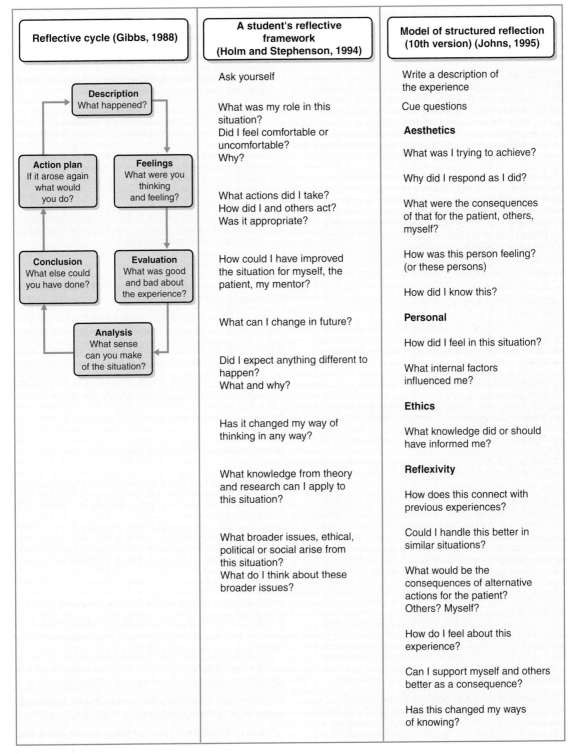

Reflective cycle (Gibbs, 1988)

Description
What happened?

Action plan
If it arose again
what would
you do?

Feelings
What were you
thinking
and feeling?

Conclusion
What else could
you have done?

Evaluation
What was good
and bad about
the experience?

Analysis
What sense
can you make
of the situation?

A student's reflective framework (Holm and Stephenson, 1994)

Ask yourself

What was my role in this situation?
Did I feel comfortable or uncomfortable?
Why?

What actions did I take?
How did I and others act?
Was it appropriate?

How could I have improved the situation for myself, the patient, my mentor?

What can I change in future?

Did I expect anything different to happen?
What and why?

Has it changed my way of thinking in any way?

What knowledge from theory and research can I apply to this situation?

What broader issues, ethical, political or social arise from this situation?
What do I think about these broader issues?

Model of structured reflection (10th version) (Johns, 1995)

Write a description of the experience

Cue questions

Aesthetics

What was I trying to achieve?

Why did I respond as I did?

What were the consequences of that for the patient, others, myself?

How was this person feeling? (or these persons)

How did I know this?

Personal

How did I feel in this situation?

What internal factors influenced me?

Ethics

What knowledge did or should have informed me?

Reflexivity

How does this connect with previous experiences?

Could I handle this better in similar situations?

What would be the consequences of alternative actions for the patient? Others? Myself?

How do I feel about this experience?

Can I support myself and others better as a consequence?

Has this changed my ways of knowing?

Figure 14.1 Frameworks to structure reflection.

Case example 14.2 Structured reflection using Gibbs's (1988) reflective cycle

Description: What happened?
My first ward as a student of nursing – it's cardiology. The first thing I am shown is how to put out an 'arrest call' and where the 'crash trolley' is. On my second day I'm left to do the 'obs'. This becomes a regular occurrence throughout my stay. I am told how important they are. I wonder why they are left to me with my inexperience and what would happen if I did them wrong.

Feelings: What were you thinking and feeling?
I felt really worried that I'd make a mistake, that I'd not count the patient's pulse and respirations properly or misread their blood pressure or temperature. My concern arose from my lack of confidence in my abilities. Did I know how to do observations correctly? No one had checked. I couldn't get these thoughts from my mind. What if important changes in the patients' condition were missed, and they died or were seriously ill? It would be all my fault – I could never forgive myself.

Evaluation: What was good and bad about the experience?
I was pleased to be trusted and at least I felt useful, but my overwhelming feelings at the time were anxiety and fear, making it rather difficult to see anything positive in the situation.

Analysis: What sense can you make of the situation?
Looking back I can understand my anxiety. I felt not only responsible for the task in hand but totally accountable too. I felt that all mistakes, omissions and their consequences would be my fault – I had the weight of the world on my shoulders.

I realise now that as a student my accountability is limited. In this situation my mentor was in charge and would be required to explain her decision to delegate the observations to me and not to check my accuracy (not that this would make me feel better if anything went wrong!). However, I also realise that if I am unsure of my ability to undertake a delegated task I must point this out. I didn't, and I think this is because I wanted to be seen as competent, to be useful and to fit in. I'm also not very good at saying 'no', probably because I want to be liked. Furthermore, my mentor and other staff always seem so busy and I didn't want to be a nuisance.

As a result of one of the lectures I received, I now also recognise that the assessment and monitoring of changes in the patient's condition consists of far more than doing their TPR and BP. Assessment has many facets and nurses look at their patients, not just their observation charts!

Conclusion: What else could have been done?
Perhaps people's expectations of me (and my own expectations of myself) were a little high considering it was only my second day. None the less, I could have improved some aspects of the situation by being less proud and admitting both my limited experience and my limited understanding of the delegated task.

Action plan: If such a situation arose again what would you do?
I have decided that in order to aid my own learning and promote safe practice, in future I will:

- practise my skills when I am unsure
- remember that I am a student and I need to learn and that this is my responsibility and that I must ask if unsure
- remember that I can say no and that I have a duty to tell my mentor if I am not yet proficient in any task
- read about observations and how to do them properly – what they are for and when to report readings immediately
- read about assessment in general and to remember that this includes consideration of the whole person not just their observation chart!

Reflection is perceived by many as forming a necessary part of our professional practice. There appears to be a general consensus that the process can enhance personal and professional learning and assist in the development of nursing knowledge (Jarvis 1992, Atkins & Murphy 1993, Palmer et al 1994, Hancock 1998, Wilkinson 1999). More specifically it is suggested that reflection:

- offers a tool to make sense of the world of practice
- can be used to help integrate theory and practice
- helps to advance learning from experience
- may increase self-awareness and insight into behaviour
- helps to facilitate the development of a critical thinking, problem-solving practitioner able to adapt to the ever changing world of health care.

However, while reflection is perceived to have a valuable role to play in the development of safe and effective practitioners, the process is not without its critics (Activity 14.4).

In response to Activity 14.4 you may have identified a number of potential problems with the process. For example, Newell (1992) suggests that reflection is flawed due to its reliance on memory. Quinn (1998) identifies three categories of concern about reflection. First, from an ethical standpoint, he suggests that there is little evidence for the

Activity 14.4

Reflective practice is popular within nursing and widely written about. However, there are some potential problems associated with the process. Can you identify any potential disadvantages or difficulties?

Case example 14.3 Using literature to improve patient care

I was working on a ward for older people and worked as part of the 'blue team', so I usually looked after the same group of patients with my mentor. One lady was constantly asking for the commode, as she was 'desperate' to pass urine. Yet when I fetched it (sometimes at 5-minute intervals) she hardly passed a drop. I started to ask if she was really sure she needed to go, indicating that I'd only just taken the commode away. I began to feel a little irritated. I even felt like ignoring the lady and walking by sometimes. I know this is awful but I had other things to do. At one point I really hoped that we would be in the 'green team' the following day!

Reflection on my practice assisted me in this case. Why was I getting so cross? Part of me was frustrated, I wanted to help, the lady seemed distressed and I didn't know what to do. The other part of me wished she would wait until she really needed to go. Remembering that my mentor had mentioned 'frequency' and 'urgency', I started by looking up these words and discovered that these were symptoms of numerous conditions such as the presence of a urinary infection or an unstable bladder. I knew that the lady didn't have an infection as they had said so in the hand-over report. Further reading revealed that if her bladder was 'unstable' we could probably help her to 'retrain' it. The key to being able to help it lies in thorough assessment of this lady's urinary problems. I discovered that many people can be cured, or at least made a lot more comfortable, but unfortunately only a limited number of individuals seek help, through embarrassment or the belief that nothing can be done. I now felt awful – I'd not understood, I'd assumed that she could wait, that she did not need to go.

I learned a great deal about myself from this incident and decided that I shouldn't be too quick to judge. The patient should guide me. Frequency and urgency are urinary symptoms with underlying causes. If my practice was to be safe and effective I not only needed to actively read to support my placement learning, but really 'listen' and respond to the patient. There was also a need to talk to other staff about the situation and agree a care plan to help this lady regain some bladder control rather than continue with just 'frequent toileting' which was achieving very little.

I also realised I like to fix things. I needed to think about this – I was sure there would be occasions when I couldn't.

effectiveness of reflection, yet individuals sometimes have little or no choice about engaging in the process. Second, from a professional perspective, it could be argued that reflection places the onus on the individual to maintain and improve standards of care (ignoring the potential role of the environment or context of care). There is also the suggestion that reflection may actually undermine confidence and morale by encouraging a constant review of practice, as if there are bound to be negative issues. Finally, pragmatic reservations include the time required and that the type of reflection discussed above is 'after the event' and of limited value.

On balance, however, this author believes that reflecting on practice is worthwhile and helpful, especially in the early stages of nursing or when encountering traumatic situations or when engaged in new activities. Reflection does not have to be a solo activity. If an incident is distressing or you are having difficulty making sense of an experience, learning and moving on from it, it may help to reflect with someone else, perhaps someone with more experience. Reading the literature associated with the area may also assist you to resolve difficult situations. See Case example 14.3 which is drawn from personal experience.

It is important to preserve the anonymity of those involved in the incidents you select for reflection. For example, when writing down events in order to reflect upon them or when discussing your reflections with your colleague or mentor, the names of individuals, hospitals or other practice areas, wards or teams should not be included. Confidentiality is an important aspect of the nurse–patient relationship and it is important that the codes of conduct governing your practice are observed throughout the reflective process.

Reflection has an important role to play in helping us to examine our practices. We need constantly to examine what we do in order to maximise the learning available to us and assure ourselves that we are safe and effective.

INFORM YOUR PRACTICE WITH UP-TO-DATE KNOWLEDGE AND EVIDENCE

INFORMED DECISION MAKING

Delivering safe and effective practice involves ensuring that what we do is based on the very best evidence. The evidence on which treatment and care decisions are based comes from a variety of sources (Activity 14.5).

In attempting Activity 14.5, you may have identified your lectures and the staff in the clinical area as major sources of knowledge. You have, no doubt, also identified other sources such as journal articles, books and research.

The term evidence-based practice entered the nursing profession's vocabulary in the 1990s. Yet nurses have endeavoured to base their practice on the very best evidence for many years. As early as 1972 the Briggs committee (DHSS 1972) recommended that nursing become a research-based profession, a sentiment reinforced many times since (DoH 1993, 1999).

Several professional and government-led initiatives have been set up to ensure that practice is informed by the best possible evidence. Examples include the Cochrane Library, the NHS Centre for Reviews and Dissemination (under the auspices of NICE) and the National Electronic Library for Health.

From the inception of the evidence-based practice movement there has been a great deal of emphasis on health care research. Moreover, certain types of research, for example that which takes the form of quantitative work (particularly randomised controlled trials), have traditionally

been viewed as more worthwhile than more qualitative, descriptive and exploratory studies. It is now increasingly recognised that both types of research evidence have a role to play in informing our practice. Even so, evidence, particularly evidence of effectiveness, is often represented in the form of a hierarchy, with the highest order, or best evidence at the top (Fig. 14.2).

While, ideally, it is recommended that the highest level of available evidence informs our practice, it must be remembered that not all research is good research and that even randomised controlled trials need to be appraised for their validity, reliability and usefulness.

However, nursing is a relatively young profession in the research stakes and this form of evidence is not available to inform all of our clinical and management decisions. It is doubtful, given the complexity of nursing practice, that this will ever be the case (see Ch. 12 for specific information on types of research and examples of effective and important nursing research). Other sources of evidence must therefore be recognised. Examples include:

- evidence based on experience
- evidence based on theory that is not research based
- evidence passed on by expert role models or through policy.

Activity 14.5

Think of a task or aspect of care you have carried out as part of your role as a student nurse. From where did you obtain the knowledge that informs this practice? How do you know that you are approaching this intervention in the correct manner? How do you know that the underpinning knowledge you have is based on the very best evidence?

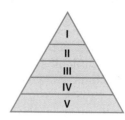

I   Systematic review in which well-designed randomized controlled trials feature

II Randomized controlled trial which is well designed and of appropriate size

III Trials without randomization or non-experimental studies (e.g. cohort or case control)

IV Qualitative studies

V   Opinions of respected authorities

Figure 14.2 A hierarchy of research evidence (based on Swage 2000).

Activity 14.6 Evidence-based decision making

Research studies are undertaken on large populations of people. Nurses and other health care professionals most frequently make decisions about individual patients or clients.

Choose a specific piece of research relevant to patients/clients in your practice area. Below is a series of questions which require you to consider in relation to evidence-based decision making at an individual patient/client level:

- What strategies does it recommend in order to help your patients/clients?
- Are some programmes more strongly recommended than others are? If so why? Is the evidence for these interventions stronger?
- Would the preferred intervention be suitable for a particular patient/client? Is it acceptable? Would it be tolerated? Can it still be employed given any other conditions or problems that the patient/client may have? Are there any risks associated with the treatments recommended? Would this patient/client be able to comply with all aspects of the treatment plan? Are there any other interventions worthy of consideration?
- What is the best way forward in this particular instance given your knowledge of the treatment/care plan and the characteristics of this particular patient/client?

Activity 14.7 Why is evidence-based practice important?

Consider the following questions. What does evidence-based practice have to offer:

- the patient/client?
- the nurse?
- the organisation, such as the NHS Trust?

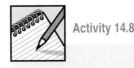

Activity 14.8

Have you noticed any tools in your practice area that help nurses and other health care professionals to decide what care to give and how that care may be best performed?

Furthermore, the right of the patient or client to make choices is also of vital importance in evidence-based decision making.

DiCenso and colleagues (1998) say that: 'in practising evidence-based nursing, a nurse has to decide whether the evidence is relevant for the particular patient. The incorporation of clinical expertise should be balanced with the risks and benefits of alternative treatments for each patient and should take into account the patient's unique clinical circumstances, including co-morbid conditions and preferences.' This illustrates the importance of assessing and negotiating with the patient or client the plan of treatment and care. It is applying the evidence from research or elsewhere to the individual being cared for that requires our professional knowledge and skill as nurses (Activities 14.6 and 14.7).

The use of the best available evidence to support practice is intended to enhance care, and lead to consistency in practice and a better-informed public. It is hoped that this in turn will contribute to an increase in the public's confidence in the health care system. From the nurse's perspective it is anticipated that the use of evidence to inform decision making will assist us to account for our practice and that the generation of such evidence will contribute to our body of knowledge as nurses. From an organisation's perspective, the use of the very best evidence to inform practice should contribute to a reduction in risk (and associated litigation), the best use of resources and an enhanced reputation.

There are many tools that provide a summary of the available evidence and help us to deliver safe and effective practice (Activity 14.8).

POLICIES, PROTOCOLS AND CARE PATHWAYS

The best available evidence is often translated locally into guidelines, protocols, principles of practice, and policies which are defined as follows:

- *Policies.* Statements that guide decision making and require employees of an organisation to work within certain parameters.
- *Guidelines.* Systematically developed statements to assist practitioner and patient decisions about appropriate health care for specific clinical circumstances (NHSE 1995).

- *Protocols.* A term often used to refer to a way of prescribing exactly what must be done in (often high risk) situations.
- *Principles of practice.* A statement which explains how things should be done.

It is important for you, as a student nurse, to ensure that you become familiar with the 'local scene' as a matter of priority. You will need to know the existence of policies and procedures in your practice placements, even if you are not expected to use them immediately. Such policies will include things such as care of drugs, patient or client control and restraint, care of patients' property, speaking out policy, patient resuscitation, fire procedures, Mental Health Act implications for patients' leave, child protection. There are many more, some examples of which are described later in this chapter or elsewhere in the book.

Care pathways

The use of care pathways has become increasingly important within health care today. A care pathway is an outline of anticipated clinical practice for a particular group of patients or clients with a particular diagnosis or set of symptoms. Successful care pathways are, normally, constructed by interdisciplinary care teams and they are derived from evidence-based practice. The National Pathways Association (1998) states that: 'An integrated care pathway determines locally agreed, multidisciplinary practice based on guidelines and evidence, where available, for a specific patient or client group. It forms all or part of the clinical record, documents the care given and facilitates the evaluation of outcomes for continuous quality improvement.'

Example of a care pathway (Appendix 1)

It is impossible in the space available for this chapter to give examples for all branches. Integrated care pathways are complex and result in the creation of large documents which constitute the patient's live record of care. The use of care pathways is still being developed in the NHS but you are most likely to see those which are for patients with conditions most often encountered.

The example shown at Appendix 1 (p. 430) is for myocardial infarction (heart attack) which is, of course, one of the most common causes of admission to the health care system today. It identifies the total care regimen, including admission to the accident and emergency department, through the coronary care unit and via a general ward to discharge into the care of a cardiac rehabilitation nurse. All aspects of the care are based on evidence-based 'best practice' for both medicine and nursing. At this stage, you will not necessarily know about all the medical treatments and drugs used, but the pathway does show the integration of all aspects of this person's care.

Important features of successful pathways include the fact that:

- they are agreed by all members of the multidisciplinary team or agencies involved in the patient's episode of care
- their focus is the patient or client rather than any one professional group
- the care contained within the pathway is based upon the very best evidence available (Activity 14.9).

Your answer to Activity 14.9 may have included the potential of care pathways to improve communication, not only between those delivering care but also between health professionals and the patient or client. This is an important benefit. Expectations are clearly mapped out in advance. Care pathway development necessitates the review of existing practice and its continual monitoring. They can also help to promote evidence-based practice and reduce unwanted variations in care delivery. You may also have identified their potential use as a teaching tool for students and new team members. In short, care pathways

Activity 14.9 The advantages of care pathways

Reflect for a moment on the descriptions of care pathways in this section of the chapter. What do you perceive to be the advantages of care pathways?

promote many of the activities required to ensure the delivery of safe and effective care.

However, care pathways are not without their critics. For example there is a belief that they will reduce clinical judgement or be used unthinkingly, resulting in poorer, rather than enhanced, care. Clearly this depends on how they are introduced. Whether care pathways are in place or not, nurses and other health care professionals are still accountable for their actions, and decisions still need to be made about the appropriateness of standard actions for individual patients and clients. Professional judgement and patient preference cannot be suspended if practice is to be safe and effective rather than routine.

Audit

Care pathways are not the only method of ensuring that practice is evidence based. Earlier we identified the use of other tools such as guidelines and protocols. Audit is another important strategy and widely used in all areas of health and social care today. Audit of practice is usually integrated within a care pathway, but it can be undertaken independently in conjunction with guidelines and standards. Audit involves reviewing practice and ensuring that it is in accordance with that defined as 'the best', and that action is taken to rectify the situation when shortfalls occur.

Delivering safe and effective care based on the very best evidence requires active efforts to keep abreast of new knowledge: national and international strategies are in place to facilitate this process. Evidence of continuing professional development (which involves keeping abreast of the latest knowledge and evidence) is a requirement to remain on the register as a nurse and is vital if we are to be accountable practitioners, able to reason for our actions. Chapter 1 provides details of the continuing professional education requirements for nurses today.

KNOW YOUR LIMITATIONS

When one considers the expectations placed on nurses in practice today, it is little wonder that they are sometimes faced with new and complex situations beyond their existing knowledge and experience. For a student of nursing this is clearly to be expected, yet given the dynamic and changing face of health care it is a situation that you can expect to face well beyond registration. Progress means that as nurses we are expected continually to learn and develop our practice, for example through reflection, further academic study and supervised practice.

As discussed in Chapter 11, nurses are accountable for their practice, that is they must be able to explain the reasoning behind their decisions and actions. The accountability of nurses and other health care professionals is primarily to the patients and clients in their care but nurses are also accountable to the employing organisation, to other members of the profession and to the professional body (UKCC).

Accountability means not only knowing how to carry out a particular aspect of care, but also being clear about the limitations of your knowledge and experience. Although as nursing students your accountability is limited, the principles still apply as listed in the Code of Conduct (described in Ch. 11). In order to be safe in practice it is vital that we are aware of our limitations as well as our strengths, and that we know when to seek advice and support. This may not always be easy, especially in the early stages of your training (Activity 14.10).

Your response to the question in Activity 14.10 may have included some, or perhaps all, of the following:

- you may have feared looking foolish
- you may have already asked once before but were unable to remember or did not grasp the response

 Activity 14.10

Although it is an important part of providing safe and effective practice that we do not undertake tasks for which we do not feel prepared and for which we are not competent, it can sometimes be very difficult to say no or seek help. Why might this be the case?

Activity 14.11

Think of a situation in which you felt unprepared to undertake the task asked of you. Use one of the frameworks provided earlier to reflect upon this incident.

What was your response? Did you undertake the task or ask for help? Why did you behave in this way? What factors influenced your judgement? Would you deal with the situation in the same way next time, or would you do things differently?

- the nurses may have looked busy and you did not wish to interrupt them
- you may have asked questions in the past and received a curt response.

It is important to understand the concept of accountability and to know how to handle situations for which you feel ill prepared (Activity 14.11).

Case example 14.4 describes a situation in which a student nurse is reflecting on facing up to her limitations and how she would act differently in future, to ensure safe and effective care.

PROFESSIONAL SELF-REGULATION

Self-regulation is a privilege granted by parliament. It is not a right. It has to be earned continually to sustain public trust and confidence in the profession. Integral to self-regulation is the onus placed on each and every member of a profession, including the nursing profession, to ensure that his or her practice is safe and effective. Chapter 11 covers this in some detail.

BE AWARE OF HAZARDS IN THE ENVIRONMENT

HEALTH AND SAFETY FOR PATIENTS AND STAFF

Environmental awareness begins shortly after birth and continues throughout life and, ideally, people make choices in the nature and style of their personal environment. This is true even for the ill or disabled, who devote much energy

Case example 14.4 Knowing my limitations

It was during my first placement on an orthopaedic ward that the incident took place. My mentor had arranged for me to attend fracture clinic, something I was looking forward to. When I got there it was suggested that I join the doctor and nurse covering clinic 'A'. I spent the first hour watching patients be booked in, called through, seen by the doctor and leave. It was interesting and a lot busier than I'd expected. I was then sent to fetch some medical notes that had been left in reception. On my return the staff nurse was nowhere to be seen and the buzzer for the next patient was sounding. I didn't know what to do, I looked around, and all staff appeared to have vanished. The doctor came out, I explained that I was unsure where the staff nurse had gone. He said 'Not to worry, you can do it. Call in the next patient or we will be running late'. I had watched the staff nurse, so I did as I thought she had done. I soon realised how difficult it was. I was unfamiliar with the abbreviations used, I had never heard of half of the words used and found it quite impossible to spell them. When I was asked for the simplest thing it took me ages to find it and I just got more and more flustered.

I felt really distressed by the time the nurse returned. She apologised immediately and told me that I should have fetched someone else. I went home and worried … what if I had heard the doctor's instructions incorrectly or if what I had managed to write down did not make sense? Would the patient get the 'wrong' care? I began to feel angry for being put in the situation. I was angry with both the doctor and the staff nurse, it was their fault!

On reflection the nurse was right – I should have persisted in my attempt to get some assistance, but I panicked and did not want to look foolish. The fact that I didn't know the staff seemed to make getting help harder; I wasn't sure how they would respond as they were clearly busy. Would they be angry? I did not want to be a nuisance.

I learned a great deal about myself from this incident. I like to be seen as competent and helpful and I find it very difficult to say 'no' when asked to do something.

However, I now recognise that I was putting my need to look good before the safe and effective care of the patients. Perhaps the staff nurse should not have left me, but this will happen occasionally. Although I recognise that as a student I do not carry full professional accountability in situations such as this, it is my responsibility to make the limitations of my knowledge and experience known. Next time, if faced with a situation I feel ill-prepared for, I will speak out. This will not only reduce my anxiety about being left in similar situations, but will be in the interests of safe patient care.

towards accomplishing tasks to fulfil their wish of being master of their personal environment. The quality of the health and safety of our environment is greatly affected by the environment itself, and never more so than in the health care setting, where patients and clients may be more vulnerable than when in their own homes. Florence Nightingale suggested that patients in health care settings may be harmed just by being there. Recent media reports about hospital acquired infection in the UK highlight the need for health care professionals to be vigilant about this and other potential hazards to patients. So, a major task for all is to promote and maintain a safe environment. Of course, the health and safety of staff is also important and the Health and Safety Commission (1992) places a general duty on employers to ensure the health and safety of employees.

Promoting a safe environment is one of the many functions of the nurse. In fact, the UKCC Code of Professional Conduct makes this explicit by requiring nurses to ensure that no action they undertake is detrimental to the safety and well-being of patients, and to ensure that they report any unsafe practice or environmental danger which might affect the safety of either patients or staff (see Ch. 11 for further details of the Code of Conduct). Within this section of the chapter only three specific nursing activities are covered and the important issue of the prevention of pressure sores is covered later.

INFECTION CONTROL AND THE ROLE OF THE NURSE

Today, disposable items such as dressings, gloves, aprons and other equipment are the norm in hospitals and in the community, and were introduced to prevent the spread of infection. It is therefore of grave concern to learn that, at the time of writing, hospital acquired infection is at its highest, with infections that cannot be cured with the present range of antibiotics (e.g. MRSA – methicillin resistant *Staphylococcus aureus*). Reasons related to the over-use of antibiotics have contributed to this problem but the role of the nurse in preventing the spread of infection remains important.

Awareness of pathogens such as the HIV virus and the more sophisticated use of chemotherapy for the treatment of cancer call for more diligence in relation to the cleanliness of the patient's environment and to preventing cross-infection.

What is infection?

An infection is caused when the body is invaded by pathogenic (disease producing) organisms, either bacteria or viruses. Infection is usually accompanied by a high temperature (pyrexia), sweating, and sometimes even causes a rigor. If the infection is associated with a wound then this will be red, hot and inflamed and the patient will complain of pain around the inflamed area. All these signs and symptoms are the body's response to the presence of a pathogen. Bacteria are smaller than the average body cell (this is why they are called microorganisms) but they are larger than viruses. They are unicellular and are often found attached to one another in clusters or chains. They are known according to their shape, for example 'cocci' are spherical, e.g. *Staphylococcus aureus* which is found in the nose and around the face, and bacilli which are straight, rod-shaped cells, e.g. *Escherichia coli* which is a common bacterium found in the gut.

As we cannot see bacteria or viruses it is difficult to understand how they cause infection and how it is spread. This of course was the problem in the past before microscopes became more powerful and microbiologists were able to identify individual organisms and discover how bacteria and viruses invaded the body and were transferred from one person to another. Box 14.1 shows how cross infection from person to person, or from implements or the atmosphere can occur.

Pathogenic microorganisms are around in the atmosphere all the time and on the body most of the time and it is almost impossible to make the air 'germ free'. Some bacteria live on the body and are not harmful (commensals) unless they gain entry, made easier if suffering from disease or following an accident or operation. The most common hospital-acquired infections are of the urinary tract (mostly in catheterised patients), the lower respiratory tract, the skin and wounds.

Box 14.1 How pathogens enter the body

- Ingestion through the mouth, e.g. ingestion of contaminated food or water.
- Inhalation through the nose, e.g. breathing in microorganisms from the atmosphere, particularly bacteria and viruses causing sore throats, coughs and colds leading to chest infections. The respiratory system may also succumb to more contagious aerobic bacteria such as *Mycobacterium tuberculosis*, which causes tuberculosis. Patients on artificial breathing machines are specifically at risk.
- Via the skin, through abrasions, wounds, including open pressure sores and 'compound' fractures, i.e. the bone has broken the skin. Burns, particularly those covering large areas of the body, are so prone to infection that these patients have to be nursed in specially designed units aimed at reducing infection to the minimum. An incision made in order to undertake an operation may be sutured afterwards, but still provides a portal of entry for infection. There is the potential for infection to occur even when the skin is broken.
- Injections of any kind, intravenous fluids, central venous pressure lines, and transfusing blood and blood products including contaminated blood.
- Invasive procedures such as catheterisation, bladder washouts, chest drainage, wound drainage.
- Changing dressings.

All bacteria can be grown in the laboratory using special culture media, and then identified under the microscope. Having cultivated a bacterium, antibiotics can then be tested on them for their sensitivity (to see if they can be destroyed). If they are sensitive to a certain antibiotic, then this will be recommended to the doctor as the drug of choice. Antibiotics have been developed against most common bacteria. However, because of the prolific use of antibiotics and, in some cases, patients not taking the full course of tablets prescribed, certain bacteria have become resistant to the antibiotics available.

This is the case with MRSA (methicillin resistant *Staphylococcus aureus*) which is now common in hospitals. Viruses are too small to be identified in this way, and do not respond to antibiotics but can be just as virulent.

Hospital infection

'Whatever the setting, *everyone* who works in health care establishments is responsible for maintaining a safe environment' (Parker 1999). Despite a great increase in the legislation governing working practice in hospitals aimed at reducing cross-infection, the situation appears to be getting worse rather than better. Parker's statement is therefore very relevant and demonstrates that such an important issue cannot be considered to be the sole responsibility of the microbiology department or the infection control nurse. One of the simplest, and probably the single most important contribution to the prevention of cross-infection, is hand washing, which nurses and all clinical staff are taught as a matter of priority and yet it is sometimes rushed or neglected altogether. *Disposable gloves may protect you, but they do not protect your patients unless you wash your hands and change your gloves between each procedure or patient.* At the time of writing, as HM Government is trying to reduce the spread of infection in hospitals, charge nurses are being urged and supported to insist that all medical and other staff wash their hands between every patient on every round and in every clinic! Knowing how to wash hands is important (Box 14.2). Figure 14.3 illustrates those areas of the hand most often missed during washing.

In the operating theatre 'scrubbing up' area, hand washing at its best can be seen.

Disposable gloves and aprons

Disposable gloves and aprons do more harm than good if they are not used and disposed of correctly. A habit of abiding by some simple principles will give greater protection to your patient, preventing cross-infection.

Aprons. Sometimes plastic aprons are supplied in different colours for different tasks, e.g. for serving meals or doing dressings. Aprons should be worn:

- for all situations where there is direct patient contact
- where there is contact with body fluids
- handling bed linen, excreta or clinical waste
- handling items that have been in contact with infectious disease, including clothes and books.

Box 14.2 Hand washing

- The hands should be washed before and after all patient contact.
- To prevent cross-infection, jewellery should not be worn, a plain wedding ring only is permissible, and it is preferable not to wear a watch on the wrist.
- A waterproof, occlusive dressing should cover any cuts or abrasions.
- A sink with elbow- or foot-operated mixer taps is best, the temperature of the water adjusted so that it is comfortable and the flow steady so that it avoids splashing the surrounding area.
- Liquid soap or antiseptic detergent hand washing solution should be used, applying sufficient to create a good lather. Scrubbing the skin with a nail-brush is *not* recommended as this causes abrasions, but the fingernails may be scrubbed.
- Wash hands thoroughly under running water and then rinse them, making sure that all traces of soap/detergent are removed.
- Turn off the taps using elbows or feet, but keeping your hands pointing upwards, to avoid water from the wrist area and above which has not been washed coming into contact with the washed area.
- Dry hands well to minimise growth of micro-organisms and to prevent the hands from becoming sore.
- Dispose of used towels in a foot-operated waste bin.

To use them:

- wash and dry hands before putting on the apron
- pull the apron over your head, trying to avoid touching the hair or uniform
- tie the apron loosely at the back so that any liquid will quickly run off
- remove the apron by pulling the neckband and the sides, thus breaking the ties, and fold the apron in on itself to prevent the spread of microorganisms
- do not allow your hands to touch your uniform, and discard the used apron into the yellow clinical waste bag
- wash and dry your hands thoroughly.

Disposable gloves (non-sterile). The use of gloves does not reduce the need to wash the hands before and after the gloves have been worn. This is because the hands sweat and create a warm, moist environment that will encourage microorganisms to thrive. Another reason for this is that the gloves may not completely protect the hands as they have been shown to develop tiny puncture holes that go undetected, but allow microorganisms to enter. Seamless, single-use

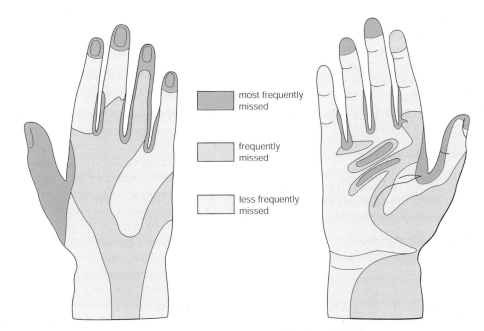

most frequently missed

frequently missed

less frequently missed

Figure 14.3 Areas most frequently missed in hand washing (Nicol et al 2000).

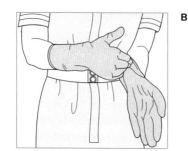
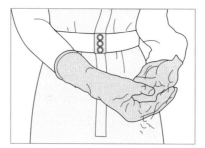
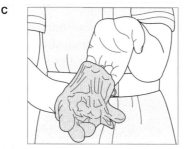

Figure 14.4 Safe removal of gloves (Nicol et al 2000).

latex or vinyl gloves are recommended. These come in three sizes and fit either hand.

Gloves:

- should be worn whenever patient care involves dealing with blood or other body fluids
- may be required when in contact with a patient who has an infection, e.g. hepatitis, HIV or MRSA
- should be worn when giving certain intramuscular drugs such as antibiotics.

Choosing the correct size of glove is important as too large or too small could impair dexterity. If gloves are required for a clean procedure these should be taken from the clean area rather than those stored in the sluice. To use gloves:

- wash and dry hands thoroughly
- take the correct size of glove from the appropriate area
- to remove the gloves, do not touch your wrists or hands with the dirty gloves. Using a gloved hand, pinch up the cuff of the other hand and pull the glove off inside out. Using

the ungloved hand, insert it behind the cuff, and pull the other glove off, turning it inside out (Fig. 14.4)
- used gloves should be discarded immediately into the yellow clinical waste bag.

The infection control nurse and infection control policies

Every hospital Trust will have an infection control team which will include a specialist infection control nurse. Infection control nurses are qualified experienced nurses, who have usually taken a further course on infection control. They are there to advise staff on how to prevent cross-infection and care for patients with infectious diseases, and to assist in the interpretation of hospital policies and procedures dealing with infection control. They are very much involved in finding and implementing the latest research on infection control, advising on new products and updating nursing procedures. They work closely with the microbiology department and the health and safety officer (Activity 14.12).

Activity 14.12

- Find out who your infection control nurse is, and how he or she can be contacted.
- Locate your infection control manual.

Policies and procedures in relation to infection control

Much can be achieved by reducing the level of pathogenic organisms in the environment by routine cleaning. With the amount of movement of personnel, visitors and the high turnover of patients, any environment where patients or clients are nursed or where they are resident can quickly become contaminated with dust, soil and debris, along with organic matter and potentially infectious organisms. A safe environment can easily be achieved by following simple guidelines on the disposal of contaminants and by introducing routine and effective cleaning. In fact, at the time of writing there is a major government initiative, with funding, to 'clean up' hospitals as part of the drive to reduce hospital acquired infections.

Chadwick & Oppenheim (1996) state that cleaning the hospital environment is a cost-effective method of controlling infection. Routine cleaning with household detergents and hot water is considered sufficient to maintain the appearance of the building and reduce the number of microbes in the environment (Collins 1988). A clean environment inspires confidence in patients, relatives and staff. It is also well known that certain organisms responsible for hospital acquired infections such as *Staphylococcus aureus* and *Escherichia coli* survive for long periods in most environments. If the environment is not cleaned regularly there will be a build-up of dust and debris that will support the growth of these and other microorganisms. The report from the Standing Medical Advisory Committee sub-group on antimicrobial resistance (SMAC 1998) states that the role of hospital cleaning staff is fundamental to controlling the spread of multiresistant microorganisms.

At the same time, the House of Lords Select Committee on Science and Technology (1998) wants infection control and basic hygiene to be placed 'at the heart of good hospital management and practice'.

All hospitals have to produce an infection control policy and this should be read and made easily accessible for all hospital personnel. Infection control policies should include the following topics:

- contact telephone numbers of appropriate personnel such as the infection control nurse and key personnel in the microbiology department who will give advice and guidance
- admissions, transfers and discharges (patients with known or suspected infection)
- cleaning, disinfection and decontamination, if necessary, of medical equipment
- how to handle outbreaks of diarrhoea, hepatitis, meningitis and other notifiable infectious diseases
- specific guidance on handling patients with MRSA and HIV infection
- handling laundry
- food handling
- waste disposal
- disposal of 'sharps' (i.e. syringes and needles) including dealing with injuries
- collection of specimens
- control of pests (e.g. cockroaches, fleas)
- control of hazardous substances and spillages.

Disposal of waste and equipment

As student nurses you will need to be aware of the exact procedures in your practice placements. If in doubt regarding the disposal of waste or equipment, ask! There is always someone to help – either the procedure will be explained in the local infection control manual or the health and safety manual or call the infection control nurse. It is important to understand what is meant by the terminology 'cleaning', 'disinfection' and 'sterilisation' (Box 14.3).

As a result of European legislation, the Medical Devices Agency (MDA) has been given full

Box 14.3 **Some definitions** (Medical Devices Agency 1996)

Cleaning
A process which physically removes contamination but does not necessarily destroy microorganisms. The reduction of microbial contamination is dependent upon many factors, including the efficiency of the cleaning process and the initial amount of microbial contamination. Cleaning removes microorganisms and the organic material on which they thrive. It is a necessary prerequisite of effective disinfection and sterilisation.

Disinfection
A process used to reduce the number of viable microorganisms but which may not necessarily inactivate some microbial agents, such as certain viruses and bacterial spores. Disinfection may not achieve the same reduction in microbial contamination level as sterilisation.

Sterilisation
A process used to render an object free from viable microorganisms including viruses and spores.

responsibility to carry out the directives required in the UK. The definition of medical devices is any instrument, apparatus, appliance or material or other article, whether used alone or in combination (including software) on human beings for the purpose of diagnosis, prevention, treatment, investigation, replacement or modification of the anatomy, control of conception, and certain pharmacological products.

The Department of Health has issued guidance on all medical devices which need to be inspected, serviced, repaired or transported, and the requirement of a declaration of contamination status (NHS Management Executive 1995). Staff should refuse to handle such equipment if it is not accompanied by documentation indicating that it has been decontaminated.

Devices are designated for single or multiple use (MDA 1996), and this should be adhered to. Recycling items such as opened packs of wound care products, unused swabs and dressings from packs, or sharing topical creams between patients, reusing nebulisers, oxygen masks, failing to change sheets, pillowcases, blankets or duvets between patients, all increase the risk of cross-contamination.

Clinical waste

Any waste generated in the health care setting that has been in contact with blood or other body fluids is classified as clinical waste and must be *incinerated*. Examples are: soiled dressings, swabs, wound drainage tubes and bags, catheters, urine drainage bags, sputum pots, incontinence pads, used gloves and aprons.

All clinical waste should be disposed of in *yellow plastic bags* for incineration.

Non-clinical waste

This is general waste that poses no risk to the public, for example packaging, dead flowers, paper hand towels. Non-clinical waste should be disposed of in *black plastic bags*.

Needles and other 'sharps'

Many clinical procedures require the use of a needle, scalpel or lancet which is capable of puncturing the skin. Consequently they become contaminated and could pose a danger to health care workers if they are not used and disposed of in a responsible manner. All sharps must be discarded into a special *yellow sharps bin*, which is rigid, puncture resistant and leak-proof. It will have a special opening that is designed to allow sharps to be dropped in, but will not allow them to be taken out or spill over should the container topple over. Sharps bins should not be used once they are three-quarters full, they should then be sealed so that they cannot be reopened.

The safe disposal of needles and sharps is the responsibility of the user, and they should not be left for someone else to clear away. Used needles should not be re-sheathed and should not be separated from the syringe. They should be disposed of as soon as possible using a sharps bin with a needle removing facility if available. If this is not possible they should be left in a rigid container. Always make sure you know where the sharps bin is before you use any sharp implement.

Linen

Used linen refers to the majority of linen that has been used but is not soiled (e.g. sheets, towels, clothing). To prevent contact with your uniform a plastic apron should be used when making beds or handling used linen. Used linen should be placed immediately into a polythene or fabric linen bag.

Soiled or *fouled* linen refers to linen that has been contaminated with blood or other body fluids or excreta. To prevent leakage, this linen should be placed in a plastic bag indicated for this purpose (according to local policy) and then placed in bag for used linen. It will then be handled separately in the laundry.

Infected linen refers to linen from patients with infectious conditions such as MRSA, salmonella, hepatitis, pulmonary tuberculosis or HIV. This linen is placed in a specific plastic bag identified for this purpose and then in another linen bag (often red or with red markings, but check your local policy). The linen is not handled by anyone as the plastic bag has special water-soluble seams which dissolve when they come onto contact with the high temperature wash at 95°+C.

General equipment

Equipment such as washing bowls, commodes, mattresses and beds must be washed with hot water and detergent and dried thoroughly between each patient to avoid cross-infection. Washing bowls in particular can be a source of infection if not cleaned correctly. Abrasives should not be used as this roughens the surface, giving a good surface for micro-organisms to adhere to and multiply. Once washed and dried, it is preferable to store them upside down in a pyramid to allow air to circulate rather than stacking them one inside the other.

Methicillin resistant *Staphylococcus aureus* (MRSA)

As mentioned above, most hospitals have a specific policy regarding patients with MRSA.

Because of the concern over the rising number of cases of MRSA it is worth considering the management of such cases. It was first reported in the UK in 1961 and has been responsible for many outbreaks of infection. As we have seen, *Staphylococcus aureus* is a common bacterium that may be carried naturally in the nose of healthy people and not cause problems. Alternatively it may cause wound or skin infections but these respond to antibiotics. It is only when the bacterium becomes resistant to certain antibiotics that it is referred to as MRSA. It has become more prevalent in the last 10 years in this country and now worldwide as a result of the increased use of antibiotics. Patients sometimes bring MRSA into hospital without their or our knowledge from other hospitals at home or abroad. For this reason it is important to screen such patients. There is no evidence that MRSA poses a risk to health care workers or their families. Similarly there is no justification for discriminating against people who have MRSA by treating them with prejudice or refusing them admission.

How to prevent the spread of MRSA (also applicable to HIV infections)

Basic infection control principles are adequate to prevent spread and protect staff from MRSA:

- Hand washing is essential and should be carried out as described in Box 14.2. This should occur after any contact with the patient or client and before contact with another patient.
- All cuts and grazes should be covered with waterproof plaster. Staff with skin problems such as eczema or psoriasis must not attend patients with MRSA.
- Wear gloves and apron for all patient contact and discard immediately on leaving the patient.
- Any equipment that comes into contact with the patient should be thoroughly cleaned with soap/detergent and water before use by anyone else.
- Linen should be bagged separately and identified as infected linen (usually a red bag).
- Cutlery and crockery should be washed as usual.

FOOD HYGIENE

Food regulations

Since the outbreak of salmonella food poisoning at the Stanley Royal Hospital in Wakefield in 1984 (DHSS 1986), in which 19 patients died, several new pieces of legislation have been passed regarding the preparation and serving of food. Despite this, outbreaks of food poisoning continue to occur. The Food Safety (General) Regulations (Department of Health 1995) document forms the basis of good practice in any catering establishment and this includes hospitals. The regulations cover the training of food handlers and details the processes required in order to provide food that is fit for consumption. Nurses are, of course, closely involved with food preparation, food handling and assisting patients with their meals. Any of these occasions could be an opportunity for a drop in food hygiene standards that could result in food poisoning. All nurses should receive instruction on food hygiene and observe the following safety points (DoH 1990):

- wash hands before touching or preparing food
- wash hands after dealing with patient's needs
- wash hands after using the toilet or seeing to a patient's toiletry needs
- cover cuts and sores with brightly coloured waterproof plaster so that it can be easily identified if it falls into food
- do not cough or sneeze over food
- do not pick your nose, touch your hair, lips or mouth when serving food, unless you wash your hands immediately afterwards
- keep equipment and utensils clean
- keep food clean and covered, and handle it as little as possible
- keep lids on waste sacks and dustbins.

Although the preparation of food is usually the responsibility of the kitchen staff and catering manager, it is useful for nurses to be aware of the commonest reasons for the outbreak of food poisoning, which are (Barrie 1996):

- preparing food too far in advance of the event
- storing food at room temperature

- cooling food too slowly before putting in the refrigerator
- not re-heating food to a temperature that would kill food poisoning bacteria
- using food that is already contaminated, especially poultry
- undercooking meat, meat products and poultry
- inadequate thawing of frozen foods
- cross-contamination between raw and cooked food
- keeping hot food below 63°C
- infected food handlers.

Nurses have a responsibility to see that all patients are appropriately fed (UKCC 1997). This will be dealt with later in the chapter but, initially, this means keeping hot food hot (above 63°C) and cold food cold (below 5°C). Meals should be served immediately they arrive and if there is any delay or the patient is out of the ward then a fresh meal should be requested. Meals should not be reheated in the microwave in a clinical area, unless it can be confirmed that the food reaches a temperature of 75°C and has been heated uniformly. All hospitals issue guidelines regarding the handling of food and failure to follow these may result in prosecution under the Food Safety Act of 1990.

MOVING AND HANDLING

The safe moving and handling of both patients and any heavy items within the workplace can obviously not be dealt with adequately in a textbook. But a consideration of hazards in the environment – to patients or staff – would be incomplete without a reference to the importance of safe moving and handling. Back injury is one of the commonest causes of time off work for nurses and still causes long-term injury and disability for some. From a patient's viewpoint, being moved and handled with care is a critical issue if you are immobile, disabled, critically ill or in pain (or any combination of these) and where movement is an essential part of your recovery or rehabilitation. All nurses must learn how to lift correctly for the sake of their patients and for themselves. It will be one of the earliest practical skills taught, and one which no nurse should enter the practice setting without having learned.

The implementation of a number of European directives in 1992 led to important changes in health and safety requirements in relation to manual handling and moving. These directives stipulate that employers have a duty to ensure the safety of all employees involved in manual handling and moving. Employers have a responsibility to make a thorough assessment and implement measures to avoid risk or minimise it to the greatest possible degree. Employees also have a responsibility to obey reasonable and lawful instructions in relation to moving and handling and to act with reasonable care and skill. These directives mean that employers have a responsibility to provide the correct and sufficient lifting aids, and appropriate training (and updating) in moving and handling; and employees have a duty to use the aids and attend all available training.

Many health care organisations are working towards safer handling or no-lifting policies. The provision of, and training in, the use of no-lifting equipment, such as hoists, transfer aids (for from trolley to bed, bed to bed, etc.) has extended considerably during the last 10 years. Not only does this help to prevent injury for the nurse, but it also ensures that patients are not damaged by bad lifting and moving which can result in shearing force on the skin of back, buttocks and heels or dislocation of shoulders by being heaved up the bed with an underarm lift. Description of the techniques involved is not possible in this book, and safe moving and lifting can only be learned in practice with a skilled instructor. But the main principles to be applied to any handling situation are seen in Box 14.4.

Moving and handling patients within an acute hospital setting, with the availability of other colleagues and lifting aids, is more easily achieved safely than trying to move a patient in their own home, in a low bed and without the support of staff and mechanical aids. Community nurses are able to obtain lifting aids and will always take a colleague to assist with lifting. The principles of safe moving and handling are still applied.

Box 14.4 Principles of safe handling

- From your first day in practice, never put yourself at risk, never lift alone, find out where all the lifting aids are.
- Assess the situation for moving the patient.
- Communicate clearly with your partner/s so that all know what to expect and do.
- Avoid tensing your muscles.
- Adopt a stable stance – this usually means having your feet about a hip-width apart.
- Keep your knees 'soft' or bent.
- Keep the load as close to your body as possible and avoid stretching.
- Avoid twisting or bending sideways.

SAFE ADMINISTRATION OF MEDICINES

It is beyond the scope of this book to go into great detail regarding the administration of medicines, but all nurses should familiarise themselves with their local nursing policy regarding this subject. It is one of the most important responsibilities of nurses, whatever branch they may pursue. This chapter is about safety, and that is the key issue in this procedure. New medicines are introduced daily and it is the nurse's responsibility to gain a sound knowledge base regarding the medicines she is dealing with, their purpose, action and side-effects, the patient's needs, the environment in which they are given. Unfortunately, prescribing or administering the wrong drug or the wrong dose can happen, as can theft of controlled drugs from the health care environment, presenting a potential hazard to patients and others. Management of drugs and their administration is, therefore, a strictly controlled process and one which all nurses need to learn in the early stages of training. Educating patients about their drug regimens is a key teaching role for the nurse, as well as evaluating the effectiveness of the drugs.

In your first year, you will almost certainly be involved in assisting with the administration of medicines. If your experience is in an acute care setting, the 'medicine round' with the 'drug trolley' will become a familiar event. In a community setting, such as a care home for people with learning disability or a rehabilitation centre for people with mental health problems, the administration of medicines may not look as formal but the principles of safe storage, administration and recording are still strictly applied. The administration of medicines is not solely a mechanistic task to be performed in strict compliance with the written prescription of a medical officer: it requires knowledge, thought and the exercising of professional judgement.

The administration of medicines is an important aspect of professional practice of all those on the UKCC's Register. The Council makes it clear in its Code of Professional Conduct (UKCC 1992a) that all practitioners, including student nurses, are responsible and accountable for the safe administration of medicines. In their *Standards for the Administration of Medicines* (UKCC 1992b), the Council recommends that all medicines should be administered by a first-level nurse or midwife.

The treatment of patients with medicines may be for therapeutic, diagnostic or preventative purposes. The term 'medicines' or 'drugs' covers not only oral tablets, pills, capsules, suppositories and drugs given intravenously and intramuscularly, but also medical gases, medicated dressings and parenteral infusions. There are specific guidelines for the administration of medication to children, and a book on nursing practice along with local policies will give details of the different types of administration. The general principles are dealt with here. The safe administration of medicines involves five main principles:

1. safe storage
2. safe prescribing
3. safe administration
4. receiving from the pharmacy
5. accurate recording.

Storage

It is a legal requirement that all medicines are safely stored, and it is part of the nurse's role to see that this is carried out according to local policy. There is different legislation for controlled drugs (drugs of addiction and poisons). The main principles are as follows:

- All medicines, lotions and reagents (except intravenous fluids and drugs used in emergency situations) must be stored in a locked cupboard. Drugs for emergency use have to be readily available and are therefore allowed to be stored in a sealed container that is replenished and resealed after use.
- All medicines should be stored at the correct temperature that is recommended by the manufacturers, e.g. particularly intravenous fluids and drugs that require refrigeration. The fridge should be one designated for this purpose and not one also used for food.
- Medicine cupboards and drug trolleys should be kept locked at all times when not in use. Drug trolleys should be secured to the wall.
- All stock should be rotated so that it is used before the expiry date.
- Labels on medicine containers must not be altered or added to. Any damaged or obliterated labels or ones that require changing in any way must be returned to the pharmacy department.
- Medicines must not be transferred from one bottle to another.
- Borrowing from other wards or departments should be discouraged except in an emergency, when it should be documented and the pharmacy department notified.
- Medicines held in wards, units and departments must only be used for the patients for whom they have been prescribed and not be issued to hospital personnel or visitors.
- For controlled drugs, these should be kept in a separate cupboard with the key kept separate from the other drug keys. A controlled drug register must be kept, and all controlled drugs given must have two signatories and be accounted for in the register. Local policies will dictate the ordering, receipt and checking procedures for controlled drugs.
- No unauthorised person must be allowed access to the drug cupboard keys.
- The security of the medicines is the responsibility of the qualified nurse in charge.

Prescribing

In any health care setting where patients or clients receive medication, a doctor must prescribe all medicines before they can be administered. Before administration takes place the nurse must ensure that the prescription meets the following criteria:

• It should be written legibly (or printed) in ink and dated. The approved generic name should be used. It should not be altered once written and should be written out again in full if it is necessary to change the dose or frequency. When a prescription is to be cancelled, it should be crossed out (indicating the start and finish of the line) and signed and dated by the doctor. The nurse should not administer the medicine if the prescription is illegible. She should not guess the name of the drug to be given.

• It should clearly and accurately identify the patient. In an acute care setting, it should match the wrist band name.

• It should specify the preparation to be given (e.g. tablets, capsules, suppositories, etc.).

• It should state the strength, the dose, the timing and the frequency. For certain drugs (e.g. antibiotics), the proposed duration that the drug is to be given should be stated.

• It should state the route of administration.

• It should be signed and dated by the doctor.

In an emergency a first-level nurse may take a telephone message for the administration of medicines. The prescription must be written and signed for by the nurse, stating that it was a verbal request, and giving the time, the date and the doctor's name. The doctor should countersign the prescription as soon as possible. No telephone orders should be repeated. Since 1999, specialist community nurses have been trained to prescribe particular types of medication. This may extend into other branches of nursing.

Administering

Medicines can only be administered by a registered nurse. In principle this means that a registered nurse 'takes charge' of the task and oversees all aspects of it. It will be reasonable to expect a student nurse to participate in the giving of medications under the supervision of a registered nurse. Student nurses can expect to give oral, intramuscular, subcutaneous and topical medicines according to the correct procedure and when trained to do so, under the direct supervision of the registered nurse.

The following principles apply to the administration of all medicines, whatever the route. Local policy may require that two nurses check certain medicines before administration. Two nurses are required to check and administer all controlled drugs. Box 14.5 gives the procedure for the safe administration of medicines.

Box 14.5   The safe administration of medicines

• Check the location of the patient before dispensing medication.
• Do not leave the unlocked trolley unattended, or medicines out on a locker or a table to be administered later.
• Make sure the patient understands the reasons for the medication being given when possible, and check whether the patient has any drug allergies.
• Wash and dry hands thoroughly.
• Prepare the medicines to be administered and the appropriate equipment for the route of administration.
• Check the prescription chart has the patient's full name and hospital number.
• Check the prescription, bearing in mind the points outlined above.
• Check it is the correct time to administer the medicine and that the patient has not already received it. Check any special observations (e.g. blood pressure) or requirements (e.g. before, with or after food) relating to the medication.
• Check the medicine container against the prescription to identify that it is the correct medicine. Check the expiry date of the medicine.
• Calculate how much is required to achieve the dose prescribed.
• Check the patient's identity, using the patient's name band, with the prescription.
• Administer the medicine as prescribed.
• Ensure the patient is comfortable and understands any instructions related to the medication.
• Sign the prescription chart according to local policy. Document if the medication was not given. This is a most important aspect of the process and contributes to the legal record of care.
• Monitor the effects of the medication and report and record any abnormal side-effects (e.g. antibiotic rash).
• Wash and dry hands thoroughly.

The safe administration of medicines gives:

- the right medication
- the right amount
- the right route
- the right time
- the right patient.

Self-administration

In some hospitals, and in many community care settings, patients are given the responsibility for taking their own prescribed medication. While this is normal in one's own home, a few principles have to be applied in hospitals or other units so that medications do not fall into the wrong hands. There must be the availability of locked cupboards for individual storage. The patient needs to be on a drug regimen that is not liable to frequent change, and the drugs need to be dispensed individually by the pharmacy department. The nurse's role is liaison with the pharmacist and the education of the patient in adhering to the drug regimen.

Receiving medicines

This refers to ordering and receiving of medicines from the pharmacy department, checking that they are correct and ensuring they are stored in the appropriate locked cupboard. Local policies will give guidance on this and on stocktaking.

Stocktaking within hospitals and in residential settings must take place at appropriate intervals. This involves recording, checking stocks and disposing of unwanted medicines according to legislation and local policy. Any discrepancies in the stock must be reported immediately to the nurse in charge and investigated.

Practical skills of giving medication

Giving injections, applying topical lotions, inserting suppositories and overseeing intravenous infusions is all part of the expected role of the nurse and skills which you will learn in the early stages of your course. They are outside the purpose of this chapter, but consult the 'Further reading' list at the end of the chapter for information and guidance. Advanced skills in relation to safe practice and medications are required for nurses working in chemotherapy units, transplant centres and possibly in community psychiatry.

There is a great deal more to safe practice in dealing with medication than just handing out pills.

REMEMBER THAT PREVENTION IS THE KEY

As referred to earlier in this chapter, the UKCC Code of Conduct calls upon nurses to promote and safeguard the well-being of patients and to ensure that no action or omission of care is detrimental to patients. This section of the chapter describes activities related to prevention of illness or disability or which alert the nurse to potential clinical problems. All of them are aspects of care which every first year nurse will encounter and they include ensuring adequate nutrition and hydration of patients and clients, preventing the complications of immobility and carrying out clinical observations. All of these nursing duties may be seen as routine; indeed they form part of the daily work of the nurse and experience of the patient, but they are far from routine and ordinary in their consequences if they are not fulfilled as required within the patient's care plan.

NUTRITION

Poor nutritional status is known to be associated with delayed recovery, a longer stay in hospital and a higher mortality rate. Therefore adequate nutrition not only promotes growth and repair of tissues but aids recovery from disease, trauma and surgery. It is well known, for instance, that patients suffering from burns may need two or three times their normal nutritional intake, according to the percentage of the body surface burned. Some patients, particularly the elderly, are admitted to hospital malnourished. Recent surveys have indicated that many people in hospital receive inadequate nourishment for a variety of reasons (McWhirter & Pennington 1994). For many patients, mealtimes are seen as highlights of the day, breaks in the relative tedium of being a patient, and for some patients eating is part of the regimen of care and therapy. It is important, then, that nurses see they have a role to play in the prevention of malnutrition by identifying patients at risk and planning care to meet the needs of undernourished patients and clients. Florence Nightingale had something to say about this when she wrote: 'If the nurse is an intelligent being and not a mere carrier of diets to and from the patient, let her exercise her intelligence in these things.'

Assessing nutritional needs

Some clinical areas and special units may have nutritional assessment tools which will help identify patients who are malnourished or at risk of developing malnutrition. Most will include the factors listed in Box 14.6, although this is not an exhaustive list.

Assisting patients with feeding

It cannot be expressed often enough that it is the nurse's responsibility to see that all patients get appropriate nourishment while in health care. Even if you have not been feeding your particular patient, it is your responsibility to know what food and fluid they have taken. All too often food and drink is left out of reach or the patient or client is not given any assistance when they need it, and consequently the patient has neither. Nutritional assessment should identify those people who need assistance with feeding and Box 14.7 gives some guidance in feeding adults. In many acute hospitals, meals are now served by kitchen or domestic staff, but it remains vital for nurses to

---

Box 14.6   Major factors involved in nutritional assessment

- Mental condition: deterioration in mental state or level of consciousness could affect the patient's desire and ability to eat or drink independently.
- Weight, build and skin condition: these will give signs of malnutrition.
- Appetite: people who do not want to eat are at risk of malnutrition.
- Physical handicap or positional difficulty: these may interfere with independence in eating and drinking.
- The ability to chew and swallow: certain conditions such as stroke and motor neurone disease make these activities difficult and leave the person at risk of malnutrition; they may well be prescribed nasogastric or parenteral (intravenous) feeding.
- The condition of the mouth, gums and teeth: these may be the underlying cause of eating difficulty.
- Special diet: this must be recognised in certain cases, e.g. diabetes mellitus, renal disease, malabsorption disorders, obesity.
- The nature of any learning disability in relation to a person's ability to make choices about food and be independent in managing food.
- Pain and distressing symptoms which interfere with eating: the timing of medication may be significant in enabling the patient to enjoy food when it arrives.
- Cultural or religious customs which may affect a person's eating habits.
- Any major illness or disorder which demands special feeding regimens: e.g. burns patients, patients with pressure sores who require high nutritional intake to aid recovery.
- Special weaning programmes for infants and the ability of parents to cope with feeding demands.
- Unusual eating habits: these may be associated with conditions such as anorexia nervosa and so require a special nutritional regimen.

Box 14.7   Feeding adults

- Establish whether the patient is on a special diet and aim to make the mealtime a pleasant experience.
- Ensure that the patient is in a comfortable position, has been offered the toilet, washed his hands and, if applicable, has a clean mouth and dentures.
- Clear a space for the tray by removing any offensive material such as urinals, sputum cartons, and position a chair beside the bed.
- Wash and dry hands thoroughly.
- Obtain the correct food, drink, cutlery and napkin, and set out the meal in a pleasing manner.
- Take the tray to the bedside and describe the food, if the patient is unable to see. Cut up the food if necessary, and protect the patient's clothing with a napkin or paper towel as appropriate.
- Sit down to feed the patient, demonstrating a more relaxed approach and that you can spend time with the patient.
- Adjust the speed and the amount of food and drink you offer, taking into account the patient's ability and giving time for him to chew and swallow the food before presenting the next mouthful, so that it is not hurried.
- Avoid asking questions while the patient is eating. This is a good time to quietly observe the patient.
- Use the napkin to remove dribbles of food or drink that may run down the chin; when giving a drink, regulate the flow by tipping the cup/glass gently.
- Encourage patients to eat and drink, but do not press this if they have indicated they have had sufficient. Little and often may produce more success.
- Assist the patient to complete oral hygiene if necessary, following eating.
- Remove tray and crockery, and wipe up any spillages.
- Ensure the patient is made comfortable and has water and belongings within easy reach.
- Wash hands and complete documentation.

oversee the meals to check that patients have the right diet and enough of it and that they eat it, or that evaluation is made if they do not. Nurses will often need to physically help the patient to eat as described in Box 14.7. Obviously, the feeding of infants and children, or those with special feeding needs such as nasogastric feeding or intravenous nutrition, will not be nursed in this way. Sometimes mealtimes are special teaching occasions for people with a learning disability, so student nurses will learn appropriate techniques during placement experiences. Patients with extreme eating disorders will have individual and special feeding regimens. At all times, it is beneficial if relatives and friends can be involved in assisting patients to eat and enjoy their food. It is often acceptable for food from home to be brought in, but it is always wise to check that this is within the agreed dietary regimen for the patient.

HYDRATION AND FLUID BALANCE

While it may seem a very unexciting activity, the role of the nurse in encouraging patients to drink (often seen in the nursing record as 'push fluids'!), preventing any patient from becoming dehydrated, is a vital activity and in some instances may be life-saving. Helping patients to take sufficient water or other fluid will often be required of the most junior nurse but it is not a negligible responsibility.

Why is water so important?

Before we discuss the importance of encouraging patients to drink, it is worth understanding why water is so essential to the normal functioning of the body. On a day-to-day basis few of us consider the composition of the body, but in medical terms it is important to do so every day. At least 70% of the body is composed of water.

The smallest unitary structure of the body is the *cell* (see Ch. 6 for details). Cells have a great liking for water. Not only is the cell the single most important structure of the body, it relies on having the correct amount of water to do its job efficiently. The cell behaves like a miniature factory, and operates 24 hours a day. In order to perform with such regularity, it is supplied with water and raw materials, while any waste products are 'removed' virtually simultaneously across the cell membrane, through the extracellular fluid, into the vascular system for excretion, mainly via the kidneys. Water is the substance of choice as the main transport system of the body and is the basic component of extracellular fluid, blood, lymph and urine, the main 'transporters'. (Ch. 6 provides more detailed explanations of all of these and the importance of them in maintaining the homeostatic stability of the body.) As a replenishing source for the body we are fortunate that water is readily available (when properly conserved) and almost free. It is also one of the simplest chemicals in the body and, in having a 'small' molecular size, it 'travels' throughout the body with ease.

Body cells can become 'selectively permeable' concerning the passage of dissolved substances (solutes) across the cell membrane so that the concentration of water in the cell is maintained at a constant level in the healthy person and the cells perform consistently well and continually. In this way the whole body is said to be 'in balance' and the person is well.

Water forms three distinct 'compartments' within the body:

1. the intracellular cellular content (30 litres)
2. the extracellular fluid content (12 litres)
3. the vascular system content (3 litres).

All of these compartments require a comparatively stable water content to do their jobs efficiently. When one compartment begins to get low in water content, the body is said to be dehydrated. The order in which the compartments become dehydrated is also very specific. The vascular system is always first, the extracellular space is next to be affected and the cellular space is always last.

There is always a loss of water from the body in 24 hours, mainly in the form of *urine*, via the kidney and the bladder. Visible sweat from the skin and insensible sweat (sweat taking place without the body feeling it), as well as water vapour we breathe out, account for approximately 3 litres

Table 14.1   Healthy water balance in a 24-hour period

Water loss	Water gain
Urine $2\frac{1}{4}$ litres	3 litres
Sweat $\frac{1}{2}$ litre (excluding exercise)	
Water vapour from breath $\frac{1}{4}$ litre	

of water lost daily which must be replaced (Table 14.1). After exercise this loss is increased, so additional water must be consumed. Water therefore is not only a transport system, it is simultaneously an excretory pathway too.

Signs and causes of dehydration

The simplest and quickest way of detecting dehydration is to inspect the patient's tongue and/or their urine. If the tongue is not completely moist, the patient is almost certainly dehydrated. The patient will find talking difficult as the tongue clings to the roof of the mouth. The urine in this case is always very dark in colour. The first *symptom* (what the patient himself feels) of dehydration, is *thirst*. People suffering from dehydration in extreme climates can quickly lose consciousness and be unable to replenish water loss for themselves, thus demonstrating that water is a powerful force in preventing loss of consciousness.

Because the vascular system is the first compartment to be affected by dehydration, the loss of water from the vascular system directly affects the body *blood pressure*. The loss of water will raise blood pressure (as the blood cell content becomes comparatively more concentrated than the plasma it needs a higher pressure to get this 'thicker' blood through the system), often causing headaches. Thus, providing everything else is equal in the body, asking a patient to drink 2, 3 or even 4 pints of water should eventually bring the blood pressure back to normal. Water can therefore act as a *treatment* as well as a transport system. Chronic, long-standing dehydration (often due to people being unwilling or unable to drink or take adequate fluids, e.g. because they are worried about problems with urinary incontinence)

may lead to constipation and renal problems. Dehydration may also decrease the ability of the mucosal membranes of the upper respiratory tract to be effective as the first line of defence against bacteria and air-borne particles, leaving the person prone to infection.

Everyday causes of dehydration are:

- alcohol
- caffeine
- sunbathing, leading to sunstroke
- central heating
- smoking
- just not drinking enough
- infection
- illness (e.g. diabetes)
- diarrhoea and vomiting.

Drinking several pints of water can remedy these matters quickly and cheaply. However, in the cases of infection and illness, further treatment is also required. This extra water would be needed over and above a normal requirement of 3 litres of water every 24 hours.

Maintaining adequate hydration

Patients' fluid intake is, therefore, a significant aspect of the preventative role of the nurse. Even minor changes in the body's fluid balance at cellular level can have major consequences for health. Where a patient is identified as being at risk of dehydration, or may have some other ailment which requires the fluid intake to be carefully maintained, the nurse's role is critical in ensuring that fluid balance is checked and recorded. Nurses may also need to work very closely with patients to encourage them to drink by checking them frequently, providing the most acceptable beverages or alternatives (e.g. ice lollies). Although they may not be receiving complicated treatments, the elderly, children, people with learning disabilities and some mentally ill patients can easily become seriously dehydrated if they are not encouraged to drink water. In extreme cases of dehydration or where the patient is unable to tolerate oral fluids, e.g. following major surgery, intravenous fluids may be given. One important aspect of care of the person with dehydration is mouth care. Enabling these patients to keep a moist and fresh mouth adds greatly to their feeling of well-being and may enable them to take oral fluids more easily.

Fluid balance charts

If a patient is suspected of being dehydrated or is having fluid any other way but orally, the total intake and output of fluids should be recorded on a fluid balance chart. Each hospital or care practice will have its own chart but they will all follow much the same format, requiring the nurse to record all types of fluid input and output, including such things as intravenous fluids, blood, plasma, vomit, diarrhoea, wound drainage as well as oral fluids and urine. Always explain to the patient why the recording is necessary and any activities that may be required of the patient (e.g. measuring his own urine), when you need to note the nature and quantity of both input and output. The fluid balance chart should be assessed regularly so that the input can be adjusted as required. Accurate recording of both intake and output is vital to be able to calculate the fluid balance. The fluid balance is totalled at the end of each 24-hour period.

THE IMPORTANCE OF NURSING OBSERVATIONS

One of the most significant nursing activities in relation to 'prevention being the key' is to keep *observing* patients. This does not always mean carrying out clinical measurements with special equipment, although of course this is carried out a great deal. It means, literally, look at your patients frequently, get used to how they appear and behave when they are stable and comfortable within their condition and do not become over-reliant on the machinery which can sometimes go wrong. You are then able to notice even very small changes in their condition and these observations can be life-saving. Case example 14.5 illustrates how a nurse noticed something a little unusual which turned out to be a very important observation.

Case example 14.5 The importance of looking at your patients

Mrs James is recovering from the abdominal surgery she had yesterday. She seems comfortable and all routine observations of blood pressure and pulse 4 hourly suggest she is stable. The ward is very busy and the nurses are well occupied with other patients. As the student nurse walks into Mrs James's bay she notices that Mrs James is slightly restless, a little sweaty and rather pale. This patient is not inclined to make a fuss or say much at any time so she does not complain. The nurse asks her if she is OK and Mrs James admits that she does feel a bit light-headed but presumed it was normal to feel like this so soon after the operation. The student reports her findings to the staff nurse, who quickly comes and checks Mrs James's blood pressure. She discovers that it is very low, she calls for the doctor and it soon transpires that Mrs James is suffering from postoperative reactionary internal haemorrhage. A regimen of care is put into place immediately to restore Mrs James's blood pressure and she eventually goes to theatre for the cause of the bleeding to be found and repaired.

The particular occurrence in Case example 14.5 is rare, fortunately, but it should highlight the need to be observant. With advancing technology and the availability of amazing equipment for keeping acutely ill patients 'under clinical surveillance', it is sometimes easy to forget to look at the person in the middle of all the tubes and wires. It is also important to remember that observing patients is especially important with children, people with learning disability, the mentally ill, some elderly people and people with speech impairment, who cannot tell you how they feel. There may also be special reasons for observing patterns of behaviour with the mentally ill or those with learning disability because changes may be signals that help is required to calm or restrain a client.

Routine clinical nursing observations and tests

It is impossible in this chapter to describe the methods of all the observations you may be asked to perform. You will probably be taught these in a skills laboratory or simulated clinical setting, and allowed to practise under supervision. You will then be expected to carry out some, or even all of them at an early stage in your practical experience. Although being asked to do 'routine observations' may seem unglamorous, it is important to know why they are being carried out, what they tell you about the patient and how they form part of the investigative or therapeutic regimen in the care pathway. The main observations to carry out are:

Temperature, pulse and respiration. These are always checked when a person is admitted to an acute care setting, as an emergency or for planned care, to ascertain base-line levels and any deviation from the normal range. Thereafter, frequency of checking will be according to the patient's condition and care plan. Sudden changes in pulse and respiration may indicate cardiovascular problems, shock, respiratory obstruction; increased temperature may indicate infection, allergic reactions to drugs, blood transfusion. Temperature recording is very significant in infants with fever and in anyone with hypothermia. Most acute care settings now use electronic thermometers, but you will still need to know how to use a mercury thermometer.

Blood pressure. This is always checked on admission to acute health care and, thereafter, if required and according to the care pathway. This is an important clinical measurement of cardiovascular function and one which denotes critical changes or potential changes in a patient's condition. Post-operatively, it is important to check and record, frequently, the blood pressure for patients with hypertension, cardiac failure, myocardial infarction, and renal and trauma patients, because of the risk of shock. It will not be a frequent observation for patients in long-stay care, mental health community care or learning disability care, unless these patients become acutely physically ill.

Peak flow measurement. This is to measure the rate of flow of exhaled breath in patients where there is, or might be, an obstructive airways disorder which reduces the effectiveness of breathing and gaseous exchange at the alveoli (see Ch. 6). This observation will be commonly required for patients with asthma, chronic bronchitis and emphysema and frequency will vary.

It is often used to check the effectiveness of treatment with nebulisers or other inhalers by carrying out before and after peak-flow tests.

Pulse oximetry. This sophisticated test enables the patient's blood oxygen level to be checked by using a sensor on the finger or ear. Patients with obstructive airways disease or cardiovascular disease will usually have this test carried out to check the severity of their condition.

Neuro-observations. These will be measured and recorded mainly for any patient who has suffered head injury, had a cerebrovascular accident, taken poisons, or is admitted unconscious for any reason; they may also be ordered for patients whose general condition and alertness is deteriorating. They include checking the person's mental orientation (if possible), pupil responses to light, responses to touch or stronger stimuli on the limbs, hands and feet if the person is unconscious, and vital signs (temperature, pulse and blood pressure and respiration) also form part of this set of observations. A conscious patient will also be checked for the level of strength in arms and legs, to see if there is any weakness and whether or not it is bilateral. Alterations from the normal range are indicators of brain damage and recordings will be taken regularly to ascertain major deterioration or recovery. Most hospitals will use a special recording chart, such as the Glasgow Coma Scale chart (Fig. 14.5). This measurement is carried out frequently within accident and emergency departments and in neurology units, and, less often, in general acute adult and paediatric care.

Skin colour and texture. The condition of the skin tells the practitioner a great deal. Pallor may indicate anaemia or shock; jaundice may be evident; swelling and pain may occur in a range of abnormalities from heart and renal failure to infection; reddening may be an early indicator of pressure damage; bruising may be a very significant finding where injury or non-accidental injury is suspected; severe dehydration affects skin texture and suppleness; the skin extremities on any splinted limb must be observed for abnormal swelling and checked for normal sensation. The need to observe and the frequency of skin observation will vary from patient to patient, but this simple detection is one of the most important in nursing.

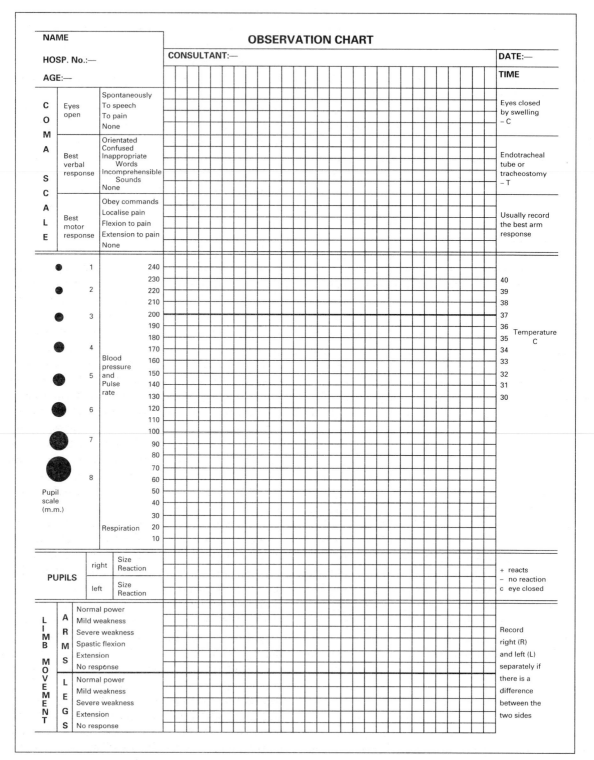

Figure 14.5 The Glasgow Coma Scale.

Urine testing. This is one of the earliest and most frequent measurements done by nursing students. Routine testing is carried out on a small sample for protein, blood, ketones, bilirubin and glucose in the urine; the urine pH, specific gravity and colour are also checked. This allows swift basic identification of abnormality and possible early diagnosis of renal, liver, and other disorders including diabetes. You will also learn how to collect mid-stream specimens for culture if infection is suspected, 24-hour specimens to check renal function, catheter or catheter bag specimens. Because urine is so easily collectible and it clearly provides a range of information about what is happening within the body as a whole, it is a very frequently used specimen.

Pain assessment. This important observation can often be overlooked in the busy world of health care, unless you are working in a specialist palliative care setting. However, it is vital in all areas of care, not just when working with cancer patients or the terminally ill. Postoperative patients, burns patients, patients with arthritis are among those who can suffer extreme pain and for whom accurate assessment of their pain and the effectiveness of analgesia is important. For full details on pain assessment, see Chapter 15.

Record the results

While this is not a complete list of all clinical measurements you may be required to undertake, these are the most common and ones which you may be expected to do in your first year. The activities themselves are very important, and so is recording the results. The charts or the appropriate place in the care plan/pathway form part of the legal record of the patient's care and may sometimes be used in cases of investigation or review of care in relation to complaints or police matters. Not only is it important to record, but it is important to record accurately.

PREVENTION OF THE COMPLICATIONS OF IMMOBILITY

This important aspect of nursing should become so much part of daily routine care that it becomes impossible to forget it. The two main complications of immobility are deep vein thrombosis and pressure sores, both of which are painful and unpleasant for the patient, costly for the organisation, and can also be life-threatening. The existence of pressure sores for patients in NHS care is taken extremely seriously and sore-free skin is one of the national Patient's Charter standards. All NHS Trusts have to send in data to the Department of Health, and report to their Trust boards regularly, about pressure sore prevalence. While the same does not apply to deep vein thrombosis, prevention is taken very seriously.

Deep vein thrombosis

Patients who are immobile, undergoing surgery or who have predisposing factors such as dehydration or hypotension are at risk of developing deep vein thrombosis (DVT). Wherever possible, patients should be encouraged to mobilise as much as possible, and as soon as possible after surgery, to reduce venous stasis in the legs and so reduce the risk of developing DVT. Patients should be taught foot and leg exercises to do and be reminded to do them. Where a period of immobility is planned, such as known surgery, the patient can be taught what to do following surgery and reminded to do it. They should be discouraged from crossing their legs in bed. If the patient is unable to do these exercises for himself, or for any unconscious patient, the nurse can carry out gentle passive leg movements on the patient. Physiotherapists will usually assist with this and other aspects of patient activity to reduce DVT risk. Deep breathing and regular fluids should also be encouraged. There are now special machines available which carry out the equivalent of these leg exercises on the patient and they are often used for patients who have had major leg and knee surgery where movement and walking is initially very painful. Many patients undergoing surgery, and almost all patients undergoing hip and leg surgery, are fitted with special anti-embolism stockings which they are requested to wear for several days, possibly weeks, after their operation.

As well as encouraging mobility, deep breathing and wearing the stockings, the nurse must, once again, observe the patient for any signs of the complication. The legs should be checked daily for signs of redness or tenderness in the calves, which are the main signs of DVT.

Pressure sores

Pressure sores are seen as one of most emotive issues in nursing and certainly serious sores are extremely painful, prone to infection and can be life-threatening. Some would say that their presence is a reflection of poor nursing care and in some cases this is true. But there are situations in which an individual will develop a sore at home and not be seen by nurses or doctors until it is already far advanced. (For detailed information about the structure of the skin and the processes of healing, see Ch. 6.)

Most patients admitted to health care are now assessed for the risk of pressure damage to their skin. A number of different assessment tools are available and each area is likely to use the one most suitable for their type of patient. One in common use is the Waterlow scoring system (Table 14.2) which most nurses find helpful. Whatever the tool, all will include assessment of most if not all of the factors seen in Box 14.8.

Each of the factors shown in the box is scored in relation to its likely impact on the risk of developing a pressure sore. The total score for all the factors is then provided as the full risk assessment. The risk score then indicates to the care team the appropriate care programme required to prevent pressure sores developing in that patient. Different wards and departments will all have developed their 'plans of care to match

Table 14.2 Waterlow pressure sore prevention/treatment policy. Ring scores in table, add total, several scores per category can be used

Build/weight for height	★	Skin type Visual risk areas	★	Sex Age	★	Special risks	★
Average	0	Healthy	0	Male	1	**Tissue malnutrition**	★
Above average	1	Tissue paper	1	Female	2		
Obese	2	Dry	1	14–49	1		
Below average	3	Oedematous	1	50–64	2		
		Clammy (temp. ↑)	1	65–74	3	e.g. Terminal cachexia	8
Continence	★	Discoloured	2	75–80	4	Cardiac failure	5
		Broken/spot	3	81+	5	Peripheral vascular disease	5
Complete/						Anaemia	2
catheterised	0	**Mobility**	★	**Appetite**	★	Smoking	1
Occasion. incont.	1						
Cath./incontinent		Fully	0	Average	0	**Neurological deficit**	★
of faeces	2	Restless/fidgety	1	Poor	1		
Doubly incontinent	3	Apathetic	2	N.G. tube/		e.g. Diabetes, M.S., CVA,	
		Restricted	3	fluids only	2	motor/sensory paraplegia	4–6
		Inert/traction	4	NBM/anorexic	3		
		Chairbound	5			**Major surgery/trauma**	★
						Orthopaedic – below waist, spinal	5
						On table > 2 hours	5
						Medication	★
						Cytotoxics, high dose steroids, anti-inflammatory	4

Score	10+ at risk	15+ at risk	20+ very high risk

Source: J Waterlow 1991 (Obtainable from Newtons, Curland, Taunton TA3 5SG)

Box 14.8   Risk assessment for pressure sores

Weight, height, build: an overweight or very thin person is at greater risk of pressure damage.

Level of mobility: any immobility increases the risk of damage.

Nutritional state: poor nutritional health, emaciation or eating difficulty can all increase the risk.

Skin condition: oedematous, dry, thin, clammy skin is all more prone to pressure sores. Any pre-existing sores or blisters should be noted.

Medical condition: vascular disorders, some cancers, diabetes, pain and a period of time on an operating table can all predispose to pressure sore development.

Mental condition: depression, apathy and lethargy can mean greater risk of pressure sore development because these patients are less likely to want to move about, eat, etc.

Any special medication: some drugs can cause sedation and increased immobility, steroids affect skin property.

Box 14.9   Preventing pressure sores

Ensure that pressure on the body is relieved regularly. For some patients, encouraging them to get out of bed, stand, walk and move about will be sufficient if done frequently enough. Postoperative patients should be encouraged to walk as soon as their condition will allow. If this is painful, following surgery or because of a painful condition such as arthritis, adequate pain relief must be administered. For the bedridden patient, the person's body must be moved at least every 2 hours, so that different parts of the body are in contact with the bed. It is now usual for every immobile patient to be nursed on a pressure-relieving mattress and the nurse must ensure that this happens. But these patients will still need turning frequently. The frequency of mobilising and turning patients will vary according to the risk assessment score and care plan.

Ensure the patient is receiving adequate nutrition and hydration to maintain healthy skin.

Keep the skin clean and dry at all times. Episodes of incontinence should be dealt with promptly, talcum powder should be used sparingly because it can become clogged and lumpy on the skin.

Check buttocks and bony prominences frequently for signs of reddening and soreness. It may be necessary to alter the care regimen slightly or add further pressure-relieving aids to elbows and heels.

Avoid shearing forces and mechanical injury to the skin. This is the result of poor lifting technique where a patient is dragged up the bed or chair, or sheets remain crinkled.

score' based on their experience and best evidence. But all care pathways will have certain features in common, as described in Box 14.9.

Pressure sores are a very serious problem. Once developed they may be very difficult to cure, they may become infected and may eventually require skin grafting. They substantially increase the length of stay in hospital or nursing home. They are avoidable by following the above guidelines.

HELPING PATIENTS AND CLIENTS TO WASH AND DRESS

Since maintaining the integrity of the skin is essential in the prevention of pressure sores, bathing and skin care is an important part of nursing the vulnerable patient. Bed-bathing or assisting with bathing or showering for the more-independent patient provides a vital opportunity to observe the skin and identify the need for possible treatment or intervention.

For the majority of people, a significant aspect of a sense of well-being and dignity is that they are clean and smart to their own standards.

Most cultures instruct children into performing their own personal cleansing and dressing activities until they can perform them independently. This is usually done in privacy and in rooms designed for this purpose and so attitudes towards cleansing both one's body and clothes are learned at an early age. Cleanliness and attention to personal hygiene are recognised in most cultures, and odour and infestation are not well tolerated. All this needs to be borne in mind for the patient or client who is confined to bed or unable to do these personal tasks because of mental or physical disability (Activity 14.13).

   Activity 14.13

Mr Watts is 43 and suffering from severe depression. On admission it is apparent that he has not carried out any personal hygiene for the last few weeks. You have run the bath but on returning to see how he is getting on, you find he is still in his clothes and gazing at the water. How would you help this client?

It is often said that it is good for a nurse to have the experience of being a patient. All too soon you realise how difficult it is to wash in a few centimetres of lukewarm water or not to be able to clean your teeth properly. In considering a patient's hygiene the following principles would apply:

- Assisting patients or clients with their personal hygiene is another occasion to use your observation skills.
- Discuss with patients whether they prefer a bath or a shower.
- Ascertain whether patients wish to use the toilet before taking them to the bathroom.
- Some hospitals/units prefer patients to use antiseptic cleansing solution rather than soap as a prophylaxis against methicillin resistant *Staphylococcus aureus* (MRSA).
- Ensure patient privacy by restricting access and closing shower curtains or doors.
- Ensure by testing that the temperature of the bath or shower is appropriate.
- Assist patients if required by using mechanical hoist or stool.
- Observe skin integrity, pressure points and any signs of inflammation, bruising, discoloration or rash.
- If assisting with washing, maintain the patient's dignity by covering with a towel.
- Remove any supportive bandage, wash the limb, and reapply or renew bandage, checking for soreness or chafing of the skin.
- If leaving the patient to wash, ensure that everything the patient needs is to hand, including access to a call bell.
- Assist with drying, using toiletries, brushing/combing hair, cleaning teeth or dentures if required. Ask patients if they require their nails to be filed or request a visit from the podiatrist.
- Clean the bath or shower afterwards ready for the next person and collect and return toiletries.
- Help with dressing and/or assist the patient to return to bed.
- Record the procedure in the patient's notes, noting how much assistance the patient required, the patient's general condition, state of skin and pressure points.

If the patient is unable to have a bath or a shower then a daily bed bath will be required. Similar principles apply as above, but the patient will require much more assistance. In the case of an unconscious patient or the very ill then they will be completely dependent on the nurse to carry out all their hygiene needs. Main points in this procedure are:

- Having removed the night clothes, always ensure that the areas not being washed are covered by a sheet or blanket to maintain warmth and dignity.
- Wash, rinse and dry the body in a systematic order, usually face, neck, arms, chest and abdomen first. Next the genital area, using a disposable flannel, legs, feet and then back. Drying the body is important, particularly where there are folds of skin and over pressure points. This prevents pressure sores, and patients will usually tell you if they feel dry, if they are able to.
- Change the water after washing the genital area or if it becomes dirty or cold.
- Remove any soiled linen and replace, and remake the bed. If the patient is totally dependent this may require assistance.
- Dress the patient in clean night clothes and assist with brushing or combing the hair, cleaning teeth or dentures and filing nails if required. Carry out mouth care and catheter care according to local policy, if required.
- Rinse flannels under running water to remove all soap and leave to dry. Discard disposable cloths into clinical waste. Wash and dry the bowl.

TAKE PROMPT ACTION IN THE CASE OF AN EMERGENCY

The two most significant emergencies with which every student nurse must know how to deal are *fire* and the *'crash call'* (where a person is expected to require resuscitation and life support). Fire safety procedures are not covered here, but all staff are required to attend fire lectures in their place of work as part of their induction and annually thereafter. The same is true for students.

Case example 14.6

Mr P was a 53-year-old man admitted to the medical assessment unit for further investigations into intermittent chest pains. On the morning following his admission he had been out to the bathroom for a wash and was sitting on his bed, looking in his locker for his book. He suddenly experienced an intense crushing pain in the centre of his chest, and cried out before slumping backwards onto the bed.

Assessment
A student nurse who had been walking towards the bed saw Mr P collapse and ran towards him. Checking that the area round the bed was safe, she approached the patient, and called his name out, shaking him by the shoulders at the same time. There was no response, and she then pulled the emergency call button to summon more help. She also pulled the curtains round the bed. By this time two staff nurses had arrived and together they laid Mr P flat on the bed, removing all pillows and the bed-head in order to gain better access for assessing him.

The staff nurses had brought with them the emergency trolley containing equipment and emergency drugs. One staff nurse lifted the patient's chin to open his airway, did a mouth sweep to check for obstruction, and checked for signs of respirations. Having established that the patient was not breathing, the staff nurse told the student nurse to run and telephone for the resuscitation team, using the emergency code number. She then gave Mr P two rescue breaths, establishing the rise and fall of his chest. The second staff nurse checked the carotid pulse to establish whether there was circulation. There was no pulse present, and she then began external cardiac compressions.

Meanwhile the first staff nurse had connected the Ambu (breathing) bag to a mask and oxygen tubing and attached it to the wall oxygen supply at 10 litres per minute and prepared a Guedel airway for insertion. After the two rescue breaths, the staff nurse inserted the airway upside-down into the mouth then turned it over into position over the back of the tongue, which ensured a clear airway. While the external cardiac compressions continued, the first staff nurse continued to give breaths, lifting the chin, holding the mask to the face, and compressing the Ambu bag. Thus cardiopulmonary resuscitation continued at a rate of 2 breaths to 15 compressions. The student nurse was, in the meantime, standing by the emergency trolley, and the first staff nurse explained what would be required next. First the patient was attached to the cardiac monitor so that any heart activity could be seen. Then some of the drugs normally used in a cardiac emergency were prepared (e.g. adrenaline, atropine).

By this time the medical team had arrived and assessed the situation and obtained a brief history of events from the staff nurse. The anaesthetist took control of the airway. Although the patient was still unresponsive, not breathing and without a pulse, the cardiac monitor indicated that his heart was fibrillating. The staff nurse prepared the defibrillator and pads, and the medical registrar administered two shocks, bringing the patient's heart back into sinus rhythm. A pulse was now present and the patient was beginning to breathe unaided, although he continued to receive oxygen via the Ambu bag until able to expel the Guedel airway.

Mr P was still seriously ill and would require several more hours of intensive treatment and observation. However, the prompt action of all the nurses in initiating cardiopulmonary resuscitation proved life-saving in this instance.

A more common emergency for nurses is the need for cardiopulmonary resuscitation. As a student you will be taught this in the early part of your course. Before giving information about the process of resuscitation, it is worth noting a few important background points which will help you:

- Know where the resuscitation trolley is as soon as you start to work in a new area.
- Know how to make the crash call wherever you are working in practice.
- Remember that prompt action, but not panic, is essential in the case of this emergency.
- If you are the first to notice a collapsed patient, do not stop to think about the cause, shout for help immediately and begin resuscitation.
- Recognise and follow instructions from whoever is the leader of the crash team. A good crash team will always nominate one leader and follow their instructions without question whatever their grade or clinical role.
- Do not worry about what looks like chaos: it isn't.
- Do not forget health and safety of staff and others around the event.
- If you are not needed at the event itself, try to provide reassurance to other patients or clients about what is happening.

THE PROCESS OF CARDIOPULMONARY RESUSCITATION (CPR)

As with all aspects of nursing, observation of the patient is significant. Noticing that a patient in

Case example 14.7

Mrs B was a 42-year-old woman who had come into the accident and emergency department with heavy p.v. (per vaginum) bleeding and cramping abdominal pain. She had been assessed by the staff nurse in triage and was waiting to be called through and be seen by the doctor. Approximately 20 minutes after being assessed, she walked out to the toilet. Another patient waiting to be seen witnessed Mrs B come out of the toilet and suddenly slump to the floor. He ran to call the staff nurse working in the triage area.

Assessment

The staff nurse could see that the patient was unresponsive and not moving. Checking the immediate area for safety, he then approached the patient, first calling out her name, and then gently shaking her shoulders. There was no response and the staff nurse asked the receptionist at the triage desk to telephone through to the main department and ask for immediate assistance. He then ensured the patient's airway was open by tilting the head and lifting the chin. He assessed whether she was breathing, looking for chest movements, listening for breath sounds, and feeling for air on his cheek. Having ascertained that she was breathing but was still unresponsive, he placed her into the recovery position. This he did by placing her on her side, with the uppermost hand under her cheek, and the uppermost knee bent to prevent her from rolling onto her stomach.

Having been reassured by the receptionist that help was coming, the staff nurse stayed with the patient, checking that she was continuing to breathe spontaneously. He also checked her carotid pulse, which indicated that she was tachycardic. By this time more help had arrived in the form of a doctor, staff nurse, porter and a trolley with an oxygen supply. The patient was carefully transferred to the trolley and kept in the recovery position, with the nurse continually observing her respirations and checking her pulse. Oxygen was administered at 4 litres per minute through a mask and she was taken to the resuscitation area of the accident and emergency department. While on her way to that area she began to move and make groaning noises and after a few more minutes had opened her eyes and was asking the staff nurse what had happened to her.

The staff nurse was able to reassure Mrs B that she had fainted in the waiting room while waiting to see the doctor, but that she was much better now, although she needed further observation and treatment from the medical team to ensure a full recovery.

bed has collapsed and become unresponsive is where the process of CPR begins. Of course, a walking person may suddenly collapse and fall to the ground, and the immediate process of care is just the same.

First, it is important to assess the patient rapidly to determine the specific course of action required. Not all collapsed individuals need all aspects of CPR and some do not need anything more than being placed in the recovery position. Case examples 14.6 and 14.7 describe two collapsed patients who required very different care.

The principles of CPR are well described in Figure 14.6. and in the case examples. In a hospital setting, the presence of trained nurses, doctors and the crash team ensures a streamlined, efficient and rapid programme of care. However, you will be trained to carry out CPR on your own in a non-clinical situation in case that is necessary. All nursing students, whatever specialist branch they choose, must know how to care in this particular emergency situation.

POSSIBLE CAUSES OF COLLAPSE

These include the following although it is not an exhaustive list:

- simple faint
- haemorrhage
- choking
- drugs which cause respiratory arrest
- cardiac arrest
- fitting
- hypoglycaemia
- febrile convulsions
- cerebrovascular accident.

In every case, the approach to the patient is the same as described in Figure 14.6, even though subsequent care for each is very different.

COMMUNICATE EFFECTIVELY

When the National Health Service investigates complaints, the majority can be traced to poor communication. Nursing and health care staff are often bad at giving patients and those who care for them sufficient information and explanation (see Ch. 9).

Patients and clients entering hospital, GP surgery, community home or being visited at home by a nurse immediately become the

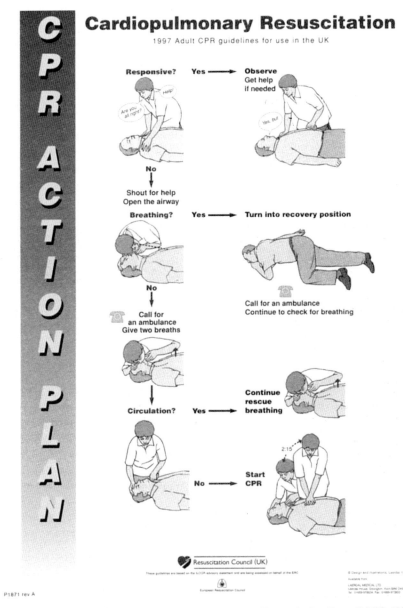

Figure 14.6 Cardiopulmonary resuscitation action plan (Resuscitation Council (UK) 1997).

responsibility of those administering the care. It is therefore of paramount importance that every nurse knows what her responsibilities are while the patient is in her care. Statutory regulations which include safe practice are covered through the UKCC Code of Conduct and these are discussed more fully in Chapter 11. It is therefore appropriate for us to look more closely at

how such responsibilities operate in practice in certain specific areas.

INFORMED CONSENT FOR PATIENTS AND CLIENTS

On the whole patients accept that that they will, at one time or another, be cared for by nursing and medical students and other health care workers in training. It is worth remembering that every patient or client has the right to refuse care from a student, and not to take this too personally should it happen. Often it is due to a misunderstanding of your role or perhaps a previous bad experience. Some hospitals issue leaflets informing patients of students in training, asking for their cooperation and support in helping to train students for their future roles, but also informing them of their rights. Examinations or treatments on patients and clients should not normally be carried out without their prior consent, which has been obtained following an explanation of the procedures involved.

The purposes of gaining the patient's consent are:

- To ensure that the patient understands the nature of the treatment or examination, including alternatives and possible potential complications or risks, thus allowing him to make an informed decision.
- To indicate that the patient's decision was made without pressure, and to protect the patient against unauthorised procedures.
- To protect the medical staff and the hospital against legal action by a patient who claims that an unauthorised procedure was performed.

The circumstances requiring *written consent* are any procedure that requires a general anaesthetic, any invasive procedure or those treatments carrying a side-effect or a substantial risk. Some drug therapy (e.g. cytotoxics) and therapy involving ionising radiation also require written consent. If in doubt always ask a qualified member of the nursing staff or the doctor.

Before consent is requested for any examination or treatment and before the patient has any sedation, it is the nurse's responsibility to ensure that the patient is told about the options available in clear and simple terms by a doctor or health professional who should be experienced and knowledgeable. The nurse can help in explaining again anything that the patient was unsure about. Remember, anxiety often hinders concentration.

The information provided should include:

- details of the diagnosis, prognosis and consequences if the condition is left untreated
- any uncertainties, including the need for further investigations
- options of treatments available, including the option not to treat
- description of the proposed treatment, any consequences, as well as substantive risks
- advice about whether the treatment is experimental or part of a research programme
- how the patient's condition and treatment will be monitored or re-assessed, the recovery period and the time involved
- the name of the clinician who has overall responsibility for the treatment and, where appropriate, the names of the senior members of the team
- whether clinicians in training will be involved
- a reminder that the patient may change his mind at any time
- a reminder that the patient has the right to a second opinion
- details of costs and charges if applicable
- a reminder of possible complications, disfigurement, or removal of parts
- an opportunity for the patient to ask any questions (if you do not know the answers the patient should be referred to either a senior member of staff or the doctor).

Obtaining consent

Consent may be implied or expressed. For the majority of procedures and treatments, including nursing procedures and treatments, only verbal consent is required. The golden rule before taking any action is to *always explain the procedure to the patient or client*. Implied consent may be by offering an arm for venepuncture or taking up the required position for the treatment, and this is taken that consent has been given. However, it should be remembered that this does not necessarily indicate that the patient has understood what is proposed. Expressed consent is that which is confirmed orally or in writing. Where there are language difficulties an official interpreter should be used. A family member or friend who does not understand medical terminology is not an appropriate interpreter. Certain religious beliefs may have an effect on the patient giving their consent, for example Jehovah's Witnesses, who do not agree with blood transfusions. Such issues need to be explored with the patient and help sought from one of their leaders if necessary.

Consent form

A different consent form should be signed for each operation or procedure. Consent for one procedure does not give any automatic right to undertake any other. If the patient is unable to write, an 'X' to indicate his signature is acceptable if there are two signed witnesses to his mark. For those with learning disabilities or with sensory deprivation, the nurse's role is essential in helping the patient to understand what is happening. The use of visual aids and drawings can be effective in getting the message across. Standard consent forms should be used and all details filled in correctly. Once the signature is obtained the form should be filed in the patient's notes.

A child between 13 and 16 years who is alone and has sufficient understanding may consent to an examination or to treatment by a doctor or other health professional but not to a surgical procedure or anaesthetic. A full note should be made of the factors taken into account when assessing the child to be knowledgeable and their capacity to give consent. A child over the age of 16 years may consent to any surgical, dental or medical treatment.

For those patients who are unconscious or irresponsible a parent or guardian's signature is required. If neither is available, the duty administrator may be authorised to give the consent. For female sterilisation, the consent of the husband or partner is preferable but not essential.

Refusal to consent can happen, and initially the patient should receive a further detailed explanation (preferably by the clinician) of the proposed treatment and why it is necessary. If the patient still refuses to agree and is deemed competent to do so, the refusal should be respected and a note,

witnessed if possible, made in the patient's medical records.

Examination or treatment without consent should only occur in exceptional circumstances, for example:

- when the patient is unconscious and the procedure would be life-saving
- in some cases where the minor is a ward of court and the court decides that the treatment would be in the child's best interests
- treatment for a mental disorder of a patient liable to be a detainee under the Mental Health Act 1983.

DOCUMENTATION

As the number of patients and clients being treated by the NHS continues to increase, careful and accurate documentation is essential, whether taken by hand or entered into the computer. Remember, anything that is entered into the patient's notes becomes part of a legal document and can be used in a court of law. Different types of documentation are dealt with more fully in Chapter 13. The NHS is trying to move to a single patient record but the majority of Trusts still have separate medical and nursing notes. Confidentiality regarding any knowledge you may acquire of a patient or client has to be observed and is both a legal and professional requirement. This subject has been discussed in more detail in Chapter 11.

Routine biographical documentation is made of any patient or client seeking care (i.e. name, address, age, date of birth). It is the nursing assessment that gives you the opportunity to meet your patient or client and practise your communication skills! It is also an ideal time to use your observation skills in assessing the patient's physiological and psychological status.

SOME PRINCIPLES OF COMMUNICATING WELL WITH PATIENTS AND OTHER PERSONNEL

- How you feel and look will influence establishing a good nurse–patient relationship and how you first approach the patient will influence

Activity 14.14

Nurse Simpson had rushed on duty on the surgical ward having had a quick lunch of garlic pâté and toast. Her uniform was rather crumpled and it was obvious that it had not been washed for several days; her hands showed that she had been gardening. Sister asked her to undertake the nursing assessment of Mrs Gill (age 65) who had just arrived and was waiting in the day room. Nurse Simpson quickly looked at the notes and noted that Mrs Gill's first name was Gladys. 'Shall we go and find somewhere quieter, Gladys?' she asked hurriedly, and was quite surprised when Mrs Gill did not respond.

How could Nurse Simpson have improved this first encounter?

how (and whether) you gain their cooperation and confidence, and this applies to any branch of nursing (Activity 14.14).

• Although it is the custom in Western countries to use the surname as the main means of identification, this may not be so in all cultures, so it is important to record the 'correct' surname. The use of first names is now more frequent for both patients and staff. However, care should be taken, particularly with older patients and those of a different culture, and it is preferable to ask *all* patients how they wish to be addressed, rather than taking it for granted that they are happy with the one you have chosen for them! Not all patients like the name they were given and may prefer that you use a different name.

• When answering the telephone your surname should be used as well as the information that you are a student or a staff nurse.

• Always keep in mind the purpose of anything you record and the audience for whom it is intended. For instance, care pathways are records to be used by a multidisciplinary team, and patients are now allowed access to their records. Facts (not opinions) must be identified and stated precisely, clearly and accurately. Bias and misinterpretation must be avoided.

• Avoid using abbreviations as these can lead to misunderstanding unless they are in common usage and well known to all those using the records.

• Observations have been discussed earlier; these should be recorded as soon as they are taken, accurately and clearly. *Never* make these up – a patient's treatment and even life may depend on what has been recorded. Always report to the person in charge if you have been unable to complete any observations. See also Chapter 9.

CONFIDENTIALITY

All patients have a right to expect that the information that they give to a doctor or nurse is treated with complete confidentiality. It may be necessary to discuss a patient's condition with other members of the health care team involved in the care of that patient but not to other staff unless specifically indicated. It is imperative that you do not talk about a patient's condition to anyone else without the permission, verbal or preferably written, of the patient. This includes giving information to the police unless the patient has given permission. However, if the police bring a patient into the casualty department, then they can be given the name, age, address and brief description of the problem to enable them to inform the next of kin.

You should be careful when giving information over the telephone, particularly if the patient may be of interest to the press. There should be no communication with the press without the permission of the patient or the patient's relatives, and all press enquiries should be directed to the organisation's public relations officer or senior manager.

Sometimes there may be an instance when the patient does not wish to communicate with relatives, and this should be respected. If you are uncertain who should be given information, it is a wise precaution to take the caller's number, then ask the patient if it is alright for them to have the information.

REPORT CONCERNS

National and local mechanisms are in place in all health and social care organisations to ensure that practice is safe and limitations are recognised. In addition to promoting continuing professional development, recent policy developments have encouraged the use of competency frameworks and personal development plans for all NHS staff. Many other employers have similar procedures. These initiatives help both individuals and their employing organisations to judge the level of support a practitioner requires in order to practise safely, and to identify their learning needs and by implication their limitations (see Ch. 1).

'Speaking out' policies are now in place in many NHS Trusts and other health and social care employing agencies. Supported through the implementation of clinical governance, individuals are encouraged to bring to the attention of the organisation their concerns about practitioners who are underperforming or, frankly, performing dangerously or harmfully to patients or the organisation. Together with clinical incident and 'near miss' reporting, this initiative is designed to ensure that action is taken promptly to prevent unsafe practice. Associated with the success of these developments is the presence of a 'no blame' culture, where learning and improvement rather than reprisal is the focus, a culture which is also expected to make acknowledging our limitations a little easier. (Ch. 11 describes 'speaking out' policies and their role in relation to the UKCC nursing Code of Professional Conduct.)

NHS organisations are also required to have anti-fraud policies in place and to have a designated fraud officer in post. Part of reporting concerns includes reporting fraud or suspected fraud within the workplace. While this will rarely affect the quality of patient care directly, unless patient property is the subject of the fraudulent act, it is important in relation to the honesty and integrity of the institution and the staff within it.

A particularly important area for reporting concern is when a nurse, or other professional, has noticed possible non-accidental injury of patients. While this is a particular issue in paediatric care (see Ch. 1), it may also be seen in other client groups, particularly the elderly or mentally frail. Employers will have policies and procedures to follow when these things are suspected and student nurses should become familiar with them.

REFERENCES

Atkins S, Murphy K 1993 Reflection: a review of the literature. Journal of Advanced Nursing 18:1188–1192

Barrie D 1996 The provision of food and catering services in hospital. Journal of Hospital Infection 33:13–33

Chadwick C, Oppenheim B A 1996 Cleaning as a cost effective method of infection control. Lancet 347:1776

Collins B J 1988 The hospital environment: how clean should it be? Journal of Hospital Infection 11(Supplement A):53–56

Department of Health 1990 Food handler's guide. HMSO, London

Department of Health 1993 Report of the task force of the strategy for research in nursing, midwifery and health visiting. HMSO, London

Department of Health 1995 Food safety (general) regulations. Stationery Office, London

Department of Health 1998 A first class service: quality in the new NHS. Stationery Office, London

Department of Health 1999 Making a difference: strengthening the nursing, midwifery and health visiting contribution to health and health care. DoH, London

Department of Health and Social Security 1972 Report of the committee on nursing (Briggs Report). HMSO, London

DiCenso A, Cullum N, Ciliska D 1998 Implementing evidence based nursing: some misconceptions. Evidence Based Nursing 1(2):38–40

Gibbs G 1988 Learning by doing: a guide to teaching and learning methods. Further Education Unit, Oxford Polytechnic, Oxford

Hancock T 1998 Reflective practice: using a learning journal. Nursing Standard 13(17):37–40

Health and Safety Commission 1992 Provision and use of equipment regulations 1992. SI 1992/2932. HMSO, London

Holm D, Stephenson S 1994 Reflection: a student's perspective. In: Palmer A, Burns S, Bulman C (eds) Reflective practice in nursing: the growth of the professional practitioner. Blackwell Science, Oxford, pp 53–62

House of Lords Select Committee on Science and Technology 1998 Report. Resistance to antibiotics and other antimicrobial agents. Stationery Office, London

Jarvis P 1992 Reflective practice in nursing. Nurse Education Today 12:174–181

Johns D C 1995 Framing learning through reflection within Carper fundamental ways of knowing in nursing. Journal of Advanced Nursing 22:226–234

McWhirter J, Pennington C 1994 Incidence and recognition of malnutrition in hospital. British Medical Journal 308:945–948

Medical Devices Agency 1996 Sterilisation, disinfection and cleaning of medical devices and equipment. Guidance from Microbiology Advisory Committee to the Department of Health Medical Device Agency. Part 2: Protocols. HMSO, London

National Health Services Management Executive 1995 Hospital laundry arrangements for used and infected linen. HSG 95 18. DoH, London

National Health Services Management Executive 1996 Clinical guidelines: using clinical guidelines to improve care within the NHS. DoH, Leeds

National Pathways Association 1998 Care pathways definition. Spring News Letter, NPA, London, www.the-npa.org.uk/fdgs.html

Newell R 1992 Anxiety, accuracy and reflection: the limits of professional development. Journal of Advanced Nursing 17:1326–1333

Nicholls S, Cullen R, O'Neill S, Halligan A 2000 Clinical governance: its origins and foundations. British Journal of Clinical Governance 5(3):172–178

Nicol M, Bavin C, Bedford-Turner S, Cronin P, Rawlins-Anderson K, 2000 Essential nursing skills. Mosby, London

Nightingale F 1859 Notes on hospitals. Longman, London

Nightingale F 2001 <http:chatna.com/author/nightingale.htm>

Palmer A, Burns S, Bulman C (eds) 1994 Reflective practice in nursing: the growth of the professional practitioner. Blackwell Science, Oxford

Parker L J 1999 Managing and maintaining a safe environment in the hospital setting. British Journal of Nursing 8(16):1053–1066

Quinn F M 1998 Reflection and reflective practice. In: Quinn F M (ed) Continuing professional development in nursing. Stanley Thornes, Cheltenham, ch 7

Resuscitation Council (UK) 2001 Basic life support resuscitation guidelines 2000. Resuscitation Council (UK), London/Laerdal Medical Ltd, Orpington

Royal College of Nursing 1994 Guidance on infection control in hospitals. RCN, London

SMAC 1998 Sub-group on antimicrobial resistance: the path of least resistance. DoH, London

Swage T 2000 Clinical governance in health care practice. Butterworth-Heinemann, Oxford

UKCC 1992a Code of professional conduct. UKCC, London

UKCC 1992b Standards for the administration of medicines. UKCC, London

UKCC 1996 Guidelines for professional practice. UKCC, London

UKCC 1997 Responsibility for feeding of patients. UKCC, London

Waterlow J 1985 Pressure sores: a risk assessment card. Nursing Times 81(48):49–55

Wilkinson J 1999 Implementing reflective practice. Nursing Standard 13(21):36–40

Wilson K J W, Waugh A 1996 Anatomy and physiology in health and illness, 8th edn. Churchill Livingstone, Edinburgh

FURTHER READING

Deeks J 1995 Pressure sore prevention: using and evaluating risk assessment tools. British Journal of Nursing 5(5):313–320
Provides readers with an overview of available risk assessment tools and their suitability in everyday practice.

National Back Pain Association and Royal College of Nursing 1998 The guide to the handling of patients, 4th edn. NBPA, London
Prepared with nurses for nurses and provides a definitive guide to safe lifting, moving and handling of patients to minimise the risk of injury to both patients and nurses.

Nicol M, Bavin C, Bedford-Turner S, Cronin, P, Rawlins-Anderson K, 2000 Essential nursing skills. Mosby, London
*Written to help student nurses carry out clinical skills safely. It uses a step-by-step approach to over 100 essential skills of foundation nursing care. Its emphasis is on the care carried out in the general nursing setting but **all** common foundation students should find it helpful in the early stages of training.*

Resuscitation Council (UK) 1997 The 1997 Resuscitation guidelines for use in the United Kingdom. Resuscitation Council(UK), London
This is a full procedure manual, of only 12 pages, for basic life support care and covers the theory and practice in lively and accessible language. Used widely in 'A and E' departments, the ambulance services and all areas where life-saving procedures are carried out.

Royal College of Nursing 1996 Code of practice for patient handling. RCN, London
Guidelines and associated safety procedures for all aspects of patient handling. Written from a health and safety perspective for the prevention of back injury to nurses.

Skinner S 1996 Understanding clinical investigations. Ballière Tindall, London
Provides information about the rationale and procedure for all major observations carried out on patients.

Snowley G, Nicklin P, Birch J 1992 Objectives for care: specifying standards for clinical nursing, 2nd edn. Wolfe, London
Emphasises the systematic approach to nursing care and embraces all care groups and care settings. Written to provide a link between theory and practice, links in with available research and accompanied by detailed bibliographies.

APPENDIX 1 MYOCARDIAL INFARCTION CARE PATHWAY

PATIENT DETAILS

Patient ID label

Preferred name ....

Home telephone number ....

Registered GP ....

....

....

Marital status ....

Religion ....

Next of kin details

Name ....

Address ....

....

....

....

Tel. Number (day) ....

Tel. Number (night) ....

Relationship ....

ICP GUIDELINES FOR USE (ICP)
Myocardial infarction (MI)

Criteria

This pathway is for all patients who have had an uncomplicated MI, with or without thrombolysis. The MI patient who has not received thrombolysis is still eligible for this pathway. MI patients on drug trials may also be included.

The reason for the pathway is to ensure that the patient receives the best care, and that it serves as a checklist for those who use it, and its tick and initial format makes it much quicker than conventional methods. *Please write all comments on the ICP.*

Doctor's guidelines

Complete all activities and associated documentation at the appropriate time period. If this cannot be done, please record the fact and the given reason. This is termed a variance.

If a patient develops complications or has a prolonged course of treatment it may be necessary to insert extra sheets into the pathway, or remove the patient from the pathway and use usual clinical notes. Reasons for discontinuing the pathway must be given.

Nursing guidelines

Complete all activities and associated documentation at the appropriate time period. If you are unable to do this then you need to document this as a variance, in the space provided. Use alphabet code to identify variance in care (there is some space for each section to document any comments, otherwise tick box and initial).

The only care plans that are needed for a patient on an MI pathway are those for additional problems (e.g. diabetes), then a care plan needs to be written as per documentation policy. Any other information should be recorded on the nursing communication sheet.

If a patient develops a complication (e.g. prolonged heart failure), which disturbs the care required on the pathway, then the patient must be removed from the pathway and usual nursing documentation commenced.

Reasons for discontinuing the pathway must be documented in the notes.

Note any problems please contact: Dr . . . .: A&E consultant Bleep 261
Dr . . . .: Consultant Physician Ext. 5492
Sister . . . .: Coronary Care Unit Ext. 4848

THIS INTEGRATED CARE PATHWAY IS THE PATIENT'S NOTES

MANAGEMENT OF MYOCARDIAL INFARCTION

Assessment
1. Brief history
2. Brief examination:
    a) Heart rate
    b) Blood pressure
    c) Rule out dissection
3. Contraindications to thrombolysis
4. ECG

Treatment
1. O^2 – 5–6 litres
2. GTN sublingually
3. i.v. diamorphine – 2.5–5 mg slow i.v.
4. i.v. metoclopramide 10 mg
5. Oral aspirin 300 mg
6. IV thrombolysis – **if not contraindicated**
7. Streptokinase 1.5 MU in 100 ml of normal saline over one hour. Or TPA 100 mg/$\frac{1}{2}$ hr (15 mg bolus, 50 mg over 30 min, 35 mg over 60 min).

Indications for thrombolysis
There is ST elevation in 2 of
    a) II, III, a VF   - OR
    b) I, a VL V5 V6   - OR
    c) VI–V6   - OR
    d) assumed new LBBB - OR

Thrombolysis may not be indicated if
1. The ECG is normal
2. There are T-wave changes only
3. There is ST segment depression only
In case of any doubt, please contact medical registrar before treating patient with thrombolysis

Possible contraindications to thrombolysis
1. Prolonged chest compression
2. Active peptic ulcer disease/severe oesophagitis
3. Stroke within 12 months
4. Surgery (including tooth extraction) within 4 weeks
5. Bleeding diathesis (? Warfarin) if INR greater than 2
6. Aortic dissection
7. Possible pregnancy
8. Recent injury and contusion (including vigorous CPR)
9. Diabetic retinopathy

Myocardial Infarction
Care Pathway

A&E DOCTOR

DOCTOR'S NAME:	DATE SEEN:
TIME OF ARRIVAL:	TIME SEEN:

HISTORY:	COMMENTS:
1. Type of pain 2. Duration of pain 3. Previous history 4. Medication 5. Allergy	

ASSESSMENT:	COMMENTS:
1. BP 2. Pulse and rate 3. ECG 4. Indication for thrombolysis 5. Contraindication for thrombolysis 6. Inform CCU of probable admission	 1. 2. 1. 2.

	Dose	Time given & signature
1. Aspirin 2. O^2 60% 3. GTN sublingually 4. i.v. diamorphine 5. Thrombolysis (specify thrombolytic drug) 6. i.v. metoclopramide		

POST-THROMBOLYTIC THERAPY 1. ECG

Referred to Medical Registrar	Time:

Myocardial Infarction
Care Pathway

ON ADMISSION

Doctor:	Consultant:

Time seen by admitting doctor:

Date of symptom onset:	Time of symptom onset:

Aspirin given? Yes ☐ No ☐

Date: Time:
If not, reason:

Thrombolysis given? Strep/TPA Yes ☐ No ☐

Date: Time:
If not, reason:

SYMPTOMS
CVS

Chest:	Pain ☐	Severity:	Mild ☐
	Tightness ☐		Moderate ☐
	Other ☐		Severe ☐
	Radiation:		
	Duration:		

Breathlessness	Yes ☐	No ☐
Dizziness	Yes ☐	No ☐
Syncope	Yes ☐	No ☐
Nausea	Yes ☐	No ☐
Vomiting	Yes ☐	No ☐
Sweating	Yes ☐	No ☐

Date ..../ ..../	Time	Signature	Bleep number ....

PLEASE PLACE PATIENT LABEL IN A&E INTEGRATED CARE PATHWAY REGISTER BOOK

Myocardial Infarction
Care Pathway

ON ADMISSION

DOCTOR'S NOTES

OTHER HPC:

AS:

CNS:

RS:

UGS:

PAST HISTORY:

Previous chest pain	Yes ☐	No ☐	Date ....
MI	Yes ☐	No ☐	Date ....
CVA	Yes ☐	No ☐	Date ....
Diabetes	Yes ☐	No ☐	Date ....
Hypertension	Yes ☐	No ☐	Date ....
Contraindications to thrombolysis	Yes ☐	No ☐	Date ....

Other: ....

Family history of heart disease	Yes ☐	No ☐

Comments:

PREVIOUS TREATMENT

Streptokinase	Yes ☐	No ☐	Date ....
Aspirin	Yes ☐	No ☐	Date ....
Anticoagulants	Yes ☐	No ☐	Date ....

Allergies:

Myocardial Infarction
Care Pathway

ON ADMISSION

DOCTOR'S NOTES

MEDICATION ON ADMISSION

SOCIAL HISTORY

Occupation: ....

Lives alone: Yes ☐ No ☐   Lives with: ....

Alcohol consumption: .... Tobacco consumption: ....
Comments:

ON EXAMINATION

General:

CVS: Pulse: Rate: BP:
                      Rhythm:
                      Volume: JVP:
                      Character: HS:

RS:

Abdomen:

CNS:

ECG:

CXR:

*Myocardial Infarction
Care Pathway*

ON ADMISSION

DOCTOR'S NOTES

PROVISIONAL DIAGNOSIS

Definite acute MI   ☐
Possible acute MI   ☐
Unstable angina   ☐
Angina   ☐

Other (specify) ....

OTHER INVESTIGATIONS

Bloods: Urea & electrolytes   ☐ ....

         Cardiac enzymes   ☐ ....

         Glucose   ☐ ....

         Full blood count   ☐ ....

         Cholesterol (within 24 hr of admission)   ☐ ....

PRESCRIPTIONS AND FORMS

Anticoagulants   ☐

Oxygen   ☐

Diamorphine i.v./2.5–5.0 mg slow i.v.   ☐

Nitrates   ☐

Anti-emetic i.v./metoclopramide 10 mg or prochlorperazine 12.5 mg i.m.   ☐

Oral analgesia   ☐

Complete routine forms: Cardiac enzymes (×2)   ☐

                                  U & Es   ☐

                                  ECG (×2)   ☐

Date ..../ ..../ .... | Time .... | Signature .... | Bleep number ....

Myocardial Infarction
Care Pathway

A&E NURSING

Named nurse in A&E
Time patient arrived
1. Attach cardiac monitor
2. O^2 therapy
3. a) Record 12-lead ECG and inform doctor of findings

b) Record observations $\frac{1}{4}$ hourly
     TPR
     BP

4. Use pain assessment tool (facing this sheet)
5. Action taken from pain assessment tool
6. Give prescribed 300 mg aspirin

7. Start prescribed i.v. therapy
   (For thrombolysis monitor $\frac{1}{4}$ pulse and BP)
   Start time
   Completion time
   Inform doctor if either drops
   Reason for stopping thrombolysis

8. Inform patient of expected transfer to CCU
9. Record post-thrombolytic ECG (immediate)
10. Inform CCU of expected admission time
Document in appropriate area personal details of patient started on ICPs and area transferred to
CCU   Length of wait ....
Ward   if not CCU; reason ....
Communication/Variance

Variance source code
1. Patient condition	5. Doctor response time	9. Data availability
2. Pt/family decision	6. Nurse decision	10. Department overbooked
3. Pt/family availability	7. Nurse response time	11. Department closed
4. Doctor decision	8. Bed availability	12. Community services

Myocardial Infarction
Care Pathway

PAIN RULER

MATCH THE WORD(S) THAT APPLY TO YOUR PAIN WITH A NUMBER ON THE SCALE WHICH CORRESPONDS TO THE SEVERITY OF YOUR PAIN

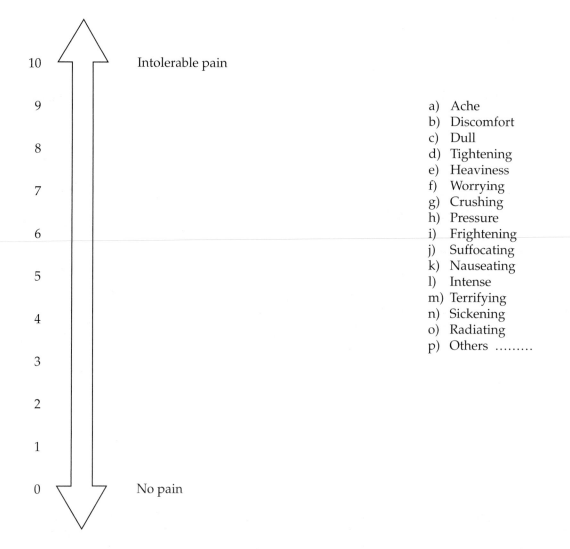

10 Intolerable pain

9

8

7

6

5

4

3

2

1

0 No pain

a) Ache
b) Discomfort
c) Dull
d) Tightening
e) Heaviness
f) Worrying
g) Crushing
h) Pressure
i) Frightening
j) Suffocating
k) Nauseating
l) Intense
m) Terrifying
n) Sickening
o) Radiating
p) Others ....

Myocardial Infarction
Care Pathway

ON ARRIVAL TO CCU

NURSING

		EARLY:
a) Named nurse in CCU:	Signature:	
b) Time of admission	Time patient arrived	
c) Attach to cardiac monitor and record rhythm strip take 12-lead ECG Document findings	Yes ☐ No ☐	Date:
d) Record observations Temperature Pulse Respirations		Time:
CCU observation chart Oxygen therapy Blood pressure Urine Capillary blood sugar (if venous blood not taken) Urinalysis		Signature:
		LATE:
e) Have you checked the Venflon site	Yes ☐ No ☐	Time:
f) Have you checked any infusions in progress and documented this	Yes ☐ No ☐	Signature:
g) Use pain assessment tool. Document if any action taken		
h) Fluid balance chart commenced	Yes ☐ No ☐	**NIGHT:**
i) Have you checked blood results (L&E, CK, cholesterol, BC)	Yes ☐ No ☐	
j) Have you explained about monitoring equipment and initial care with patient/carer/relative and documented this	Yes ☐ No ☐	Time:
k) Have you documented in admissions book that patient is on ICP	Yes ☐ No ☐	Signature:
l) CCU information leaflet given Given to whom	Yes ☐ No ☐	

Communication/Variance

Variance source code
1. Patient condition	5. Doctor response time	9. Data availability
2. Pt/family decision	6. Nurse decision	10. Department overbooked
3. Pt/family availability	7. Nurse response time	11. Department closed
4. Doctor decision	8. Bed availability	12. Community services

Myocardial Infarction
Care Pathway

UP TO 24 HOURS IN CCU

DOCTOR

Doctor:	Consultant:

Reassess clinical status
Reassess drug therapy
CPK 5–6 hours after first sample
Repeat U & Es/cardiac enzymes
Review 12-lead ECG
? CXR
? Glucose

Date ..../ ..../	Time	Signature	Bleep number ....

Myocardial Infarction
Care Pathway

24 HOURS OF ARRIVAL

NURSING IN CCU

a) Named nurse:	Signature:			
b) Assess frequency of observations required (2–4 hourly) and document. CCU observation chart	Yes ☐	No ☐		**EARLY:**
c) Use pain assessment tool				Date:
d) Check ECG recorded and document findings and actions	Yes ☐	No ☐		
e) Record rhythm strip and ECG if arrhythmias occur and document findings and actions				Time:
f) Continue with fluid balance chart	Yes ☐	No ☐		Signature:
g) Record i.v. therapy and when stopped	Yes ☐	No ☐		
h) Explain reasons for bed rest to patient/carer/relative	Yes ☐	No ☐		**LATE:**
i) Explain average length of stay in CCU to patient/relative/carer	Yes ☐	No ☐		Time:
j) Check blood results				Signature:
U&E	CK			**NIGHT:** Time:
Clotting	Cholesterol			Signature:

Communication/Variance

Variance source code

1. Patient condition	5. Doctor response time	9. Data availability
2. Pt/family decision	6. Nurse decision	10. Department overbooked
3. Pt/family availability	7. Nurse response time	11. Department closed
4. Doctor decision	8. Bed availability	12. Community services

Myocardial Infarction
Care Pathway

DAY 2

DOCTOR

Doctor:	Consultant:

Clinical status: Assess for transfer to a ward area		
Set provisional discharge date		
Repeat cardiac enzymes if diagnosis in doubt		
Review 12-lead ECG		
Consider likely need for exercise tests as an in-patient	Yes ☐	No ☐
Consider likely need for Echo as an in-patient	Yes ☐	No ☐
Check rehabilitation consent form signed		

Date ..../ ..../	Time	Signature	Bleep number ....

Myocardial Infarction
Care Pathway

DAY 2

NURSING IN CCU

a)	Named nurse in CCU:	Ward:				
b)	Review frequency of observations (1–4 hourly) Assess need to change to 4 hourly chart	Yes ☐	No ☐	**EARLY:**		
c)	Check 12-lead ECG	Yes ☐	No ☐	Date:		
d)	Use pain assessment tool					
e)	Fluid balance chart – assess need to continue	Yes ☐	No ☐	Time:		
f)	Record weight as part of admission policy	Yes ☐	No ☐			
g)	Record when i.v. therapy stopped	Yes ☐	No ☐	Signature:		
h)	Re-assess Venflon site	Yes ☐	No ☐			
i)	Refer to cardiac rehab nurse and check consent form signed	Yes ☐	No ☐	**LATE:**		
j)	Refer to rehab nurse section/intervene as necessary	Yes ☐	No ☐	Time:		
k)	Inform patient/carer/relative of possible transfer out of CCU	Yes ☐	No ☐	Signature:		
l)	Inform bed manager	Yes ☐	No ☐			
m)	Sit in chair	Yes ☐	No ☐			
n)	Prepare thrombolysis card and give to patient when leaving CCU	Yes ☐	No ☐	**NIGHT:**		
o)	Check provisional discharge date set Date:	Yes ☐	No ☐	Time:		
p)	Social work referral	Yes ☐	No ☐	Signature:		
q)	Assess need for dietician referral	Yes ☐	No ☐			
r)	Check blood results U&E ☐ CK ☐ Clotting ☐					
s)	Check whether patient's bowels have opened	Yes ☐	No ☐			
t)	Give shared care card	Yes ☐	No ☐			

Communication/Variance

Variance source code
1. Patient condition
2. Pt/family decision
3. Pt/family availability
4. Doctor decision
5. Doctor response time
6. Nurse decision
7. Nurse response time
8. Bed availability
9. Data availability
10. Department overbooked
11. Department closed
12. Community services

Myocardial Infarction
Care Pathway

DAY 3

DOCTOR

Doctor:	Consultant:

Reassess clinical status:
Assess for transfer to a general ward – if still in CCU
Assess need for i.v. access
Plan date for discharge
Beta blockers
Ace inhibitors
Oral nitrates Consider simvastatin

Date ..../ ..../	Time	Signature	Bleep number ....

Myocardial Infarction
Care Pathway

DAY 3

NURSING

a)	Named nurse:	Ward:		
b)	Assess frequency of observations needed. Discontinue chart and use 4 hourly chart			**EARLY:**
c)	Discontinue fluid balance chart	Yes ☐	No ☐	
d)	Remove Venflon if not being used	Yes ☐	No ☐	Date:
e)	Record date and time of transfer and name of ward in admissions book. Ensure carer/relative informed. Update PAS	Yes ☐	No ☐	Time:
f)	Discuss short- and long-term self-care aspects providing written information. Use patient wise information. Document here.	Yes ☐	No ☐	Signature:
g)	Cardiac rehab nurse: see own section Named nurse to read this	Yes ☐	No ☐	**LATE:** Time:
h)	Mobilise around bed area	Yes ☐	No ☐	Signature:
i)	Walk out and supervise in bathroom	Yes ☐	No ☐	
j)	Check whether need a 3rd ECG	Yes ☐	No ☐	
k)	Social work referral	Yes ☐	No ☐	**NIGHT:**
l)	Inform patient/relative/carer of professional discharge date	Yes ☐	No ☐	Time:
m)	Give patient/carer patient wise information and explain	Yes ☐	No ☐	Signature:
n)	Ensure thrombolysis card given to patient	Yes ☐	No ☐	
o)	Discontinue cardiac monitoring	Yes ☐	No ☐	

Communication/Variance

Variance source code
1. Patient condition
2. Pt/family decision
3. Pt/family availability
4. Doctor decision

5. Doctor response time
6. Nurse decision
7. Nurse response time
8. Bed availability

9. Data availability
10. Department overbooked
11. Department closed
12. Community services

Myocardial Infarction
Care Pathway

DAY 4

DOCTOR

Doctor:	Consultant:

Reassess clinical status:
Reconsider use of Ace inhibitors
Reconsider use of beta blockers
Write up TTAs if possible (even if only provisional)
Check rehabilitation nurse's notes/consent form (colour code)

Date ..../........../	Time	Signature	Bleep number ....

Myocardial Infarction
Care Pathway

DAY 4

NURSING

a) Named nurse:	Ward:			**EARLY:**
b) Assess frequency of observations	Yes ☐	No ☐		
c) To mobilise around ward and walk to wash room	Yes ☐	No ☐		Date:
d) Check cardiac rehabilitation nurse has met with patient Check details on rehab nurse section	Yes ☐	No ☐		Time: Signature:
e) Reinforce rehabilitative information with patient/carer/relative	Yes ☐	No ☐		
f) Assess need for referral to physiotherapy for stair assessment	Yes ☐	No ☐		**LATE:** Time:
g) Plan with medics definite date for discharge and inform patient/carer/relative	Yes ☐ Date ...../......./..........	No ☐		Signature:
h) Advise patient to arrange transport for discharge date (check arrangements made) Or provisionally book transport	Yes ☐ Yes ☐ Date ...../......./.......... Time	No ☐ No ☐		**NIGHT:** Time:
i) Send TTA request to pharmacy	Yes ☐	No ☐		Signature:

Communication/Variance

Variance source code
1. Patient condition
2. Pt/family decision
3. Pt/family availability
4. Doctor decision

5. Doctor response time
6. Nurse decision
7. Nurse response time
8. Bed availability

9. Data availability
10. Department overbooked
11. Department closed
12. Community services

Myocardial Infarction
Care Pathway

DAY 5

DOCTOR

Doctor:	Consultant:

Reassess clinical status:
Complete discharge letter for general practitioner
Request OPA (4–6 weeks) unless going for an angiogram
Reconsider need for exercise test in OPD? Book if required   Yes ☐   No ☐   Date ....
Hepatitis B if going for an angiogram (summary needed for – Hospital) MRSA screening forms Check whether consent form for rehabilitation signed

| Date ..../........./......... | Time .... | Signature .... | Bleep number .... |

Myocardial Infarction
Care Pathway

DAY 5

NURSING

a)	Named nurse:	Ward:		**EARLY:**
b)	Reassess frequency of observations	Yes ☐ No ☐		
c)	Check consent form signed for rehabilitation if patient is participating	Yes ☐ No ☐		Date:
d)	Ensure TTAs have been sent from pharmacy	Yes ☐ No ☐		Time:
e)	Check discharge letter has been completed	Yes ☐ No ☐		Signature:
f)	Has a stair assessment been prepared with the physiotherapist, if needed	Yes ☐ No ☐		
g)	Book OPA Date ....../......../........ Time .... Book transport for OPA if needed (before 12:00) Request car if appropriate	Yes ☐ No ☐		**LATE:** Time: Signature:
	Give OPA card to patient	Yes ☐ No ☐		**NIGHT:**
h)	Commence discharge checklist/plan	Yes ☐ No ☐		Time:
i)	Ensure appropriate patient wise information given to patient/relative/carer	Yes ☐ No ☐		Signature:

Communication/Variance

Variance source code
1. Patient condition
2. Pt/family decision
3. Pt/family availability
4. Doctor decision
5. Doctor response time
6. Nurse decision
7. Nurse response time
8. Bed availability
9. Data availability
10. Department overbooked
11. Department closed
12. Community services

Myocardial Infarction
Care Pathway

DISCHARGE DAY – DAY 6

DOCTOR

IF PATIENT IS NOT TO BE DISCHARGED PLEASE DOCUMENT REASON. ADDITIONAL SHEETS TO BE ATTACHED TO ICP

Doctor:	Consultant:

Reassess clinical status before discharge

Summary to be dictated

Final diagnosis

1.

2.

3.

4.

On aspirin   Yes ☐   No ☐
If no, state reason

Date ..../ ..../	Time	Signature	Bleep number ....

Myocardial Infarction
Care Pathway

DAY 6

NURSING

a)	Named nurse:	Ward:		**EARLY:**
b)	Check Venflon has been removed	Yes ☐	No ☐	
c)	Check thrombolysis card given	Yes ☐	No ☐	Date:
d)	Check patient has cardiac rehab number	Yes ☐	No ☐	
e)	CCU direct line number given	Yes ☐	No ☐	Time:
f)	Discuss TTAs with patient/carer/relative	Yes ☐	No ☐	Signature:
g)	Check patient has written information about his/her condition	Yes ☐	No ☐	
h)	Has the patient wise information been given	Yes ☐	No ☐	**LATE:**
i)	GP letter given to patient	Yes ☐	No ☐	Time:
j)	Give a copy of last 12-lead ECG to patient and explain why	Yes ☐	No ☐	
k)	Check whether MRSA screen needed if going for an angiogram as an outpatient	Yes ☐	No ☐	Signature:
l)	Date and time screened if yes Date .... Time			**NIGHT:**
m)	Check OPA given	Yes ☐	No ☐	
n)	Check sick certificate given if needed	Yes ☐	No ☐	Time:
o)	Complete discharge checklist/plan	Yes ☐	No ☐	Signature:
p)	On patient's discharge, place this ICP document in the patient's medical records folder			

Communication/Variance

Variance source code
1. Patient condition
2. Pt/family decision
3. Pt/family availability
4. Doctor decision

5. Doctor response time
6. Nurse decision
7. Nurse response time
8. Bed availability

9. Data availability
10. Department overbooked
11. Department closed
12. Community services

*Myocardial Infarction
Care Pathway*

CARDIAC REHABILITATION NURSE

Patient assessed – Cardiac rehabilitation interventions are appropriate for this patient	Yes ☐	No ☐	

Cardiac rehabilitation nurse	Bleep number	Date........./........./..........

	Yes	No	N/A	Date	Time	Initial
a) Education/information (re cardiac condition)	☐	☐	☐			
b) Relative/partner involved	☐	☐	☐			
c) Post discharge activity advice	☐	☐	☐			
d) Work related advice	☐	☐	☐			
e) Driving related information	☐	☐	☐			
f) Psychological readjustment	☐	☐	☐			
g) Sexual activity advice	☐	☐	☐			
h) Social activity advice	☐	☐	☐			
i) Smoking cessation	☐	☐	☐			
j) Exercise recommendations	☐	☐	☐			
k) Dietary recommendations	☐	☐	☐			
l) Cholesterol/lipids information	☐	☐	☐			
m) Weight control advice	☐	☐	☐			
n) Stress management	☐	☐	☐			
o) Hypertension	☐	☐	☐			
p) Diabetes	☐	☐	☐			
q) Genetic predisposition	☐	☐	☐			
r) Chest pain response/management	☐	☐	☐			
s) Medication	☐	☐	☐			
t) Cardiac tests	☐	☐	☐			
u) Cardiac surgery/PTCA	☐	☐	☐			
v) Assess need for post discharge support	☐	☐	☐			
w) Provide contact phone number	☐	☐	☐			
x) Assess for the cardiac rehabilitation programme	☐	☐	☐			
y) Will patient be: Attending ☐ Not Attending ☐ Still Undecided ☐						
Variances:						

MEDICAL CONSENT: For the Patient to Attend the **CARDIAC REHABILITATION PROGRAMME**

The exercise component for this patient will be set at: Normal Intensity ☐
Moderate Intensity ☐
Low Intensity ☐

Date ..../.........../	Time	Signature	Bleep number ....

15

Caring for the person with pain

Linda Husband

CHAPTER CONTENTS

Introduction 458

Classifying the experience of pain 459
Acute pain can become chronic pain 460

The physiology of pain 460
Nociceptive pain 460
The transmission of nociceptive pain
stimuli 461
Treating nociceptive pain 462
Non-pharmacological approaches 462
Pharmacological approaches 462
Neuropathic pain 465
Drugs used in the management of
neuropathic pain 465
Post-herpetic (shingles) neuralgia 466
Phantom limb pain 466
Other types of phantom pain 467
Cancer pain 467
Managing cancer pain 468
The WHO analgesic ladder 469

Assessing pain 470
Assessing pain in adults 470
Assessing pain in infants and children 471
Physical cues 472
Behavioural cues 472
CRIES 472
Assessing pain in people with learning
disability or severe communication
difficulty 473
Assessing and managing pain in elderly
people 474
Managing pain with non-pharmacological
interventions 474

Transcutaneous electrical nerve stimulation
(TENS) 475
Other non-drug interventions 477
Additional pain-relieving strategies 477
So, what does it take to ensure good pain
assessment and management? 478

References 479

Further reading 480

Internet 481

The successful management of a patient's pain is one of the most challenging and satisfying aspects of nursing practice. However, few outcomes require such a refined integration of knowledge and skill to achieve. The nurse must have not simply a sound working knowledge of the nature of pain and the pharmacological and non-pharmacological interventions useful in its relief, but must also have good communication skills, be astute in the assessment of verbal and non-verbal cues and have an understanding of the patient as a person with a unique personal and social history.

After reading this chapter the student should be able to:

- classify different pain experiences (acute and chronic, nociceptive and neuropathic)
- describe the physiology of pain
- give an account of how the pain pathway can be blocked using pharmacological and non-pharmacological means
- describe the management of pain in different types of illness, including cancer
- give an account of how to assess pain in adults and children, including those with learning disability or severe communication difficulty
- describe the assessment and management of pain in elderly people
- describe the use of various complementary therapies in pain control.

INTRODUCTION

Pain has been defined as the unpleasant sensory or emotional response to injury or to the perceived threat of injury (International Association for the Study of Pain 1979). It is a complex phenomenon that encompasses not just our physical responses to actual tissue damage but also the emotional and intellectual reactions that arise when we feel ourselves to be at risk of harm. The multidimensional nature of pain is of great use to the professional nurse because it provides an equal number of avenues of pain management; pain may be alleviated through physical measures, through emotional support and through educational input that empowers.

Pain is, by its very nature, a deeply personal experience. McCaffery (1968, p. 95), an internationally recognised expert in the nursing care of patients in pain, emphasised this fact when she defined it in this way: 'Pain is whatever the experiencing person says it is, existing whenever he says it does.' A number of assessment tools for pain are described later in this chapter, but it is important to appreciate that nothing can replace the self-report of the patient, when available. However, communicating the pain experience is not easy. It is not a simple matter of description of a physical phenomenon; pain only makes sense when it is understood in context (Activity 15.1).

In carrying out Activity 15.1 you will probably have found that in your attempt to share your experience you provided your colleague with a description that conveyed not just the physical symptoms, but also how you felt about it and what your thoughts were at the time. Indeed you will probably have found that it was inadequate to give a description merely of a physical symptom: the actual experience of pain encompassed far more. If your colleague was able, in return, to relate a story of pain of the same nature, you may have found that her description was in some ways similar but in some ways very different from your own. Pain, in short, is unique to each person and has a physical, emotional and intellectual dimension.

Activity 15.1 The personal experience of pain

Talk with a colleague and share a pain experience that each of you has had. Perhaps you have had a dental abscess, a sprained ankle, broken bone, or an operation. How would you describe the pain you experienced as a result? Has your colleague had the same source of pain? If so, was her experience the same as your own? How was your pain assessed and managed?

CLASSIFYING THE EXPERIENCE OF PAIN

Pain is usually classified in terms of its duration or its source but there are many other important factors to be considered in the professional management of the person in pain. A pain that lasts a short time is usually labelled as *acute* whereas one that continues beyond 6 months is termed *chronic*. Acute pain often makes sense to us in a way that chronic pain does not. It may safeguard us by signalling when tissue is being damaged and thus allow us to take avoiding action or give an injury time and protection to heal. By contrast, chronic pain has little protective value but has tremendous potential to destroy not only the person's quality of life but also, untreated, the person himself.

When the source of the pain is considered, pain is defined as being either *nociceptive* or *neuropathic*. If a pain originates from stimulation outside the nervous system it is termed nociceptive and if it originates or is sustained from actions within the nervous system it is defined as neuropathic. Nociceptive literally means 'of a noxious or harmful nature' and in this case the nerve ending, termed a nociceptor, is picking up information about a stimulus that is able to damage tissues. Neuropathic refers to dysfunction within the nervous system (*neuro* = nerve and *pathic* = disordered).

Acute and chronic pain may be either nociceptive or neuropathic but acute pain tends to be nociceptive. Examples of acute nociceptive pain would include injuries incurred from falls or from a tear of the skin on your arm while pruning the roses. Acute pain has an important function as a body defence, even though experiencing it can be very distressing. Painful sensations usually stimulate movement away from the source of damage or bring about investigation for a cause. Where pain sensation is impaired, for example when nerve pathways have been damaged (as in paraplegia, diabetic neuropathy), the person can be severely damaged by developing sores or other lesions.

Chronic pain of a nociceptive nature might come from ischaemic disorders such as arterial leg ulcers in which case the pain would be the result of ongoing inflammatory reactions and tissue damage. Neuropathic sources of chronic pain would include phantom limb pain and postherpetic (shingles) neuralgia. In these cases the pain would originate from activity within the nervous system.

Before considering how pain is handled within the nervous system it is important to consider how acute and chronic pain differ in terms of presentation. Think about a patient you have cared for who was in acute pain following trauma, then think about a person with chronic pain from a condition such as degenerative vertebral disc disease, cancer pain or arthritis and you will recall very different physiological and behavioural expressions of pain. The key differences are summarised in Table 15.1.

Table 15.1 shows how and why it is easy to miss a diagnosis of chronic pain in particular. What you can see is not what the patient is experiencing at all. The potential problems for the patient are more far-reaching, however, than our failing to recognise and help with pain management. A lack of appreciation of the physiology of pain and of the differences between acute and chronic pain presentation can lead to interpersonal conflict between health care workers and patients.

Consider the case history shown in Case example 15.1, which may be a familiar one. Knowing more about the nature of pain should immediately have made two points clear in relation to Mrs Smith. First, Mrs Smith is the expert on her own pain assessment so her request is totally appropriate and should be treated as

Table 15.1 Differences between acute and chronic pain	
Acute	**Chronic**
Rapid pulse	Normal pulse
Raised blood pressure	Normal blood pressure
Dilated pupils	Normal pupil size
Quiet, rubbing part, guarding painful area	Normal activity, perhaps limited in nature
Reports pain	May not even mention pain unless questioned

Case example 15.1 Mrs Smith's pills

Mrs Smith rings her bell and asks you for 'my pain pills'. You ask her about her pain and she tells you that it's her back, 'as usual', that it's very painful and it is a gnawing type of pain. You know she has a prescription written up and you promise to get back to her as soon as you can. You are then delayed in getting her medication due to an emergency admission to your ward. In the meantime visitors come onto the ward. Mrs Smith's niece, whom she loves to see, arrives as you are hurrying to dispense the tablets you promised her half an hour ago. When you arrive at the doorway of her room, Mrs Smith is sitting up and happily chatting and laughing with her niece. She does not appear to be in any pain at all. She thanks you for the tablets, takes them and you walk away feeling somewhat exasperated. There you were rushing to meet what you thought was a legitimate need only to find that she is just fine!

Table 15.2 Differences in function between Aδ and C nerve fibres

Aδ	C
Myelinated: fast transmission	Non-myelinated: slower transmission
Small receptive field	Large receptive field
High threshold	Lower threshold
Sharp, well localised	Dull, aching, burning pain in a general area
Unimodal: mechanical or heat	Polymodal: mechanical, heat, chemicals
25% of nociceptors	75% of nociceptors

(Hayes & Molloy 1997). For nurses to provide sensitive, timely and appropriate help to a person experiencing pain of any kind, it is extremely important to understand the physiology of pain.

accurate. Second, a knowledge of the differences between acute and chronic pain can assist in the true interpretation of patient behaviour. There is a third aspect of this situation that is covered later in the chapter: how pain is modulated within the nervous system to give temporary relief.

Acute pain can become chronic pain

The importance of effective postoperative pain relief has been highlighted by a number of recent studies. Research has shown that acute pain can become chronic pain in some patients who have had poor pain management in their early postoperative period. The results of a study of 93 women who had undergone surgery for breast cancer found that those who recalled their postoperative pain as being more severe tended to develop chronic pain (Tasmuth et al 1996). It seems that brief acute pain is handled in a straightforward way within the central nervous system but the response within the spinal cord alters significantly if the pain continues for even a few hours (Dickenson 1995). The changes that occur under these conditions may well lead to the patient experiencing chronic pain. It has been suggested that effective management of acute pain may prevent or reduce the changes occurring and thereby decrease the incidence of chronic pain states

THE PHYSIOLOGY OF PAIN

NOCICEPTIVE PAIN

A nociceptor is a nerve that has the function of alerting the brain to the presence of 'noxious' (i.e. harmful) stimuli. Pain is transmitted to the brain along myelinated Aδ nerve fibres and/or along unmyelinated C fibres (see Ch. 6 for information about the nervous system, in particular the function of myelin to allow for the speedy transmission of nerve impulses). Because of this, information carried on Aδ fibres reaches the brain before those carried along the unmyelinated C fibres.

There are a number of other important differences in how these two types of nerves respond and these are shown in Table 15.2. Fast pain and slow pain pathways are shown diagrammatically in Figure 15.1.

In stating that an Aδ fibre has a small receptive field, this means that it gathers information about a very small area of the body. As a result, when the information reaches the somatosensory cortex of the brain it gives precise (sharp) information about the location. As an example, think what happens when you place your hand on a hot surface in your kitchen. You respond immediately by

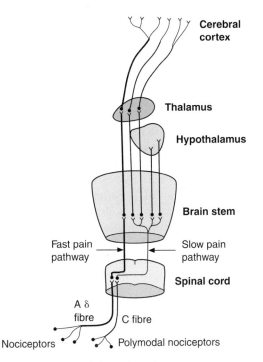

Figure 15.1 Fast and slow pain pathways.

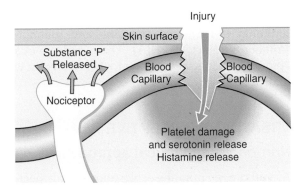

Figure 15.2 The inflammatory response and substance P release.

withdrawing your hand. Your nervous system has responded to a noxious stimulus with exactness. The C fibres, however, activate adjacent nerve cells in the reticular formation of the brain stem so that more areas of the cortex are activated and so the source of the signals cannot be exactly localised. Therefore, slow pain via the non-myelinated C fibres is not well localised.

Being unimodal or polymodal means that the nerve fibre responds to a single (i.e. *uni* modal) type of stimulus or to many (*poly* modal) stimuli. The Aδ fibres being unimodal respond to specific stimuli such as heat or mechanical pressure, but the C fibres can respond to a variety of different stimuli.

The transmission of nociceptive pain stimuli

Nociceptive pain results from the injury of tissues and is mediated by the inflammatory response. This response (described in Ch. 6) is an intricate and highly organised one. Figure 15.2 illustrates

this simply in relation to the nociceptor. In this diagram an arrow indicates the source of injury. Once the skin is punctured a number of chemicals are released from the tissues and are present in the exudate that permeates the injured area. One chemical responsible for making the capillary increasingly permeable to fluid is histamine and as a result the area becomes swollen. Some of the numerous other chemicals involved in the inflammatory process are: serotonin which comes from damaged platelets, substance P which is released from nociceptor terminals, bradykinin and prostaglandins.

Having been sensitised to the harmful stimulus, the nociceptor will transmit the pain message to the point at which it terminates in the dorsal horn of the spinal column (see Fig. 6.18 in Ch. 6 where the sequencing of nervous regulation is shown). What happens beyond this point needs further elaboration in relation to pain physiology. The pain at this point requires a neurotransmitter, that is, a chemical substance that will enable the impulse to move across the synapse and onto the next neurone of the dorsal horn (Box 6.14 gives further information on transmission at the synapse). Substance P is a key neurotransmitter at this point. If the transmission is successful, the message will ascend to the part of the brain that localises and notes the nature of the incoming information, that is, to the somatosensory cortex. The brain next activates a descending pathway that modulates or alters the pain impulses being relayed in from the dorsal horn. The descending neurones release substances such as the body's own opioids, known as endorphins, and also serotonin (5-HT), noradrenaline and gamma-aminobutyric acid (GABA). These endogenous opioids are especially secreted when the body is undergoing stress.

TREATING NOCICEPTIVE PAIN

Non-pharmacological approaches

As you can see from the explanation of how nociceptive pain is transmitted, there are a number of ways in which to block the pain pathway. Starting at the skin surface, superficial cooling may be a useful way to numb the skin and decrease the firing of the nociceptor. In addition the vasoconstriction that will result will act to prevent further swelling which could increase pain. Such measures are in common use: when you burn or scald your hand you know that placing it under the cold tap will help, and if you have ever sprained your ankle you will know that an ice pack will decrease the pain you feel coming from the area of injury. Similarly, elevating the site of injury if appropriate will allow the oedema to drain away more easily, as might compression bandaging. Care must always be taken in applying compression to a limb, however, as adding a physical support to the area might also threaten the blood supply. This is particularly relevant in the case of the patient with ischaemic disease who incurs physical injury to the limb: compression must never be applied to an ischaemic limb until the appropriate tests of perfusion are carried out under the care of a consultant.

Pharmacological approaches

There are three groups of analgesic drugs available to treat pain: these are the non-opioids, the opioids and the adjuvants. The non-opioids include paracetamol and the NSAIDs (non-steroidal anti-inflammatory drugs). These will be considered before turning to the opioids. Adjuvant analgesics are drugs that are not classified as analgesics, but which may be used to treat pain in certain situations. The adjuvants will be considered later in the chapter when neuropathic

pain is presented because they are most often seen in that pain management context.

NSAIDs

This group of drugs is used for pain that is inflammatory in nature. As you have seen, the pain response is mediated by a number of chemicals such as histamine, prostaglandins, bradykinin and serotonin. These are inflammatory agents and they can be dealt with by NSAIDs (or through the use of corticosteroids). Perhaps the commonest NSAID in general use is ibuprofen. As well as dampening the inflammatory response, NSAIDs are also unfortunately a threat to the lining of the stomach and this is sometimes given as a reason for not prescribing them, particularly to elderly people (Box 15.1).

Paracetamol/acetaminophen

Paracetamol is not an NSAID and needs to be classified separately within the non-opioid group. Although it has very little anti-inflammatory action it seems to be effective in managing the pain in many inflammatory conditions. It seems to act centrally within the nervous system where it has analgesic and antipyretic (fever reducing)

Box 15.1 **NSAIDs and the elderly**

The action of NSAIDs on the gastric mucosa has often been used as a reason not to prescribe these drugs for the elderly. Certainly, the risk of adverse side-effects increases with age, and in those 60 years and older the risk of gastrointestinal (GI) bleeding is 3–4% (the average in the general population is 1%). For older people with a history of GI bleeding the risk increases to about 9% (Greenberger 1997). A drug that can be used to help protect the stomach lining, misoprostol, is only partially effective and it does nothing for the other often troublesome side-effects in this client group. The American Geriatrics Society (1998) has suggested that the risk/benefits ratio be carefully considered before these drugs are used at high doses on a chronic basis. Alternatives available include acetaminophen (paracetamol) for mild to moderate pain and opioids for moderate to severe pain of a chronic nature. Low dose steroids are also useful for pain of an inflammatory nature.

action. It has the advantage over NSAIDs of not causing gastric irritation and in addition can safely be used in patients allergic to aspirin or other NSAIDs (McCaffery & Pasero 1999).

Opioids

The second major group of drugs available for use in the management of nociceptive pain is the opioids. A number of misconceptions are held by nurses, doctors and the public that limit the use of this group of drugs. Box 15.2 itemises the major misconceptions and gives the true versions regarding treatment. It will be appreciated that there is a real need for further professional and client education if pain is to be effectively managed and the quality of life enhanced for a number of patients who are subject to pain by the nature of their conditions.

Mode of action of opioids

Opioids act on both the central and peripheral nervous system. They do this by binding to opioid receptors which are located in the central nervous system, particularly in the dorsal horn of the spinal cord, in the gastrointestinal tract, on the peripheral terminals of sensory nerves and on cells of the immune system. They then block the transmission of substance P across the synapse and so pain is reduced or eliminated (Fig. 15.3). The body's own endogenous opioids, the endorphins, enkephalins and dynorphins, produced within the central nervous system, are pharmacologically related to morphine. This means that opioid drugs such as morphine and endogenous opioids are able to bind at the same receptor sites.

There are three types of opioid receptors, mu, kappa and delta, and although binding at all three types will produce analgesia, each has a somewhat different profile and will produce other effects as well (Table 15.3).

Opioids such as morphine, the mainstay of pain management in situations of acute and cancer pain, are termed 'mu agonists' or 'pure agonists' and this means that they produce analgesia by binding to the mu receptors. Other drugs in this category that have a strong affinity for the mu

---

Box 15.2 Major misconceptions about opioids

1. Misconception
The use of opioids in pain management will lead to addiction.

Truth
Addiction occurs in under 1% of those taking opioids for pain relief. However, so widespread is this misconception that the term 'opiophobia' has been coined (Zenz & Willweber-Strumpf 1993).

2. Misconception
Some pain is not opioid responsive.

Truth
All pain responds to opioids to a greater or lesser extent.

3. Misconception
Opioids cause respiratory depression.

Truth
If the dose of opioid is prescribed correctly, respiratory depression is rare. It is most likely in patients whose pain has never before been managed with opioids, that is, in those termed as 'opioid naïve'. However, even in this group of patients, careful dose management and monitoring of respiratory side-effects will avoid life-threatening respiratory depression. It is noteworthy that tolerance to the respiratory depression effects of opioids occurs in about 72 hours so that patients taking opioid analgesics long term are at less risk when their dosage needs to be increased.

4. Misconception
Opioids should be avoided in the early stages of a disease so that adequate analgesia will be available later on 'when it is really needed'.

Truth
There is no ceiling to the analgesia offered by opioids. If pain escalates, the dose can be adjusted to compensate. Opioids should not be withheld for fear of meeting tolerance (i.e. decreasing effectiveness of the same dose).

5. Misconception
If you are prescribed opioids you must be considered to be terminally ill and the end must be near.

Truth
As will be appreciated by the informed patient and health care professional, opioids are useful in the management of pain in general and are particularly useful in the management of pain of an inflammatory nature. They are no longer reserved for the longer-term pain management of those who are terminally ill or for short-term use by those who have just had surgery.

---

receptors include codeine, fentanyl, pethidine and propoxyphene.

Some opioids, however, are termed 'agonist–antagonist' and this means that they bind at one

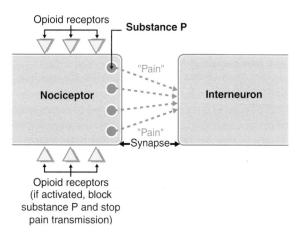

Figure 15.3 Neurotransmitter P at synapse.

Table 15.3	Opioid receptors and their effects

Receptor	Effects
Mu	Analgesia, euphoria, respiratory depression, constipation
Kappa	Analgesia, dysphoria
Delta	Analgesia without respiratory depression, euphoria

Activity 15.2 Managing Mrs Jones's pain

You are visiting Mrs Jones, an elderly lady, in her home with her district nurse. Mrs Jones has been prescribed morphine for her chronic pain, and she takes her sustained release morphine morning and night. She has recently developed rheumatoid leg ulcers. They are very badly infected and dressing changes cause her considerable pain. The district nurse points out that the doctor has prescribed Temgesic (buprenorphine) for 'breakthrough pain' and Mrs Jones has, on her advice, started taking these sublingual tablets half an hour before the dressing is due to be changed.

Questions
How effective will the Temgesic be in dealing with Mrs Jones's pain at dressing changes?
Is it an appropriate choice for this patient?

Points to help in your reflection
Temgesic has a partial agonist action at the mu receptors.
Morphine is a strong agonist at the mu receptors.
What will be the effect of taking these two drugs together?
NOTE: Temgesic/buprenorphine sublingual has an onset of action of 5 minutes but it peaks at 3 hours.

or more opioid receptors to produce analgesia but at other opioid receptors they compete with morphine and so block analgesic effects. An example of this is a drug called pentazocine which has antagonist action at the mu and delta receptors, and an agonist action at the kappa receptors. What is the clinical relevance of this sort of information? Try Activity 15.2 which allows you to use your knowledge of the physiology of pain and of pharmacology to help Mrs Jones.

In the case of Mrs Jones (Activity 15.2), the doctor was asked to visit while the nurse was doing the dressing. He approved the request for a swab to be taken for culture and sensitivity and he discussed the analgesia. He changed the prescription and ordered that another preparation of morphine be taken prior to dressing changes for as long as was required. The end result for the patient was improved comfort and quality of life. Her district nurse continued with her care as necessary to deal with the ulcers – in this lady's case, a long-term problem that was less amenable to resolution than her pain. From the information given earlier in the chapter, you were perhaps able to realise that Temgesic and morphine should not have been prescribed together because they compete for the same receptors in the central nervous system. The easiest and most sensible solution was to give her an oral immediate release dose of morphine before her dressing change. This has an onset of action of about 15 minutes, peaking between 30 minutes and 1 hour, which made it ideal. The activity also illustrates the role the nurse can play in discussing options with the patient and her other professional carers.

To complete this section, one drug classed as a pure antagonist should be mentioned. Naloxone acts as a strong antagonist at the mu, kappa and delta receptors and for this reason it is useful clinically in dealing with opioid induced respiratory depression. It binds to the receptors and blocks access to them by opioids and this causes reversal of all opioid effects (see Table 15.3).

NEUROPATHIC PAIN

Neuropathic pain is pain that originates from pathology within the nervous system tissue. It differs from nociceptive pain in two other important ways: it does not appear at the time of injury but rather may take weeks or even months to appear and it has no protective value. The pathophysiology is essentially unknown although a number of theories have been put forward over the years. What seems to be commonly accepted is that this type of pain arises from damage or malfunctioning of the nervous system and it differs from nociceptive pain in presentation and management in the following ways:

- Typically, neuropathic pain is associated with altered sensory function. This means that stimuli that would normally be experienced as pleasant or at least innocuous, may cause pain. This situation is known as allodynia.
- The area of the body affected usually feels different to the patient. Sensations such as burning and shooting pains are common.
- These types of pains do not usually respond well to opioids and other analgesic drugs. However, as has been said, all pain is essentially opioid responsive and opioids and other drugs may have a place in selected patient management.

There are a number of important pain syndromes that are associated with this type of damage but the most familiar are post-herpetic neuralgia and phantom limb pain (see later in this chapter).

Drugs used in the management of neuropathic pain

Opioid analgesics are usually not the sole answer or even the best choices for pain of neuropathic origin. Antidepressants and anticonvulsants are the mainstay of management.

Antidepressant drugs

It is not known how these drugs work to relieve neuropathic pain. It is believed that their action alters the balance of certain neurotransmitters and causes changes perhaps in the endorphin levels. What we do know, though, is that their action against pain differs from their action against depression in four main ways:

1. They are much more quickly effective in their pain relieving action than in their antidepressant action.
2. Lower doses are needed for pain control than for management of depression.
3. They are successful for pain control in people who have no depressive illness.
4. Not all antidepressants are analgesic in action.

It is particularly important to explain the prescription of this group of drugs to a patient being treated for pain because there still tends to be a stigma attached to anyone who is diagnosed as being mentally ill. As irrational as this may be, it is a fact of life, and health care professionals need to appreciate this in order to give professional care (Activity 15.3). Patients can become very worried about this specific drug treatment which can give rise to responses such as: 'the doctor gave me an antidepressant: he must think it's all in my mind' and 'the doctor gave me an antidepressant: if my family see this prescription they will think I am mentally ill'.

It is therefore imperative that we explain to the patient the four key differences between antidepressant drugs and drugs prescribed as 'adjuvant analgesics' – that is, drugs that have an analgesic action against some types of pain but which are usually prescribed for other conditions. Unless the patient and the appropriate family/significant others know why drugs are being prescribed, a great deal of unnecessary distress may be caused.

Activity 15.3 Antidepressants for pain?

What might be significant immediate reactions from a person who has been prescribed antidepressants for the treatment of neuropathic pain?

Anticonvulsant drugs and pain relief

Pains described as 'shooting' in nature often respond to carbamazepine. How it acts to manage pain in these situations is not clearly understood. What is known is that it is a drug that can increase brain levels of a chemical called 5-hydroxytrypt-amine (5-HT for short, also known as serotonin). Carbamazepine is, interestingly enough, chemi-cally derived from tricyclic antidepressant drugs. It has been found effective in such conditions as trigeminal neuralgia, post-herpetic neuralgia, diabetic neuropathy and phantom limb pain. If the patient has 'lancinating' (i.e. shooting type) pain, then carbamazepine is likely to be a useful drug in pain management.

Post-herpetic (shingles) neuralgia

Shingles can occur only in someone who has previously had chickenpox because it is caused by the reactivation of the varicella-zoster virus. After the initial episode of chickenpox, the virus retreats to one or more dorsal root ganglia in the spinal cord and remains dormant until something untoward stimulates its reappearance. It is not known exactly what needs to change for the virus to re-emerge and its development can be spon-taneous from middle age onwards, but we do know that it is more common in patients who have a reduced general immunity from condi-tions such as HIV and certain cancers.

Shingles can be a very painful experience. Typically, the patient notices a burning pain before the rash erupts, then the vesicles appear along the course of the nerve affected. The skin lesions crust over in 2–3 weeks and are well on the way to heal-ing in about 6–8 weeks. For many patients, the need for analgesia will end as the lesions heal. However, for a significant minority, the complica-tion of post-herpetic neuralgia will ensue.

Age is the most important predictor of which patients will go on to develop post-herpetic neu-ralgia – over half of the patients who are aged over 65 who have shingles will go on to develop it. The pain will be truly debilitating for some. Byas-Smith (1997, p. 108) describes the situation in this way: 'Patients describe the pain as jabbing,

electric, shooting, or burning to name a few. Wearing clothing over the painful area may be impossible without inducing considerable pain and discomfort. Sleeping at night is problematic and sexual activity is nearly impossible.'

It is extremely important to take this pain seri-ously because it is the main reason of patients over 80 taking their own lives (Byas-Smith 1997).

Aggressive management of the pain of the herpes zoster itself is considered now to be of the utmost importance in decreasing the incidence of post-herpetic neuralgia. This is usually accom-plished by the use of opioids, antiviral agents, and nerve blocks. You will recall that opioids were dis-cussed as being appropriate for nociceptive pain and this is precisely their use here during the inflammatory phase of this acute illness. Again you will note the importance of treating acute pain in order to decrease the incidence of chronic pain syndromes: this cannot be overstated.

Treatment of post-herpetic neuralgia

If the patient goes on to develop post-herpetic neuralgia, then the tricyclic antidepressants will be the drugs of choice for this neuropathic pain syndrome; in fact a review of the literature con-ducted by Volmink et al (1996) concluded that this class of drug is the only one with a proven benefit to patients with established post-herpetic neural-gia. However, as it is older people who are likely to suffer from this syndrome it is important to note that they often do not get adequate pain management because of fears that the side-effects of sedation and dizziness might put this group of people at risk. Stitzlein Davies (1999) has pointed out that the key to successful management in these situations is a low starting dose that is grad-ually increased and carefully monitored. Being older is not a reason to be left in pain, and special-ist health care intervention should be available for this very debilitating condition.

Phantom limb pain

This is pain in a part of the body that has been removed either surgically or through the trauma of injury. This is a particular problem after the removal of a limb. All patients who have an amputation may have some sensations apparently from the area that has been removed, and pain is a problem for up to 85% of them. Nikoljsen and colleagues (1997) found a correlation between pre-amputation pain and post-amputation stump and phantom pain. In fact now it is widely recognised that phantom pain can largely be prevented by dealing adequately with the pain before the time of the surgery (Jahangiri et al 1994, Ovechkin et al 1996, Baron et al 1998). In patients who have this syndrome for longer than a year, the success in managing the pain decreases. Once again, the importance of preventing acute pains from tripping over into chronic pain syndromes is highlighted.

Treatment of phantom pain

This type of pain can be very difficult to treat, but it is important for the nurse to show that she believes the patient's pain is *real* and not imaginary. Phantom limb pain causes extreme suffering for the patient. Treatments which are helpful include antidepressants, anticonvulsants, transcutaneous electrical nerve stimulation (TENS) (dealt with later in this chapter), anaesthetic nerve blocks and topical capsaicin (Baron et al 1998).

Other types of phantom pain

Another presentation of phantom pain you may see is phantom breast pain. This is unfortunately far more common than is generally realised. A study reported by Wallace and colleagues in 1996 gathered data on women having four types of breast surgery:

- mastectomy
- mastectomy with reconstruction
- cosmetic augmentation
- breast reduction.

Pain was reported a year later in 31% of those who had a mastectomy, 49% who had mastectomy plus reconstruction, 38% who had breast augmentation and 22% who underwent surgery to reduce the size of their breasts. Surgery to the breast is clearly not without dangers. For women who have cancer of the breast, there may be no option but surgical intervention. They are most at risk of injury to the intercostobrachial nerve when axillary dissection is done. This nerve serves the axilla and the medial aspect of the arm and that is where the neuropathic pain is felt. This is a serious problem for the women affected who may, as a result, not be able to wear a breast prosthesis or even close fitting clothing over the area because of the pain that is triggered by such contact. Newer surgical techniques that prevent the need for axillary dissection altogether may decrease this problem over time but in the meantime, antidepressants, capsaicin cream and TENS may be used. In every sense, this is a most distressing condition requiring the most sensitive nursing care.

CANCER PAIN

It might seem odd to consider pain from cancer as a separate category because, like other pains, it is either nociceptive or neuropathic. However, cancer pain is often considered separately because there are a number of distinct features about it that are important to note and which influence its management. Most importantly, we need to remember that pain caused by cancer is likely to change in intensity and location over time. Frequent evaluation of current treatment and holistic assessment of the patient are of paramount importance if pain is to be adequately managed and the patient's quality of life maintained at its maximum level.

Pain in patients with cancer is usually discussed under three headings:

1. pain arising from the presence of a tumour
2. pain caused by diagnostic procedures or by treatment
3. other pains unrelated to the cancer.

We are used to dealing with pain from diagnostic procedures such as biopsies and from treatments such as surgery, but cancer also presents us with unexpected sources of pain because cancerous cells can be located throughout the body and can give rise to a variety of pains and to pain syndromes. The nociceptive pain of cancer may be *somatic* or *visceral* in origin. If the nociceptive pain is somatic it means that it is caused by damage to the tissues of the body such as bone, muscle, skin or blood vessels as the tumour invades. If it is visceral, it arises from damage or injury to the pleura, peritoneum or organ capsules. Examples of visceral pain include the stretching caused by bowel obstruction or by the pressure on the liver capsule from a tumour within the liver.

Neuropathic pain associated with cancer might arise from a variety of sources such as damage to the nerves during surgery or from chemotherapeutic agents or radiotherapy. Some chemotherapeutic drugs, such as vincristine, are actually neurotoxic and directly affect the nerves.

So it is important to make these additional distinctions when considering cancer pain. The precision with which we can assess the locations and causes of pain in patients with cancer helps us to target interventions. Some pains associated with cancer will be directly linked to inflammation and tissue destruction or to pathology within the nervous system and will respond to the analgesic approaches described earlier. However, sometimes the experience of pain is compounded because of the location of the tumour and in these cases special approaches may be necessary.

Pains caused by pressure. Consider the patient who has liver cancer or a brain tumour. In these situations the tumour is growing within a confined space and may at some point cause pain from pressure against other tissues. Analgesics will be useful but it is also helpful to reduce the size of the mass. Surgical 'debulking' may be an option. If part of the mass can be removed, the pressure is relieved and the problem reduced or resolved. But sometimes surgery is not an option because of the location of the tumour or the condition of the patient. In these situations it is helpful to reduce the overall size of the mass by one of two means: reducing the inflammation surrounding the tumour or targeting the tumour with radiotherapy or chemotherapeutic agents. Tumours commonly have an area of inflammation around them so anti-inflammatory agents are appropriately used in these situations. It is

important to note that drugs used in this way do not shrink the cancerous mass, but only the inflammation around it. They act directly on the area of inflammation and by decreasing the swelling, they relieve the pain. Anti-inflammatory agents include both non-steroidal and steroidal drugs. Corticosteroids, such as dexamethasone, are powerful anti-inflammatory agents and are often used in these circumstances (Twycross 1994, p. 441). When used this way the steroid is classed as an 'adjuvant analgesic', that is, as a drug that is used primarily for a purpose other than pain relief but which, in certain circumstances, may be useful in managing pain.

The use of corticosteroids in the resolution of bowel obstruction caused by gynaecological and gastrointestinal cancers has been evaluated by Feuer & Broadley (2000) and their abstract appears in the Cochrane Collaboration Website (see the end of this chapter). Feuer & Broadley (2000) found that reducing the obstruction does not appear to be linked to longer survival times but that corticosteroids appear to be able to resolve pain caused by cancers invading these areas. Corticosteroids are not without their side-effects though, and it is important to be aware that they are only used in certain situations.

Another approach to pain caused by pressure in confined spaces, such as bones, is radiotherapy. Radiotherapy has its greatest effect on dividing cells and therefore will destroy reproducing cancer cells as well as bone cells. An evaluation of the use of radiotherapy in the palliation of painful bone metastases (the secondary spread of cancer) was undertaken by McQuay and colleagues (2000). They found that radiotherapy produced complete pain relief at 1 month in 25% of patients and some relief in 41% at some point in the trial periods they evaluated. It is a useful intervention and used in this way it is referred to as palliative radiotherapy, that is, radiotherapy used to decrease or to ease rather than to cure.

MANAGING CANCER PAIN

Cancer pain is not always as straightforward to manage as other sources of pain. Take, for example, the situation of the patient with a broken leg.

You would anticipate that, if healing were progressing well, his pain would diminish over time. Similarly, in a patient who has an arthritic condition, apart from periods when the condition might be unstable and flare up, you would expect the patient's pain to be handled using a more or less predictable range of drugs and with little variation in dosage. But would you expect the same to hold true for the patient with cancer?

This is another way in which pain from cancer differs from pain from other causes: it is unpredictable. In the patient who is experiencing the disease as an acute or chronic condition, variation in the nature of the pain requires a varied approach to treatment and care. Simply because cancer is in many cases a chronic disease it needs to be approached from a chronic illness perspective. That means that symptoms should be handled in a way that allows the patient maximum control over his own pain management and thus minimises the impact of the illness and its treatment on his life. The keys to effective management of pain in cancer are:

- assessing the patient's pain holistically
- giving drugs to manage the pain around the clock and not as necessary
- preventing the occurrence of pain: when pain can be predicted, prevent it
- using the oral route for medication if at all possible
- treating predictable side-effects proactively.

The WHO analgesic ladder

The World Health Organization in 1982 produced a guide for the management of pain in cancer. It is a clear three-step approach that is illustrated in Figure 15.4. It is important to appreciate that all patients do not necessarily progress through the steps from one to three. Some patients may have moderate or severe pain at the outset whereas others may only have mild pain.

Step one deals with mild pain and non-opioid analgesics are suggested with the possibility of combining them with an adjuvant. Here, 'adjuvant' may also mean drugs added to reduce the side-effects of the analgesic. If pain is managed

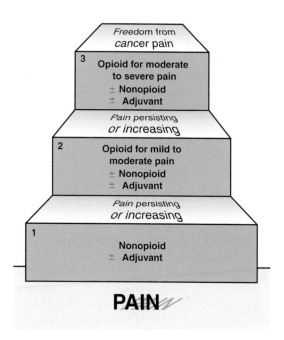

Figure 15.4 The WHO analgesic ladder. (Adapted from WHO (1996).)

with a non-opioid such as aspirin or ibuprofen, for example, then the patient is maintained on this level. If the pain increases, however, the professional managing care would be aware that there is a so-called 'ceiling effect' with these drugs – that is, there is a dose beyond which increased pain management is not obtained.

Step two deals with moderate pain. Note here, however, that there is no difference in the types of drugs included in this and in step three. The only reason for having a step two is to highlight the fact that many of the opioid plus non-opioid combinations prescribed for moderate pain are not necessarily appropriate choices for severe pain or pain that may be increasing in severity. This is because of the way the drugs are linked in the usual prescribed combinations. In situations where more pain relief is required the patient needs to be switched to step three.

Step three is the level for pain that has not been adequately managed in step two. The pain here is often severe and because of this the pharmacological requirements are quite different than those found in step two. In step two analgesics with a duration of action of 4–6 hours are almost

Activity 15.4 Morphine, its effects and side-effects

Look up the drug data on morphine and find out why it meets the criteria for stage three pain control. What are its main side-effects and what adjuvant drugs would you expect to see prescribed? What are the nursing implications of caring for a patient receiving morphine?

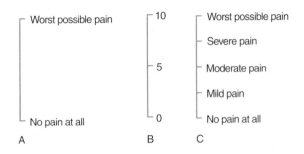

Figure 15.5 (A) Visual analogue scale (VAS). (B) Numerical rating scale (NRS). (C) A simple 5-point verbal descriptor pain scale (VDS).

the norm. But when you are trying to manage pain that is severe in intensity you really need drugs that act very quickly and have a short half life so that you can adjust the dosage easily and quickly to obtain maximum control. As you would imagine, it would also be advantageous if the same drug were available in a sustained release formulation so that once you had the pain under control, the patient would have less need to be encumbered by a frequent dosing schedule (Activity 15.4).

An important feature of morphine is that there is no ceiling dosage for this drug of choice for stage three pain management. As McCaffery & Pasero (1999, p. 122) point out, it is important to assess the effect and not to focus on the milligrams. Constipation is the entirely predictable side-effect that needs to be treated proactively. If a patient is prescribed morphine, he needs to be prescribed a medication to prevent constipation and the discomfort and pain that constipation can entail. Remember: constipation is not a side-effect that affects some patients on morphine; it is the norm for them all.

ASSESSING PAIN

Knowledge of the physiology of pain and the pharmacology of its treatment is entirely useless unless it is linked to the professional practice of nursing that ensures that patients receive the best possible care. No effective pain relief is possible until an accurate assessment of the pain and its cause has been made. This can only be achieved through discussion with, and observation of, the person with the pain. Obviously, this poses

particular problems when the person is a young child, a disorientated adult or a person with a learning disability. The skilled pain assessor is patient, observant, a good communicator and willing to embrace a variety of pain assessment aids, adapting them to the specific needs of different patients. However assessment is carried out, it is vital for the assessor to remember the subjective nature of pain, and that everyone reacts to it, describes it and perceives it differently. But it is important to gain an initial or baseline measurement of pain against which the effectiveness of pain-relieving measures can be evaluated.

ASSESSING PAIN IN ADULTS

Figure 15.5A and B shows two related pain assessment tools. These scales are usually printed on small pieces of card or plastic. They are highly effective if correctly used and if the appropriate tool is used for each patient. Figure 15.5A shows a visual analogue scale (VAS) which consists of a vertical or horizontal line with a brief pain descriptor at each end. The patient is asked to mark on the scale the point that represents the pain he is currently experiencing. The scale can then be used for comparison with further readings during administration of drugs or other pain relieving interventions. The numerical rating scale (NRS) shown in Figure 15.5B is similar to the VAS; it has numbers instead of descriptors but is used in the same way. These assessment scales may not be suitable for all patients; for the scale to be effective the patient has to be capable of representing his pain experience on it and to see a connection between a number and the awfulness of his pain. Figure 15.5C shows the verbal descriptor scale (VDS). This is more popular with some patients but for others it is not sensitive enough because it may be impossible to pick a spot between two descriptors. In this respect, slight changes in the pain experience (for example, following analgesia) cannot easily be demonstrated.

It seems reasonable to think that dealing with pain in adult patients would not be a problem. However, numerous studies indicate that nurses are poor at assessing and managing adults' pain. Surprisingly, we tend not to be knowledgeable enough about pain management (Hamilton 1992 Ryan et al 1994, Coyne et al 1999). Often nurses simply fail to ask patients about their pain and patients fail to tell us about it. In an interesting study of postoperative patients McDonald and colleagues (2000) found that patients described avoiding or delaying telling nurses about their pain because they did not want to complain, or take the nurse away from other patients.

Sometimes nurses seem to act as though if they know the source of the pain they need to take no further action. The author recalls overhearing a nurse on a surgical ward saying to a patient: 'Of course you're in pain; you've just had major surgery!'. Often, nurses demonstrate unfounded fears of causing addiction and the under-administration of drugs as prescribed by the doctors is a misguided attempt to protect patients. Then, too, patients may have the same worries and therefore refuse analgesia (Clarke et al 1996).

Nurses also often fail to do the obvious when they have assessed the pain and administered the prescribed intervention: they just do not go back to check to see if it has worked and take appropriate action!

Sometimes health care professionals make judgements about the pain of their patients. Almost invariably, we underrate the pain experienced. Larue and colleagues (1997) found in a study of patients with HIV disease that when doctors were asked to assess their patients' pain, they underestimated pain 52% of the time. In patients who reported moderate to severe pain, 57% did not receive any analgesic treatment. In

another study, 14 nurses were asked to assess the pain of 31 surgical patients. In all, they conducted 114 pain assessments. The researchers found that the nurses consistently underrated the pain of their patients and the dose of opioid analgesia they administered was more often linked not to the patients' ratings, but to their own (Puntillo et al 1997).

ASSESSING PAIN IN INFANTS AND CHILDREN

First of all, look at Activity 15.5. Can you see the problem encountered when considering the situation of this infant? First, the infant cannot describe his pain in words. Second, previous definitions of pain assume that the person experiencing pain can associate it with previous experience: this will not be the case for the infant. It has therefore been suggested that pain in infants be defined as the response to noxious stimuli and the subsequent processing of that data within the nervous system. Assessing the pain experienced by a baby is very difficult, although it is probably easier to recognise general distress.

But do infants feel pain? The answer is simply and definitely: yes they do. However, you may still hear it argued that infants have an immature nervous system and that, because fibres are incompletely myelinated, noxious stimuli are not transmitted into the central nervous system. The answer to these misconceptions is that by 20 weeks' gestation the fetal sensory receptors are present in the skin and mucous membranes, the neonatal cerebral cortex has a full system of neurones, and myelination of nerves is not a prerequisite of pain perception: the system is indeed ready

 Activity 15.5 Assessing pain in children

Your patient is an infant who has just had surgery for the repair of a hernia. How would you know if he were in pain?

to note noxious stimuli from a point earlier than birth. Porter and his colleagues (1999) have shown, without doubt, that pain and stress induce significant physiological and behavioural reactions in newborn infants. In fact, Anand & Scalzo (2000) among other researchers are looking for a possible link between early insults to the infant, such as pain, and subsequent behavioural problems in adults.

Returning to the infant who has had the surgery described in Activity 15.5, your list of pain indicators might have included physical and behavioural cues as listed below:

Physical cues

These might include:

- increased heart rate
- increased breathing rate
- increased intracranial pressure, shown by dilated pupils
- decreased transcutaneous oxygen saturation, shown by pallor of the skin
- nausea, vomiting.

Behavioural cues

These might include:

- crying
- facial expression
- changes in sleep and eating patterns
- body movements that indicate trying to get away from the harmful stimulus.

It is important always to look carefully at the face of the infant or child: there is a phenomenon known as the 'silent cry' and it means that you have all the signs except the sound. This might happen if the child is intubated as is often the case in intensive care baby units.

There are several assessment tools to help recognise and measure pain in both infants and young children. The tool that is appropriate to use varies with age and the situation. Assessing a child's pain presents particular problems for nurses and doctors, both in hospital and in the home. A young teenager may well be able to complete an assessment tool, as shown in Figure 15.5, but a child of 4 or 5 cannot do this. A parent may be able to spot signs of general distress – the child may be crying and red-faced, unable to stay still, or pale-faced, silent and lying absolutely still. Some appropriate pain assessment tools to help nurses and others are described below.

CRIES

CRIES is a postoperative pain measurement tool for the neonatal patient. It is similar to the APGAR score you may see used in assessing the condition of a newborn infant. The letters stand for:

Crying
Requires increased oxygen
Increased vital signs
Expression
Sleeplessness.

It is a valid and reliable tool (see Krechell & Bildner's (1995) article which is listed in the references for this chapter).

A helpful pain assessment tool for children uses printed faces, some smiling and happy, others

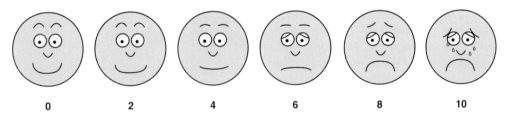

| 0 | 2 | 4 | 6 | 8 | 10 |

Figure 15.6 'Wong–Baker faces' pain assessment scale.

Box 15.3   **The Eland Color Tool and instructions for its use** (Eland 1985)

1. Ask the child: 'What kinds of things have hurt you before?'
2. If he doesn't answer, ask: 'Has anyone ever stuck your finger for blood? What did that feel like?'
3. After discussing several things that have hurt the child in the past, ask: 'Of all the things that have ever hurt you, what was the worst?'
4. Give the child 8 crayons and ask him: 'Of these colours which is like the thing that hurt you the most?' Important: name the painful incident specifically.
5. Place the crayon representing severe pain to one side.
6. Ask 'Which colour is like a hurt, but not as bad as your worst hurt?' (Again, specifically name the hurt.)
7. Place the second crayon next to the one representing severe pain.
8. Continue in this way, choosing crayons that represent just a little hurt and no hurt at all.
9. Give the 4 chosen crayons to the child along with the body outlines. Write the child's name above or below the outline.
10. Ask the child to use his crayons to show you on the outline where he hurts a lot, a middle amount, just a little, or not at all.
11. Ask: 'Is this hurt happening right now, or is it from earlier today? Does it happen all the time or on and off?'
12. Remember to include a colour key on the tool.
13. Document all the child's responses, using his own words.

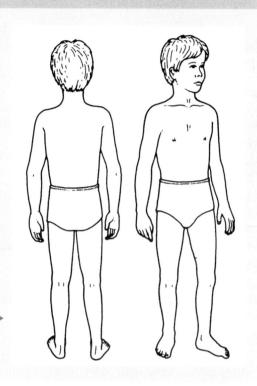

frowning. The child is asked to point to the face whose expression seems closest to that of his own feelings. An example of such a tool is shown in Figure 15.6. This has proved popular with adults as well as children! Other assessments use simple drawings representing the shape of the body and the child is encouraged to point to which part hurts. A modification of this method is the Eland Color Tool which is shown in Box 15.3.

ASSESSING PAIN IN PEOPLE WITH LEARNING DISABILITY OR SEVERE COMMUNICATION DIFFICULTY

This is particularly challenging because if a person lacks the normal abilities to communicate verbally with us he can be even more at risk of poor pain management. A study of older cognitively impaired people in Canada found that they were prescribed significantly less medication than those who were cognitively intact (Kaasalainen et al 1998). The problems of assessment were highlighted by Wynne and her colleagues (2000). They attempted to determine which of three pain severity and location instruments were most useful for pain assessment with this group of people. They used body pain charts, a doll, and also asked the patients to point to the source of pain on their own bodies. They found that pointing to themselves was the most frequently used method. Their work indicates how important it is to have a variety of assessment approaches and a commitment to communication and patient comfort. However, we currently need to accept that there has been little work done to help the professional in this area and much remains to be researched. In the meantime it is essential that we realise that these patients are at particular risk and do our utmost to ensure their safety and comfort. McCaffery & Pasero

(1999) give the following list of behaviours that are possibly indicative of pain:

- *Facial expressions:* frown (wrinkled forehead), grimace, fearful, sad, muscle contraction around mouth and eyes
- *Physical movements:* restlessness, fidgeting, absence of movement, slow movements, cautious movements, guarding, rigidity, generalised tension (not relaxed), trying to get attention (beckoning someone)
- *Vocalisations:* groaning, moaning, crying, noisy breathing.

Using these factors, we can at least attempt to make accurate assessments for our patients who cannot communicate well with us. Assessing their responses following interventions and managing pain will help to ensure their comfort.

ASSESSING AND MANAGING PAIN IN ELDERLY PEOPLE

Look at Activity 15.6.

Gordon (1999) pointed out that one of the difficulties, particularly with older surgical patients, is that we often need to manage both acute and chronic pain. This requires considerably more knowledge and skill than many nurses are able to achieve in their first-level training. In these situations there is a need to involve specialist nurses and other health professionals specialised in pain management, and to demonstrate a commitment to comfort for each patient.

Desbiens & Wu (2000) reported that in their sample of patients over 80 years of age who were hospitalised, pain was a major problem. They recommended that routine monitoring of pain should be undertaken and that the concerns of elderly people regarding side-effects from their

Activity 15.6 Pain and the older person

Older patients are at risk of poor pain management. Can you think of reasons to explain this fact?

essential pain-relieving drugs should be addressed. This is a factor we sometimes fail to consider: patients may not want the side-effects they associate with pain relief. Another concern sometimes voiced by older people is that they think there is only a limited amount that can be done for pain relief. You hear this reflected in such comments as 'Oh, no, I can cope with this pain. I don't want to take drugs now in case I get something more serious and need help later'. In other words, they have a mental set that might have been accurate years ago before we had more drugs available, more understanding of drug action, and more appreciation of the options we can use to ensure that for the vast majority of people, pain should never be something they 'just have to put up with'.

MANAGING PAIN WITH NON-PHARMACOLOGICAL INTERVENTIONS

Drugs are only one approach to pain management. Because pain is multidimensional and has cognitive, emotional and physical components, this means that we can use any one approach or a combination of approaches to help our patients. There is a tendency to consider that drugs are the mainstay of pain management; certainly they are important, but they are not the only intervention and their action can often be enhanced by combining them with other approaches.

Respect for using a combination of approaches is very common now. A few years ago complementary approaches to pain management were considered cranky, but the research base has grown steadily over recent years and some of the previous 'alternative' approaches have gained a place in our armoury of weapons against pain. Acceptance of these approaches is not limited to one centre or country: the use of a variety of techniques in the management of acute paediatric pain is discussed and advocated by Rusy & Weisman (2000) in the USA, the use of aromatherapy in managing the symptoms, including pain, of mothers in labour is being explored in Oxford (Burns et al 2000), and in Sweden, for example, acupuncture has been found to be more effective than physiotherapy in the

Activity 15.7 Complementary therapies and pain control

Why might our patients find alternative approaches to pain management attractive? What might they gain from them, either used alone or in combination with analgesics?

This question may not be easy to explore unless you have experience of one or more of the complementary therapies. If you have not, ask family or friends who have used them and try to discover what led them to complementary therapies/therapists and what benefits they felt they gained.

management of low back and pelvic pain in pregnant women (Wedenberg et al 2000). We know that in the UK about 20% of the population has used a complementary therapy within the last year and that herbalism, aromatherapy, homeopathy, acupuncture/acupressure, massage and reflexology were the most popular treatments used (Ernst & White 2000). The complementary approaches are ones we as health care professionals need to be knowledgeable about if we are to advise and protect our patients (Activity 15.7).

People go to complementary therapists for so many reasons. For many it may be because they are not getting the level of symptom control that they desire, or perhaps they find the more collaborative approach attractive or the more holistic view better suited to the management of their chronic illnesses overall. Perhaps they want to do something themselves and have a sense of control over their illness and its management within this framework.

Ann Gill Taylor (1999, p. 282) summarises the situation succinctly when she writes: 'The philosophy of many CAM (complementary, alternative medicine) therapies is one that fosters a sense of well-being, human integrity and healing the person rather than curing the disease. These factors have a potentially important role in relieving pain.'

Transcutaneous electrical nerve stimulation (TENS)

This is one of the most frequent non-drug interventions you will see deployed within the health care setting. In TENS, small electrodes are moistened and fastened to the skin above the painful area and are connected to a control box (containing batteries) by wires. A switch, activated by the patient, turns on a small electrical current whose power can be adjusted, again by the patient. As the power increases, the patient feels a tingling sensation from the electrodes. If this sensation turns to one of pain, or if the muscles under the skin start to twitch, the power is too high. The electrodes should not be placed over areas of damaged skin or over a bony prominence.

Gate control theory

How, then, can an electrical stimulation of the skin cause pain perceptions to be reduced or absent? At first it seems an entirely fanciful intervention. However, Melzack & Wall (in 1965) proposed what is known as the 'gate control theory of pain' (Melzack & Wall 1982) to explain why it is that sometimes the central nervous system registers noxious stimuli and sometimes, despite tremendous tissue damage, it ignores them. They postulated that there was a 'gating' mechanism in the dorsal horn of the spinal cord and that it could be closed by, among other things, stimulating the Aβ nerve fibres. The Aβ fibres are large myelinated nerve fibres that respond to light pressure on the skin and to electrical stimulation. They conduct impulses into the central nervous system much faster than either the Aδ or the C fibres. The pain messages coming into the dorsal horn can be overridden and the gate closed if the Aβ fibres are activated. Aβ fibres can be stimulated by gentle skin massage, movement, and transcutaneous electrical stimulation (see Case example 15.2 and Figures 15.7A, B and C for a simplified explanation of the gate control mechanism at work in a patient whose foot pain is relieved by gentle massage and diversion from conversation with the nurse). In non-physiological language, rubbing the skin over an affected area, or applying electrical stimulation to the area, keeps the brain 'busy' and prevents it being too bothered about the impulses arising from the source of the pain. The diagrams also show that pain inhibition is assisted by descending impulses from the brain,

Case example 15.2

Miss Philips is awakened every night by the pain in her foot. She has long been a cigarette smoker, and now, as a complication of this, she has gangrene in the toes of her left foot. She is currently in hospital awaiting an operation to remove the foot. Last night she asked the nurse for some painkillers, which were only partially effective.

Tonight, there is a different nurse on duty, who brings her not only two tablets but a cup of tea. The nurse then sits down by Miss Philips and they talk about their families and the holidays they have enjoyed.

'Will you rub that awful leg for me?', asks Miss Philips, and the staff nurse gently massages the left leg as the two of them converse.

After half an hour, Miss Philips is feeling drowsy and thinks she will try to get off to sleep once again. 'You know, my foot feels so much better now. Pity you aren't on duty every night.'

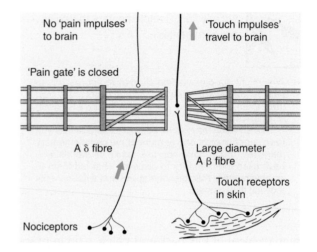

Figure 15.7B (Highly figurative.) Nerve impulses from touch receptors in the skin pass through the spinal cord and ascend to the brain, but the spinal 'gate' is closed to the

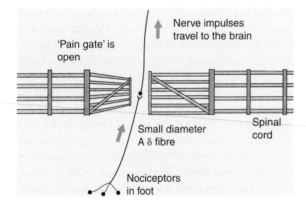

Figure 15.7A The 'gate' is open to nerve impulses from nociceptors, and the person feels pain.

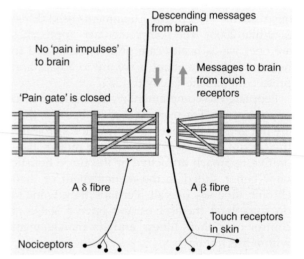

Figure 15.7C Descending impulses from the brain inhibit the transmission of pain impulses in the spinal cord; the pain 'gate' is closed, and the person feels no pain.

such as would arise from a person's sense of well-being from, say, a pleasant conversation, beautiful music, seeing loved ones – all of which constitute strong, positive psychological inputs.

Does TENS work?

A review of the use of TENS in patients with low back pain was undertaken by Gadsby & Flowerdew (2000). They found that there is evidence, albeit from limited data, to support the view that TENS and ALTENS (acupuncture-like

transcutaneous electrical stimulation) reduces pain and improves range of movement in patients with chronic back pain. This reference is the most significant one to date.

In addition there is a very interesting nursing study. Hidderley & Weinel (1997) applied TENS to acupuncture sites in an attempt to relieve pain in patients with head and neck cancers (that is patients for whom it would be difficult to apply TENS in the usual fashion). The dosage of analgesia for three of the four patients remained unchanged but it is significant that the pain scores came down. As the consultant was reluctant to give large doses of opioid analgesia to these patients, one may assume that the level of pain relief was not good enough without this alternative approach.

TENS cannot be used successfully for all types of pain but its success is well known in many areas, particularly neuropathic pain. TENS also causes the secretion of the body's own endogenous opioids discussed earlier, so even when the current is switched off the analgesic effect can continue for many hours. An important feature of TENS therapy is that it is under the patient's own control so that he can feel he is making a positive contribution to the control of his pain, rather than just enduring it. There are very few problems involved in using TENS provided the instructions are followed carefully.

Other non-drug interventions

Aromatherapy

Aromatherapy uses essential oils. It is thought to work through inducing the relaxation response, through actual physiological changes and at a cellular level. The evidence base has yet to be established. However, there are some very useful studies that should be discussed. Wilkinson et al (1999), for example, undertook a study of aromatherapy massage in patients receiving palliative care. They studied 103 patients and randomly allocated them to either massage with simple carrier oil or to massage with Roman chamomile oil. They found significant reductions in anxiety, improved scores in relation to symptom (pain) experience, and improvements in quality of life measurements in those treated with the Roman chamomile.

Reflexology

Reflexology is a form of treatment involving the massage of pressure points in the feet. It is said to be a 'focused pressure technique' that is 'based on the premise that zones or reflex areas exist in the hands and feet that correspond to all organs, glands and systems of the body' (Bisson 2000). At present the research base is absent in this area of pain relief. However, in a therapy that purports to work by helping the body to rid itself of toxins, specific symptom relief measures would be hard to obtain.

Reiki

Reiki is a touch healing system that usually involves a qualified practitioner placing the hands in a set pattern of positions on the body. It involves energy transfer of the life force energy through the practitioner to the client. Olson & Hanson (1997) carried out a fascinating study of the use of Reiki as an adjuvant to opioid therapy in the management of pain. Using 20 volunteers experiencing pain from a variety of causes, including cancer, they measured outcomes using the visual analogue scale and a Likert scale questionnaire immediately before and after Reiki. Both instruments found a statistically significant reduction in pain following Reiki treatment.

Without doubt complementary therapies afford some relief to those who use them. Our difficulties as health care practitioners is that, in general, the evidence base is lacking to support their effectiveness in pain management. This does not mean that they do not work: it simply means that the solid research base is only now being developed.

Additional pain-relieving strategies

Drugs, TENS and the therapies described above all have vital roles to play in the reduction of both acute and chronic pain. They are, however, not the only measures that can be used to reduce the distressing experience of pain. Other methods which may appear simple and obvious contribute to high quality nursing care and are, sadly, often overlooked in the face of 'high-tech' management of pain. These methods may include any or all of the following.

Positioning, rest and sleep. For many patients, whether at home or in hospital/hospice, pain seems worse at night. Changing the position of the pillows, smoothing the bottom sheet, bringing drinks and talking to the patient are all simple measures which can make such a difference in combination with the right analgesia. During sleep, pain is forgotten.

Rubbing and massage. On banging an elbow or knee, the almost automatic response is to rub the affected part to reduce the pain. The gate theory, described above, helps to explain how this works. The same applies to massaging, which can involve lightly stroking the skin or may be more intense in applying firm pressure to the underlying muscle. Specialists in therapeutic massage have a role to play in the general care of people in pain and many nurses now undertake the relevant training. An important factor in massage is the physical contact. To be massaged by someone in order to reduce pain is to know that someone else cares and is actively doing something about the pain.

Diversion and meditation. Sometimes, one's mind can be taken off pain by some external factor – conversation, the television, human company in general. Being in hospital can often be a very boring experience for the patient and when the person is in pain he has little else to do but dwell on his pain. Having a nurse take an interest by listening and chatting can be very effective. Once again the gate control theory explains why. Diversion is, of course, something that the patient's relatives and other visitors can carry out. They often feel helpless at the bedside, but to be encouraged to fill the person's time with conversation, perhaps read to him, look at photographs, will help them to feel more useful in helping to reduce their loved one's pain.

Meditation is often helpful to those who have regularly practised it. It is not a technique which can be suddenly switched on when a person has pain but to the experienced meditator it can provide calm and deep relaxation which may enable him to distance himself from the pain experience. The nurse can be aware of this and make space and quiet available for someone who wishes to meditate.

The topical use of heat, cold and ointments. People suffering from some forms of arthritis sometimes find that heat, in the form of a hot water bottle or an electric heat pad, can be very soothing to their joints. Some ointments, rubbed into the skin above a painful joint, provide the sensation of warmth by causing dilation of the local blood vessels. It is thought that the soothing effect of warmth is, again, due to the gate control mechanism. In some cases, cold packs may be used to reduce inflammation in some painful conditions such as sprains, sports injuries and, of course, cold water poured over burns is very effective in reducing pain.

SO, WHAT DOES IT TAKE TO ENSURE GOOD PAIN ASSESSMENT AND MANAGEMENT?

Hopefully, this chapter has provided the necessary basic knowledge and examples of good care practices to enable the new nursing student to approach the nursing of a patient in pain with confidence. The underlying principles of nursing the patient in pain are:

- a commitment to the premise that the patient is the expert on his own pain experience
- the routine and systematic use of a pain assessment tool (a variety of these has been shown in this chapter: check which are used in your area)
- a sound knowledge of pharmacological and non-pharmacological approaches to pain management
- good communication between the patient, his carers and the health care professionals
- a commitment to managing the patient's pain using sound practice guidelines or agreed approaches to care that involve the multidisciplinary team.

Patients in pain are patients who are vulnerable. There are numerous studies to indicate how damaging the experience of pain is in physiological and psychological terms, but in closing we should consider how pain can do more than destroy the body: it can also destroy the person who suffers it.

It is time for all nurses to act as if we believed that freedom from pain is a human right. If it is a human right, then each of our patients should rest assured that when he defines himself as being in pain, relief will be given. If freedom from pain is his right, then we as health care professionals have a moral duty to protect him from it wherever possible.

Cicely Saunders gave us the concept of 'total pain', that is, the idea that pain involves far more than the physical: pain encompasses the spiritual, the emotional and the social aspects of our being as well. As nurses we must attend to the total experience of our patients' personal pain if we are to provide professional care.

We have a professional duty to act as advocates for our patients. When they are vulnerable through disease and pain we have the duty to protect them and ensure their comfort. Through education, training and commitment we can respond positively to the challenge that Laurel Archer Copp made to us in 1993: 'Our colleagues in hospices have made the moral judgement to relieve their patients' pain unconditionally and within the parameters of sophisticated pain management and nursing care. Can we accept the challenge in hospitals, nursing homes, outpatient clinics and in the home to manage pain as an ethical and professional imperative?'.

REFERENCES

American Geriatrics Society Panel on Chronic Pain in Older Persons 1998 The management of chronic pain in older persons. Journal of the American Geriatrics Society 46:635–651

American Pain Society 1992 Principles of analgesic use in the treatment of acute and cancer pain, 3rd edn. Glenview, Illinois

Anand K J, Scalzo F M 2000 Can adverse neonatal experiences alter brain development and subsequent behavior? Biology of the Neonate 77(2):69–82

Baron R, Wasner G, Lindner V 1998 Optimal treatment of phantom pain in the elderly. Journal of Drugs and Aging 12(5):361–376

Bisson D A 2000 Reflexology. In: Novey D W (ed) Clinician's Complete Reference to Complementary and Alternative Medicine. Mosby, St Louis

Bowsher D 1997 The management of post herpetic neuralgia. Postgraduate Medical Journal 73(864):623–629

Burns E E, Blamey C, Ersser S J, Barnetson L, Lloyd A J 2000 An investigation into the use of aromatherapy in intrapartum midwifery practice. Journal of

Alternative and Complementary Medicine 6(2):141–147

Byas-Smith M 1997 Common pain syndromes. In: Moreau D (ed) Expert pain management. Springhouse, Pennsylvania, pp 87–123

Clarke E B, French B, Bilodeau M L, Capasso V C, Edwards A, Empoliti J 1996 Pain management knowledge, attitudes and clinical practice: the impact of nurses' characteristics and education. Journal of Pain and Symptom Management 11(1):18–31

Copp L A 1993 An ethical responsibility for pain management. Guest Editorial. Journal of Advanced Nursing 18:1–3

Coyne M L, Reinert B, Cater K, Dubuisson W, Smith J F, Parker M M, Chatham C 1999 Nurses' knowledge of pain assessment, pharmacologic and nonpharmacologic interventions. Clinical Nursing Research 8(2):153–165

Desbiens N A, Wu A W 2000 Pain and suffering in seriously ill hospitalized patients. Journal of the American Geriatric Society 48(5 Supplement):S183–S186

Dickenson A H 1995 Central acute pain mechanisms. Annals of Medicine 27(2):223–227

Ernst E, White A 2000 The BBC survey of complementary medicine use in the UK. Complementary Therapies in Medicine 8(1):32–36

Feuer D J, Broadley K E 2000 Corticosteroids for the resolution of malignant bowel obstruction in advanced gynaecological and gastrointestinal cancer. Cochrane Review. Cochrane Library. Issue 2, 2000. Update Software, Oxford

Gadsby J G, Flowerdew M W 2000 Transcutaneous electrical nerve stimulation and acupuncture-like transcutaneous electrical nerve stimulation for chronic low back pain. Cochrane Database Systematic Review 2000; (2) CD 000210. Update Software, Oxford

Gordon D B 1999 Pain management in the elderly. Journal of Perianesthesia Nursing 14(6):367–372

Greenberger N J 1997 Update in gastroenterology. Annals of Internal Medicine 12:827–834

Hamilton J 1992 A survey examining nurses' knowledge of pain control. Journal of Pain and Symptom Management 7(1):18–26

Hayes C, Molloy A R 1997 Neuropathic pain in the perioperative period. International Anesthesiology Clinics 35(2):67–81

Hidderley M, Weinel E 1997 Effect of TENS applied to acupuncture points distal to the pain site. International Journal of Palliative Nursing 3(4):185–191

International Association for the Study of Pain 1979 On a taxonomy of pain terms: a list with definitions and notes on usage. *Pain* 6:249–252

Jahangiri M, Jayatunga A P, Bradley J W, Dark C H 1994 Prevention of phantom pain after major lower limb amputation by epidural infusion of diamorphine, clonidine and bupivacaine. Annals of the Royal College of Surgeons of England 76(5):324–326

Kaasalainen S, Middleton J, Knezacek S, Hartley T, Stewart N, Ife C, Robinson L 1998 Pain and cognitive status in the institutionalised elderly: perceptions and interventions. Journal of Gerontological Nursing 24(8):24–31

Knott C, Beyer J, Villarruel A, Denyes M, Erickson V, Willard G 1994 Using the Oucher developmental approach to pain assessment in children. MCN

American Journal of Maternal Child Nursing 19(6):314–320

Krechel S W, Bildner J 1995 CRIES: a new neonatal postoperative pain measurement score: initial testing of validity and reliability. Paediatric Anaesthesia 5(1):53–61

Larue F, Fontaine A, Colleau S M 1997 Underestimation and undertreatment of pain in HIV disease: multicentre study. British Medical Journal 314(7073):23–28

McCaffery M 1968 Nursing practice theories related to cognition, bodily pain, and man–environment interactions. University of California, Los Angeles

McCaffery M, Pasero C 1999 Pain: clinical manual, 2nd edn. Mosby, St Louis

McDonald D D, McNulty J, Erickson K, Weiskopf C 2000 Communicating pain and pain management needs after surgery. Applied Nursing Research 13(2):70–75

McQuay H J, Collins S L, Carroll D and Moore R A 2000 Radiotherapy for the palliation of painful bone metastases. Cochrane Review. Cochrane Library. Issue 2, 2000. Update Software, Oxford

Melzack R, Wall P 1982 The challenge of pain. Penguin, London

Nikoljsen L, Ilkjaer S, Kroner K, Christensen J H, Jensen T S 1997 The influence of preamputation pain on postamputation stump and phantom pain. Pain 72(3):393–405

Olson K, Hanson J 1997 Using Reiki to manage pain: a preliminary report. Cancer Prevention and Control 1(2):108–113

Onghena P, Van Houdenhove B 1992 Antidepressant-induced analgesia in chronic non-malignant pain: a meta-analysis of 39 placebo controlled studies. Pain 49:205–219

Ovechkin A M, Gnezdilov A V, Arlazarova N M, Savin I A, Fedorova E V, Khmelkova E I 1996 Preventive analgesia: true of preventing the postoperative pain syndrome. J Anesteziol Reanimatol (Anesteziologiya I Reanimatologiya) (4):35–39

Pendas S, Dauway E, Cox C E, Giuliano R, Ku N N, Schreiber R H, Reintgen D S 1999 Sentinel node biopsy and cytokeratin staining for the accurate staging of 478 breast cancer patients. American Surgeon 65(6):500–505; discussion 505–506

Portenoy R K 1996 Basic mechanisms. In: Portenoy R K, Kanner R M (eds) Pain management: theory and practice. F A Davis, Philadelphia, pp 19–39

Porter F L, Grunau R E, Anand K J 1999 Long term effects of pain in infants. Journal of Developmental and Behavioral Pediatrics 20(4):253–261

Puntillo K A, Miaskowski C, Kehrle K, Stannard D, Gleeson S, Nye P 1997 Relationship between behavioural and physiological indicators of pain, critical care patients' self-reports of pain, and opioid administration. Critical Care Medicine 25(7):1159–1166

Rasmussen K G, Rummans T A 2000 Electroconvulsive therapy for phantom limb pain. Pain 85(1–2):297–299

Rusy L M, Weisman S J 2000 Complementary therapies for acute pediatric pain management. Pediatric Clinics of North America 47(3):589–599

Ryan P, Vortherms R, Ward S 1994 Knowledge, attitudes of pharmacologic management. Journal of Gerontological Nursing 20(1):7–15

Stitzlein Davies P 1999 Herpes zoster and postherpetic neuralgia. In: McCaffery M, Pasero C Pain: clinical manual, 2nd edn. Mosby, St. Louis

Tasmuth T, Estlanderb A, Kalso E 1996 The effect of present pain and mood on the memory of past post operative pain in women treated surgically for breast cancer. Pain 68(2–3):343–347

Taylor A G 1999 Complementary/alternative therapies in the treatment of pain. In: Spencer J W, Jacobs J J (eds) Complementary/alternative medicine: an evidence based approach. Mosby, St Louis

Twycross R 1994 Pain relief in advanced cancer. Churchill Livingstone, Edinburgh

Volmink J, Gray S, Silagy C, Lancaster T 1996 Treatments for post herpetic neuralgia: a systematic review of randomised controlled trials. Journal of Family Practice 13(1):84–91

Wedenberg K, Moen B, Norling A 2000 A prospective randomised study comparing acupuncture with physiotherapy for low back and pelvic pain in pregnancy. Acta Obstetrica Gynecologica Scandinavica 79(5):331–335

Wilkinson S, Aldridge J, Salmon I, Cain E, Wilson B 1999 An evaluation of aromatherapy massage in palliative care. Palliative Medicine 13(5):409–417

Wong D L, Baker C M 1988 Pain in children: a comparison of assessment scales. Pediatric Nursing 14(1):9–17

World Health Organization 1996 Cancer pain relief, 2nd edn. WHO, Geneva

Wynne C F, Ling S M, Remsburg R 2000 Comparison of pain assessment instruments in cognitively intact and cognitively impaired nursing home residents. Geriatric Nursing 21(1):20–23

Zenz M, Willweber-Strumpf A 1993 Opiophobia and cancer pain in Europe. Lancet 341:1075–1076

FURTHER READING

American Geriatrics Society Panel on Chronic Pain in Older Persons 1998 The management of chronic pain in older persons. Journal of the American Geriatrics Society 46:635–651
This article presents the best discussion of the issues of pain relief in the older adult. It is a clearly written, accessible and authoritative source of information. In it you will find a good discussion of the relative dangers of NSAIDs to certain groups of older people and sound advice on the use of opiates in this age group.

Carter B 1998 Perspectives on pain: mapping the territory. Arnold, London
This book explores pain from a personal and a professional perspective. It will stimulate you to reflect upon the nature of pain and how it is viewed across a range of ages and in a number of conditions. It covers, among many other topics, the social and the psychological aspects of pain management and the relationship of pain and suffering.

McCaffery M, Pasero C 1999 Pain: Clinical Manual, 2nd edn. Mosby, St Louis
*Margo McCaffery is **the** nurse expert on the subject pain. This is a reasonably priced book and invaluable resource. If you buy just one book on this subject, make it this one. It is comprehensive and will provide you with the answers to most of your nursing problems in relation to pain or it will give you the lead you need to find the answers for your patients.*

Melzack R, Wall P 1996 The challenge of pain. Penguin Paperback, Middlesex
This is an amazingly engaging book on the topic of pain. It explores the physiology of pain, pain theories and the control of pain through a wide variety of approaches. It discusses some of the pain syndromes you will encounter such as at phantom limb and cancer pain.

Wall P 1999 Pain: the science of suffering. Weidenfeld & Nicolson, London
This is one of the most up to date and readable books on this subject for the healthcare student. Patrick Wall is one of the worlds leading experts on pain and in this book he presents the latest medical findings. He helps us to explore many aspects of the subject including: our experience of pain, the placebo response, the use of complementary, psychological and pharmacological approaches to pain.

INTERNET

http://hiru.mcmaster.ca/cochrane/default.html

The use of corticosteroids for the relief of pain due to pressure from tumours particularly in the bowel or gynaecological tumours.

16

Palliative care and care of the dying

Linda Husband   Christine L. Henry

CHAPTER CONTENTS

Causes of death in the UK today   484

History of care of the dying   484

The palliative care approach   486
Palliative care education   487
Models of palliative care and the
multidisciplinary team   487
Hospital-based services   487
Home care   488
Day hospices   488
Children's hospices   488
Extended home nursing services   488
Hospice in-patient care   488

Facing the possibility of death   489
Reacting to the prospect of death   489
Stages of adjustment   490
Stages or phases?   493
To tell or not to tell?   493

**Palliative care and managing the
symptoms   495**
Pain   495
Breathlessness   496
Fatigue   496
Constipation   496
Nausea and vomiting   497
Mouth problems   497

Managing the last days of life   497
Keeping the patient comfortable   498
Family support   499
Last offices   499

Bereavement   500
The stages of loss   500
Children and bereavement   502

Special types of loss   502
Miscarriages, abortions and
infant death   502
Deaths due to suicide   503
Complicated grief   504
Spiritual issues   505

The stress of caring for the dying   505

References   506

Further reading   507

Internet   507

Palliative care is defined as the 'active total care of patients whose disease is not responsive to curative treatment. Control of pain, of other symptoms and of psychological, social and spiritual problems is paramount' (European Association for Palliative Care 1989). 'The goal of the palliative care approach is the achievement of the best possible quality of life for patients and their families' (World Health Organization 1990, p. 11). Not all death is expected or timely. The families and loved ones of those who have died suddenly (e.g. stillborn or cot-death babies, suicides, victims of trauma and sufferers of myocardial infarction) have special needs, but, whatever the circumstances, nurses must develop the resources to give the best possible care for the dying and the bereaved.

With this in mind this chapter aims to:

- provide an understanding of the development of attitudes towards, and care of, the dying
- explore the emotions encountered in adjusting to the prospect of one's own or another's death
- consider the physical, emotional and spiritual needs of the dying person
- examine the concepts of, and feelings involved in, bereavement, loss and grief
- draw attention to the stress produced by nursing the dying.

It should be noted that throughout this chapter the term 'family' refers not only to actual relatives but also to other key people who are important to the patient.

CAUSES OF DEATH IN THE UK TODAY

Kenneth Calman, as Chief Medical Officer, in his last report, *On the State of the Public Health* (DoH 1997), reflected upon how far we have come in terms of improving the health of our nation: infant mortality is at its lowest ever rate at

Table 16.1 Causes of death for all ages over 28 days in England and Wales, 1999

	Male (%)	Female (%)
Cancers	26	22
Ischaemic heart disease	24	17
Cerebrovascular disease	7.8	12
Chronic obstructive pulmonary disease	5.9	4.3
Accidents (injury and poisoning)	3.9	2
Suicide	1	0.3
HIV	0.4	0.007

Source: based upon figures from the ONS Mortality Statistics 2000
Office for National Statistics 2000 Mortality Statistics: Cause: 1999 England and Wales. DH2, No 26. Office for National Statistics, London

5.9/1000 live births, post-neonatal mortality has fallen to 2 per 1000 live births and in general our life expectancy has risen to be 74.6 years for men and 79.7 years for women. In fact, he noted that mortality rates for men had fallen by 11% and for women 7% in just the 6 years up to the report.

Improvements such as these have led to a changing pattern of disease such that our major causes of death are no longer acute infections but chronic illnesses, mental health problems and accidents. Table 16.1 shows the major causes of mortality for all ages over 28 days in 1999.

HISTORY OF CARE OF THE DYING

A century ago the care of the dying and the bereaved would have been very different. Infant mortality was far higher, life expectancy in general was considerably lower, and acute diseases were the main threats to survival. Today, when we talk about the care of the dying we are more likely to be discussing the care of adults who have become ill during their middle years from cancers and from heart disease. How have these changes altered the way we deliver palliative care?

During the last century it is argued that death was a far more 'normal' and everyday experience within the local community. In fact, if you were to ask an older person in your area you might hear stories of how each locality had a woman who was responsible for laying out the dead, and of others who notified those in the community of 'the passing' of one of its members, and you would perhaps find information about a number of traditions that would have acted to support the bereaved in their mourning. A very interesting account of the changes that have occurred in one community, Staithes in Yorkshire, is found in an article by Clark (1982).

It is easy to forget how relatively recent the development of modern medicine and surgery is and how it has transformed the face of health care and the way care is provided in our communities. Antiseptics, anaesthetics, the use of radium in diagnosis and therapy, the development of the National Health Service, chemotherapeutic agents, antibiotics, insulin, modern heart surgery, organ transplants, a plethora of powerful drugs for virtually every ill: all of these and more have come to be so taken for granted. During the time of the rapid expansion of health care it is easy to understand how much hope and faith people came to have in the medical profession; with accurate diagnostic technology and increasingly effective or promising treatments, those with major illnesses came to be cared for increasingly in high tech hospitals. The 'medicalisation' of health and illness became commonplace.

Since the 1950s there has been a trend for people to die in hospital rather than at home. This result is not what the majority of people appear to want, but rather a reflection of how society and health care have changed. With an increasing number of older people, an increasing number of whom live alone, it is not always possible for care to be given in the home. Terminally ill patients are most likely to be admitted to hospital from a combination of three factors: the inability to achieve adequate palliation of symptoms in the community setting, a lack of carers to look after them at home and a lack of primary care and community resources to provide adequate care.

Is an acute care hospital the right place for palliative care to be delivered and for terminally ill people to spend their final days? The answer is not a simple one. What the patient deserves is care that matches his needs and this may place him in any number of settings. However, unless

highly technical and specialised interventions are required, then usually one could say that acute wards – where the pace is fast, the staff are pressed for time and the emphasis is on active/curative treatment – are not ideal places for those requiring care in the final stage of life. Care for this group of patients is perhaps better delivered in a setting where the focus is more holistic and where the patient and his carers can be given the time, privacy and total support they require to deal with the major issues that facing death raises: the hospice movement emerged as a response to these needs.

It is a commonly held misconception that the hospice movement in the UK started with the work of Dame Cicely Saunders. There were in fact a number of hospices before the opening of St Christopher's in London in 1967. Her pioneering work and charismatic leadership, however, are arguably the force that led to the development of the modern hospice movement and subsequently the concept of the palliative care approach.

From the outset, the hospice movement has aimed to provide sound medical care that is based upon quality research and the dissemination of information through education: this, one could argue, is the ideal approach to all sick people. Robert Twycross, an internationally recognised medical leader in palliative care, argued that the hospice movement was not so much a radical shift from the medical model as a redressing of the balance between cure and care: 'We are witnessing,' he said, 'an attempt to re-emphasise that doctors, nurses and paramedics are in the business to cure sometimes, relieve often, to comfort always' (Ajemian & Mount 1981).

The transition from curative to palliative care is often a difficult one. What we do know is that when the last study was undertaken asking people where they wished to spend their final days, the majority (58%) replied that they wished to die at home, 20% indicated a preference to be cared for in hospital another 20% in a hospice and 2% elsewhere (Townsend et al 1990).

In the final analysis patients need to have comprehensive care delivered across a variety of settings and aimed at providing the best quality of life possible in a manner acceptable to them. This is the basis of the palliative care approach: an approach that should be available to all patients in the NHS.

THE PALLIATIVE CARE APPROACH

In recent years we have seen concerted efforts within the UK to ensure that a uniformly high quality of care is available for every patient with cancer. However, there is growing recognition that patients suffering from other life-threatening illnesses such as AIDS/HIV, respiratory, cardiovascular, cerebrovascular and motor neurone disease and multiple sclerosis may also require periods of palliative care. The Health Service Circular (HSC) 1998/115 (NHS Executive 1998) stated that 'the principles and practice of palliative care for all those facing life-threatening illnesses need to be integrated into the whole of NHS practice'. In short, there is an awareness of need and commitment to deliver this to all who require it.

The National Council for Hospice and Specialist Palliative Care Services (1997b), in their Occasional Paper II, paved the way for this statement when it set out the two vital principles for the provision of palliative care:

1. 'It is the right of every person with a life-threatening illness to receive appropriate palliative care wherever they are.'

2. 'It is the responsibility of every health care professional to provide palliative care, and to call in specialist colleagues if the need arises, as an integral component of good clinical practice, whatever the illness or its stage.'

The palliative care approach aims to promote both physical and psychosocial well-being. The key principles underpinning palliative care which should be practised by all health care professionals wherever the patient is being cared for are shown in Box 16.1. Not all patients with palliative care needs will require specialist palliative care services, but the care principles should be available to all patients wherever they are.

Box 16.1 **Key principles of palliative care**
(National Council for Hospice and Specialist Palliative Care Services 1999)

- A focus on quality of life which includes good symptom control
- A whole-person approach which takes into account the person's past life experience and current situation
- The provision of care which encompasses both the person with life-threatening disease and those that matter to that person
- Respect for patient autonomy and choice (e.g. over place of care, treatment options, access to specialist palliative care)
- An emphasis on open and sensitive communication, which extends to patients, informal carers and professional colleagues

---

Table 16.2 The spectrum of palliative care provision (National Council for Hospice and Specialist Palliative Care Services, March 1999)

General palliative care	Hospice palliative care	Specialist palliative care
Provided for: Patients with least complex/acute needs	*Provided for:* Patients with moderately complex/acute needs	*Provided for:* Patients with the most complex/acute needs
Provided by: Some nursing homes Some community hospitals	*Provided by:* All hospices	*Provided by:* Some hospices Specialist palliative care units and teams
A workforce skilled in the palliative care approach — in primary care — in hospitals — in nursing homes		

NOTE: In practice, the boundaries between the three segments of palliative care provision will overlap.

Therefore a range of services is available to meet all patients' needs (Table 16.2).

PALLIATIVE CARE EDUCATION

Having the palliative care approach available throughout the NHS and accessible in any setting means that health care professionals need to have additional skills in order to give professional care to a wide range of patient groups. In relation to this, the World Health Organization has suggested that palliative care education and training should be:

- compulsory in courses leading to a basic professional qualification
- accepted as a suitable subject for testing by examination boards
- recognised by universities and professional bodies as an appropriate subject for study, dissertations, certificates, diplomas and advanced degrees
- included in postgraduate programmes of continuing professional education
- recognised as an appropriate subject for scholarships, fellowships and grants by academic institutions and research funding bodies (WHO 1989).

There is well researched evidence of previous educational deficiencies in the professional training of doctors, nurses and social workers in palliative care (Thorpe 1991, Doyle 1992). However, today palliative care education is widely available to all members of the multidisciplinary team including doctors, nurses, social workers, the clergy, volunteers, etc. There are many degree and diploma courses in palliative care for both nurses and doctors, some special programmes for social workers and some courses are multiprofessional. Palliative medicine was recognised as a speciality with its own training programme by the Joint Committee on Higher Medical Training in 1987 and by the Medical Council of Ireland in 1995 and there are now many well-qualified specialist nurse practitioners in palliative care.

MODELS OF PALLIATIVE CARE AND THE MULTIDISCIPLINARY TEAM

In the UK, palliative care, with its roots in the hospice movement, developed an anti-authoritarian model of care. Although led by doctors, the emphasis was on a multidisciplinary approach to care which also included volunteers. The idea was to support rather than replace the existing hospital and primary care services. It is now recognised that 'hospice care' is a philosophy of care rather than a service or building. It encompasses a wide range of skills and expertise that can be delivered through a variety of models. Most areas will have all or some of the services supplied by specialist hospital in-patient teams, hospice in-patient and day centre provision and specialist home care teams (Table 16.3).

Hospital-based services

Hospital-based palliative care teams were initiated in the UK at St Thomas's Hospital in the late 1970s (Bates et al 1981). They are usually multidisciplinary and include doctors, nurses, and often other professions allied to medicine, social workers and chaplains. They provide an advisory and

Table 16.3 Level of palliative care team services across the UK in 2000 (Directory 2000)

	Home care	Extended home care	Day care	Hospital support teams	Hospital support nursing services
England	258	48	195	165	96
Wales	29	5	16	23	2
Scotland	42	7	19	21	14
N. Ireland	9	1	4	6	6
Eire	26	3	6	11	4
Channel Islands and Isle of Man	3	2	3	0	1
Total	367	66	243	226	123

education service to their colleagues in the hospital on symptom management and assist with psychosocial and spiritual support to patients and counselling for the bereaved. In some smaller hospitals, advice and support is offered by specialist nurses and/or medical consultants who work alone and not within a designated multidisciplinary team.

Home care

Palliative care services within the home vary enormously depending on local need and resources. However, in most areas the major burden of care falls on the patient's family (Bosanquet & Salisbury 1999). The primary health care team is the main provider of professional care at home and often in residential care as well. In most areas the members of the primary health care team will be supported by specialist nurses, often funded by the Macmillan Cancer Relief charity and known as 'Macmillan nurses'. Their role is very similar to the hospital specialist nurses. There are now about 1800 Macmillan nurses working in hospitals, hospices and in the community, usually as part of the NHS specialist teams. The Marie Curie Cancer Care charity also supports over 5000 part-time, specially trained Marie Curie nurses throughout the UK. These nurses provide hands-on, round the clock nursing care for patients in their own homes. Access to Marie Curie nurses is usually through the NHS district nurse.

Day hospices

Day care is an important supplement enabling many patients to continue living at home while having access to important palliative care services. They may include medical and nursing care, spiritual support, and social care such as hairdressing and chiropody. Day care also offers the patients an opportunity to meet with others who are going through similar experiences and provides some respite for family carers.

Children's hospices

At the time of writing, there are 21 in-patient hospices for children in the UK, with a total of 159 beds. They offer medical and nursing care (often respite care) for children with a life-threatening illness.

Extended home nursing services

Many areas now provide extended nursing care at home, sometimes referred to as 'hospice at home' or 'respite care at home'. This includes practical nursing (day or night) to enable patients to stay at home longer. Some services also have ready access to expert medical advice.

Hospice in-patient care

Originally, these in-patient services in free-standing units in the UK were supported by voluntary contributions or charitable organisations (e.g. Macmillan Cancer Relief, Marie Curie Cancer Care, Sue Ryder Foundation). Increasingly the NHS has become involved in supporting these units. All units follow a multidisciplinary team approach to care and many rely heavily on volunteers. The philosophy of care is quite distinct from that of hospitals and involves a personal non-institutional approach (Bosanquet & Salisbury 1999). An important principle in hospice care is that no one care giver can meet the needs of a patient with a life-threatening illness and the multitude of issues they and their family have to face. To understand and be capable of helping to meet the physical, psychosocial and spiritual needs requires a range of skills from different team members.

The multidisciplinary composition of teams varies according to local needs and resources. At the heart of any team is the patient and the patient's family. Their uniqueness and response to the illness should be the foundation for developing their care plans. Other members of the team will include doctors, nurses, social workers, chaplains and volunteers. Other disciplines such as physiotherapists, occupational therapists, psychologists, pharmacists, dieticians, etc. form part of the extended team who may be involved as the need arises.

Today there are over 200 hospice and palliative care in-patient units in the UK (Table 16.4 and Activity 16.1).

Table 16.4 Hospice and palliative care in-patient units in UK, 2000 (Directory 2000)

	Total units	Total beds	NHS units	NHS beds	Voluntary units	Voluntary beds
England	158	2514	36	446	122	2068
Wales	13	124	10	68	3	56
Scotland	24	345	10	86	14	259
N. Ireland	4	65			4	65
Eire	10	136			10	136
Channel Islands and Isle of Man	3	21			3	21
Total	212	3205	56	600	156	2605

Activity 16.1

Establish what services exist in your area and how palliative care is delivered for the patients you are caring for.

Activity 16.2

Think about the subject of death for a few moments. Jot down any examples of images of death that you have seen during the last week from the television, cinema, etc. Also think about what conversations you have had about death recently. Did you discuss a news story or the death of a loved one? Perhaps capital punishment, war, the plot of a film or play? Consider, too, how we refer to death: we have so many euphemisms to cover the reality. We 'kick the bucket', 'snuff it', 'fall off our perches', we 'pass away' – so many ways simply to avoid saying that a person has died. What language did you use in your discussions?

FACING THE POSSIBILITY OF DEATH

The subject of death is often seen as a taboo subject in our society. We learn as we grow up to avoid discussing it – at least in a personally relevant way. As a society we seem to have little trouble in discussing violent deaths or mass tragedies as portrayed in films and novels, but we do not appear to handle the natural process of death with any degree of ease (Activity 16.2).

Few of us grow up viewing death as a normal part of life. Our society has changed and we now expect the process of health care to be medicalised: science and technology are the bedrock of everyday living and our belief in their power has usurped more spiritual values. Dealing with life-threatening illness is a medical challenge, a battle to be waged and won. When the battle is lost, a doctor certifies death and a professional funeral director deals with the body. Gone are the days when living and dying were easily a part of the same continuum and where the social fabric of our lives was automatically contained in the circle of known members of our communities. As

an eminent researcher puts it: 'The more we are achieving advances in science, the more we seem to fear and deny the reality of death…we make the dead look as if they were asleep, we ship the children off to protect them from the anxiety' (Kubler-Ross 1969, pp. 6–7).

Reacting to the prospect of death

One of the first doctors to focus research attention on the reactions to the prospect of dying was Elisabeth Kubler-Ross. In the mid-1960s she began to ask patients to tell her what it was like to be dying. In her own words: 'We have asked him [the patient] to be our teacher so that we may learn more about the final stages of life with all its anxieties, fears and hopes' (Kubler-Ross 1969, pp. 6–7). Activity 16.3 asks you to consider your own possible reactions.

Activity 16.3

Think about what your reaction would be to learning that you had a life-threatening illness. What would change for you if you were given a diagnosis of AIDS or of motor neurone disease or cancer? Jot down a few points about your feelings and thoughts. Then follow on and see how your own reaction might agree with or differ from those discussed in this chapter.

Stages of adjustment

Kubler-Ross developed a five-stage model to describe the process of adjustment to the prospect of death. Her model was developed after interviews with hundreds of patients. She gathered their stories and looked for the common threads and the sequence of events for them. Her model is well grounded in her data but it must be remembered when the model was developed and consider what later changes in palliative care might have influenced her findings.

The stages in the process of adjustment she found were:

1. denial and isolation
2. anger
3. bargaining
4. depression
5. acceptance.

Stage 1: denial and isolation

Hundreds of patients who spoke to Dr Kubler-Ross said they were sure that there had been a mistake: tests were mixed up, it couldn't possibly be the right diagnosis. Their denial led some of them to seek second opinions. 'Denial functions as a buffer after unexpected shocking news, allows the patient to collect himself and, with time, mobilize other, less radical defenses' (Kubler-Ross 1969, p. 35). Reality can be too difficult to face at times and in those periods we may deny in order to remain sane. It is the retreat into denial that is isolating for the individual because as long as he needs/chooses to remain there, communication is impeded. It must always

be remembered, though, that the patient sets the pace at all times and it is not appropriate for us to attempt to force a patient into 'facing the facts'.

How can you help? Learning to break bad news well

Those who feel the need to withdraw into denial are often those who have been told of their diagnosis too quickly or too abruptly. Consider the impact of being given this type of diagnosis: the patient needs a careful and a gentle approach that respects the level of threat the news represents to him. Breaking bad news will not be your job as a beginning practitioner, but it is an important skill and one that you will need to learn as you progress in your nursing career. It is important that bad news is broken well because:

- it supports trust between the health professional and the patient
- it reduces uncertainty
- it prevents inappropriate hope
- it allows eventual adjustment
- it prevents the 'conspiracy of silence' and collusion that can deny a patient his right to be informed of his situation and take an active and informed part in decisions relating to his treatment (Kaye 1996, p. 3).

How do nurses learn this skill? This is achieved by reading, by discussion with colleagues who have greater experience, by taking courses in communication, by watching and listening to expert nurses and doctors in the clinical setting (Activity 16.4).

Activity 16.4

Think about how would you like to be told bad news. If you were in your doctor's surgery and she had bad news to deliver to you, what would you feel was important to you? How do you think you might handle this situation? Jot down a few points before reading on.

You might have considered some of the following points in Activity 16.4:

• Having a family member or friend with you for emotional support as well as being someone who could help you explore issues then and later on.

• Having a longer appointment than the usual one. You might want quite a long time in order to assimilate, consider, reflect on key issues raised.

• Perhaps you would want to discuss difficult issues with a particular doctor: one you felt you had good rapport with and someone who knew you that little bit better than the rest.

• You might want to know just what the probable outcome of the test results and standard treatments would be. Or you might want a wealth of information on alternative approaches and sources of knowledge on which to base your considered opinion.

• You might want just the bare minimum immediately but with opportunity to come back in a day or so to go over the results again.

Stage 2: anger

Once the shock has worn off, as it does for the majority of patients, the reaction changes from 'No, not me' to 'Why me?'. This is a difficult stage for those people around the patient and indeed for the patient. Imagine what the patient might focus his anger upon: the doctors who should have diagnosed him sooner, the hospital for not having the treatment facilities he needs, the diet he has to adhere to, the treatments that cause such distressing reactions, the surgery necessitating prolonged hospitalisation, the nurses for not bringing the medications quickly, etc. The list is endless.

Where does this anger come from? It may come from the loss of possibilities, from the loss of abilities, from the loss of a future. However, this anger is so hard to be around when it erupts. 'The real tragedy is perhaps that we do not think of the reasons for the patient's anger and take it personally, when it has originally nothing or little to do with the people who become the target of the anger' (Kubler-Ross 1969, p. 46). Anger

responded to personally escalates into more anger and the patient's hostile behaviours may well increase.

How can you help? Try to allow the angry person to just be himself and ventilate his feelings without you getting caught up in the need to judge, defend or blame. Once the burden has been laid down through expression, the patient will be able to move on. Sometimes you may think that the anger being expressed is not linked to the present situation; this is anger at its most dangerous because you and the people around the patient might be tempted to try to intervene rather than just honouring the person's emotional response.

Stage 3: bargaining

'Bargaining is really an attempt to postpone; it has to include a prize offered "for good behaviour"; it also sets a self imposed "deadline" and it includes an implicit promise that the patient will not ask for more if this one postponement is granted' (Kubler-Ross 1969, p. 73). This may be viewed as plea bargaining by a person who has acknowledged the finality of the situation. However, there is hope in this stage and it is the hope that tries to find a way to exist within the reality without succumbing to despair.

How can you help? Most bargains are made with God as the patient knows Him and this leads Kubler-Ross to suggest that when we hear the patient expressing his bargaining we listen sensitively. He may be expressing guilt. If this is the case he may only need this to be heard by another person or he may need referral to someone else in the multidisciplinary team.

Stage 4: depression

Depression arrives when the person faces the loss of the past and anticipates the losses that the future will entail. The patient now is fully aware of what he has lost: possibly his job, the income he once enjoyed, the social life he happily took for granted, the ability to undertake favourite pastimes and hobbies, the ability to fulfil his role in his family or social group. This type of

depression could be labelled as 'reactive' in nature. But the patient also has losses to anticipate as he views his future and this type of depression Kubler-Ross calls 'preparatory depression'. She wisely helps us to see how we might respond helpfully to those of our patients suffering both types:

Our initial reaction to sad people is usually to try to cheer them up … . We encourage them to look at the bright side of life, at all the colourful, positive things around them. This is often an expression of our own needs, our own inability to tolerate a long face over any extended period of time. This can be a useful approach when dealing with the first type of depression in terminally ill patients … [but] When the depression is a tool to prepare for the impending loss of all the love objects, in order to facilitate a state of acceptance, then encouragements and reassurances are not as meaningful. (Kubler-Ross 1969, pp. 76–77)

Think about these ideas for a few minutes. Kubler-Ross is not saying reactive depression is a minor problem or one we can simply 'jolly' our patients out of. She is saying that it may, for example, help a mother to know that her children are settled well with a child minder or in a nursery, that they play happily with their friends, and that they take part in school activities with enthusiasm. In helping a patient to see such facts, the losses of the past may be balanced with hope and reassurance that in spite of the loss of her presence right now, her children are doing reasonably well. However, faced with the loss of a future with her children, this approach cannot help. What comfort can be offered to balance the fact that this mother will not be there for her daughter's wedding, or for a graduation? Against such losses there is no comfort available in the present: there is often a quiet grief that seems deeper than words can adequately express.

How can you help?

With reactive depression there is sometimes the opportunity to help the patient to find a balance between loss and life lived in the present. Information about the family or friends or groups with whom the patient is integrally linked may help. With preparatory depression the nurse is perhaps most helpful as a presence, as someone who can be with the patient in silence. This is a time when touch may say more than words. The resolution of this phase will be personal and unique. The nurse's role is to allow the patient to express his feelings of loss and anguish, to listen, to be present and to be aware of the other resources of the multidisciplinary team to help the patient navigate this most painful phase and be ready to refer as appropriate.

Stage 5: acceptance

If a patient has sufficient time and the help he needs to work through the previous stages, Kubler-Ross indicates that he will reach the stage of acceptance. This, she hastens to say, is not a happy state but a time almost devoid of feelings. This is also a time of quiet and of peace when the patient often just wants to 'be' and not to engage in a lot of news and problems coming in from the outside world. It is a period when non-verbal communication may continue to be the norm and quietly sitting with the patient, holding a hand, listening to music or the sound of the birds in the garden, may be all that is wanted and needed.

How can you help?

If this stage is experienced in this way then the family may need more from you than the patient who has settled and found this sense of peace. To those around him, it may look as though he has lost the will to live, or the desire to fight, or even lost hope. It is indeed important that this state is clearly and accurately differentiated from the withdrawal of depression and here the other members of the multidisciplinary team can help.

Summarising the stages of dying

Kubler-Ross has given us a very useful model that is helpful in assisting us to understand the process that some patients may go through in their terminal illness. However, what needs to be considered carefully is whether the five stages represent the path that all patients will travel in a progressive fashion. Will the patient necessarily

move through anger and onto bargaining never to return to the former phase? Is anger only an early stage experience? Do all patients respond in this fashion? Might there be some patients who, rather than being in shock and denial, respond with relief to finally having an accurate diagnosis? All of these are possible.

The Kubler-Ross model has been seen as useful in any situations where a person faces significant loss or threat. It has, for example, been adopted for use in bereavement work. It is a seminal contribution to our understanding of dying and if used appropriately it can help people to map the territory of terminal illness. However, as with any map, it is only a guide to possible destinations and possible routes. The patient is the expert on what he feels and thinks and there is never any substitute for direct communication with him in order to determine where he locates himself in the personal process of his terminal illness.

Stages or phases?

Dr Kubler-Ross conducted her initial studies over 30 years ago in the USA. A more recent work considers that what the dying person goes through is not so much stages along a clear pathway, but phases in which there might be many reactions. In his book *I Don't Know What to Say: How to Help and Support Someone Who is Dying* Dr Rob Buckman (1988) puts forward an alternative 'map' and he discusses it in relation to that of Dr Kubler-Ross. He thinks that what she describes as 'stages' should perhaps be considered as 'reactions' to the threat of terminal illness. He goes on to state that, in his experience, there are far more reactions than those listed by Dr Kubler-Ross. He develops his theme by discussing the reactions that are most likely to occur at the beginning, the middle or at the final stages of the illness journey. Buckman (1988) gives us a simple and very helpful three-phase model which charts the progress of a person from perceiving himself as a well person, through considering himself as someone who might die, to the final realisation that he will die: there are in each phase, likely reactions but no suggestion that the patient is anything but a unique individual navigating his own unique course. The 'transition' consists of:

1. A beginning phase when the person faces the threat of death. This is the time of diagnosis and his reaction to it.

2. An illness phase during which the person has to adjust to the changes brought about by his physical decline from the disease. This phase is marked by the illness experience and by uncertainty. Initially he might feel very well and this in itself adds to the difficulty in dealing with the situation. However, inevitably, during this phase there is a loss of control over a number of important areas of the person's life: the experience of the illness becomes an ongoing and difficult grind and the future is unknown.

3. A final phase when the person approaches his death. This is the period when the patient may come to accept the inevitability of his own death. However, in contrast to the emotional void of the 'acceptance stage' in the Kubler-Ross model, this can become a time when the patient is living life to the limit of his ability. It can be a time of tremendous engagement with life in sorting out last wishes, organising one's affairs, perhaps making memory boxes for children and friends, perhaps even getting married.

The contrast between the two models is pronounced but we need to consider the differences that time has made to palliative care and the quality of life for terminally ill patients. When Kubler-Ross was conducting her initial interviews there were far fewer options for pain control, there were no specialist palliative care nurses and analgesics were not generally administered around the clock, there were no syringe drivers. Powerful anti-emetics had not been developed and radiotherapy techniques were less refined. Perhaps it was a period when the achievement of acceptance that was marked by peace and disengagement was all that could have reasonably been expected.

To tell or not to tell?

All patients may either give informed consent to treatment or refuse it. The NHS Management

Executive (1991) issued guidelines for consent and stated that: 'Patients are entitled to receive sufficient information in a way that they can understand about the proposed treatments, the possible alternatives and any substantial risks, so that they can make a balanced judgement' (NHS Management Executive 1991). However, the guidelines go on to say: 'A doctor will have to exercise his or her professional skills and judgement in deciding what risks the patient should be warned of and the terms in which the warning should be given'.

So, while there is backing for the concept of informed consent, in the UK there is clearly acceptance of a more paternalistic approach that allows doctors to use their discretion and to act in what they consider to be the patient's best interests. In clinical practice you will most often see approaches to patient care that respect the patient's ethical right to know, but you should be aware of the wider professional and legal situation. The Open University study materials for the K260 programme (particularly Workbook 2, section 2, and the suggested readings in the course reader) are excellent sources of information on this subject (Activity 16.5).

In this situation in Activity 16.5 the daughter is asking the consultant to collude with her in keeping the truth from her father. She may have good reasons for wanting to try to protect her father from the diagnosis. Requests like this one are

usually attempts to protect a loved one from bad news or a shock: they are made in all good faith and often with great love. However, each of us has the right to be treated as self-determining and autonomous. We can only make reasoned judgements for ourselves when we have all the relevant facts at our disposal. The daughter is actually asking that her father does not have those facts and this cannot be justified ethically. But what should the consultant do in the actual situation? How could he handle it to respect the position of the daughter and also honour the right of the father to the information he needs to make informed choices? Peter Kaye (1996) suggests a four-step approach in which the patient is the focus and the person who has control of the agenda and the pace. According to Kaye, the health care professional would approach this situation by:

1. Talking to the patient and dealing with his questions and concerns and then gaining his permission to speak to the relatives.
2. Talking to the relatives in order to:
   — determine what they know of the situation. Often fears come from incomplete information.
   — ask why they do not want the patient to know the truth. The family are often experts in knowing the patient, but not always. It is important to understand why they have asked for the truth to be withheld because that holds valuable information for you as the health care worker.
   — discuss what the consequences of not being open might be.
   — reassure the relatives that you will be talking to the patient only to give him information that he wants to know and not forcing the issue or giving him information he cannot or does not want to handle.
3. Talking to the patient alone and checking to see if he is in denial. If he is, then deal with the communication blocks.
4. Talking to the patient and family together. This final step gives resolution and allows the patient and his family to be open and aware of what they each know and how they are handling the information (Activity 16.6).

Activity 16.5 'Please don't tell my father – he won't be able to cope'

Mr Smith is a 60-year-old man on your ward. He has been having tests for changed bowel habits and a low haemoglobin. On the day the test results come back his daughter asks the consultant what they show. The consultant tells her that her father's situation is serious and that he will speak to her after he has seen her father. The daughter begs the consultant not to tell her father the whole truth 'if it's cancer' because he just wouldn't be able to cope with it.

- What should the consultant do?
- Has the daughter the right to try to block full disclosure of information from her father?
- Why might she be asking this of the consultant?

Activity 16.6

Try to role-play the scenario as described in the text and Activity 16.5 with two or three fellow students. You could ask a Macmillan or other nurse with specialist skills to help you play out this scene in the classroom setting. It is in practising such skills in safe settings that you will gain familiarity with approaches and begin to develop skills that you will later be able to take into the clinical setting under the supervision of a senior colleague.

PALLIATIVE CARE AND MANAGING THE SYMPTOMS

In terminal illness the individual's quality of life fluctuates. Good palliative care demands detailed attention to the physical, emotional, social and spiritual components of symptom control. A multidisciplinary team approach is essential as no one discipline possesses all the skills required. But nursing is usually the one discipline which can establish the supportive relationship with the patient and family that is necessary to identify their needs and initiate and monitor interventions, because nurses spend the greatest amount of time with the dying patient (Jenkins 1997). The following are some of the more common physical problems patients may suffer and ones in which nurses can make the biggest difference. For control of other symptoms please see the Further reading list at the end of the chapter.

Pain

The need for cancer pain relief was identified as a major public health problem in the mid-1980s (WHO 1986). At diagnosis 20–50% of patients report pain as a symptom. This rises to 75% in those patients with advanced disease (Bonica 1990, Donnelley & Walsh 1995). The World Health Organization (1997) states that pain management should be available to all patients with cancer at whatever stage they are in their disease. They suggest that patients who are pain free are

Activity 16.7

Consider your own experiences of nursing patients with cancer. Was their pain controlled to their satisfaction? If this was not the case what do you think were the possible reasons for this?

better able to withstand aggressive cancer treatments and should therefore have their pain managed prior to anti-cancer treatments. In 1990 the World Health Organization suggested: 'The greatest improvements in quality of life for cancer patients and their families could be effected by implementation of existing knowledge of pain and symptom control' (Activity 16.7).

While you were thinking about the questions in Activity 16.7, did you consider the doctors' concerns and reluctance to use morphine and other strong opiates; or the nurses who are too afraid to challenge the doctors' decisions or act as the patients' advocates; or the patients' acceptance of their pain and their unwillingness to complain for fear of being seen as a nuisance?

Pain related to cancer can be classified as somatic, visceral and neuropathic in type (Payne & Gonzales 1996) (see Ch. 15 on how to manage these types of pain). The important factor is to try and establish what is causing the pain so that the appropriate treatment choices can be made. Pain is one of the most feared consequences of cancer and many people believe that cancer and pain are synonymous. It is the role of the nurse to reassure the patient that most pains can either be completely alleviated or greatly eased and that they do not have to experience intolerable distress.

Accurate assessment of the type and severity of the pain is an important part of good pain management because no effective treatment is possible until this is done. There are many different assessment tools available and most hospital wards and community nursing teams will use one (Activity 16.8). (Chapter 15 gives detailed information about the assessment and treatment of pain.)

Activity 16.8

Which pain assessment methods are used in your area?

Breathlessness

Breathlessness is an unpleasant sensation of being unable to breathe easily (Davis 1998). It is important to remember that, as with other symptoms, breathlessness is not just a physical problem. It is a particularly frightening experience for both patients and their families. Emotions such as fear and anxiety can make the situation worse. As a calming presence to offer reassurance to both the patient and family, the nurse can be enormously beneficial. As with all symptoms, assessment of the cause is the first line of management. Explanation to patient and family of the cause and treatment may help to alleviate some of their fears. A cool stream of air such as a fan or open window is usually necessary. The physiotherapist can help with advice on positioning in bed, adapting the patient's activities of daily living, control of breathing and relaxation techniques.

Fatigue

Fatigue is a major symptom in 78–96% of patients with cancer and is particularly common in those undergoing treatment (Irvine et al 1991, Vogelzang et al 1997). This chronic fatigue differs from what might be called 'simple' or 'acute' fatigue. If a person becomes tired through overwork or simply not getting enough sleep, the solution is simple: a good night's sleep will be restorative. But for the patient suffering from chronic fatigue this is not the case: some other mechanism is acting. It is a type of fatigue that just does not lift, that takes enjoyment out of life, that makes ordinary things seem a struggle. Imagine feeling tired all the time and having to make decisions, shop, cook, study, socialise, care for a family. This is a major quality of life issue.

Fatigue may have many causes including anaemia, drugs, prolonged stress, changes within the nervous system, depression, nutritional disorders, infections, sleep disturbance. It is important that a thorough assessment of the patient is undertaken when this symptom presents. Patients may be able to experience considerable relief by having medication altered, or through learning to prioritise and pace themselves through their activities. Gentle exercise is sometimes helpful in increasing the feeling of well-being and in reducing the fatigue simply because it breaks the downward spiral of fatigue – more rest – less functional strength and endurance – more fatigue. There is an excellent resource on the internet that you might wish to explore: the National Cancer Institute has a web-site where information on a number of topics, including fatigue, is available. The web-site address can be found at the end of the Further reading list for this chapter.

Constipation

Most ill patients will suffer with constipation at some time. Nearly all patients on strong analgesics will become constipated unless they are given laxatives prophylactically.

Constipation can cause nausea and vomiting, abdominal pain, bloating, headache and confusion. Remember constipation can present as diarrhoea (due to faecal overflow).

The management of constipation should, first, include prevention (i.e. asking the patient about bowel activity and recording the information). Care must include prompt response to a patient's request to go to the toilet and, if possible, for the patient to use a commode instead of a bedpan with his feet on a footstool to help brace the abdominal muscles. Diet is an important aspect of managing constipation, trying to tempt the patient's failing appetite with small well-presented meals of his choice, adding bran to the diet if possible and increasing the fluid intake. Regular laxatives will be required by most patients receiving palliative care and many of these patients will also need rectal measures as well (i.e. suppositories or enemas).

Nausea and vomiting

Nausea and/or vomiting can make the dying person feel miserable and exhausted. Can you remember the last time you felt nauseated? Try to imagine what it must be like to feel like that for hours or even days. Often the only relief is to vomit when you may feel slightly better for a period of time.

Vomiting is what the nurse sees but the patient may have felt nauseated for many hours before this. It is just as important to treat constant nausea as it is to treat vomiting. Talking to patients and encouraging them to tell you how they feel may be the only way you will learn about their nausea. Many patients dislike complaining and do not want to bother the nurse or to be seen as a nuisance.

There are many causes of nausea and vomiting and, just as when treating pain, an assessment of what the cause is will help in choosing the correct treatment. Anti-emetics should be prescribed and given regularly for those patients who have constant or frequent nausea and/or vomiting. It is cruel and unnecessary to give such drugs only on a when-needed basis as this means the patient often has to earn his treatment by vomiting first!

Mouth problems

The main mouth problems experienced by terminally ill patients are dry mouth, dirty mouth, infection, pain and halitosis (Jenkins 1997).

Dry mouth. This is a common problem for any ill patient. There are many possible causes but the most common are drug induced (e.g. opiates, diuretics), dehydration or infection. The management should include a review of the patient's drug regimen to see if any drugs can be changed, together with frequent sips of water, sucking boiled sweets or chewing gum. Sucking ice cubes, fresh pineapple chunks or the use of artificial saliva may also help.

Dirty mouth. Jenkins (1997) suggests that dirty mouths are best cleaned using a small soft toothbrush and toothpaste and rinsing the mouth with water. However, a very dirty and coated tongue may require the use of sodium bicarbonate solution (1 teaspoon to 1500 ml warm water), effervescent vitamin C (tablet dissolved directly on the tongue) or sucking fresh pineapple chunks.

Infections. Many very ill patients are susceptible to fungal infections, particularly those who have had cytotoxic treatments, corticosteroids or antibiotics. The treatment of choice is a topical antifungal (e.g. Nystatin) – remember the patient must be taught how to rinse and hold this in the mouth before swallowing. Dentures need to be removed prior to treatment and cleaned and treated before re-insertion otherwise treatment will fail. Systemic antifungal treatments may be needed for some patients.

Pain. Oral pain may be due to local tumours, infections or certain treatments (e.g. cytotoxic or radiotherapy). Treatments may consist of systemic analgesia as well as topical (e.g. gel applied to the mouth or mouthwash).

Halitosis (unpleasant or foul smelling breath). The causes in ill patients may include severe infection, gastric stagnation, dirty mouth or possible necrosis of the mouth, pharynx, nasal sinuses, lungs, etc. Whatever the causes for any of the above problems, they can lead to unnecessary distress for the patient. Meticulous regular mouth care is a vital component of good nursing care. Ask yourself how you would feel with a painful, sore or offensive mouth.

MANAGING THE LAST DAYS OF LIFE

Unless death occurs suddenly or unexpectedly, there is usually a terminal phase when it is recognised by the health professionals that death is inevitable. This phase can last for days or even weeks. It is important to remember that patients and their relatives may not have recognised what is happening as treatment goals are redefined and the nature of the primary illness becomes less important. Patients and relatives may feel we have 'given up' or 'abandoned them'. Control of symptoms and psychological support for all those involved takes priority. If the nurse believes in the value of the individual and the sanctity of life, which should be the case, then

caring and concern must continue at the highest level as death approaches. Recognising and understanding the characteristics of the dying process will enable the nurse to respond to dying patients and their family needs. The reasons for any changes in treatment must be explained in a sensitive manner to patients and family to prevent further distress.

The National Council for Hospice and Specialist Palliative Care Services (1997a) suggests that the aims of management at this stage should be to relieve distressing symptoms and fears in the patient – as far as possible. It is also very important to provide support for the family, to enable the patient to die in the place of their choice, if feasible, and to minimise the morbidity associated with bereavement.

KEEPING THE PATIENT COMFORTABLE

An analytical approach to symptom control should continue but must rely much more on clinical findings rather than investigations. Drugs should be reviewed regularly and only those needed to keep the patient comfortable continued. The route of administration needs assessing regularly; some patients will manage oral medication until near to death but others may need an alternative route. When this time arises all medication should be given via the subcutaneous route. Intramuscular injections are cruel and unnecessary for the terminally ill patient. Ask yourself which kind of administration you would prefer. The rectal route is an alternative but this is less convenient and most patients dislike it. To prevent misunderstandings about the rationale for these changes, clear, open and sensitive communications with the patient and family are essential.

Terminal restlessness

Restlessness is often seen in the last hours of life. The threshold for discomfort is often lowered in very ill and anxious patients. It is therefore important to pay attention to the patient's surroundings. If possible the patient should be in a quiet and peaceful environment with soft lighting and people they know. The presence of a member of the family who should be encouraged to hold the patient's hand and speak gently to them (even if the patient seems unresponsive) can have a calming effect. Both patient and family will need reassurance.

As with all symptoms, there are many possible causes of terminal restlessness. Treatable causes should be excluded (e.g. unrelieved pain, full bladder or rectum, breathlessness). Immobility can lead to bed-bound patients suffering joint stiffness, bedsores and frustration. Simple nursing measures such as pressure relieving mattress, regular turning and careful positioning are vital for the terminally ill patient. Some drugs may cause terminal restlessness and if possible they should be discontinued or changed. Metabolic disorders (e.g. liver failure, renal failure, hypercalcaemia, hyponatraemia, and hypoglycaemia) are possible causes. If it is not appropriate to treat the cause (for example it would be cruel and unacceptable to start treating metabolic disorders in the last hours of life), or if the cause is not apparent, then a sufficient dose of an anxiolytic or tranquilliser should be given either subcutaneously on a regular basis, or constantly via a syringe driver.

Noisy 'bubbly' breathing

Noisy breathing, often referred to as the 'death rattle', usually occurs because the patient is unable to cough up or swallow their secretions from the oropharynx and trachea (Faull 1998). The patient is often not aware of the problem but the family can find it very distressing. Drugs are the mainstay of management and need to be commenced as soon as the problem arises. If appropriate, gentle physiotherapy may help and it is always worth asking a physiotherapist for an opinion. Careful positioning of the patient may also help.

Emergencies

Emergencies in the last days of life are rare except for severe haemorrhage and respiratory

obstruction, both of which should be treated promptly with a fast acting sedative. Haemorrhage is distressing for both patients and relatives: dark coloured towels or blankets to make the view less traumatic will aid comfort for all those involved.

Dehydration

Most patients will stop eating in the terminal phase and in the last few days of life very few continue to take fluids. This can cause enormous distress to the family who feel the patient is being allowed to die of dehydration. Giving fluids either intravenously or subcutaneously has not been shown to be of any benefit at this stage of a patient's life and for some patients may make the situation worse by causing peripheral or pulmonary oedema (National Council for Hospice and Specialist Palliative Care Services 1997c). Again the family need help to come to terms with the changing situation and reassurance that everything is still being done to keep the patient comfortable.

FAMILY SUPPORT

Most relatives will be distressed and frightened at this time. It is the responsibility of the health professional to offer as much support as possible to the family. If the patient is in hospital, the nurse should make a conscious effort to approach the family to speak to them and not expect the family to seek them out. They are often afraid of being seen as a nuisance or interrupting a busy schedule. Many relatives complain of not been kept up to date or informed of the patient's condition. This may be because there is no change and nothing to report but they should be told that and given the opportunity to ask questions and express their feelings.

Wherever the patient is being cared for the family should be given the opportunity to assist in the care of the patient if they wish to. This may be simple tasks such as keeping the mouth moist but the nurse should always ask the family if they would like to help in other ways, e.g. washing the patient or helping with pressure area care.

The knowledge that they have helped to keep their loved one comfortable can be enormously beneficial in the family's bereavement.

During the last few days of life many relatives wish to keep a vigil by the patient. They should be encouraged and supported to do this but not made to feel guilty if they find it too hard to do. If the person you love most in the world was dying where would you want to be? If the patient is at home, it maybe that a Marie Curie nurse is staying during the night to care for the patient and allow the family to rest knowing the nurse will alert them to any changes. In hospitals and nursing homes there should be somewhere close by for the family members to sleep. Some relatives may choose to stay by the patient's bed so, if at all possible, a folding bed or recliner chair should be in the room with the patient to allow the relative to rest. Relatives can become totally exhausted both physically and mentally during this very difficult period and the nurses should be alert to the family's needs. Patients rarely want to be left alone to die – if the family is unable to be with them, every effort should be made to ensure that someone else is. This will usually be the nurse.

LAST OFFICES

A respectful and correct procedure of last offices is integral to the holistic care of the patient. It is the last nursing act that practitioners can carry out for their patients. Once the death has occurred the family, or significant others, must be informed. Each member of the family who wishes it should be allowed private time with the deceased person. They must not feel as though they are being rushed, as this may be their last opportunity to be with the person they love. A quiet room should be provided away from the bed for the family to be together, and refreshments should be offered. The nurse should make herself available to talk to the relatives and answer any of their questions and concerns and to offer support and comfort.

The body of the deceased should be attended to according to local policy which will include addressing any cultural and religious requirements. If appropriate a family member may like to be involved in the washing and dressing of the deceased and should be given the opportunity to do so. The nurse should also honour any family requests for special clothing for the deceased.

Arrangements for the registration of the death need to be explained, with sensitivity, to the next of kin. In some settings this is carried out by the nursing staff but in others there may be a special administrative office for such matters. If there is property to be collected by the relatives, this should be carefully managed since these articles may represent special memories of the deceased.

BEREAVEMENT

The experience of bereavement and loss is a common one throughout our lives and it is likely that you will already have experienced loss of some kind (Activity 16.9). In each case you probably faced the feeling of missing the person or thing lost and you had to change in some way to accommodate your loss. How severe your reaction was will have depended upon many factors including the nature of the relationship you had with the person, the permanence of the situation and your ability to change appropriately to handle the loss.

THE STAGES OF LOSS

Colin Murray Parkes (1988, p. 56), one of the key contributors to our understanding of loss and grief, has developed a theory of psychosocial

Activity 16.9

Think of the losses you have experienced, for example the death of a person you loved, the ending of a special relationship, the death of a pet, the loss of a favourite toy or book, the loss of friends who went away to other schools and cities. What sort of emotions did you go through when these losses happened? Jot down some of the things that you felt and did, then discuss these with one or two colleagues.

transitions to explain the challenges we face in situations of loss. He talks about the 'assumptive world' we inhabit each day. Think about the hundreds of things you took for granted, or assumed would be the case when you awoke this morning. You might have assumed that you would meet certain people, or that you would be able to contact them. You might have entered today assuming that certain events would take place, that you would eat certain foods, enjoy certain sights and sounds and interact with friends who would respond in certain reasonably predictable ways. In short, you assumed that you could navigate your way through the day with a certain degree of assurance of who would be there and what the day would be like.

The loss of a loved one would have shattered so many of your expectations. Because we each expect the day to unfold in reasonably known ways we would react to such a major loss with shock and disbelief. We would be disorientated and feel dazed. Next we would suffer the feelings of missing that person and move into grief which might be marked by such strong feelings as loneliness, anger, guilt or despair. We might feel absolutely overwhelmed by our sense of loss. Eventually we would reorganise our assumptive world to accommodate the absence of that person, at least in ways that allowed us to function and re-engage in our normal lives.

There are many models of grief and many attempts have been made to chart the tasks the bereaved person must successfully complete in order to deal with his loss. Katz & Sidell (1994, pp. 16–17) summarise the stages listed by most writers on the subject of grief in the following way:

1. shock and disbelief
2. pining
3. reorganisation and reintegration.

When you look at this list of reactions you see how similar they are to the Kubler-Ross stages of response to the prospect of loss of life.

If these are the stages, what are the tasks to be undertaken? Worden (1991) is one of the most cited authors whenever 'grief work' is discussed. He summarised the Harvard Bereavement Study (the Omega Project) and stated that grief resolution involves the following:

1. acceptance of the reality of the loss
2. experiencing the pain and grief
3. adjustment to an environment in which the deceased is missing
4. withdrawal of emotional energy and reinvestment into another relationship.

How can bereaved people be helped in their grief work?

Stage 1: accepting the reality of the loss

People who have not been prepared for a death will have a natural reluctance to believe that a loved one has died and may have greater difficulty in this stage than those who anticipate it. The shock can be profound.

This stage can be helped by such practices as viewing the body and in this regard the last offices are very important. Seeing the body of a loved one carefully prepared in a pleasant setting can be a great comfort and afford the time and privacy the family want to say their personal goodbyes. The reality of loss is also helped by talking about the person and the death, by sharing experiences and stories, by looking at photos. Dealing with the personal effects of the deceased person and distributing them among the friends and family also makes the loss more real.

Stage 2: experiencing the pain and grief

Murray Parkes (1975, p. 57) states: 'The most characteristic feature of grief is not prolonged depression but acute and episodic "pangs". A pang of grief is an episode of severe anxiety and psychological pain. At such a time the lost person is strongly missed and the survivor sobs or cries aloud for him.' The shock and numbness can soon give way after a death to feelings of total anguish. In this period a number of things are common: the survivor may sense the presence of the deceased, smell a particular scent associated with the person, and dream of him and thus re-enter the acute pain of loss.

It is also a time of guilt and of anger: 'Perhaps if I hadn't done X this wouldn't have happened.' and 'How could he have left me now? What am I supposed to do without him?!' are not unusual reactions at this time.

At this stage, the most important work for the nurse is to show unconditional positive regard to the bereaved person and engage in active listening.

Stage 3: adjustment to an environment in which the deceased is missing

When a person dies, patterns of everyday life change forever for those who mourn. Perhaps one partner has always handled the finances or attended to the servicing of the car, another may have done all the domestic tasks such as cooking, ironing or always dropped the children off at school or taken them to sports events. Successful adjustment to a person's death will require that the survivors take on new tasks and new roles in order simply to keep life running relatively smoothly. This phase does not require the bereaved person to fill all the gaps personally: other family members or friends might take over some tasks and ease the adjustment. The important issue is that the bereaved person does not withdraw from life but finds ways to make life work.

People can be helped during this phase by family and friends who are willing to assist them in learning new skills or in supporting them as they face new challenges. Health professionals can help at this time by simply monitoring how the adjustments are being made and offering support and help as necessary.

Stage 4: withdrawal of emotional energy and reinvestment into another relationship

Eventually the bereaved person will come back into the mainstream of life and will be able to take the risk of loving again. Loss is the price we pay for love: without connection and commitment there would be no mourning. It takes time and considerable optimism and courage to reconnect with life after losing a loved one but most of us will manage this task successfully at some point in our lives. This stage is, in many ways, a natural progression from the third stage where the bereaved person adjusts in terms of tasks and roles. This is a daunting phase but we should remember that those best placed to help are usually family and friends who can gently and persistently encourage the bereaved person to re-engage with life in all its richness.

Health professionals can help by being sensitive to the feelings bereaved people have at this time. Many feel it is disloyal to even consider falling in love again and remarrying or re-committing to another and they may need time and space to consider these feelings in order to move on. Others may feel that they cannot possibly consider another significant relationship because they just do not want to face another loss of this magnitude. So much that happens in this stage is dependent upon the nature and the quality of the previous relationship and the support and love the person feels in dealing with these feelings. In the end, to reinvest in life in its fullness means accepting that one is vulnerable and this is never easy. Does 'reinvesting' mean that the bereaved person is 'over' the loss of a loved one, that they now no longer miss that person or think of them? Not at all. To complete 'grief work' well means that they find a way of dealing with their loss and reinvesting in life. The memories, both sad and joyful, of the person they have lost are part of the fabric of their life, part of the person they are and therefore taken with them into a richer future.

CHILDREN AND BEREAVEMENT

Children can be deeply affected by grief. If they have been robbed of a parent or sibling they are capable of responding with anger and guilt. The need to help children to deal with their own grief adds to the weight of a bereaved parent's burden. If children do not get help with anger and guilt, these emotions may surface in the form of restlessness, learning difficulties, truancy, vandalism, withdrawal and depression. The nurse can help by befriending and supporting the whole family.

SPECIAL TYPES OF LOSS

In the ordinary course of events we expect that we will lose older friends and relatives: it is the painful but natural order of life. When the losses occur through the advances of age or through a known illness then they may be easier in some respects to deal with. That is not to say that loss and grief will be easy but simply that they will be anticipated. There are some situations, though, in which we would all probably have far more difficulty in dealing with bereavement: the death of a baby or infant, the sudden loss of a person through an accident or the death of a person through suicide. What differentiates these types of losses seems to be the degree to which they are anticipated and the apparent 'sense' these deaths make to the survivors.

Miscarriages, abortions and infant death

The loss of a child is considered to be one of the worst possible losses to deal with largely because it is not what anyone anticipates: people are supposed to live increasingly long lives and losses in the prenatal period or in infancy are not the norm. In short, losing a baby goes against the order of things we have come to expect.

The subjects of stillbirths, neonatal and sudden infant deaths are too large to be dealt with properly here. However, you may want to explore these areas through personal study and through reflection. Some helpful web-site addresses are given at the end of this chapter.

Opinion has changed considerably in recent years about how we can best help parents in their grief following miscarriage or other prenatal death. Not so many years ago, when parents lost a baby they were encouraged to 'get over it' quickly and have another child as soon as possible. The situation was treated as though their loss was somehow less acute and real because the child was a stillborn baby or of an age when it was presumed they would be less attached to the child. Losses are experienced in relation to the meaning ascribed to them and health professionals must treat each loss individually. To one mother or couple a miscarriage might spell the end of their chances of ever having a child of their own and the grief might be acute. To another person, to whom the timing of the pregnancy was poor in terms of her health or family finances, it might be less distressing. As Kohner (1993) said: 'It is the personal significance of the loss, not the gestational age of the baby, which determines the extent of parents' bereavement and their need to grieve.'

Although we now appreciate the importance of acknowledging the loss of a newly delivered baby there are particular difficulties in making the death 'real' for the parents because certain key factors are absent from this situation. An older infant or child would have a name, for example, but a newly delivered baby or stillborn baby might not, so helping a mother to grieve might be facilitated by naming the baby. Similarly, unlike the grieving parents of an older child, these parents may not have any photographs apart from a scan image and so opportunities to take photos may be helpful in keeping these memories intact. Just as another parent would be able to see, hold and spend time with the newly delivered baby, so these things are important for the mother and father of a baby who was stillborn or who died very soon after birth. Similarly, the rituals that help us mark the transitions in life are equally important here and some sort of memorial service/funeral may be very significant. What is most important is that we treat each loss individually and allow those who mourn to decide on what is best for them, give them information and time to reflect. If you wish to explore this important subject in more detail you might like to read *Loss and Bereavement in Childbearing* by Dr Rosemary Mander (1994), a midwife with tremendous expertise in this area.

Deaths due to suicide

Recent data available from the Samaritans 2000 web-site (address at the end of the chapter) shows that suicide accounts for 18% of all deaths of young people. The suicide rates in older people have dropped in recent years but still remain high in comparison to the general population.

Suicide in older people (over 64 years of age) accounts for 15% of all suicide deaths. There is a rising trend in attempted suicide and in the case of young men, suicide attempts have risen by 172% since 1985. Some factors linked to suicide in the young include: alcohol and substance abuse, family problems, physical and sexual abuse. In older persons the following factors are linked to suicide: depression, physical pain or illness, living alone and feelings of hopelessness and guilt. It is clear from the statistics that the UK has one of the highest rates of attempted suicide in Europe. It is therefore likely that you will come across friends and families grieving for a loved one who has died through suicide. You will certainly care for patients who are in hospital because of attempted suicide. The stigma attached to suicide is great and there continues to be a tendency to ascribe the death to other causes and to ignore it as a social issue of considerable importance. The stigma comes from a variety of sources. Some people feel that a person must be mentally ill to attempt suicide, others see it as something that is prohibited by religion. The guilt that family and friends feel can be immense as they search their memories for clues in the days or hours leading up to the suicide and blame themselves for not realising that the person was close to taking his own life. There are no easy answers here. Each person who takes his own life has very individual reasons and the bereaved have complex grief work to accomplish (Activity 16.10).

A study carried out by Grzybowska & Finlay (1997) tried to determine the incidence of suicide in patients in palliative care units. They surveyed 43 units and asked for data covering the years 1990–94. Thirty-four units replied and between them they had 72 633 referrals during that 5-year

Activity 16.10 Suicide and people receiving palliative care

How common is suicide among patients receiving palliative care? An odd question? Think about it for a few minutes. Under what circumstances might someone wish to control his death when suffering from a terminal illness?

period and between them reported 21 suicides and 37 attempted suicides. Their sample included only patients who had cancer as a diagnosis. Although the figures appear small in relation to the overall referrals in this study and no firm conclusions can be drawn from it, it is important to note that international data suggest that patients with cancer have higher suicide rates than those found in the general population. Some of these patients might attempt suicide because of depression, or uncontrolled pain, or their perception that they have lost their dignity as people because of their illnesses.

COMPLICATED GRIEF

Given time, most of us will re-engage with life after a death. The time it will take each of us will vary. We may never be the same again but we will emerge as people who are secure in the hard earned knowledge that being involved with others is worth the risks and the costs. However, some people will not emerge whole from their grief and our question now must be how do we recognise these people and how can we help them?

Complicated or abnormal grief reactions are unhelpful or maladaptive patterns arising from loss. The function of grief is to help us to deal with our losses in a way that recognises their importance but also allows us to move on into a future where we can function normally and find happiness in engaging with other people and activities.

How long should this take us? It is commonly believed that 1–2 years is 'normal'. But we cannot use time alone as a guide: we are each unique and one loss does not equate with another. I may take 6 months to adjust to the loss of a pet I have loved for 12 years and to come to the point where I contemplate finding another one, but I may take a number of years to fully engage again in a life where my partner is now forever absent.

So if time is not on its own an indicator, how would you recognise complicated grief (Activity 16.11)?

Abnormal grief at its most extreme is illustrated in the character Miss Havisham in Charles Dickens's novel *Great Expectations*. Jilted at the altar on her wedding day years earlier,

Activity 16.11 Abnormal grief

Think of people whom you consider have grieved in abnormal ways and list what it was about their reactions that made you think their grieving was unusual/unhelpful in returning them to an active and full life.

Miss Havisham had kept her home exactly as it was on that day, as if time had stopped at that moment. She became a recluse, locked into the past because she could not bear to contemplate a future that had gone so badly wrong. She is truly a picture of abnormal grieving!

You may have made some notes about a person you knew who had suffered from depression or anxiety following a loss. You may have noted that the person felt suicidal. Or perhaps in contrast you made notes on someone who did not appear to grieve at all. You may have jotted down points about the person living months afterwards as if the person were still alive and physically real and whose memory influenced current decision making. These are indications that the grieving process is not moving forward towards resolution. Box 16.2 indicates those individuals who are most at risk of having difficulty with their bereavement.

The role of the health care professional here is, first, to recognise that the person is not progressing in their grief work. If someone is 'stuck' in his grief then it is important that it is handled properly by professionals competent to help in these situations. Talking to family, friends, the general practitioner, other health professionals who are involved may alert those with special skills that their care is required. There are a number of organisations that help those who are bereaved:

• CRUSE is a counselling service available to anyone who is bereaved and is finding it hard to deal with. There are a number of internet sites run by local groups and you may wish to explore their resources.

• The Samaritans operate a phone line staffed by trained people able to help those in distress from whatever cause.

Box 16.2	**Factors indicating high risk for abnormal grief resolution** (Parkes 1990, Worden 1991)

1. *A severe reaction to the loss.* The manifestation of severe distress, anger or self-reproach.
2. *An ambivalent relationship.* Where the individuals involved had ambivalent feelings towards each other, often with unexpressed hostility or in situations when the relationship was highly dependent.
3. *Circumstances surrounding the death.* Sudden deaths where there was less than 2 weeks to adjust to the loss, and unnatural deaths, such as suicide or murder, or when confirmation of the death is uncertain and the body never found.
4. *Previous unresolved grief.* One of the complications of bereavement is unresolved grief, and when a subsequent death occurs, it is much harder for the bereaved person to adjust.
5. *Multiple life crises.* If the bereaved person has many additional problems or losses to cope with, this may inhibit normal grief resolution.
6. *Personality factors.* People with a strong self-concept are usually better able to cope with crisis situations, including bereavement, by using their own coping mechanisms more appropriately.
7. *Low socioeconomic status.* Although this was found to be a factor in the early period in the study of Parkes & Weiss (1983), grief resolution had returned to normal after 2 years for those in the low socioeconomic group.
8. *Poor social support.* Those who have a close family and supportive friends cope better with bereavement. At risk would be those individuals who have recently moved house or whose families live at a distance. Probably as important as the amount of support an individual has is his perception of that support. Those who perceived themselves to be unsupported had more problems with their bereavement.
9. *Age.* Young adults have more difficulty adjusting to bereavement than do older people.

- There are counselling services available through the general practitioner's surgery or accessible privately.
- There are community psychiatric nurses available to assess and recommend treatment options.

SPIRITUAL ISSUES

Spiritual issues are all important in caring for those who face life-threatening illness, death, grief and distress. It is important not to mistake religious issues for spiritual ones. Religion provides a framework for some of our spiritual beliefs but seldom encompasses the wholeness of our values. In an increasingly secular society it is spiritual rather than religious values that inform and support more and more of us as we search for the meaning and face our own and others' deaths.

We are all individuals and need to have our spiritual and religious needs assessed and solutions to our specific needs explored. For those who are members of certain religious groups, the needs may be specific. You will be able to find a guide to the religious care of patients who belong to various faiths from the hospital chaplains but never assume that because your patient belongs to a particular faith you know what his needs are: you only know when you have explored these issues with your patient.

Spiritual assessment is often regarded as a difficult task. The North American Nursing Diagnosis Association (NANDA) (Carpenito 1997) is very helpful in giving both definition and direction to our exploration of patient needs. NANDA defines 'spiritual distress' as 'the state in which the individual or group experiences or is at risk of experiencing a disturbance in the belief or value system that provides strength, hope and meaning to life'. By their definition, a person is in spiritual distress when the way in which he usually views his world is shaken. The definition includes factors such as questioning the meaning of life, not practising one's usual rituals, feeling spiritually empty, detached, despairing or being discouraged. They also state that a key factor in diagnosing this problem is asking for assistance with your problems in your belief system.

You might like to consult Carpenito's (1997) text on the application of nursing diagnosis to clinical practice because it provides a wealth of information on the various religious faiths and gives suggestions for both assessment and intervention which you might find useful.

THE STRESS OF CARING FOR THE DYING

Working with dying patients and their families brings nurses into contact with the distressing situations of grief and loss. With those patients and families for whom you have cared over a length of time you will have some degree of emotional involvement and will feel the grief yourself.

Coping with another person's anguish and despair is one of the most difficult aspects of being a nurse. Experiences of significant stress and feelings of being inadequate are not uncommon among even the most senior nurses at such times. There are many reasons for this, such as inadequate training in communication skills and age – there is evidence to suggest that the younger the caregiver, the more stressful they find caring for the dying (Vachon 1987). Other stressors could be as a result of particular death experiences in your own life or unresolved personal grief, stress within your job or low job satisfaction. Whatever the reason, it is nothing to be ashamed of.

A good working environment is one where colleagues support each other, where time is set aside for team meetings and team building. Many teams use debriefing sessions for staff to discuss difficult issues or problems. Many employers now offer a counselling service for their employees. Why not look into what supportive services are available locally for you. Remember that being a good colleague means supporting fellow colleagues around you as well as looking for support yourself.

No one could ever say that caring for the dying is easy but there is an enormous amount of satisfaction in knowing that you have helped to make the last few days or weeks of a human being's life more comfortable, both physically and emotionally.

REFERENCES

Ajemian I, Mount B 1981 The adult patient: cultural considerations in palliative care. In: Saunders C (ed) Hospice: the living idea. Edward Arnold, London

Bates T, Hoy A M, Clark O G, Laird P P 1981 The St Thomas Hospital terminal support team. Lancet 1:1201–1203

Bonica J J 1990 The management of pain, 2nd edn. Lea and Febiger, Philadelphia

Bosanquet N, Salisbury C 1999 Providing a palliative care service: towards an evidence base. Oxford University Press, Oxford

Buckman R 1988 I don't know what to say: how to help and support someone who is dying. Macmillan, London

Carpenito L J 1997 Nursing diagnosis: application to clinical practice, 7th edn. Lippincott, Philadelphia

Clark D 1982 Death in Staithes. In: Dickenson D, Johnson M (eds) 1993 Dying and bereavement. Sage, London

Davis C L 1998 Breathlessness, cough and other respiratory problems. In: Fallon M, O'Neill B (eds) ABC of palliative care. BMJ Books, London

Department of Health 1997 On the state of the public health: the annual report of the chief medical officer of the Department of Health for the year 1997. DoH, London

Department of Health 1999 Saving lives: our healthier nation. Stationery Office, London

Directory 2000 Hospice and palliative care services in the United Kingdom and the Republic of Ireland. Hospice Information Services, St Christopher's Hospice, London

Donnelly S, Walsh D 1995 The symptoms of advanced cancer. Seminars in Oncology 22(Supplement 3):67–72

Doyle D 1992 Nursing education in terminal care. Nursing Education Today 2(4):4–6

European Association for Palliative Care 1989 Newsletter No 1. Milan

Faull C, Carter Y, Woof R 1998 Handbook of palliative care. Blackwell Science, Oxford

Grzybowska P, Finlay I 1997 The incidence of suicide in palliative care patients. Palliative Medicine 11:313–316

Irvine D M, Vincent L, Bubela N, Thompson L, Graydon J 1991 A critical appraisal of the research literature investigating fatigue in the individual with cancer. Cancer Nursing 14(4):188–199

Jenkins R 1997 Nursing care. In: Kaye P (ed) Tutorials in palliative medicine. EPL Publications, Northampton

Katz J, Sidel M 1994 Easeful death: caring for dying and bereaved people. Hodder and Stoughton, London

Kaye P 1996 Breaking bad news: a ten step approach. EPL Publications, Northampton

Kohner N 1993 The loss of a baby: parents' needs and professional practice after early loss. In: Dickenson D, Johnson M (eds) Death, dying and bereavement. Sage, London

Kubler-Ross E 1969 On death and dying. Tavistock, London

Mander R 1994 Loss and bereavement in childbearing. Blackwell Scientific, Oxford

National Council for Hospice and Specialist Palliative Care Services 1995 Specialist palliative care: a statement of definitions. Occasional paper No 8. NCHSPCS, London

National Council for Hospice and Specialist Palliative Care Services 1997a Changing gear: guidelines for managing the last days of life in adults. NCHSPCS, London

National Council for Hospice and Specialist Palliative Care Services 1997b Occasional Paper II. Dilemmas and directions: the future of specialist palliative care. NCHSPCS, London

National Council for Hospice and Specialist Palliative Care Services 1997c Ethical decision making in palliative care: artificial hydration for people who are terminally ill. NCHSPCS, London

National Council for Hospice and Specialist Palliative Care Services 1999 Palliative care 2000: commissioning through partnership. NCHSPCS, London

NHS Management Executive 1991 A guide to consent for examination or treatment. HMSO, London

NHS Executive 1998 Health Service Circular 1998/115 Palliative care. Stationery Office, London

Parkes C M 1975 Determinants of outcome following bereavement. Omega 6(14):303–323

Parkes C M 1988 Bereavement as a psychosocial transition: process and adaptation to change. Journal of Social Issues 44(3):53–65

Parkes C M 1990 Risk factors in bereavement: implications for the prevention and treatment of pathological grief. Psychiatric Annals 20(6):308–313

Parkes C M, Weiss R S 1983 Recovery from bereavement. Basic Books, New York

Payne R, Gonzales G 1996 Pathophysiology of pain in cancer and other terminal diseases. In: Doyle D, Hanks G W C, MacDonald N (eds) Oxford textbook of palliative medicine. Oxford University Press, Oxford

Thorpe G 1991 Palliative care to United Kingdom medical students. Palliative Medicine 5(1):6–11

Townsend J, Frank A, Fermont D, Dyer S, Karran O, Walgrove A, Piper M 1990 Terminal cancer care and patients' preference for place of death. British Medical Journal 301:415–417

Vachon M L S 1987 Occupational stress in the care of critically ill, the dying and the bereaved. Hemisphere, New York

Vogelzang N J, Breitbart W, Cella D et al 1997 Patient, caregiver, and oncologist perceptions of cancer-related fatigue: results of a tripart assessment strategy. Seminars in Hematology 34 (3 Suppl 2):4–12

Worden J W 1991 Grief counselling and grief therapy. Tavistock/Routledge, London

World Health Organization 1986 Cancer pain relief. WHO, Geneva

World Health Organization 1989 Expert Committee on Palliative Care. WHO, Geneva

World Health Organization 1990 Cancer pain relief and palliative care. WHO, Geneva

World Health Organization 1997 Looking forward to cancer pain relief for all. CBC, Oxford

FURTHER READING

Twycross R 1995 Introducing palliative care. Radcliffe Medical Press, Oxford and New York
This book emphasis the needs of the whole person, examine the systems of care in hospice and home, the ethics of palliative care, symptom management and communicating with dying patients and their relatives in order to meet their psychological and spiritual needs.

Clark D, Seymour J 1999 Reflections on palliative care. Open University Press, Buckingham
This is essential reading for anyone concerned about the care of the dying patient. It looks at the development of palliative care and the organisation of death and dying in modern society.

Twycross R 1997 Symptom management in advanced cancer, 2nd edn. Radcliffe Medical Press, Oxford and New York
This book offers practical and up to date information and advice on symptom management. It is useful for doctors and nurses involved in the care of cancer patients both in hospital and in the community.

Sheldon F 1997 Psychosocial palliative care. Good practices in the care of the dying and bereaved. Stanley Thornes Ltd, Cheltenham
This book is a comprehensive handbook for anyone involved in the care of the dying and their families. It shows the importance of the cultural and social aspects of caring for these venerable patients.

Singh K D 1998 The grace in dying: how we are transformed spiritually as we die. Harper, San Francisco
This is a beautiful book that cannot be recommended highly enough. Kubler-Ross gave us such insight into the physical and psychological aspects of dying but Singh provides us with insight into the spiritual transformations that can occur as we face death.

Levine S 1988 Who dies? Investigation of conscious living and conscious dying. Gateway Books, Bath
This is a book that will encourage you to explore how we live and how we die. It is written in a very accessible style and covers such issues as children and death, working (not simply dealing with) pain and working with the dying. This book can change the way you live each day if you can open to its message.

Rinpoche S 1992 Tibetan book of living and dying. Rider Books, London
This is a book by a great Buddhist Master. Based upon the Buddhist perspective, it has much to offer us all. Sogyal Rinpoche hoped in writing his book that he would change the way we looked at death and cared for the dying. I think he has accomplished this. The book is particularly strong to the Westerner in discussing compassion.

Regnard C F B, Tempest S 1998 A guide to symptom relief in advanced disease, 4th edn. Hochland and Hochland, England
This is an indispensable companion for doctors and nurses involved in the care of people with advanced disease. It includes sections on: managing pain, psychological symptoms, emergencies and a drug formulary.

Fallon M, O'Neill B (eds) 1998 ABC of palliative care. BMJ Books, London
This is a booklet aimed at all health professionals who care for patients requiring palliative care. It starts from the assumption that good palliative care should be available to patients at all stages of their illness regardless of location. It is an excellent introduction to the field.

Regnard C, Hockley J 1995 Flow diagrams in advanced cancer and other diseases. Edward Arnold, London
This is based on algorithms that first appeared in the journal of Palliative Medicine. It takes the reader through the key clinical decisions in a logical and step by step progression. Recommended as an excellent guide to general problem solving.

INTERNET

National Cancer Institute
  http://www.nci.nih.gov/cqancerinfo/index.html
  For information on symptom control, especially fatigue.

Stillbirth and Neonatal Death Society
http://www.cafamily.org.uk/Direct/s57.html

Foundation for the Study of Infant Death
http://www.sids.org.uk/fsid/

Sudden Infant Death Syndrome Alliance
http://sidsalliance.org/

Samaritans 2000
http://www.samaritans.org/sams.html/suistats.html

Index

Page numbers in **bold** indicate main discussions.

A

Abbreviations, 430
Aβ nerve fibres, 475, 476
ABO blood group system, 175
Abortion, **117–118**
  conscientious objection, 117–118,
    135, 318
  grief reaction, 502–503
Abortion Act (1967), 117–118
Absorption, **184**
Acceptance
  of loss, 501
  stage of dying, 492
Access to Health Records Act (1990),
  127, 320, 388
Access to Medical Reports Act (1988),
  127
Access Modification (Health) Order
  (1987), 320
Accident and emergency departments
  health promotion and, 300–301
  waiting times, 59
Accidents, 288
  childhood, 15–16, 299–300
  reports, 127
  statistics, 300
Accommodation, cognitive, 208
Accountability, **312–313**, 401–402
  student nurses, 323
Acetaminophen (paracetamol),
  462–463
Acetylcholine, 189
Acheson Report (1998), **287**, 289
Achondroplasia, 157, 158
Action
  research, 338
  taking, **264–265**
  theory of reasoned, **291**

Action for Sick Children (formerly
  National Association for the
  Welfare of Children in
  Hospital, NAWCH),
  14–15, 16
Activities of daily living, 372–373
Activity/rest, 378, 379
Act of Parliament, 114
Acupuncture, 140–141, 474, 475, 476
Acute sector, 10, 44
  future trends, 28
  independent provision, 69
  shorter in-patient episodes, 14, 255
  terminal care, 485
Adaptations
  physical, 303
  in Roy's model of nursing, 374–375
Aδ nerve fibres, 460, 461, 476
Adenosine triphosphate (ATP), 163
Adolescents, 18
  consent by, 121
  health education, 300
  pregnancy, 294, 303
  see also Children; Young people
Adrenal cortex, 192, 221
Adrenaline, 192, 221
Adrenal medulla, 192, 221
Adrenocorticotrophic hormone
  (ACTH), 192
Adults
  consent by, 121–122
  feeding, 415
  nursing, **10–14**
  pain assessment, 470–471
  see also Elderly; Young people
Advertising, 322
Advice, giving, **265–266**, 269
Advisory Committee on Training of
  Nurses, 328
Advocacy, 265

patients in pain, 481
role of nurse, 312, 315
services, 61, 62
Aerobic reactions, 163
Affective learning, 292–293
Afferent nerves, 190
Afro-Caribbeans, meals in hospitals,
  143
Agammaglobulinaemia, 157
Agapistic ethics, 99
Age
  for giving consent, 121
  grief reaction and, 505
Age Concern, 244, 248
Agglutination, 175
Aggression, 267
AIDS/HIV infection, 28, 195
  antenatal testing, 302
  in children, 281
  infection control principles,
    406–407
  labelling patients, 82
  prevention, 290, 302, 303
  UKCC code of conduct, 318
Air, 378, 379
Airedale NHS Trust v. *Bland* [1993], 114
Albinism, 157
Alcohol
  consumption, 288
  metabolism, 185
Aldosterone, 187, 192
Alimentary canal
  motility, 182–183
  structure, 181–182, 183
Allodynia, 465
Alternative therapy, *see*
  Complementary/alternative
  therapies
Altruistic ethics, 99
Alveoli, 179

Amino acids, 185
Amputation, limb, 466–467
α-Amylase
   pancreatic, 184
   salivary, 184
Anaerobic respiration, 163
Analgesics, **462–464**
   adjuvant, 462, 465, 468
   in neuropathic pain, 465–466
   non-opioid, 462–463
   opioid, *see* Opioids
   WHO ladder, **469–471**
Anaphylactic shock, 194
Androgens, 192
Aneuploidy, 162
Anger, dying patients, 491
Anoxia, 163
Antenatal care, 299, 303
Antenatal diagnosis, 159
Anthropology, 132, 136–137
Antibiotics, 403, 404
   resistance, 407
Antibodies, **193**, 194
Anticonvulsant drugs, 466
Antidepressants, 23, 25
   for neuropathic pain, 465, 466
Antidiscriminatory nursing practice, **104–105**
Antidiuretic hormone (ADH), 187, 192
Anti-embolism stockings, 421
Anti-emetics, 497
Antifungal drugs, 497
Antigens, 174, 193
Anti-inflammatory agents, 468
Anti-psychiatry movement, 24
Anxiety, posture in, 260
Anxiolytics, 498
Appearance, 260–261
Appraisal
   primary, 222
   secondary, 222
Aprons, disposable, **403–404**, 408
Arbitration and Conciliation Advisory Service (ACAS), 116
Aristotle, 4, 100
Army Medical School, 6
Aromatherapy, 474, 477
Arterial system, 172, **176**
Ascorbic acid, 166
Asian cultures, 237
   diet, 143
   health promotion, 306
   personal hygiene and washing, 143–144
Assaults, on nurses, **119**
Assertiveness, 267
Assessment
   integrated care pathways, 384
   needs, **241**, 295
   nursing, 370–371
      Casey's model, 380
      cultural dimension, 134, 135–136, 141

Orem's self-care model, 378, 379
   psychological aspects, **213–216**
   Roper et al model, 373
   Roy's adaptation model, 376–377
nutritional, 415
pain, *see* Pain, assessment
spiritual, 505
Assimilation, 208
Assistant nurse, 8
Asthma, 12, 15, 179
Asylums, 21
ATP (adenosine triphosphate), 163
Attention, **213–214**
   giving, 273–274
Attitudes
   changing, 293
   health behaviour and, 291
Attribution
   covariance model, 215–216
   theory, **215–216**
Audit, **401**
   clinical, 57–58
   committees, 57–58
Audit Commission, 64, 248
Authenticity, 272
Authoritative approach, teaching, 267
Authority, moral expertise and, 83
Autoimmunity, 195
Autonomic nervous system, 221
Autonomy, 96, 200, **201–202**, 209
   constraining factors, 201–202
   respect for, 95, 102
   working with, 104
Autosomal inheritance, 157, 158, 159
Autosomes, 153
Autotrophic organisms, 181, 182
Axons, 188–189

B

Back injury, 410–411
Back pain, 476
Bacteria, 403–404
Badness, moral, 79–80
Bad news, breaking, 490–491
Bargaining stage, dying, 491
Barnet v. *Chelsea & Kensington HMC [1969]*, 124
Barristers, 116
Bartlett, Sir Frederick, 217
Bathing, 423
Battery, 119
Bed baths, 423–424
Bedford Fenwick, Dr, 7
Bedford Fenwick, Mrs (formerly Ethel Gordon Manson), 7, 8, 328
Beds
   extra, 60
   intermediate care, 60, 69
Behaviour

changing, **290–291**
   theory of reasoned action, 291
Behaviourism, **205–207**
Beliefs
   health, *see* Health beliefs
   moral, **80**
Beneficence, 95
Bentham, Jeremy, 93–94
Bereavement, 484, **500–505**
   children, 502
   helping organisations, 504–505
   historical aspects, 484–485
   special types, 502–504
   spiritual issues, 505
   see also Death; Grief
'Best interests', patients', 118, 119
Better Government for Older People (1998), 248
Better Services for the Mentally Handicapped, 21
Bevan, Aneurin, 43, 44
Bile, 183–184, 185
Bioethical model, 91
Biographical details, 385, 386, 429
Biomedical model, 229–230, **372**
   see also Medical model
Biotin, 166
Bisexual patients, 82
Black Report (1980), 63, 287
Bladder emptying, 188
Blair, Tony (Prime Minister), 58
   five challenges, 58, 59
Blaming
   in ethical reasoning, 83
   victim, 305
Bland, Tony, 114, 118–119
Blinding, 344
Blood, **172–176**
   cellular components, 174–176
   clotting, 168, 169, 174
   groups, 174–175
   liver functions, 185
Blood pressure, 284
   arterial, 176
   in dehydration, 417
   measuring, 419
Blood transfusion, refusal, 135, 429
Boards of directors, 45, 49, 62
Body, dead, 499–500, 501
Body temperature
   checking, 419
   controlling, 373
   regulation, 171, 173
Bolam test, 123–124
Bolam v. *Friern Hospital Management Committee [1957]*, 120, 123
Bone metastases, painful, 468
Bovine spongiform encephalopathy (BSE), 28
Bowel obstruction, in cancer, 468
Bowlby, John, 16
Bowman's capsule, 186, 187
Brain, pain pathways, 461–462
Branches, nursing, 9, **10–27**

Breaking bad news, 490–491
Breast
 cancer, 302, 467
 phantom pain, 467
Breathing, 180–181
 noisy 'bubbly', 498
 in Roper et al model, 373
Breathlessness, 496
Briggs Report (1972), 323, 333, 398
British Association of Counselling, 271
British Journal of Nursing, 7
Bronchitis, chronic, 179
Bronchogenic carcinoma, 179
BSE (bovine spongiform
  encephalopathy), 28
Buckman, R., 492
BUPA, 69
Burford Hospital, Oxford, 14
Burns, 414
Butterworth Report (1994), 27
Butyrophenones, 24–25

C

Cadets, 31
Caesarean section, refusal of consent,
  122
Calciferol, 165
Calcitonin, 192
Cancer
 childhood, 15, 337, 338
 inheritance, 160
 pain, **467–469**
 pain management, 468–469, 495
 prevention, 302
 service development, 61
 suicide, 504
 symptom management, 495, 496
 targets, 287
Capacity, to give consent, 120, 122–123
Capillaries, 172, **176–178**
Carbamazepine, 466
Carbon dioxide, 179, 181
Cardiac cycle, 177
Cardiac muscle, 176
Cardiopulmonary arrest, 218–219
Cardiopulmonary resuscitation (CPR),
  218–219, **423–425**, 426
Cardiovascular system, **172–179**
Care
 ethical dimensions, **85–86**
 nursing, 366–367
 philosophy, 368
 standards of, 312
 see also Health care
Care coordination team, 241
Career, nursing, **27–33**
 history and development, 7, 8
 modern framework, **30–31**, 71
 options, **28–29**
Care management, **241**
Care manager, 241

Care pathways, 367, 371, **400–441**
 definitions, 382–383
 example, 400, 434–457
 integrated, **381–384**, 385
Care plan, 371
 Casey's model, 381
 Orem's self-care model, 378
 Roper et al model, 373
Care programmes, 381
Care protocols, 381
Carers
 educational role of nurse, 268
 sick children, 16–17
 support services, 64
Caring, **80–81**
 as basis for nursing ethics, **97–100**,
  109
 dimensions, 80–81
 virtuous, 98–99
Caring for People (1989), 240, 241, 244
Carriers, X-linked disorders, 158, 160
Casey's model of nursing, **380–381**
Catecholamines, 221, 222
Catharsis, 204
Catholicism, 4–5
Ceiling effect, pain management, 469
Cell, **151–163**, 416
 chemistry, enzymes in, **164–167**
 division, 154–155
 genetic material, 152–154
 membrane, 151–152
 respiration, **163–164**
Central nervous system (CNS), 189,
  190
Centre for Reviews and
  Dissemination, University
  of York, 52, 398
Cerebrovascular accident, *see* Stroke
Chadwick, Sir Edwin, 5
Challenging, **266–267**
Changing behaviour, **290–291**
Charge nurse, 8, 30, 31, 73
Chemoreceptors, 181
Chemotherapy, cancer, 468
Chest pain clinics, 61
Chief executives, 45, 48, 49
Chief medical officer (medical
  director), 48, 51–52
Chief nursing officer (director of
  nursing), 45, 48, 51–52
Child abuse, 18
Child protection, 18
Children
 accidents, 15–16, 299–300
 AIDS/HIV, 281
 'at risk' register, 18
 bereavement, 502
 cancer, 15, 337, 338
 Casey's model of nursing, 380–381
 consent by, 121, 428
 dental health, 299
 developmental screening, 302
 with diabetes, 296
 health care provision, 16

health inequalities, 286
health promotion, 288
hospices, 488
 as interpreters, 142
 negligence actions, 124
 nursing care, 317
 pain assessment, 471–473
 patterns of health and illness,
  15–16
 socialisation, 233
 United Nations list of rights, 14, 15
 value formation, 87–88
Children Act (1989), 380
Children's nurse, role of, 16–17
Children's nursing, **14–18**
 in community, 16
 future, 18
 in hospital, 16
 other aspects, 18
 special skills, 17
Choices, health, 283–284
Cholecystokinin–pancreozymin (CCK-
  PZ), 184
Christianity, 4–5
Chromatin, 152
Chromosomal abnormalities, 156, 157,
  158–159
 numerical, 158–159, 161, 162
 structural, 159
Chromosomes, 152–153
 translocations, 159
Chronic illness, 10, 14
 health education, 303
Chronic obstructive airways disease
  (COAD), 179
Chymotrypsin, 184
Circumcision, female, 130
Cleaning
 environmental, 407, 408
 mouth, 497
Cleansing, personal, 373, 429–431
Client-centred approach, 26
Clients, **10**
 see also Patients
Clinical governance, **50–52**, 219
 ethical aspects, 82
 nursing practice and, 392–393
 nursing research and, 332
 practitioner perspective, **57–58**
 professional regulation and, 54, 55
 reporting concerns and, 431
 support agency, 62
Clinical grading, 30
Clinical indicators, 57
Clinical Negligence Scheme for Trusts
  (CNST), 54
Clinical nurse specialists, 31
Clinical service development, 61
Clinical Standards Board, 53
Clinical supervision, **268–269**, 312, 322
Clotting, blood, 168, 169, 174
C nerve fibres, 460, 461
Cobalamine, 166
Cochrane Centre, 343, 398

Cochrane Database, 52, 363
Code of conduct, 235
    International Council of Nurses, 132, 313
Code of Professional Conduct (UKCC), 86, **311–321**, 367
    administration of medicines, 412
    applying, 313–321
    clause by clause interpretation, 315–321
    confidentiality, 102, 125, **319–320**
    environmental safety, 403
    legal aspects, 115
    purpose, 313
    students and, 313
    text, 314
    transcultural care, 132, 317–318
Co-factors, enzyme, 164
Cognition, 207
Cognitive-behavioural approach, mental illness, 24
Cognitive-behaviour therapy, 26
Cognitive impairment
    pain assessment, 473–474
    see also Dementia
Cognitive learning, 292
Cognitive processing, 207
Cognitive psychology, 200, **207–209**
Cognitive theory, moral development, 100–101
Cold therapy, 462, 478
Collapsed patients, 424–425
Colorectal cancer, 306
Colostomy, 13
Colwell, Maria, 18
Commensal organisms, 404
Commercial interests, promoting, 322
Commission for Health Improvement (CHI), 47, 52, 53
Commitment, in counselling, 273
Commonalities, between people, 200, **201**
Common Foundation Programme (CFP), 9
    UKCC competencies, 9–10, 35–39
Common law, **115**
Communication, **253–277**, **425–431**
    channels, 258
    complexity, 256–257
    components, 257–261
    in different contexts (TACTICS), 263–276
    dimensions, 257
    in health education, 291–292
    importance in nursing, 254–256
    inevitability, 255
    modes, 259
    non-verbal, 258, **259–261**, 262
    personal flexibility, 257
    principles of good, 428–429
    problems, 256–257
    record-keeping and, 385–386
    reflection on, 263
    in Roper et al model, 373

    self and, 261–263
    in transcultural care, **142**
    verbal, 258
Communications technology, 27
Community care, 14, **240–244**
    children, 16
    communication aspects, 255
    elderly, 64, 241, 242–244, 245
    future trends, 28
    inter-agency cooperation, 242, 245–246
    in learning disability, 21–22
    in mental illness, 25, 26–27
    nursing models, 375
    political aspects, 50
    services, **242–244**
Community health councils (CHCs), **50**, 61
Community nurse, 31
    manual handling and moving, 411
    paediatric, 16, 17
    specialist, 29
Community plan, 65, 66
Community psychiatric nurse (CPN), 25, 29, 505
Competence
    awareness of limitations, 316, **401–402**
    Common Foundation Programme, 9–10, 35–39
    definition, 9
    maintaining, 316
    pre-registration, 35–39, 72
Complaints, 62
Complementary/alternative therapies, 232
    in mental illness, 26
    pain management, 474–475, 477
Computed tomography (CT) scanners, 61
Computers
    data analysis, **353–355**
    patient records, 385–386
Conditioning
    classical, 206
    operant, 206
Confidentiality, **102–103**, **125–126**, 430
    action for breaching, 125, 126
    breach of, 103, 125
    justifiable breach of, 104, 125–126
    patient records, 388
    in reflective practice, 397
    UKCC code of conduct, 102, 125, **319–320**
Conflict, 227
Confrontation, 266
Congenital disorders, 156–160
Congruence
    in communication, 258
    in counselling, 272
Conscientious objection
    to abortion, 117–118, 135, 318
    UKCC code of conduct, 318
Conscious mind, 200, **202**, 261–262

Consent, **119–123**
    by adults, 121–122
    by children, 121, 428
    criteria for validity, 120
    in elderly care, 122
    ethical aspects, 85–86
    expressed, 427
    form, 120–121, 429
    implied, 125, 429
    informed, **103**, 120, **427–429**, 493–494
    in mental illness, 122–123
    nurse's responsibility, 427
    obtaining, 428–429
    to research participation, 357–358
    to sharing of information, 103, 104, 125, 320
    verbal, 428
    voluntariness, 120
    written, 120–121, 428
    by young people, 121
Consequentialism, 93
Conservative governments (1979–1997), 43, 49–50, 245
Constipation, 470, 496
Containers, medicine, 412
Continuing education, 326
Continuing professional development, 32, **52–53**, 73, 401
Control
    group, 343, 345
    locus of, **212**
    taking, for others, 265
Coping, 221, 222
Coronary heart disease
    genetics, 160
    housing and, 281
    prevention, 282, 288, 300, 305
Coroner, 116
Corticosteroids, 468
Cortisol, 192
Counselling, **271–275**
    bereavement, 505
    commitment, 273
    defining, 271
    focusing on patient, 272–273
    from dependence to independence, 272
    genetic, 299
    listening and responding skills, 273–275
    in mental illness, 26
    requirements for effective, 271–272
    staff, 506
    within nursing context, 271
County court, 119
Courts, 116, 117
Covariance model of attribution, 215–216
Cox case, 118
Crash calls, 423–424
Credit Accumulation and Transfer Scheme (CATS), 316
Creutzfeldt–Jakob disease (CJD), 28

CRIES, 472–473
Crimean War, 5–6
Criminal Injuries Compensation
  Authority, 119
Criminal law, **116–119**
Critical care nursing, **12–13**
Critical pathways, 381
Crockery, 409
Cross-cultural care, 132
  see also Transcultural care
Cross-over designs, 343
Crown court, 117
Crown Prosecution Service, 117
CRUSE, 504
Cry, silent, 472
Cultural brokerage, 135
Cultural diversity, 107–108, **129–145**,
  238
  UKCC code of conduct, 132,
    317–318
  use of touch, 259–260
Cultural heritage, 237–238
Cultural sensitivity, 133–134,
  138–141
Culture, **130–132**, **237–238**
  assessment, 134, 135–136, 141
  changing behaviour and, 291
  concepts of health and, 132,
    230–231
  definitions, 130–131, 237
  as dimension of care, 134
  health care and, 131–132
  nursing care and, 132
  universal, 238
  versus ethnicity, 136
Cupboards, medicine, 412, 413
Cutlery, 409
Cystic fibrosis, 15, 157, 159

D

Darwinism, social, 357
Data
  analysis and interpretation,
    353–356
  collection methods, 347–351
  collection and recording, 351–353
Data Protection Acts (1984 and 1998),
  127, 319, 354, 388
Day-case surgery, 12, 27–28, 61
Day centres, **242**
Day hospices, 487, 488
Death
  causes of, 484
  customs and beliefs about, 318
  last offices, 499–500, 501
  legal aspects, **118–119**
  place of, 485
  rattle, 498
  reactions to impending, 489–493
  registration, 500
  sudden, 502, 505
  see also Bereavement; Dying;
    Terminal illness
Decision-making
  on behalf of patients, 106
  evidence-based, **218–219**, 398–399
  informed, **398–399**
  moral, *see* Moral decision-making
  patient empowerment, 312
Deep vein thrombosis (DVT), **421–422**
Defecation, **185**
Defence mechanisms
  immune, 191–192
  mental, 204–205
Dehydration, 187, 416
  signs and causes, 417
  in terminal illness, 499
Delta opioid receptors, 463, 464
Dementia, 284–285
  consent to treatment, 122
  pain assessment, 473–474
Demographic trends, 28, 84, 255
Demonstration, learning from, 293
Denial, 204, 490
Dental health, 299
Deontology, **91–93**, 97–98
  act, 92–93
  rule, 93
  versus utilitarianism, 95
Deoxyribonucleic acid (DNA), 150,
  152, 153, 335
Departmental sister, 30
Department of Health, 46, 48, 59, 363
  Research and Development
    Strategy, 333–334
Department of Health and Social
  Services (Northern Ireland),
  46, 48
Dependency, nursing home residents,
  243
Depression, 301
  posture in, 260
  preparatory, 492
  reactive, 492
  stage of dying, 491–492
Descriptive studies, **344–345**
Design, research study, 343–347
Detoxification, 185
Developmental screening, 302
Devi v. *West Midlands RHA* [1981], 119
Diabetes mellitus, 12, 15, 185
  health education, 296
  inheritance, 160
Diagnosis, nursing, 371
Dialysis, renal, 188
Diaphragm, 180
Diaries, communication, 265
Diarrhoeal diseases, 15
Diet
  healthy, 295
  in palliative care, 496
  transcultural issues, **143**
  see also Eating; Food
Differences, individual, *see* Individual
  differences
'Difficult' patients, 81, 315
Diffusion, 152
  facilitated, 152
Digestion, 181–182
Digestive enzymes, 183–184
Digestive system, **181–185**
Director of nursing (chief nursing
  officer), 45, 48, 51–52
Disability adjusted life years, 84
Disabled people
  community care, 242–244
  discrimination against, 106
  health promotion, 282–283, 303
  negative labelling/stereotyping, 82
Disaccharidases, 184
Disadvantage, social, 286–287
Disinfection, 408
Displacement, 204
District nurse, 29
Diversion, in pain, 478
DNA, 150, 152, 153, 335
Dobson, Frank, 42, 70, 72, 246
Doctors
  assessment of performance, 56, 62
  clinical governance and, 51–52
  numbers, 60
  nurses as subordinates to, 311
  power relationships, 101
  professional self-regulation, **55–56**
  research by, 359–360
  revalidation, 55–56
Documentation, *see* Record-keeping
Dogma, preaching, 83
Dominant inheritance, autosomal, 157,
  158
Donabedian, A., 338
Donohoe v. *Stevenson* [1932], 123
Double blinding, 344
Down's syndrome
  inheritance, 157, 159, 161, 162
  nursing research, 337–338
  Orem's self-care model, 378, 379
Dressing, 373, **423–424**
Dressings, changing, 404
Drinking, 415, 417
  in Roper et al model, 373
  transcultural issues, **143**
Drug misuse, 63, 288, 292
Drugs, 412
  analgesic, *see* Analgesics
  controlled, 412, 413
  for emergency use, 412
  for mental illness, 23, 24–25
  metabolism, 185
  in terminal illness, 498
  see also Medicines
Drug trolleys, 412
Dual ethnocentrism, simultaneous,
  134
Duchenne muscular dystrophy, 157
Duty
  of care, 123–124
  professional versus legal, 115
  sense of, 93

Dying, 484, **489–494**
    history of care, 484–485
    legal aspects, **118–119**
    phases, 493
    reactions to, 489–493
    in Roper et al model, 373
    spiritual issues, 505
    stages of adjustment, 490–493
    stress of caring for, 505–506
    telling the truth, 493–494
    see also Death; Palliative care;
            Terminal illness

E

Eating
    assisting patients, 415, 416
    disorders, 415
    healthy, 231, 280–281
    in Roper et al model, 373
    transcultural issues, **143**
    see also Diet; Food
ECG (electrocardiogram), 177
Economics, health care provision, 28
Eczema, 409
Education
    health, *see* Health education
    medical, *see* Medical education
    nursing, *see* Nurse education
    palliative care, 487
    teenage pregnancy and, 294
Educational cycle, 295
Educational role (of nurse), **267–269**
    clinical supervision, 268–269
    with colleagues, 268
    with patients and carers, 268
    UKCC code of conduct, 323–325
Edward's syndrome, 162
Efferent nerves, 190
Egalitarianism, 96
Egypt, ancient, 4
Eland Colour tool, 473
Elderly, 11, **14**, 255
    community care, 64, 241, 242–244,
            245
    consent to treatment, 122
    demographic trends, 28, 84
    discrimination against, 106
    ethical aspects of care, 82, 84
    future care, 28, 70
    health education, 247–248
    independent sector provision,
            69–70
    intermediate care, 69, 70
    long-term care, 242, **246–247**
    national service frameworks, 66
    negative labelling/stereotyping, 82
    NSAIDs and, 462
    nutrition, 414–415
    pain assessment and management,
            474
    post-herpetic neuralgia, 466

rights, 106
    suicide, 503
Electroconvulsive therapy (ECT), 25,
        467
Electronic mailing, 259
Elimination
    Orem's self-care model, 378, 379
    Roper et al model, 373
Email, 259
Emergencies, **424–426**
    drugs for use in, 412
    legal aspects, 121–122, 124–125
    in terminal illness, 498–499
Emotional health, 285
Emotions, facial expression, 260
Empathy, 267, **271–272**
Emphysema, 179
Empirical knowledge, 82, 83
Employers
    counselling services, 506
    health and safety issues, 403
    negligence, 123
    policies on assaults, 119
    reporting concerns to, 320–321, 431
    safe handling and moving, 411
    vicarious liability, 124
Employment
    contracts, 126
    teenage pregnancy and, 294
Employment tribunals, 116
Empowerment
    model of health education, 305–306
    patient, 312
Encouraging, 274
Endocrine glands, 183, 191
Endocrine system, **190–191**
Endocrinological disorders, 11
Endorphins, 462, 465
Energy, 181, 182
    from cellular respiration, **163–164**
    processes requiring, 163
England
    National Board, 326–327
    NHS organisation, 46, 48
Enterokinase, 184
Environment
    care, 320
    cleaning, 407
    hazards, **402–414**
    maintaining a safe, 373, 404
    physical, 261
Environmental health, 286
Enzymes, **164–167**
    digestive, 183–184
    factors affecting action, 164–167
Equilibrium, 208
Equipment
    disposal, **407–409**
    investment in, 61
    safe use, 409–410
Equity, 10, 104–105, 316
Erythrocytes, 174–175
Erythropoietin, 188
Escherichia coli, 407

Ethics, **77–112**
    decision-making, *see* Moral
            decision-making
    issues in nursing, **104–108**
    Kantian, 93
    medical, **91–95**
    normative, 79
    nursing, **78–87**
        caring as basis, **97–100**, 109
        case study file framework, 109,
                110
        code of, *see* Code of
                Professional Conduct
        common errors in reasoning, 83
        context of health care and,
                84–85
        dimensions of care, 85–86
        ethical enquiry process, 79–84,
                109
        medical ethics as basis, **91–97**
        in practice, 84–87, **100–108**
        principles of biomedical, **95–97**
        research, 357–358
        theory, 91–97
        virtue, 97, 98–100, 109
Ethics committees, 357
Ethnicity, 130
    versus culture, 136
Ethnic minorities, 73, 130
    health care, 131–132
    health inequalities, 286–287
    health promotion, 283, 306
    negative labelling/stereotyping, 82
    rights, 106
    understanding difference, 107–108
Ethnocentrism, simultaneous dual, 134
Ethnography, 336, 349, 351
Ethnomethodology, 349–350
European Community (EC), 324,
        325–328
European Directives, 114
    manual handling and moving, 411
Euthanasia, 118
Evaluation, nursing, 372
Evidence
    hierarchy, 398
    sources, 398
Evidence-based practice, 52, 312,
        398–401
    decision making, **218–219**,
            398–399
    ethical aspects, 82–84
    nursing models and, 381
    policies, protocols and care
            pathways, 399–401
    research and, **331–363**
    see also Research
Excretion, 185
    by kidneys, 187–188
    by skin, 171
Exercises, foot and leg, 421–422
Exhaustion, 222
Exocrine glands, 183–184
Expectancy effects, in research, 344

Experience
    awareness of own limitations, 316,
        401–402
    learning from, 208
    learning values through, 89
    versus expertise, 220
Experimental groups, 343, 345
Experimental studies, **343–344**
Expertise
    definition, 219
    developing problem-solving, 220
    problem solving and, 219–220
    self-evaluation, 219–220
    see also Knowledge
Expiration, 180
Explanatory models, patients', **142**
Extended role of nurse, 60, 316–317
Eye contact, 260

F

Face-to-face contact, 259
Faces pain assessment scale, 472
Facial expression, 260, 474
Facilitative approach, teaching, 267
Facts, moral decisions based on, **82–84**
Fairness, 10, **104–105**
Family
    assisting patients to eat, 415
    in bereavement, 501
    deceased patient, 499–500
    dying patient, 494, **499**
    involvement in child's care,
        380–381
    palliative care, 488
    sick child, 16–17
    in socialisation, 233
    see also Parents
Family-centred care, 380
Family-friendly policies, 73
Family Law Reform Act, 121
Fatigue, dying patients, 496
Fats
    absorption, 184
    digestion, 185
    energy production from, 163–164
Favours, acceptance of, 322
Fear, mental illness, 24
Feedback
    in communication, 270
    in living systems, 167–168
    negative, 168
    positive, 168
Feeding, *see* Eating
Female genital mutilation
        (circumcision), 130
Female sterilisation, consent to, 428
Feminist moral philosophy, 97, 98, 100
Feminist perspective, nursing
        research, **345–347**
Fibrin, 169
Fibrinogen, 169, 174

Fires, 423
*A First Class Service: Quality in the New
        NHS (1998)*, 51, 381
First person, writing in, 357
Fitness to practice, doctors, 55–56
Fitness for Practice (UKCC 1999), 9, 324
Five challenges, Prime Minister's, 58,
        59
Fluid
    balance, 185–186, **416–418**
    balance charts, 418
    compartments, 416
    intake, 417–418
    in terminal illness, 499
    see also Water
Fold Housing Association, 244
Folic acid, 166
Folk illnesses, 230
Follicle stimulating hormone (FSH),
        192
Food, 181
    cultural diversity, 238
    hygiene, **410**
    liver function, 185
    obtaining, 181
    Orem's self-care model, 378, 379
    poisoning, 410
    regulations, **410**
    reheating, 410
    see also Diet; Eating
Foot exercises, 421–422
Force, in ethical reasoning, 83
Forums, patient, 61
Foundation for the Study of Infant
        Death, 507
Fragile X syndrome, 159
Frankl, V., 88
Fraud officer, 431
Freedom, 87
    negative, 96
    positive, 96
*Frenchay Healthcare NHS Trust v. S
        (1994)*, 114
Freud, Sigmund, 203–204, 205, 262
Function, structure and, 150
Fundholding, general practitioner, 50
Funding
    joint local government/NHS
        working and, 65
    National Health Service, 43, 44
    nurse education, 326
Funerals, 503
Further education and training, **29–30**

G

Gametes, 154
Gametogenesis, 161
Gamma-aminobutyric acid (GABA),
        462
Gastric inhibitory peptide (GIP), 184
Gastrin, 184

Gastrointestinal (GI) bleeding,
        NSAID-induced, 462
Gastrointestinal hormones, 183, 184
Gastrointestinal system, **181–185**
    secretions, 183–184
Gate control theory, 475–476
Gay patients, 82
Gaze, 260
Gender issues, 106
    nursing research, 334–335
    use of touch, 260
General adaptation syndrome (GAS),
        222
General management, 44–45
General Medical Council (GMC), 47,
        55–56, 312
General Nursing Council (GNC), 8
General nursing (nursing adults),
        10–14
General practitioners (GPs), 50, 245
    access to, 59
    fee for consultation, 44
    fundholding, 50
    notes, 385
Genes, 153, 157
    mutations, 157
Genetic code, 152–153
Genetic counselling, 299
Genetic disorders, 15, **156–160**
Genetic modification (engineering),
        162–163
Genetic predisposition, 156, **160**
Genetics, 28, 150, 155–156, 162–163
Genome, 156, 160
Genuineness, 272
Germ cells, 153
Gestures, 260
Gibbs (1988) reflective cycle,
        394, 395, 396
Gifts, 322
*Gillick v. West Norfolk and Norwich
        AHA [1985]*, 121
Glasgow Coma Scale, 419, 420
Glomerular filtration, 186
Glomerulus, 186
Gloves
    disposable, 404, **405–406**, 409
    safe removal, 406
Glucocorticoids, 221
Glucose (sugar)
    blood, regulation, 168
    in cellular respiration, 163
    transport, 152
    tubular reabsorption, 186
Glycogen, 185
Goals, setting, 371
Good, common, 93–94, 95
Goodness, moral, 79–80
Government, *see* Labour government
        (1997); Local government;
        Policy/policies, government
Grandparents, 380
Grants, local government/NHS
        partnership, 66

Great Ormond Street Hospital,
London, 16
Greece, ancient, 4, 230
Grief
complicated, 504–505
pangs, 501
special types, 502–504
stages, **500–502**
work, 500–501
see also Bereavement
Griffiths Report (1988), 44–45, 241,
242
Grounded theory, 349, 351
Groups
'in' and 'out', in nursing research,
346
learning in, 297
self-help, 304
Groupwork, in mental illness, 26
Growth hormone (GH), 192
Guardians, consent by, 121
Guidelines, 219, 399
Guidelines for Professional Practice
(UKCC 1996), 313, 322
Guillebaud Committee, 44
Gut, *see* Alimentary canal

H

Haemoglobin, 174
Haemophilia, 157, 160
Haemorrhage, in terminal illness,
498–499
Hair, 171
Halitosis, 497
Hall Report (1996), 299
Halo effect, 214
Handling, safe, **410–411**
Hand washing, 404, 405, 409
Happiness, 93–94, 95
Harm, avoidance of, 315–316, 392
Harvard referencing system, 340
Hawthorne effect, 344
Hazards
environmental, **402–414**
prevention of, 378, 379
Health, **284–287**
behaviour, changing, **290–291**
choices, 283–284
concepts, **229–231**
cross-cultural differences, 132,
230–231
defining, 284–285
environmental, 286
for everyone, 306
holistic, 285
inequalities, 66, 68, **286–287**
locus of control, **212**
as quality of life, 285–286
socially constructed concept,
230–231
social problems and, 239

Health Act (1999), **47**, 65
main elements, 47
professional self-regulation and,
47–48
Health action zones, 66
'Health for all by the year 2000' (WHO
1978), 280
Health authorities, **48–49**
in National Plan, 62
nursing home regulation, 69–70
primary health care focus,
244–245
public health strategy, 66
Health beliefs, **231–232**
diversity, 210, 211
model, 232, **290–291**
Health care, 366–367
access to, 59
changing patterns, 323
context, 84–85
culture and, 131–132
place of, 366–367
primary, **244–248**
Health care assistants, 31, 325
Health care professionals
collaboration with other, 317
as cultural group, 130
educational role of nurses, 268
pain assessment, 140, 471
reporting concerns about other,
320–321, 431
see also Doctors; Nurses
Health care provision
children, 16
economics, 28
ethical context, 84–85
political context, **42–75**
Health care resources
adequacy, 321
for clinical governance, 57
National Plan, 59, 60
rationing, 84, 85, 94, 95–96
Health education, 229, 289, **291–298**
definition, 291
getting message across, 295
holistic, 294–295
implementing, 296–297
models, **298–306**
empowerment, 305–306
preventative, 298–303
radical, 304–305
opportunistic, 296
planning, 296
primary, 298–301
primary health care groups and,
247–248
secondary, 301–302
strategies, 297–298
tertiary, 303
see also Health promotion
*Health Improvement Programmes:
Planning for Better Health and
Better Health Care* (1998),
66–68

Health improvement programmes
(HImPs), 49, 65, **66–69,
289–290**
The Health of the Nation (1992), 67,
299
Health promoting hospital, 282
Health promotion, 229, **279–308**
elderly, 248
health education and, 291–298
integrated approach, 284–290
new strategies, 281–284
principles, 280
psychology and, 290–291
settings approach, 282
Health Quality Service (HQS), 57
Health and safety, 402–403, 411
Health and Safety Commission, 403
Health visitor consultants, 30, 31
Health visitors, 16, 29
government policy, 70–73
new career framework, 30, 31
recruitment and retention, **71**
Healthy eating, 231, 280–281
Healthy neighbourhoods, 248
Healthy schools, 288, 301
Healthy workplace, 288–289
Heart, 172, **176**, 177
sounds, 176, 177
valves, 176
Heart disease, 11
see also Coronary heart disease;
Myocardial infarction
Heat
generation, 173
loss, 173
therapy, for pain, 478
Helping strategies, nurses', 264
Henle, loop of, 186, 187
Herbert, Sidney, 6–7
Hereditary disorders, human, **156–160**
Herpes zoster (shingles), 466
Heterotrophic organisms, 181, 182
High court, 119
HIMP, *see* Health improvement
programme
Hinduism, 143–144
Hippocrates, 4
Histamine, 461
History
learning disability care, 21–22
mental health care, 23–24
National Health Service, 5, **43–45**
nursing, **4–10**
HIV, *see* Human immunodeficiency
virus
Holism, 226
Holistic health, 285
Holistic health education, 294–295
Holm & Stephenson (1994) reflective
framework, 394, 395
Home
bathing service, 64
care services, **243–244**, 245
extended nursing services, 487, 488

palliative care, 487, 488
  visiting, 319
Home care assistants, 244
Homelessness, 27
Homeostasis, 150, **167–195**
  cardiovascular system and,
    172–179
  digestive system and, 181–185
  endocrine system and, 190–191
  immune system and, 191–195
  mechanisms, 167–169
  nervous system and, 188–190
  renal system and, 185–188
  respiratory system and, 179–181
  Roy's adaptation model, 374
  skin and, 169–172
Homocystinuria, 157
Hormones, **191**, 192
  gastrointestinal, 183, 184
  local, 191
Horns effect, 214
Hospice movement, 485
Hospices, 486, 487, **488**, 489
  children's, 488
  day, 487, 488
  at home, 488
Hospital acquired infections, 403,
    404–406, 407
Hospital consultants, 44, 60–61
Hospitality, acceptance of, 322
Hospitals, 44
  children in, 16
  children's, 16
  cleaning up, 61, 63, 407
  dying in, 485
  future trends, 28
  health promoting, **282**
  history, 4, 5
  independent sector, 69
  long-term care, 242
  in National Plan, 60, 61, 62
  nursing adults, 11
  nutrition in, 414–416
  palliative care, 487–488
  shorter stays in, 14, 255
Housing, 64, 287
  health and, 281
  problems, 239
Human chorionic gonadotrophin
    (HCG), 192
Human Fertilisation and Embryology
    Act (1990), 117
Human Genome Project, 156, **160–162**
Human immunodeficiency virus
    (HIV), 335–336
  infection, see AIDS/HIV infection
  testing, 302
Humanism, 24
Humanistic existential ethic, 99
Humanistic psychology, 201, **209–210**
Humanistic therapies, 26
Human nature, **203–210**
Hume, David, 82–83
Huntington's chorea, 157, 158

Hydration, **416–418**
5-Hydroxytryptamine (5-HT,
    serotonin), 462, 466
Hygeia, 230
Hygiene
  food, **410**
  personal, 143–144, 423–424
Hypothesis, 341

I

Ibuprofen, 462
Idiographic enquiry, 201
Immobility
  preventing complications, **421–423**
  in terminal illness, 498
Immune system, **191–195**
Immunisation, **193–195**, 298
Immunity, 171, **193–195**
  active, 193–195
  passive, 193
Implementing stage, nursing process,
    371
Incident reports, 127, 431
Incineration, 408
Incongruence, see Congruence
Independent (private) sector, **69–70**
  career options, 28–29
  intermediate care provision,
    69, 70
  in national plan, 61
  residential and nursing homes,
    242–243
Individual differences, 201
  acknowledging, **210–212**
  humanistic perspective, 209
  understanding, **106–108**
Individualised care, 132, 138
Individualism, 84
Induction, 82
Inductive reasoning, 336
Inductive research, see Research,
    qualitative
Inequalities
  ethical aspects, 84
  health, 66, 68, **286–287**
Infant mortality, 484
Infants
  death of, 502–503
  pain assessment, 471–473
  see also Children
Infection control, 298–299, 318,
    403–409
  nurse, 406–407
  policies, 406–407
  principles, 409–410
Infections, **403–407**
  hospital acquired, 403, 404–406,
    407
  mouth, 497
Infectious diseases, 11, 15
  immunity to, 193–195

Inflammation, 193, 194, 463
  in cancer, 468
Influenza, 195
Information
  disclosure, 103, 104, 125–126, 428
    bad news, 490–491
    consent to, 103, 104, 125, 320
    justifiable grounds, 104,
      125–126, 319–320
    see also Confidentiality
  giving, **269–270**
  retrieval, 339–340
  withholding, 104, 120, 319–320
Information technology (IT), 259,
    353–355
Informed consent, **103**, 120, **426–428**
Informed decision-making, **398–399**
Ingestion, 181, 404
Inhalation, 404
Inheritance, **155–163**
  autosomal, 157, 158, 159
  multifactorial, 160
  sex, 153–154
  sex-linked, 157–158, 160
Injections
  entry of pathogens via, 404
  in terminal illness, 498
Injuries
  childhood accidental, 299–300
  from assaults, 119
  non-accidental, 431
Inquests, 116
Inspiration, 180
Institutional care
  in mental illness, 25
  rights of patients, 106
Insulin, 168, 192
Insurance, private, 69
Integrated care pathways, **381–384**,
    385
Intellectual ability, assessing, 20
Intelligence
  artificial, 209
  quotient (IQ), 21
Intensive care units, paediatric, 18
Interactional approach, 222–223
Inter-agency cooperation, 242, **245–246**
Intercostal muscles, 180
Intercostobrachial nerve injury, 467
Interdependence, Roy's adaptation
    model, 374, 376, 377
Intermediate care, 60, 61, 69, 70
Internal market, 43, 45
International Council of Nurses (ICN),
    328
  Code of Conduct, 132, 313
International Nursing Review, **328**
International setting, **328**
Internet, 27, **354–355**, 363
Interpretative sociology, 227–229,
    233–234
Interpreters, 131, **142**, 270
  for obtaining consent, 428–429
  working with, 291–292

Interviews
in-depth, 345–346, 352–353
tape-recorded, 353
Introspection, personal, 199, 220
Invasive procedures, 404
IQ (intelligence quotient), 21
Ischaemic disease, 462
Islets of Langerhans, 192
Isolation, 204, 490
'Is/ought' distinction, 83

J

Jargon, 270, 387–388
Jehovah's Witnesses, 429
Johari window, 210–211, 212
Johns (1995) model of structured
reflection, 394, 395
Journalists, 126
Journals, learning, 265
Judges, 116, 117
Jury, 117
Justice, 80, **96–97**
egalitarian view, 96
libertarian view, 96
in nursing practice, 104–105
rights view, 96–97, 105

K

Kaccha, 144
Kant, Immanuel, 93
Kantian ethics, 93
Kappa opioid receptors, 463, 464
Kennedy Report (2000), 116
Ketones, 185
Keyhole surgery, 12, 27–28
Key words, 339
Kidneys, 186–188
excretory function, 187–188
importance of healthy, 188
urine formation, 186–187
Kinesics, 260
King's Fund, 64, 68–69, 268
Klinefelter's syndrome, 157, 161, 162
Knowledge
absolute, 200–201
affective, 219
awareness of own limitations, 316,
401–402
cognitive, 219
empirical, 82, 83
maintaining professional, 316
negotiated, 200–201
personal, 81–82
psychomotor, 219
scientific, 82
sources, 398–399
up-to-date, **398–401**
see also Expertise

Kohlberg, L., 100–101
Kubler-Ross, Elisabeth, 489–493

L

Labelling, 81–82, 214–215
Labour government (1997)
on contribution of nursing, 70–73
initial policies, 42–43, 45, 47, 50
inter-agency cooperation, 245–246
more recent policies, **50–58**
National Plan, *see National Plan
(2000)*
see also Policy/policies,
government
Lactic acid, 163
Language, 258
problems, 131, **142**, 270, 427–428
research articles, 356–357
technical, 270
using accessible, 270
Last offices, 499–500, 501
Law, **113–128**
civil, 119–126
common, 115
criminal, 116–119
forums, 115–116
importance, 113–114
natural, 91
sources, 114–115
UKCC compared to, 115
see also Legislation
Lawyers, 116
Laxatives, 496
Leadership, 30–31, 73
centres, 62
Learning, **292–293**
from experience, 208
in groups, 297
in health education, 295, **296–298**
journals, 265
lifelong, **31–32**
outcomes, assessing, 297–298
readiness for, 269
rote, 216
styles, 268
through reflection, 263, 295
types, 292–293
see also Teaching
Learning disability, 10
causes, 20
collective responsibility, 312
defining and assessing, 19–20
ethical aspects, 85–86
future trends in care, 22, 28
health education, 295
history of care, 21–22
holistic approach, 285
incidence and prevalence, 20–21
independent sector care, 69–70
joint health and social care, 10
nurse, role, 22

nursing, **18–22**
nursing models, 378
nursing research, 337, 357–358
nutrition, 415
obtaining consent, 428–429
pain assessment, 473–474
psychomotor skills learning, 293
terminology, 18–19
Legal executives, 116
Legal issues, **113–128**
documentation, 126–127
see also Law
Leg exercises, 421–422
Legislation, **114**
human rights, 106
patient records, 126–127
secondary, 114
Leininger, Madeleine, 132, 133
Sunrise model, 136, 137
Letters, 259
Leucocytes (white blood cells), 174,
175, 193
Leukaemia, 15
Liability, vicarious, 124
Libertarianism, 96
Life
expectancy, 484
sustenance of, **163–167**
Lifestyle, healthy, 280–281, 290
Lifting
aids, 411
safe, 410–411
Likert scales, 347
Limb amputation, 466–467
Limitations, awareness of own, 316,
401–402
Linen, **409**
infected, 409
soiled or fouled, 409
used, 409
Lipase, 184
Listening skills, **273–275**
Literature
review, 340, 341
searching, 339–340
Litigation, 54, 114
Liver, 185
Local adaptation syndrome (LAS),
221–222
Local government (local authorities),
241, 245
nursing home regulation, 70
partnership with NHS, 65–66
public health strategy, 66
teenagers brought up by, 294
White Paper (1997), **65–66**
Locke, John, 205–206
Locus of control, **212**
London Dance Safety Campaign, 292
Long-term care, 242, **246–247**
Loop of Henle, 186, 187
Loss
special types, 502–504
stages of, 500–502

see also Bereavement
Luckes, Miss, 7
Lung(s)
cancer, 179
collapse, 181
disorders, 11
gas exchange, 179
mechanisms of ventilation, 180–181
smoking-related damage, 179
Luteinising hormone (LH), 192
Luteotrophic hormone, 192
Lymphatic system, 178–179
Lymphocytes, 193

M

Macmillan Cancer Relief, 488
'Madhouses', 23
Magistrates court, 117, 119
Magnetic resonance imaging (MRI)
scanners, 61
Majority, appeal to, 83
Making a Difference: Strengthening the
Nursing, Midwifery and
Health Visiting Contribution
to Health and Health Care
(1999), 9, 32, **70–73**, 324
Malnutrition, 15, 415
prevention, 414–415
Management
general, 44–45
nursing, 8
risk, **53–54**
Manpower, nursing, 323
Manslaughter, 118
Manson, Ethel Gordon (Mrs Bedford
Fenwick), 7, 8, 328
Marie Curie nurses, 486
Marshall v. *Curry* [1993], 119
Marx, Karl, 227
Massage, therapeutic, 478
Mastectomy, 13, 467
Matching, 343–344
Matrons, 5, 9, 73
Mead, George Herbert, 227
Meals, 143, 410
'Meaningless phrases', 388
Media, mass, 233
Medical consultants, 44, 60–61
Medical devices, 408
Medical Devices Agency (MDA), 408
Medical director (chief medical
officer), 45, 48, 49
Medical education
access of nurses to, 62
future plans, 60
history, 5
standards board, 63
Medical model, 200, 201, **229–230**
mental illness, **24–25**
versus social care model, 64–65
Medical notes, 385

Medical nursing, 11
Medical practitioners, *see* Doctors
Medicine
hierarchical structure, 311
professional self-regulation, **55–56**
Medicines, **411–414**
administering, 413, 414
containers, 412
cupboards, 412, 414
practical skills of giving, 414
prescribing, 413
receiving, 414
self-administration, 414
storage, 412
see also Drugs
Medicines Act (1968), 114
Meditation, 478
Meiosis, **154–155**, 156
Melanocyte stimulating hormone, 192
Melanoma, 302
Membranes
cell and nuclear, 151–152
transport across, 152
Memorial services, 503
Memory, **216–218**
construction, 218
registration, 216–217
retrieval, 217–218
storage, 217
Memos, 259
Mendel, Gregor, 155
'Mental defective', 21
Mental defence mechanisms, 204–205
Mental Deficiency Act (1913), 21
Mental handicap, 19
Mental health, 285
approaches to, 24
health education, 300–301
national service frameworks, 66
nursing, **22–27**
research, 359
targets, 288
Mental Health Act (1959), 21
Mental Health Act (1984), 122–123, 265
Mental health care
future trends, 28
historical overview, 23–24
NHS and social sector
partnerships, 10
nursing models, 374, 375
settings, 25
Mental health nurse, 23
communication skills, 254
role, **25–26**
Mental illness, 10
approaches to, 24
community care, 25, 26–27
consent, 122–123, 428
cultural differences and, 108
health promotion, 283, 295, 303,
304
human rights, 106
images, 24
independent sector care, 69–70

medical model, **24–25**
nursing research, 357–358
psychological treatments, 25, 26
Mental incapacity, 122–123
Mental retardation, 19
Mental sub-normality, 21
Mentor, 32
Mentorship, 268
Menzies' social defence mechanisms,
205
Metabolism, drug, 185
Meta-ethics, 79
Methicillin resistant *Staphylococcus*
aureus (MRSA), 403, 404,
409–410
prevention of spread, 409, 430
Microbiology department, 407
Micro-organisms, pathogenic, 403–404
Micturition, 188
Midwife consultants, 30, 31
Midwifery, 29
education, 72–73
government policy, 70–73
new career framework, 30, 31
recruitment and retention, 71
Milburn, Alan (Secretary of State for
Health), 42, 58
Mill, John Stuart, 93–94
Mini-matrons, 73
Miscarriage, 502–503
Misoprostol, 462
Mitochondria, 164
Mitosis, **154**, 155
Mnemonics, 216
Mobilising, 373
Monoamine oxidase inhibitors
(MAOIs), 25
Monocytes, 193
Monogamy, 238
Monosomy, 162
Moores, Dame Yvonne, 70
Moral decision-making
facts and values in, 82–84
influences on, 101
in nursing practice, **100–108**
power relationships and, 102
prescription for, **108–110**
Moral development, **100–101**
Moral judgement, 79–80
Moral philosophy, 91, 97–98
feminist, *see* Feminist moral
philosophy
Moral thought/action
caring as basis, **97–100**
ethical theory as basis, **91–97**
in nursing practice, **100–108**
values as basis, **87–90**
Moral treatment, 23
Morphine, 463, 464, 470
Mortality rates, 484
Motor vehicle accidents, 299, 300
Mouth
care, 418, 497
dirty, 497

Mouth (*continued*)
  dry, 497
  problems, **497**
Moving, safe, **410–411**
MRSA, *see* Methicillin resistant
    Staphylococcus aureus
Multicultural Information File
    (MCRIC), 131, 143
Multidisciplinary notes, 385
Multidisciplinary team, *see* Team,
    multidisciplinary
Multifactorial inheritance, 160
Multiple sclerosis, 188
Mu opioid receptors, 463, 464
Muscle cramps, 163
Muslim patients, 144
Mutations, 157
Myelin sheath, 188, 189
Myocardial infarction, 11, 176
  care pathway, 400, **433–456**

N

Nails, 171
Naloxone, 464
Named nurse, 317
Names, using, 428
National Association for the Welfare
    of Children in Hospital
    (NAWCH, now Action for
    Sick Children), 14–15, 16
National Boards, 325, **326–327**
  UKCC and, 327
National Cancer Institute, 496, 507
National Care Commission, 247
National Care Standards Commission,
  66
National Council for Hospice and
    Specialist Palliative Care
    Services, 486, 498, 499
National Electronic Library for Health,
  398
National Health Service (NHS), **45–50**
  career options, 28–29
  continuing professional
    development, 32
  funding, 43, 44
  government policies, **42–50**
  history, 5, **43–45**
  local government partnership,
    65–66
  National Plan, see National Plan
    (2000)
  organisation, 45–46, 47
  primary health care focus, 244–245
  professional regulation and, **54–55**
  reorganisation, 8–9
  social sector partnership, **63–69**
National Health Service Act (1946), 44
National Health Service and
    Community Care Act (1990),
    21, 64, 240, 242

National Health Service Executive
    (NHSE), **48**
National Health Service (NHS) Trusts,
  49
  management, 45
  in National Plan, 62
  professional regulation and, 54–55
  underachieving, 59
National Institute for Clinical
    Excellence (NICE), 52, 62,
    219
National performance fund, 61
National Plan (2000), 43, **58–63**, 73
  announcement, 58–59
  background, 58
  concluding comments, 63
  key elements, 59–61
  reaction to, 61–62
  resourcing, 59, 60
  structural changes embodied in,
    62–63
National service frameworks, 66, 219
National Vocational Qualifications
    (NVQs), 325
Natural law, 91
Nature, human, **203–210**
Nausea, 497
'Near miss' reporting, 431
Needles, safe disposal, 408
Needs assessment, **241**, 295
Negligence, 115, **123–125**
Negotiation, nurse–patient, 134
Neighbourhoods
  healthy, 248
  unhealthy, 286–287
Neonate, severely handicapped, 118
Nephron, 186, 187
Nerve impulses, 188–189
Nervous system, **188–190**
  components, 189
  regulation, 190
Neurofibromatosis, 157, 158
Neurones, 188, 189
Neuro-observations, 419, 420
Neurotransmitters, 189
  pain, 461, 462
The New NHS: Modern, Dependable
    (1997), 47, 245
NHS, *see* National Health Service
NHS Direct, 71
NHS Plus, 63
NHS Trusts, *see* National Health
    Service (NHS) Trusts
Niacin, 166
Nicotinic acid, 166
Nightingale, Florence, **5–6**, 7, 44, 368,
    392, 403
  cultural diversity and, 132
  nursing research and, 332–333
  on nutrition, 414–415
Nightingale Nursing School, **6–7**
Nitrogenous waste products, 187–188
Nociceptors, 460, 461
  unimodal and polymodal, 461

Nomothetic enquiry, 201
Non-accidental injury, 419, 431
Non-disjunction, 162
Non-maleficence, 95
Non-steroidal anti-inflammatory
    drugs (NSAIDs), 462
Noradrenaline (norepinephrine), 189,
    192, 221, 462
Normality, promotion of, 378, 379
North American Nursing Diagnosis
    Association (NANDA), 505
Northern Ireland
  National Board, 325–326
  NHS organisation, 46, 48
Norton, Doreen, 333
NSAIDs (non-steroidal anti-
    inflammatory drugs), 462
Nuclear membrane, 151–152
Nucleoli, 152
Nucleus, **152–154**
Nuffield Health Care, 69
Numerical rating scale (NRS), pain,
  470
Nurse consultants, 30, 31, 62, 71
Nurse education, 9–10, **72–73**
  branch programmes, **10–27**
  Common Foundation Programme,
    9–10
  funding, 327
  further qualifications, 29–30
  history, 6–7
  post-registration, 29–30, 31–33, 73,
    326
  pre-registration, 9–10, 72–73, 323,
    325
  research and, 358
  role of UKCC, 323–325
  see also Student nurses
Nurse–patient negotiation, 134
Nurse–patient relationship, 255
  research, 359
  UKCC code of conduct, 315,
    318–319
Nurses
  changing role, 28, 310–311
  extended role, 60, 316–317
  numbers, 60
  recruitment, **71**, 323
  subordination to doctors, 311
Nurses, Midwives and Health Visitors
    Act (1979), 8, 115, 310,
    322–323
Nurses, Midwives and Health Visitors
    Act (1992), 115, 326
Nurses, Midwives and Health Visitors
    Act (1997), 114, 115
Nurses Registration Act (1919), 7–8
Nursing, **3–39**
  branches/specialities, 9, **10–27**
  care, 366–367
  concepts, 367, **368**
  future changes, **27–28**
  government policy, **70–73**
  hierarchical structure, 311

history and development, **4–10**
'new', 358
notes, 385
political context, **42–75**
safe practice, **391–433**
Nursing development units (NDUs),
   358–359
Nursing Ethics, 357
Nursing homes, 69–70, **242–243**, 245,
   247
Nursing and Midwifery Council, 86,
   326
Nursing models, 367, **369–381**
   biomedical, 372
   Casey's, 380–381
   limitations, 382
   Orem's self-care, 375–380
   Roper, Logan and Tierney, 372–374
   Roy's adaptation, 374–375, 376–377
   sociocultural elements, 136
Nursing officer, 8
Nursing process, 336, 338, **369–372**
   assessment, 370–371
   diagnosis, 371
   evaluating, 372
   implementing, 371
   planning, 371
Nursing Record, 7
Nursing theories, 358, 367, **368–369**
   deductive, 369
   inductive, 369
   sociocultural elements, 136
Nurture, 203
Nutrition, **414–415**
   assessing needs, 415
   feeding patients, 415, 416

O

Observation
   learning values through, 89–90
   participant, 352–353
   schedules, non-participant, 349
Observations, nursing, **418–421**
   importance, 418–419
   recording, 421, 429
   routine clinical, 419–421
Occupational nurse, 319
Oestrogens, 192
Ointments, pain-relieving, 478
Oogenesis, 161
Operant conditioning, 206
Opioid receptors, 463, 464
Opioids, **463–464**
   antagonists, 464
   in cancer pain, 469, 470
   endogenous, 461–462, 463, 477
   misconceptions about, 463
   mode of action, 463–464
   in neuropathic pain, 465
Orem's self-care model, 268, **375–380**
Osmoregulation, 185–186

Osmosis, 152
Ottawa Charter for Health Promotion
   (1986), 280–281, 304
Outpatient appointments, waiting
   times, 59
Outreach, 284
Ovaries, 192
Ovum, 154, 161
Oximetry, pulse, 419
Oxygen, 179, 181
   deficit, 163
   in energy production, 163
   transport in blood, 174
Oxytocin, 192

P

Pacemaker, cardiac, 176
Paediatric community nurse, 16, 17
Paediatric nurses, 16–17
Paediatric nursing, *see* Children's
   nursing
Paediatric units, 16
Pain, **457–480**
   acute, 459, 460
   assessment, 421, **470–474**, 495
      in adults, 470–471
      in elderly, 474
      by health care professionals,
         140, 471
      in infants and children, 471–473
      in learning
         disability/communication
         difficulty, 473–474
      principles of good, 478–479
   behaviours, 139–140, 472, 474
   biocultural model of perception,
      139
   cancer, **467–469**
   chronic, 459, 460
   classification, 459–461
   culture sensitive care, **138–141**
   definition, 458
   gate control theory, 475–476
   lancinating, 464
   management
      in cancer, 468–469, 495
      cross-cultural research, 140–141
      in elderly, 476
      non-pharmacological, 462,
         474–478
      phantom limb pain, 467
      pharmacological, 462–464,
         465–466
      post-herpetic neuralgia, 466
      postoperative, 460
      principles of good, 478–479
      in terminal illness, 495
   neuropathic, 459, **465–467**
      in cancer, 468
      drug treatment, 465–466
      TENS, 477

nociceptive, 459, **461–462**
   in cancer, 468
   transmission pathways,
      461–462
   treatment, 462–464
oral, 497
physiology, 460–470
somatic, 468
'total', 479
visceral, 468
Palliation, 222
Palliative care
   approach, 484, **486–488**
   definition, 484
   education, 487
   history, 484–485
   hospital-based, 487–488
   models, 487–488
   principles, 486
   services, 486, 487
   symptom management, 495–497,
      498–499
   see also Dying; Terminal illness
Pancreas, 192
Pantothenic acid, 166
Paracetamol, 462–463
Paralanguage, 261
Paraphrasing, 274
Parathyroid gland, 192
Parathyroid hormone, 192
Parent held records, 385
Parents
   bereavement, 502–503
   consent by, 121
   involvement in child's care,
      380–381
   sick child, 16–17
   transcultural issues, 135
Parkes, Colin Murray, 500, 501
Parson, Talcott, 227
Partnership in Action (1998), 247, 248
Passivity, 267
Patau's syndrome, 162
Paternalistic approach, 265
Pathogenic organisms (pathogens),
   403–404
Patient held records, 385
Patients, **10**
   access to records, 320, 388
   advocacy, *see* Advocacy
   assaults by, 119
   autonomy, *see* Autonomy
   availability of information to, 27
   'best interests', 118, 119
   categorisation, 81, 315
   as central focus, **87**, 272–273
   as cultural informants, 134
   educational role of nurses, 268
   explanatory models, 142
   feeding assistance, 415, 416
   health and safety, 402–403
   involvement in own care, 317, 371
   labelling and stereotyping, 81–82,
      235–236

Patients (*continued*)
  moving and handling, **410–411**
  non-accidental injury, 431
  rights, **106**, 114
  self-administration of drugs, 414
Patients' Charter (1992), 106, 317
Patients' organisations, 304
Patriarchical system, 311
PAUSE project, 298
Pavlov, Ivan, 206
Pay, nurses', 8, 71
Peach Report (1999), 324
Peak flow measurement, 419
Peer group, 233
Peer review, 312
Pentazocine, 464
Pepsin(ogen), 184
Peptidases, 184
Perception, **214**
  person, **214–216**
Peripheral nervous system, 189
Peristalsis, 182
Persistent vegetative state, 114, 118–119
Personal care, 246
Personal development plan, 32, 33
Personality, grief reaction and, 505
Personal professional portfolio, **32–33**
Personal space, 260
Personal value choices, 81–82
Phagocytic cells, 193
Phagocytosis, 152
Phantom pain
  limb, **466–467**
  other types, 467
Pharmaceutical companies, 322
Phenomenology, 349, 350–351
  sociological, 351
Phenothiazines, 24–25
Phenylketonuria, 157
Philosophy
  care, 368
  moral, 91, 97–98
Photocopies, 388
Photographs, dead baby, 503
Phylloquinone, 165
Physical environment, 261
Physical health, 286
Physiological adaptation, Roy's
    model, 374, 376, 377
Physiology, **149–195**
  pain, **460–470**
  principles, 150–151
  sustenance of life, 163–167
Physiotherapy, in terminal care, 498
Piaget, Jean, 207, 208
Pilo-erection, 173
Pilot study, 347
Pinocytosis, 152
Pituitary gland, 192
Placebo group, 344
Placenta, 192
Planning, 371
Plasma, 174
  proteins, 174, 185

Plasma membrane, 151–152
Plastic bags
  black, 408
  yellow, 408
Platelets (thrombocytes), 174, 175–176
Platt Report (1959), 16
Playing, 373
Pleural cavity, 180
Pneumothorax, 181
Poisonings, childhood, 299
Poisons, 185
Police, 117, 126, 430
Policy/policies
  government, **42–75**
    contribution of nursing, 70–73
    developments since 1997, 50–58
    independent sector, 69–70
    National Health Service, 42–50
    social care sector, 63–69
    see also National Plan
  health care, 399
  healthy public, 289–290, **304–305**
  implementation, 248
  infection control, 406–407
  social, 226, **238–240**
  stagnation, 248–249
Polydactyly, 157
Polygamy, 238
Polymorphs, 193
Polyploidy, 162
Poor Law Act (1601), 5
Poor Law Amendment Act (1834), 5
Porphyria, 157
Portfolio, personal professional, **32–33**
Positioning, in pain, 477–478
Positivist view, 200–201
Post-herpetic neuralgia, 466
Postoperative pain relief, 460
Post-registration education and
    practice (PREP), **32–33**, 326
Posture, 260
Poverty, 239, 286–287
  health status and, 68
  local government/NHS
      partnerships, 66
  teenage pregnancy and, 294
Power relationships
  ethical decision-making and, 101,
    102
  in nursing research, 346
Preceptorship, **32**, 268, 312, 322
Pregnancy
  HIV testing, 302
  refusal of treatment, 122
  teenage, 294, 303
  termination of, *see* Abortion
Pressure
  effects on skin, 173
  effects of tumours, 468
Pressure sores, 173, **422–424**
  prevention, 423
  risk assessment, 423
Preventative model, **298–303**
  primary health education, 298–301

secondary health education,
    301–302
  tertiary health education, 303
Prevention, **414–423**
  complications of immobility,
    421–423
  dehydration, 417–419
  in elderly, 248
  of hazards, 378, 379
  malnutrition, 414–415
  primary, 298–301
Primacy effect, recall of information,
    269
Primary care groups (PCGs), **49–50**, 65
  health education and, 247–248
Primary care Trusts (PCTs), **49–50**
  in National Plan, 61
Primary health care, 59, **244–248**
Principles of practice, 400
Prisons, mental illness in, 27
Private finance initiative (PFI), 43, 60, 65
Private health care insurance, 69
Private sector, *see* Independent
    (private) sector
Probability theory, 353
Probationer nurses, 5, 7
  special, 7
Problem solving, **218–220**
  approach, 311
  circle, 370
  developing expertise in, 220
  evidence-based decision-making
      and, 218–219
  expertise and, 219–220
Procedures
  infection control and, 407
  written, 259
Process, 338
Profession
  key elements, 310
  nursing as, 310
Professional conduct
  code of, *see* Code of Professional
      Conduct
  standards, 56, 310, 326
Professional Conduct Committee,
    UKCC, 310, 326
Professionalism
  changing concepts, **310–312**
  development, 7–8
Professional organisations, 327–328
Professional role of nurse, **310–328**
Professional self-regulation, 312, 402
  1999 Health Act and, **47–48**
  medical profession, **55–56**
  NHS organisations and, **54–55**
Professional socialisation, 233–234
Progesterone, 192
Project 2000, 8, 323, 325
Projection, 204
Property, patients', 318–319
Proteins
  energy production from, 164
  enzymes as, 164

excretion, 187–188
plasma, 174, 185
Protestantism, 4–5
Prothrombin, 169
Protocols, 399
Proxemics, 260
Psoriasis, 409
Psychiatric care, see Mental health care
Psychiatric illness, see Mental illness
Psychoanalysis, 24, 204
Psychodynamic psychotherapy, 26
Psychodynamic theory, **203–205**
Psychogeriatric hospital beds, 242
Psychological treatments, 25, 26
Psychology, **197–224**
    contribution to nursing, 199–203
    definition, 199–200
    health promotion and, 290–291
    making assessments, 213–216
    relevance, 202–203
    themes, 200–202
    theories of human development,
        203–210
Psychomotor skill learning, 293
Public health, strategic context, 66
Public inquiries, 116
Public interest, disclosure of
        information in, 125–126, 320
Public Interest Disclosure Act (1998),
        320
Pulse, 419
Pulse oximetry, 419
P values, 353
Pyridoxine, 165

Q

Quality of care, 57, 338
Quality of life, 285–286
Quality Patient Care Scale, 349, 350
Queen's Counsel (QC), 116
Questioning approach, adopting a,
    393
Questionnaires, developing, 347–349
Questions
    open versus closed, 274–275
    reflective, 264, 334
    research, 341

R

Race, 130
Racism, 73, 106, 107–108
    institutional, 131
Radical model, health education,
        305–306
Radiotherapy, 468
Randomised controlled trials (RCTs),
        343–344, 346–347

Random selection (sampling),
        343–344, 347
Rathbone, William, 7
Rating scales, 344–345
Rationalisation, 204
RCN, see Royal College of Nursing
Reaction formation, 204
Re A (male sterilisation) [2000], 123
Reasoned action, theory of, **291**
Reasoning
    common errors in ethical, 83
    inductive, 336
    learning values through, 89–90
Re C [1989], 118
Re C [1994], 123
Recessive inheritance, autosomal, 157,
        159
Record-keeping (documentation),
        384–388, 428, 429
    guidelines, 386–388
    importance, 385–386
    legal aspects, **126–127**
    nurse's responsibility, 315–316
    nursing observations, 421, 429
Records, **384–388**
    legal aspects, 126–127
    parent held, 385
    patient access to, 320, 388
    patient held, 385
    style, 386
    types, 384–386
Recovery position, 425
Recruitment, **71**, 323
Red blood cells, 174–175
Referencing systems, 340
Reflection, **263**, 264, **393–397**
    dimensions, 264
    in empathic responding, 274
    getting started, 393–394
    learning through, 263, 295
    models, 394–396
    potential problems, 396–397
    in practice (action), 263, 311
    on practice (action), 263, 311
    research mindedness and, 334
Reflective practice, 220, **311**
Reflective questions, 264, 334
Reflexology, 477
Refrigeration, medicines, 412
Refusal of treatment, 121, 122, 123, 429
Regard, unconditional positive, 272
Regional authorities (offices), 45, 46,
        48
Registered mental nurse (RMN), 25–26
Registered midwife, 31
Registered nurse, 31, 314, 316, 323
    administration of medicines, 413
    newly qualified, 31, 32
Register, UKCC, 310, 325
Registration
    medical, 56
    nurse, 31–32
        history, **7–8**
        UKCC competencies, 35–39, 72

Regression, 204
Regulatory bodies, coordinating body
        overseeing, 62
Rehabilitation, nursing models, 375
Reiki, 477
Reinforcement, positive, 206
Relationships, **255–256**
    nurse–patient, see Nurse–patient
        relationship
    nurse's, 257
    reflection on, 263
    reinvesting in, by bereaved,
        501–502
    research, 359
Relatives, see Family
Reliability, 351
Religion, 141, 142
    bereavement/dying and, 505
    dietary aspects, 143
    obtaining consent and, 429
Renal failure, 188
Renal system, **185–188**
Renal tubules
    reabsorption, 186–187
    secretion, 187
    synthesis, 187
Reporting concerns, 320–321, **430–431**
Reports, 259
Repression, 204
Re-registration, nurse, 31, 32
Research
    action, 338
    awareness, 332
    ethical issues, 357–358
    evidence, 398
    mindedness, 332, 334, **360**
    nurse education and, 358
    nursing, **332–335**, 359–360
        definition, 334
        historical perspective,
            332–334
    nursing practice and, 358–359
    process, **338–357**
        analysing and interpreting
            data, 353–356
        collecting and recording data,
            351–353
        data collection methods and
            instruments, 347–351
        identifying research topic,
            339–341
        presenting results, 356–357
        selecting approach, 342–343
        study design, 343–347
    qualitative (inductive), **336–338**,
        342–343
        data analysis and
            interpretation, 355–356
        data collection methods,
            349–351
        data collection and recording,
            352–353
        ethics, 357
        study design, 345–347

Research (*continued*)
quantitative (deductive), **335–336**, 342–343
data analysis and interpretation, 353–355
data collection methods, 347–349
data collection and recording, 351–352
study design, 343–345
questions, 341
triangulation, 338
types, 335–338
see also Evidence-based practice
Research Assessment Exercise (RAE), 360
Residential homes, **242–243**, 247
Resources, health care, *see* Health care resources
Respiration, **443**
anaerobic, 163
cellular, **163–164**
Respiratory depression, opioid-induced, 463
Respiratory system, **179–181**
Respite care, 64, 221
at home, 488
Responding skills, **273–275**
Responsibility
nurse's, 313, 315–316
specialisation and, 312
Rest, in pain, 477–478
Restlessness, terminal, 498
Resuscitation, cardiopulmonary (CPR), 218–219, 425–426
Re T [1992], 121
Retinoblastoma, 157
Retinol, 165
Retreat, York, 23
Revalidation, doctors, 55–56
Re W [1992], 121
Reward systems, 206
Rhesus blood group system, 175
Rheumatoid arthritis, 11
Riboflavin, 165
Ribonucleic acid (RNA), 152, 153
Ribosomes, 153
Rightness, moral, 79–80
Rights
to good pain relief, 478–479
legal, 106
patients, **106**, 114
universal human, 105
upholding, **105–106**
view of justice, 96–97, 105
Risk management, **53–54**
Rituals, 318, 503
RNA, 152, 153
Road traffic accidents, 299, 300
Rogers, Carl, 87, 271–272, 275
Role
conflict, 235–236
function, 374, 376, 377
sets, **234–237**

sick, 227, **236–237**
strain, 235
Role-appropriate behaviour, 234
Romans, ancient, 4
Roper, Logan and Tierney model of nursing, 136, **372–374**
Royal College of Nursing (RCN), 71, **327**
Institute, 328
nursing research and, 332, 333, 357
Steinberg Collection, 359
Royal College of Physicians, 357
Royal Commission on Long Term Care (1999), **246–247**
Roy's adaptation model of nursing, **374–375**, 376–377
Rubbing, in pain, 475, 478
Rules, written, 259
R. v. Salford Health Authority ex p. Janaway (1988), 118

S

Safe environment, maintaining, 373, 403
Safe nursing practice, **392–432**
Safety
environmental, 402–403
patient, 316
St Bartholomew's Hospital, London, 7
St George's Healthcare NHS Trust v. *S* [1998], 122
St Thomas's Hospital, London, 7
Saliva, 183
Salmon Report, 8
Samaritans, 503, 504, 507
Sampling
purposive, theoretical, 345
random, 343–344, 347
Saunders, Cicely, 479, 485
Saving Lives: Our Healthier Nation (1999), 66, 67, 282, **287–290**, 300
Schemas, 207–208, 216
Schizophrenia, 24–25, 160, 304
Schools, 287
health education, 301
healthy, 288, 301
sex education, 298
snacks, 301
in socialisation, 233
The Scope of Professional Practice (UKCC 1992), 316–317
Scotland
Clinical Standards Board, 53
National Board, 326–327
NHS organisation, 46, 48
Scottish Health Technology Assessment Centre (SHTAC), 52
Screening
criteria, 302

developmental, 302
health, 301–302
Seacole, Mary, 6
Search, literature, 339–340
Secretin, 184
Self
communication and, **261–263**
knowledge, 81–82
learning through reflection, 263
Self-awareness, 210, **262**
definition, 263
increasing, 262–263
own limitations, 316, **401–402**
Self-care
deficits, 378
requisites, 378–380
Self-concept, **210–212**
Roy's adaptation model, 374, 376, 377
Self-defence, 119
Self-efficacy, 212
Self-esteem, 211–212
Self-help groups, 304
Senior nursing officer, 8
Senior registered practitioners, 31
Sensation, skin, 171
Sense organs, special, 189
Sensory receptors, 167, 190
Serotonin (5-HT), 462, 466
Service and Financial Framework (SAFF), 66
Sex chromosomes, 153–154
disorders, 162
Sex determination, 153–154
Sex education, school-based, 298
Sex-linked inheritance, 157–158, 160
Sexual health, 288, 290–291
Sexuality, expressing, 373
Shaping, behavioural, 206
Sharps
bin, 408
disposal, **408–409**
Sheltered accommodation, 244
Shingles, 466
Shivering, 173
Shock, 168, 170–171
anaphylactic, 194
cardiogenic, 170, 171
haemorrhagic, 170
hypovolaemic, 170, 171
neurogenic, 170, 171
Showers, 430
Sickle-cell disease (anaemia), 157, 174
Sick role, 227, **236–237**
Sidaway v. *Board of Governors of Bethlem Royal Hospital* [1985], 120
Significance tests, statistical, 353, 354
Sikhism, 144
Silence, 274
Single gene disorders, 156, **157**
Sisters, ward, 8, 30, 31, 73
Skin, **169–172**
colour and texture, 419
cuts and grazes, 408

disorders, 409
effects of pressure, 173
entry of pathogens via, 404
functions, 171–172
rubbing, in pain, 475, 478
structure, 172
wound healing, 173
Skinner, B.F., 206
Sleeping, 373
in pain, 477–478
Smoking
attitudes to, 291
cessation advice, 283, 294, 296, 297, 300
lung damage, 179
Social care model of services, 64
Social care sector, **63–69**
career options, 28–29
local government/NHS partnership, 65–66
Social change, 5, 228–229
Social class
childhood accidents and, 299–300
health inequalities, 287
Social comparison theory, 139
Social convention, 79, 80
Social defence mechanisms, Menzies', 205
Social disadvantage, 286–287
Social exclusion, 66, 68
Social Exclusion Unit, 68, 294
Social health, 285
Social incompetence, in learning disability, 19–20
Social intervention, 378, 379
Socialisation, **232–234**
anticipatory, 233
primary, 233
professional, 233–234
secondary, 233
Social learning theory, 139
Social networks, 287
Social policy, 226, **238–240**
definition, 239
universality and selectivity, 240
Social problems, health and, 239
Social roles, **234–237**
Social sciences, inductive research, 336
Social services, 241, 242
see also Social care sector
Social support, grief reaction and, 505
Social welfare, 239–240
Socioeconomic status, grief reaction and, 505
Sociological approach, mental illness, 24
Sociological phenomenology, 351
Sociology, **225–250**
interpretative, 227–229, 233–234
levels of analysis, 226–227
structuralist approach, **227–229**, 233–234
theory, 226–229

Sodium (Na⁺), tubular reabsorption, 186–187
Solicitors, 116
Solitude/social intervention, 378, 379
Special care baby units (SCBUs), 18
Specialisation, collective responsibility and, 312
Specialist nurses (practitioners), 29, 312
Special needs, children with, 18
Special probationer nurse, 7
Sperm, 154
Spermatogenesis, 161
Spinal cord, pain pathways, 463
Spiritual distress, 505
Spiritual health, 285
Spiritual needs, **142**
in bereavement/dying, 505
Staff
counselling services, 506
health and safety, 402–403
Standards for the Administration of Medicines (UKCC 1992), 412
Standards of care, 312
maintaining, 320–321
Staphylococcus aureus, 409
methicillin resistant, see Methicillin resistant *Staphylococcus aureus*
Starling equilibrium, 178
Starvation, 164
State enrolled nurse (SEN), 8
State registered nurse (SRN), first, 8
Statistical tests, 353–354
Statute, 114
Statutory bodies, **322–326**
Steinberg Collection, Royal College of Nursing, 359
Stereotyping, 81–82, **235–236**
cultural aspects, 138, 140
nursing research and, 334–335
Sterilisation, 408
Stigma, 82
mental illness, 24
suicide, 503
Stillbirth, 117, 502–503
Stillbirth and Neonatal Death Society, 507
Stocktaking, 414
Stomach, motility, 182–183
Storage, medicines, 413–414
Stress, **221–223**
caring for dying, 505–506
composite explanation, 223
environmental approach, 221
interactional approach, 222–223
in nursing, 321
physiological approach, 221–222
Stroke (cerebrovascular accident), 14, 288, 300, 383–384
Structuralism, **227–229**, 233–234
Structure, and function, 150
Student nurses, 5, 9, **10**
administration of medicines, 413

changes in status, 323–325
refusal of care by, 427
UKCC Code of Professional Conduct and, 313
see also Nurse education
Study design, 343–347
Subcultures, 130, 238
Sublimation, 204
Subsidiarity, 59
Substance abuse, 28
Substance P, 461, 463, 464
Substrate, 164
Sudden Infant Death Syndrome Alliance, 507
Suffering, 88
Sugar, see Glucose
Suicide, 301
assisted, 117
attempted, 503
deaths due to, **503–504**
Suicide Act (1961), 117
Summarising, 274
Sunrise model (Leininger), 136, 137
Supervision, clinical, **268–269**, 312, 322
Supporting, **275–276**
Suppression, 204
Surgery
cancelled operations, 59
cancer, 468
deep vein thrombosis prevention, 421
future changes, 27–28
independent sector, 69
pain relief after, 460
service development, 61
waiting times, 59
Surgical nursing, 11–12
Surnames, 430
Surveys, descriptive, 344–345
Sutherland, Sir Stewart, 246
Swallowing, 182
Sweat, 173, 417
Symptom management, in palliative care, 495–497, 498–499
Synapses, 189

T

TACTICS acronym, 264
Taking action, **264–265**
Teaching, **267–269**
in health education, **292–293**
implementing, 296–297
strategies, 297–298
see also Educational role of nurse; Learning
Team
care coordination, 241
health care
collaboration within, 317
patient confidentiality, 125
home care, 244

Team (*continued*)
multidisciplinary, 28, 382
integrated care pathways and, 383–384
palliative care, 487–488
Technological changes, 27–28
Teenage pregnancy, 294, 303
Tele-medicine, 27
Telephone, 259
answering, 430
giving information over, 430
Television, 233
Temgesic, 464
Temperature
body, *see* Body temperature
drug storage, 412
indoor, 281
Temperature, pulse and respiration (TPR), 419
TENS, *see* Transcutaneous electrical nerve stimulation
Terminal illness, 10–11, **497–500**
in children, 18
refusal of treatment, 121
suicide and, 503–504
symptom management, 498–499
well-being in, 285
see also Dying; Palliative care
Termination of pregnancy, *see* Abortion
Testes, 192
Testicular cancer, 302
Testicular feminising syndrome, 157
Testosterone, 192
Thiamin, 165
Third person, writing in, 357
Thirst, 417
Thoracic cage, 180
Thrombin, 169
Thrombocytes (platelets), 174, 175–176
Thrombosis, deep vein (DVT), **421–422**
Thyroid gland, 192
Thyroid stimulating hormone (TSH), 192
Thyroxine (T$_4$), 192
Time limits, negligence actions, 124
Tissue fluid, 150, 176–178
Tocopherols, 165
Torture, 105
Total Quality Management (TQM), 57
Touch, **259–260**
expressive (therapeutic), 259, 260
instrumental, 259
Tracheostomy, 13
Trades Union Congress (TUC), 327
Trade unions, 327–328
Training
nursing, *see* Nurse education
teenage pregnancy and, 294
Tranquillisers, 498
major, 23, 24–25
Transactional approach, 222–223
Transcultural care, **132–138**
components, 134

definition, 130–131
goal, 136
good practice, **141–144**
implementing, 135–137
models, 136–137, 138
problems with, 138
UKCC code of conduct, 132, 317–318
Transcultural nurse, 133
Transcutaneous electrical nerve stimulation (TENS), **475–477**
acupuncture-like (ALTENS), 476
effectiveness, 476–477
Translocations, chromosomal, 159
Transplantation, 195
Transport
across membranes, 152
active, 152
policies, 281
Treatment
emergency, legal aspects, 121–122, 124–125
futile, 119
information about risks, 120
refusal, 121, 122, 123, 428
withdrawal, 114, 118–119
without consent, 428
Triangulation, 338
investigator, 338
Tribunals, employment, 116
Tricyclic antidepressants, 25, 466
Tri-iodothyronine (T$_3$), 192
Trisomy 13, 162
Trisomy 18, 162
Trisomy 21, *see* Down's syndrome
Trolleys, drug, 412
Truth, telling, 493–494
Trypsin(ogen), 184
Tubules, renal, *see* Renal tubules
Tuke, William, 23
Turner's syndrome, 157, 161, 162
Twycross, Robert, 485

U

UKCC, *see* United Kingdom Central Council for Nursing, Midwifery and Health Visiting
Unconditional positive regard, 272
Unconscious mind, 200, **202**, 261–262
Unconscious patient
consent to treatment, 121–122, 429
neuro-observations, 419
taking action for, 265
Uniforms, 261
Unison, 71, 326, **328**
United Kingdom Central Council for Nursing, Midwifery and Health Visiting (UKCC), 8, 47, 310, **322–326**
administration of medicines, 412

admission to Register, 325–326
Code of Professional Conduct, *see* Code of Professional Conduct (UKCC)
on communication, 254
Education Commission, 72
European Community and, 325, 328
further training, 326
improving standards of training, 323–325
main functions, 323
minority groups within nursing, 326
National Boards and, 327
Professional Conduct Committee, 310, 326
professional versus legal duty, 115
standards of professional conduct, 326
United Nations
rights of the child, 14, 15
Universal Declaration of Human Rights, 105
Universal Declaration of Human Rights (UN 1948), 105
Universities
nurse education within, 9, 325
nursing research, 360
'Unpopular' patients, 81
Urea, 186, 188
Ureter, 188
Urine, 417
emptying from bladder, 188
formation, 186–187
testing, 421
Uterine contractions, 168
Utilitarianism, **93–95**, 97–98
act, 94
general, 94
rule, 94–95
versus deontology, 95

V

Vaccines, 194–195
Validity, 351
Values, **80**
as basis for moral thought/action, **87–90**
caring as key, **80–81**
definition, 87
formation, 87–90
learning, in nursing, 89–90
model for clarification, 90
moral decisions based on, **82–84**
personal, 81–82, 88–89, 109
professional, **86**
Vancouver referencing system, 340
Variances, 382
Varicella-zoster virus, 466
Vasoactive intestinal peptide (VIP), 184

Vasomotor centre, 173
Vegetative state, persistent, 114, 118–119
Venous system, 172, **178**
Ventilation, 180–181
Verbal descriptor pain scale (VDS), 470, 471
Vicarious liability, 124
Violence, against nurses, 119
Virtue ethics, 97, 98–99, 109
   revival, 98, **99–100**
Virtues, 99–100
Viruses, 403, 404
Visual analogue scales (VAS), 470
Vitamin A, 165
Vitamin B$_1$, 165
Vitamin B$_2$, 165
Vitamin B$_6$, 165
Vitamin B$_{12}$, 166
Vitamin C, 166
Vitamin D, 165, 172
Vitamin E, 165
Vitamin K, 165
Vitamins, **165–166**
Vocalisations, in pain, 474
Voluntary Aid Detachment (VAD) nurses, 7–8
Voluntary services, 244
Vomiting, 497
Vulnerable groups (of patients)
   negative labelling/stereotyping, 82
   protecting, 320–321
   research ethics, 357–358

W

Waiting times, 59
Wales
   National Board, 326–327
   NHS organisation, 46, 48

Ward Learning Environment Rating Questionnaire, 347, 348
Ward sister, 8, 30, 31, 73
Washing
   bowls, 409
   dead body, 500
   hand, 404, 405, 409
   patients, 429–431
   transcultural issues, **143–144**
Waste
   clinical, 408
   disposal, **407–409**
   non-clinical, 408
Water
   balance, 185–186
   importance, 416–417
   Orem's self-care model, 378, 379
   tubular reabsorption, 186
   see also Fluid
Waterlow pressure sore scoring system, 422
Web-sites, research, 363
Welfare, social, 239–240
Well-being, 239–240, 284–285
   promoting and safeguarding patient, 315
Well man/woman clinics, 302
West, Dr Charles, 16
'Whistleblowing', 320–321, 431
White blood cells (leucocytes), 174, 175, 193
White coat syndrome, 206
WHO, *see* World Health Organization
Wills, 127
Withdrawal of treatment, 114, 118–119
Witnesses, 127
Women
   discrimination against, 106
   healing role, **4–5**
Wong–Baker faces pain assessment scale, 472
Workhouses, 5

Working, 373
Working for Patients (1989), 240, 241
Workplace, healthy, 288–289
World Health Organization (WHO), 230, 244, 328
   analgesic ladder, **469–470**
   health targets, 280, 288
   palliative care, 487, 495
World War I (1914–1918), 7–8
World Wide Web (internet), 27, **354–355**, 363
Wound
   care, 368–369
   healing, 173
   infection, 403
Wrongness, moral, 79–80
W v. Edgell [1990], 126

X

X chromosome, 153, 154
Xeroderma pigmentosum, 157
X-linked inheritance, 157–158, 160

Y

Y chromosome, 153, 154
Young people
   consent, 121
   suicide, 503
   see also Adolescents; Children